Psychological Interventions for Psychosis

Juan Antonio Díaz-Garrido
Raquel Zúñiga • Horus Laffite • Eric Morris
Editors

Psychological Interventions for Psychosis

Towards a Paradigm Shift

Springer

Editors
Juan Antonio Díaz-Garrido
Hospital Universitario de Gran Canaria
Dr. Negrín
Las Palmas de Gran Canaria
Las Palmas, Spain

Horus Laffite
Hospital Universitario de Gran Canaria
Dr. Negrín
Las Palmas de Gran Canaria
Las Palmas, Spain

Raquel Zúñiga
Hospital Universitario de Canarias
Santa Cruz de Tenerife
Sta. Cruz Tenerife, Spain

Eric Morris
Faculty of Psychology and Public Health
La Trobe University
Melbourne, VIC, Australia

ISBN 978-3-031-27002-4 ISBN 978-3-031-27003-1 (eBook)
https://doi.org/10.1007/978-3-031-27003-1

This Springer imprint is published by the registered company Springer Nature Switzerland AG
The registered company address is: Gewerbestrasse 11, 6330 Cham, Switzerland

Foreword: From Pathologizing to Meeting with Full Human Beings

In psychiatry, during the last decade, more openness has appeared towards psychotherapeutic orientation concerning the recommendations of care in psychotic crises. During the previous two decades, the neurobiological paradigm has prevailed and psychotherapeutic interventions have been neglected. For people in psychotic crises, this period was unfortunate because it meant that they only were introduced to neuroleptic medication as the standard of care. Psychotherapy was abandoned by the belief seeing psychosis as a neurotoxic condition, and neurobiological intervention became the only relevant care recommended. Emphasizing the medication as the principal care, the experiences of the persons with psychotic experience were disacknowledged as non-relevant because they were seen to be speaking from the ill brain position. Unfortunately, psychotherapists seemed to adopt the neurobiological explanations and on a large scale ceased to introduce psychotherapy in psychotic crises. This happened in individual psychotherapy but also in family therapy, which is my special interest.

People with psychotic experiences in a way were abandoned by the system of care and by psychotherapists as well. Their voices were not taken seriously, because the experts knew better what actually the problem is. This may seem like an overly critical definition of the situation, but it is actually what people with psychotic experiences say. I receive emails every day from patients and from family members all over the world and they repeat the message: "No one listens to me". No one takes it seriously. People tell stories, in which I can read that they have been put as targets of terror and bullying from professionals who deny the valour of their experiences. In many instances, professionals who used to have psychotherapeutic interest stopped working psychotherapeutically. In practice, this meant that they were no longer interested in listening to and taking seriously the accounts of the person who had psychotic experiences, because in the clinical practice professionals started to adopt the "truth" that psychotic experiences illustrating schizophrenia really would be a neurobiological illness.

All that happened for two decades was unfortunate also because professionals in clinical practice adopted the new neurobiological explanation and stopped to rely on meeting their clients with empathy. Thus, psychotherapists also became a part of the movement of abandoning the clients and their families. The sad part of the story is that the new explanation of the background of psychotic experiences was not based on reliable scientific evidence. Claims of the deterministic neurobiological quality of psychosis were based mainly on myths and studies that mostly did not clarify the issue that they were told to explain. If some study would show that a group of psychotic patients using neuroleptics during the very first weeks would recover faster from their symptoms compared to the one who did not use them, it is not a confirmation that schizophrenia is caused by structural changes in the brain and thus the medication is needed immediately. But this was the story. Poor scientific evidence was repeated in the treatment of excellence guidelines overemphasizing the importance of neuroleptic medication as the treatment of choice and disacknowledging the importance of psychosocial approaches.

Although this has been the main story, this book is an illustration that all the way through there have been clinicians who have continued the psychotherapeutic work with their psychotic clients. They have kept the flame of psychotherapy alive until the climate has become more plausible for humanistic practice in psychotic problems. Climate change started to happen in the studies, in which it was found that the use of neuroleptic medication can be related to shrinkage of the brain, they can cause structural changes in the brain and they can increase mortality especially if using multiplicity of drugs. These results encouraged to look for more human practice. While in the medication the emphasize is on removing the symptoms, the psychotherapeutic approaches have the interest to meet the full human beings, not only their symptoms.

This shift is groundbreaking, moving the focus on all the voices respecting the unique individual experience. This type of humanistic perspective is the basis of any psychotherapeutic method. But it is not a new one. In psychotic crises, psychotherapy used to have an essential role a long time ago since the 1930s. First in psychodynamic psychotherapy and in family therapy and later in several different methods of cognitive and cognitive behavioural therapies. During the last decades, we have seen the enormous growth of different psychotherapy methods including the variations of therapies emphasizing the importance of embodiment. The new arising paradigm has also been supported by new research showing the effects of psychotherapies producing more permanent results in life in comparison to only using medication.

I have been involved in developing Open Dialogues in most serious crises including psychotic problems. The special element of open dialogues is to mobilize the resources of the families and other parts of social network of the clients in crises, and the outcomes have been promising. In one study of 19 years of follow-up after the first psychotic crisis, it was found an enormous difference in comparison to treatment as usual in Finland. In the case of those who had been in open dialogue care 19 years ago during their first crises, 28% needed contact to care, 33% were using neuroleptic medication and 33% were living on disability and the rest of the patients working actively. All these mean that about two-thirds of the ones having psychotic crisis 19 years ago were doing well with having a full responsibility of their lives. What happened to the patients in medication-oriented care? Out of them, 49% were in contact with psychiatry, 81% were using neuroleptics and 63% were living on disability. The reader may remember that in the 1980s it was told a story that one-third of schizophrenia patients will recover, another one-third would become better but are in need of support and the rest one-third would be chronic. Now, more than 30 years thereafter, the outcomes are the same in medication-based care. Decades of the neurobiological hegemony the outcomes have not improved, perhaps the opposite. The results of care have become worse.

It really is the time to start to invest in psychotherapeutic approaches. What makes me glad while reading this book is the variety and beauty of the different methods. If you have an interest of starting psychotherapy with people suffering from psychotic problems, you really have a variety of approaches and thus the possibility to find the style of work that fit your interest.

What is the basis of psychotic experience? To understand psychotic behaviour as a response to what has happened in one's life seems to be the most important starting point. Usually, psychotic experiences emerge in an extreme stress situation, which may be obvious, but it also may be hidden in many small hints of life. The multiplicity of the stressors in a way put the person in a dead-end situation, in which hallucinations may be found as a solution, as an outcome of the impasse. In these hallucinations or delusions, people speak about real issues in his/her life and he/she should be taken seriously because this may be the first time ever when words are shared about the most important memories without any other words than psychotic ones.

Psychotic experiences many times include a sense of terror, which may be related to relationships with those nearest to the key person. This may lead to a sensation that others become too close and thus individual space is needed to protect oneself. This often leads to the unfortunate conclusion to isolate oneself from human relations. In isolation, people easily start to generate non-constructive strategies to survive the extreme situation. These type of non-constructive survival strategies are often visible in the behaviour of the protagonist, and we often think that they are the core of his/her illness. But instead of thinking of the behaviour style as a sign of illness or psychopathology for me, it is more fruitful to think of them as being responses of the embodied mind. Therefore, an appropriate professional response to psychotic crisis should include two important elements: Firstly, to introduce help immediately by organizing crisis intervention services; secondly, to include the family and other relevant parts of the social relationship immediately to stop the isolation and to help to see the human relationships potentially helpful.

In meetings with a person having psychotic experiences and with his/her family what is needed is to respect everyone's point of view without conditions. In different approaches, this is done in a unique way to each approach but is essential to mobilize everyone's own resources to meet with the challenging experience that perhaps never has been spoken about openly. The dialogical practice focuses on seeing things in the relational context in the life of the one having psychotic experiences. It seems to be important to have space for speaking about the emotional part of everyone's experience instead of having argument about whose observations are more real. In the end, what seems to be important is to be awake in the conversation, because while someone starts to speak about incidents of life in a psychotic way, this may be the moment to open the window more to the part of his/her experiences that never has been spoken before.

Shortly said, for me, these are the main guidelines to meet with the person and the family. In different approaches, I can easily see most of these elements. For the therapists this is challenging, and new skills are needed. I hope that with the help of the chapters in this book, we all will have more skills to be present and to be available for those who really need help more than ever in their lives.

Jaakko Seikkula

Professor Emeritus for Psychotherapy at the University of Jyväskylä, Jyväskylä, Finland
Professor at the University of Agder
Kristiansand, Norway
Clinical Psychologist and Family Therapist
Vice President of the Finnish Society for Family Therapy
Helsinki, Finland

Preface: Towards a Paradigm Shift in Psychosis – Models of Change

We are honoured as the editorial team to present a range of models and approaches that we believe reflect a broader change in how people with psychosis can be supported in their personal recovery. The chapters in this book reflect shifts in understandings: about recovery from psychosis, in how people make sense of their worlds, and increasing recognition that our efforts to help people should be guided by recognising common human needs for connection, purpose and autonomy and working collaboratively and creatively to help people meet these needs. We believe these shifts reflect important changes in how care and support for people with psychosis are considered and offered.

The chapters in this book provide the reader with a diversity of viewpoints on how psychological and social interventions may help people with psychosis. The chapter collection provides a sense of contemporary intervention models, with reflections, strategies and practical guidelines demonstrating how these models can inform practice.

Across the models presented in the chapters, we hope the reader will see the common purpose reflecting the shift in paradigm we believe is happening in psychosis care. The chapters present person-centred models that lead to a way of seeing, understanding and accompanying psychosis that is very different from the traditional biomedical model. Current authors and approaches are revolutionising an outdated model trapped in purely pharmacological actions and tautological explanations of a biological nature, where symptom control is the basic and fundamental form of approach, and in which psychotherapeutic actions take second place as a subsidiary to the former.

Approaches such as Acceptance and Commitment Therapy, Acceptance and Recovery Therapy by Levels, Open Dialogue, Compassion-Centred Therapy or the Hearing Voices movement, to name but a few of those presented in this book, represent a journey of self-knowledge and learning for those recovering from psychosis and have an intense transformative potential for the therapeutic team.

The reader can also see that working from the perspectives shared by the contributors implies abandoning the position of expert and being open to learning alongside the person recovering from psychosis through shared discoveries and finding common humanity. The approaches presented in this book have the potential to transform the professionals who participate whether through processes such as mindfulness and acceptance, the cultivation of self-compassion, new relationships with unusual experiences, or finding ways to communicate in open dialogue. This is why we feel the need to bring this collection of models and interventions in the book, and learn from contributors, to improve and guide the lives of all, professionals and people who experience psychosis, towards meaningful goals.

The fundamental principle that guides this book is to share models belonging to psychology that aim at personal development while respecting the needs, values and goals of each person, and that are capable of integrating any professional or student of clinical psychology, psychiatry, nursing, social work or any other discipline who is motivated by finding the pool of common humanity and wants to dive in and drink from these waters.

As experienced therapists, we see every day how difficult it is to intervene with people affected by psychotic spectrum disorders (PSD). These serious problems affect people globally, in each of their vital spheres (self, family, context, etc.) that make their definition a highly complex challenge. Throughout the history of psychiatry (whose object of study has always been traversed by the social context), there have been many attempts to conceptualize schizophrenia, with efforts to reach consensus around nosological criteria set out in diagnostic manuals such as the ICD and DSM. The efforts at definition have not necessarily led to greater precision and effectiveness in interventions, and there is as much disagreement as ever about the nature of psychosis. It can be argued that at worst the diagnostic conceptualizations of psychosis imply a disease model and stigmatising labels that are supported by biased pathognomonic interpretations far removed from scientific rigour. In the meantime, people recovering from psychosis may continue to have many needs under-served by mental health systems built on the assumptions of the disease model.

In these systems, it is unfortunately common for professionals to forget to "listen" to what people with psychosis tell us about what matters, to disassociate their life history from their symptoms, to disregard their most pressing needs, and to fail to take their needs into account when defining what is most important to them. This may not be deliberate but rather an outcome of these systems reducing complex lived experiences of psychosis occurring in the social and personal contexts to disorders to be treated. These systems can also result in professionals acting in paternalistic ways or from an expert position, rather than adopting a genuine "helping" position.

At present, transdiagnostic models, or new developments such as "The Power Threat Meaning Framework", together with new ways of understanding PSD are making their way from different origins and very distant theoretical-practical perspectives. With their new approaches, they show how diagnostic manuals, commonly used in the Western mental health system, do not take into account what happens to people, their suffering or their particular needs, and how they are associated with a standardized treatment that does not respond to the demand for accompaniment, respect, empathy, listening and dedication of time that people need in order to recover.

Positioning ourselves on the theoretical bases and principles of these psychological models, we have decided to write this book. The contributions in this book provide a sense of contemporary thinking and practice on psychological and social approaches to support the recovery of people with psychosis, including those models built from empirically validated knowledge and those yet to be validated. The reader will also see how these models can be demonstrated in practice with case material presented that has been elaborated by authors who intervene with PSD in its different manifestations and stages.

In addition, we delve into the importance of a paradigm shift that gives priority to the person's decisions, takes into account the traumatic history that accompanies their suffering, their personal circumstances, gives importance to psychotherapy and presents critiques of biologically reductionist approaches, which are currently widely questioned by authors who also contribute to this work. With all this, in the different chapters, we will have the opportunity to work with the social, family and individual contexts of people in an integral and holistic way.

Based on this working hypothesis, and throughout the different approaches presented in the book, we will try to bring our psychotherapeutic models to the applied environment, both public and private. We will take an interdisciplinary approach drawing on lessons from different parts of the world, with a perspective based on the individual, imbued in values and principles, committed to warm and humanistic care.

Melbourne, VIC, Australia — Eric Morris
Las Palmas de Gran Canaria, Las Palmas, Spain — Juan Antonio Díaz-Garrido
Madrid, Spain — Silvia Parrabera

Contents

1 **Toward a Change of Paradigm in Psychosis: A Contextual Phenomenological Approach** 1
Marino Pérez-Álvarez and José Manuel García-Montes

2 **Eppur si mouve** 23
Juan Antonio Díaz-Garrido, Raquel Zúñiga, Horus Laffite, and Eric Morris

3 **Rethinking Antipsychotics: Evidence-Based Medicine Calls for a Dramatic Change in Their Use** 37
Robert Whitaker

4 **Neuroleptics Do Much More Harm Than Good and Should Not Be Used** 59
Peter C. Gøtzsche

5 **Advocating for Integrated Therapy in the Social Environment to Treat Schizophrenia Problems** 77
Luis Valero-Aguayo, Miguel Valenzuela-Hernández, Sara Oneca de Miguel, Juan José Ruiz-Sánchez, and Juan Antonio Díaz-Garrido

6 **Contextualizing 'Psychosis' Behaviors and What to Do About Them** 105
Bernard Guerin

7 **Culturally Adapted CBT for Psychosis** 125
Farooq Naeem, Saiqa Naz, and Peter Phiri

8 **The Power Threat Meaning Framework and 'Psychosis'** 141
Matt Ball, Gareth Morgan, and Maria Haarmans

9 Cognitive Behavioural Therapy for Psychosis 171
Rachel Manser and Louise Johns

10 Person-Based Cognitive Therapy for Psychosis 191
Lyn Ellett

11 The Phenomenological Perspective and Metacognitive Psychotherapy in Addressing Psychosis 201
Gabriel Ródenas-Perea, Susana Al-Halabí, Félix Inchausti, and Eduardo Fonseca-Pedrero

12 Acceptance and Commitment Therapy (ACT): Contextual Therapy in the Approach to Psychosis 225
Bárbara Gil-Luciano, Francisco J. Ruiz, and Carmen Luciano

13 Acceptance and Commitment Therapy for Recovery from Psychosis 249
Daniel D. Simsion, Emma Caruana, and Eric M. J. Morris

14 Acceptance and Commitment Therapy for Psychosis in an Inpatient Context 285
Mårten J. Tyrberg and Brandon A. Gaudiano

15 Using Acceptance and Commitment Therapy Within a Functional Analysis Informed Therapy for Hearing Voices 307
Neil Thomas and Kim Morris

16 The Use of Therapist Self-Disclosure in Acceptance and Commitment Therapy for Psychosis 323
Julia Nicholls, Ellie Newman, and Eric Morris

17 Acceptance and Recovery Therapy by Levels for Psychosis (ART): A Context-Centred Model 347
Horus Laffite, Juan Antonio Díaz-Garrido, Raquel Zúñiga, María Francisca Martínez-Huidobro, and José Luis Hernández-Fleta

18 About Hobbits, Jedi, Goddesses and Magical Energies: Clinical Cases from ART 381
Raquel Zúñiga, Juan Antonio Díaz-Garrido, Horus Laffite, and Maria del Rosario Cejas-Mendez

19 Psychosocial Rehabilitation: An ART Approach – Clinical Cases ... 423
María Francisca Martínez-Huidobro, Hiurma Gil-Santiago, María Jesús Peña-Pérez, Virginia Martín-Santana, and José Luis Hernández-Fleta

20 The "Incluyete" (*Get Involved*) Program: A Socio-educational Experience for Social Inclusion in Mental Health 453
Adolfo J. Cangas, Eduardo Sánchez, Manuel López de Lemus, and Andrés López-Pardo

21 **Attention Centred on What Is Important for the Person (ACIP) Approach to a First-Episode Psychosis (FEP)** 465
Carlos Francisco Salgado-Pascual

22 **An Approximation to a Relational Approach for Psychosis: Functional Analytic Psychotherapy (FAP)** 485
María Marín-Vila, Carmen Ortiz-Fune, and Jonathan W. Kanter

23 **Dialectical Behavior Therapy (DBT)-Informed Interventions for Psychosis** 509
Maggie Mullen

24 **Personality or Psychosis, a Complex Binomial** 525
Fernando Rodriguez-Otero, Tamara del Pino Medina-Dorta, Karen Codana-Alcántara, Casimiro Cabrera-Abreu, Miguel Acosta-Ojeda, and Jose Luís Hernández-Fleta

25 **Mindfulness and Compassion as a Path to Recovery and Personal Discovery: A First-Episode Schizophrenia Case Study** 539
Gerardo Rivera, Reiner Fuentes-Ferrada, Edwin Krogh, and Álvaro I. Langer

26 **Compassion-Focussed Therapy for Voices and Unusual Experiences** 559
Andrew Fleming and Charlie Heriot-Maitland

27 **Clinical Case: Compassion-Focused Therapy** 587
Maria João Martins and Marta Alonso Maynar

28 **The Wall of Disconnection** 613
Olga Runciman

29 **Learning to Relate Differently to Hearing Voices** 637
Rufus May and Kerry Middleton

30 **Psychological Intervention with Relatives of Patients with Psychotic Disorders** 659
Gloria Roldán-Maldonado, Gloria María Bonilla-Roldán, and Rosalia Guardia-García

31 **Family Intervention in Psychosis: A Case** 699
Ernesto Baena, Carol Harvey, Cristina Abelleira, Jaime A. Fernández, and José A. Sánchez

32 **The Transformative Power of the Open Dialogue Approach in the Mental Health Field** 731
Teresa Abad-Sierra and Sara Toledano-Márquez

33 Raúl, Be Noise Amidst the Din, and Silence in the Murmur: Open Dialogue and First Episodes of Psychosis 745
Silvia Parrabera-Garcia and María Chico González

34 Conflicted Stories: A Case of Expanded Reality 787
Isabel Clarke and Tilda

35 Epilogue: Overcoming Adversities 801
Emilio Gotera-Sosa

Index 805

Chapter 1
Toward a Change of Paradigm in Psychosis: A Contextual Phenomenological Approach

Marino Pérez-Álvarez and José Manuel García-Montes

1.1 Introduction

In times that clamor for evidence, few things are more evident than the need for a change in paradigm in psychosis. On one hand, unsustainability of the dominant paradigm, presided by the biomedical model in which psychosis would be a brain disease and medication the treatment to be selected, is becoming more and more obvious. However, so-called mental diseases are not brain diseases (Borsboom et al., 2019; Ioannidis, 2019), nor is antipsychotic medication really a treatment that could correct etiological conditions. In fact, what medication really does is produce the same neurochemical and structural alterations (Whitaker, 2015; Yang et al., 2021) with psychotropic effects that can alleviate symptoms (Moncrieff, 2013; Pérez-Álvarez, 2021, Chap. 11), but not innocuously. As a symptomatic treatment, medication may be a useful resource, but it would not properly be a curative treatment. This is not to say that psychosis is not a disease, but perhaps more than a disease: a way of being-in-the-world.

On the other hand, the sustainability of an alternative paradigm, such as the phenomenological approach to schizophrenia in this case, is also more and more obvious (Sass & Parnas, 2003, 2007). Thus, the way is opening to a variety of aids in a contextual perspective (Díaz Garrido et al., 2021). Perhaps it is time to propose a contextual phenomenological approach beyond, in fact, cognitive behavioral therapy (Fuchs, 2019; Nelson et al., 2021; Pérez-Álvarez et al., 2011; Sass, 2019). A contextual phenomenological approach represents an alternative to the biomedical

M. Pérez-Álvarez (✉)
University of Oviedo, Oviedo, Spain
e-mail: marino@uniovi.es

J. M. García-Montes
University of Almería, Almería, Spain
e-mail: jgmontes@ual.es

J. A. Díaz-Garrido et al. (eds.), *Psychological Interventions for Psychosis*,
https://doi.org/10.1007/978-3-031-27003-1_1

model. At least a contextual phenomenological approach concentrates on the person and his circumstances. Nothing about psychosis can be understood without referring to the person. The person, and in this case, the self or the subject, is the level of analysis, the "thing itself" (remember the phenomenology slogan "back to the things themselves") that clinicians find themselves with. While a statistical focus dilutes individuals in supraindividual structures (averages), a neurobiological focus reduces them to subpersonal mechanisms.

A radical change in global mental health focused on the person is demanded by the World Health Organization (WHO), not without recriminating promotion of the biomedical model. The WHO follows in the steps of the United Nations Convention on the Rights of Persons with Disabilities. Not in vain, the WHO document is entitled *Guidance on community mental health services: Promoting person-centered and rights-based approaches* (World Health Organization, 2021).

The term psychosis has recently become generalized as the most appropriate denomination for a variety of disorders with their own name, such as schizophrenia, manic depressive psychosis, psychotic depression, melancholia, and mania. Manic depressive psychosis has experienced its own transformation into bipolar disorder. Bipolar disorder includes depression, melancholia, and mania now seen as a manic-depression tandem. The brilliant idea of the bipolar spectrum ends up extending bipolar disorder not only horizontally (including several categories) but also vertically, including subclinical and clinical aspects in the same dimension with no apparent solution of normal-pathological continuity (Haslam, 2016; Paris, 2021).

The notion of spectrum also came to schizophrenic psychosis, leading to the psychotic spectrum. Psychotic spectrum similarly extends horizontally and vertically. Now the psychotic spectrum and the bipolar spectrum partly overlap and each extends on its own. The remaining disorders, autistic spectrum, anxiety, addiction, etc., would be separate. The "clinical spectrum" is projected over the general population. The notion of spectrum, which has solved the problem of lack of definition of diagnostic categories, certainly without precise edges, in favor of a dimensional, less stigmatizing conception, ends up, however, overdimensioning clinical categorization and thus extending the territory of pathologization. The clinical spectrum looms over normality, converting ordinary misfortunes into "spectrum disorders" of something.

Another problem with the handy notion of spectrum that fully affects any psychopathology that values its name is that it dilutes possible differences between what happens to people, now liquified and liquidated in the abovementioned spectrum as if, for example, the world as lived in schizophrenia, melancholia, and mania were the same or eccentricities and changes in mood were already enough for a psychotic spectrum or bipolar spectrum diagnosis. In the end, psychotic spectrum or bipolar disorder is a "false friend" serving the biomedical model more than understanding of individuals according to their circumstances.

The change in paradigm in psychosis requires going beyond the mainstream established around the biomedical model, including the psychotic spectrum disorder. It also requires going beyond the standard science that sustains the biomedical model.

Standard science is no other than a positivist, statistical science "based-on-evidence", practically, randomized controlled trials and meta-analysis. It is not a matter of leaving science, but seeing which science best corresponds to the nature of clinical psychological and psychiatric problems. Progress could be made based on the discussion above that a holistic-contextual science would be more appropriate than the statistical-mechanistic science in use, not discarding it, but putting it in its place (Pérez-Álvarez, 2021; Pérez-Álvarez & García-Montes, 2019). Thus, for example, it is not proposed to avoid statistical analyzes when they are pertinent, but to direct their object towards the meaning that phenomena may have for people, who are always in a lived situation. Statistics could be, in its case, a way of extracting structures in which people's experience is organized just as, for example, it is, from a qualitative strategy, the "grounded theory". However, in practical terms, this holistic-contextual science, focused on individuals and their circumstances, becomes a qualitative methodology and clinical method. The clinical method, consisting of research in psychological phenomena in case studies, at one time was the scientific method of psychology by antonomasia. Some authors of important innovations in psychology may be recalled, who, although not clinicians, used the clinical method as their research method: Mary Ainsworth and attachment theory, Lawrence Kohlberg moral development, Jean Piaget and cognitive development and Burrhus Skinner and behavior analysis, and so many others.

In view of the above, the change in paradigm in psychosis would therefore involve going beyond the mainstream (biomedical model, positivist science) in the direction of a person-centered approach based on a holistic-contextual science shaped by the clinical method and qualitative methodology. This book of case studies is a true example of this change in paradigm, and this chapter theorizes and reasons about such a change. After all, the most practical, decisive, and hardest change is probably paradigmatic: a change in theory, viewpoint, worldview, and way of thinking. The change in paradigm is not merely a cognitive change, but one of inhabiting, thinking, and doing, a *habitus*.

The argument is developed under three headings. The first shows the need for a change in paradigm based on exhaustion of the biomedical paradigm, even though now very much currently in use. Second, a possible new paradigm for rethinking schizophrenia in a person-centered context is shown. Finally, some implications of the contextual phenomenological "turn" are highlighted as the new paradigm is identified.

1.2 Need for a Change in Paradigm: How Schizophrenia Exposes Mainstream Psychiatry

Psychiatry, like psychology, is an unstable science, in permanent crisis, always in tension due to the two souls or cultures that it is made up of, whether as positivist-naturalist sciences or human sciences (holistic-contextual). This tension is particularly evident between the biological (biomedical, neuroscientific) orientation, which is the mainstream psychiatry and hermeneutic psychiatry (phenomenological, interpersonal, contextual), which in turn, criticizes the mainstream. Critical psychiatry – criticism precisely of neurobiological psychiatry – epitomizes this tension. The same tension that also occurs in psychology between the positivist-natural psychology adhering to the biomedical model (typically second wave cognitive-behavioral therapy, Cougle et al., 2017) and phenomenological contextual, person-centered psychology, also criticizes the biomedical model (Pérez-Álvarez, 2021).

1.2.1 Intellectual Crisis in Psychiatry

The fact is that, in spite of the buoyant neuroscientific research, the main current of psychiatry is going through as much of an intellectual crisis as ever (Fava, 2020; Pérez-Álvarez, 2021, Chap. 10) and faces growing strong criticism by eminent scholars, published in the high-impact journals (van Os & Kohne, 2021). Table 1.1, taken from Jim van Os and Annemarie Kohne, presents some citations of these criticisms.

Schizophrenia and psychosis in general are like the sacred cow and the battle field of neurobiological psychiatry, as supposed brain diseases, charged to future discoveries for over a century. The so-called precision psychiatry criticized by Os and Kohne (Table 1.1) would really be a thing of the future. As their believers say, with more faith than evidence, "Precision psychiatry will eventually provide results because there is no doubt, in our opinion, that mental disorders are brain disorders, and as such, can be traced through biological clues, which may be complex, but are still there, waiting to be discovered" (Salagre & Vieta, 2021, p. 1413). About as much could be said of the Research Domain Criteria Project (RDoC). The litany that disorders are multifactorial and complex, while still true, in the neurobiological context, could mean that nothing of what they are looking for has ever really been found.

Meanwhile, schizophrenia is the abandoned illness of our time (The Schizophrenia Commission, 2012). It seems that the more is known about the brain and genome (neurotransmitters and polymorphisms included), less real flesh and blood people, reduced to a bunch of symptoms that qualify for a diagnosis and the "corresponding" antipsychotic medication, are understood. Ironically, it could be said that nothing is better than not to talk to the patients, except to confirm symptoms, if one wants to anchor schizophrenia as a brain disease. Experiences undoubtedly strange, bizarre, apparent nonsense, that seem to suddenly spring up as hallucinations, delusions, disorganized thought, duly decontextualized from the life of the person who suffers from them, will seem to be symptoms of a damaged brain to clinicians trained on the biomedical model. The consequential antipsychotic medication easily turns into an antipsychotic race, some would say, "against psychotic", insofar as what antipsychotics do is produce sedation, indifference, weakness, and thereby alleviate the symptoms. Thus, antipsychotics would better continue to be called neuroleptics or major tranquilizers.

Table 1.1 Examples of criticisms of psychiatry in high-impact journals

"There is enormous investment in basic neuroscience research and intensive searches for informative biomarkers of treatment response and toxicity. The yield is close to nil. Much of the mental-health-related burden of disease may be induced or prevented by decisions in areas that have nothing to do with the brain. Our societies may need to consider more seriously the potential impact on mental health outcomes when making labor, education, financial and other social/political decisions at the workplace, state, country, and global levels."	Ioannidis (2019)
"Ironically, although these limitations [of "biologic treatments"] are widely recognized by experts in the field, the prevailing message to the public and the rest of medicine remains that the solution to psychological problems involves matching the "right" diagnosis with the "right" medication. Consequently, psychiatric diagnoses and medications proliferate under the banner of scientific medicine, though there is no comprehensive biologic understanding of either the causes or the treatments of psychiatric disorders."	Gardner and Kleinman (2019)
"We suggest that clinical psychiatry's taken-for-granted, everyday beliefs, and practices about psychiatric disease and treatment have narrowed clinical vision, leaving clinicians unable to apprehend fundamental aspects of patients' experiences."	Braslow et al. (2021)
"The main message delivered to lay people, however, is that mental disorders are brain diseases cured by scientifically designed medications. Here we describe how this misleading message is generated. Biomedical observations are often misrepresented in the scientific literature through various forms of data embellishment, publication biases favoring initial and positive studies, improper interpretations, and exaggerated conclusions. These misrepresentations are spread through mass media documents. Exacerbated competition, hyperspecialization, and the need to obtain funding for research projects might drive scientists to misrepresent their findings. These misrepresentations affect the care of patients."	Dumas-Mallet and Gonon (2020)
"Mental disorders are not brain disorders. To the extent that mental disorders arise from the causal interplay between symptoms, as represented in network models, it is highly unlikely that the symptomatology associated with psychopathology can ever be conclusively explained in terms of neurobiology. Therefore, sticking to the idea that mental disorders are brain disorders may be counterproductive and can lead to a myopic research program, because it assumes the implausible position of explanatory reductionism a priori. As we have purported to show in the present paper, this position does not stand up to empirical and theoretical scrutiny."	Borsboom et al. (2019)
"The implicit premise of precision psychiatry is that phenomena of the mind are physically represented and that these representations are relevant to our understanding of mental suffering. This belief is so strong that it does not require explicit reflection, let alone further examination. To belong to the traditional academic psychiatric community is to reiterate the self-evident nature of the belief. To seriously entertain the hypothesis that, for example, schizophrenia may not be a self-evident disorder of the brain is dismissed as 'antipsychiatry'".	van Os and Kohne (2021)

1.2.2 *How the Biomedical Model Is Not Up to Schizophrenia*

Nobody goes crazy for no reason: without motivation and without method. Perhaps the worst part of the biomedical model is that it closes off exploration of possible reasons or motives for the psychotic crisis and excuses understanding of psychotic experiences ("symptoms") as if they lacked reasons, sense, or method. Recalling

Chesterton's famous saying: "A madman is not someone who has lost his reason, but someone who has lost everything but his reason." "Losing everything" may mean somehow *ontological insecurity* (mentioned by Laing in the *Divided Self*) such as traumatic childhood experiences, adolescent existential crisis, social defeat, or migration, conditions often found among the antecedents of psychosis. Also recalling what Polonius says about Hamlet's mad ideas, "Though this be madness, yet there is method in't." "Method" refers here to sense and function. Hallucinations and delusions make sense in the person's context, and disorganized thought also has its internal logic, far from being random products of a broken brain or something like that. The biomedical model cancels out the person and their circumstances with those of someone who is going mad.

Beyond the biomedical model (symptoms of a malfunctioning brain), schizophrenia assumes a peculiar alteration of the way of being-in-the-world. The lived world of people with schizophrenia is a break with the common conventional world and with themselves (Kusters, 2014). Even when a psychotic crisis does not spring suddenly from nothing, but has its history, probably counting on a certain way of being with its eccentricities and oddness (schizoid or schizotypy type), the truth is that the psychotic crisis is both an interpersonal rupture with others, and intrapersonal with oneself. While, for example, the voices mean strangeness of one's own thoughts or internal language experienced as voices from outside, delusion is an ontological transformation of reality in which everything now seems different, strange, altered, without any of its usual familiarity. No matter how much delusion may be a defensive "arrangement", avoiding, explaining, and protecting from anomalous experiences (such as threatening voices), it is still a "psychotic" arrangement, deranged, illusory, and delusional. Although a psychotic crisis may remain just a passing crisis, it may also lead to a "mystic psychotic path" (Kusters, 2014) and a whole existential crisis of nihilism (Klar & Northoff, 2021).

A person, typically adolescent or young adult, experiences an existential crisis and loses contact with reality, and the world taken for granted is shaken. In such a crisis, evolution is not necessarily heading toward a worsening course (*dementia* praecox as Kraepelin thought, full schizophrenia, chronification), but open to recovery, although not discarding either a certain way of being "vulnerable", eccentric, unconventional, creative, and paranoic-critical in the Dalian sense. A particular way of being "psychotic" (conventionally, "schizoid", eccentric, odd) could already be involved in the crisis itself, although it could still survive it.

In the end, schizophrenia does not stick to the person from outside, nor spring from nothing, as suggested by the expression "person *with* schizophrenia", but somehow, person(ality) may be involved. A "schizoid" style or personality has often been mentioned, perhaps due to experiences, situations, circumstances, models, to which this style would be adaptive. Although its use is understandable by reason of its stigma, the expression, "person with schizophrenia", does not remove a certain quality of being a "schizophrenic person". According to Louis Sass, "we should listen to the person's specifically schizophrenic qualities more closely and as sympathetically as possible. It may be precisely in their schizophrenia that such an individual – in a certain sense, a schizophrenic person – could embody viewpoints that challenge and profoundly enrich our own points of view" (Sass, 2007, p. 415).

The more colloquial notion of "madness" is also used as an alternative to "schizophrenia", as is "normalized madness" in Lacanian contexts.

It is not a matter of romanticizing schizophrenia at all; after all, it is an alteration of the lived world that involves great suffering, alienation, and incomprehension.

1.3 Possibility of a New Paradigm: Rethinking Schizophrenia in the Context of the Person and the Person's Circumstances

Given the need, the possibility for a new paradigm of schizophrenia beyond the biomedical model that thinks of it as a brain disease also exists. The problem with a new paradigm is that it has to open the way in a terrain colonized by the biomedical model already the default way of thinking, without having to think. When you do not think, the biomedical model thinks for you. That is why we talk about rethinking, because we have to go back and think again – weigh and weight – the preconceptions another way, somehow upstream, against the current.

Human science may even be more appropriate than natural science (often scientism more than really science) for understanding human subjects, including schizophrenia (Pérez-Álvarez, 2021, Chap. 2 and 10). The change in paradigm is beyond the mainstream, but not outside of science, but within a conception of contextual holistic human science.

In particular, the phenomenological tradition offers today a whole new way of conceiving schizophrenia (Sass & Parnas, 2003, 2007). The phenomenological paradigm opens a new field common to psychiatry and psychology (Irarrázaval, 2020; García-Montes & Pérez-Álvarez, 2010).

1.3.1 The Phenomenological Paradigm, Beyond Symptoms

The term phenomenology is common in clinical practice with regard to the description of signs and symptoms by which a nosological category of the type of the DSM (Diagnostic and Statistical Manual of Mental Disorders by the American Psychiatric Association) or ICD (International Statistical Classification of Diseases and Related Health Problems by the World Health Organization) is defined.

However, phenomenology as a psychopathological approach is different. It refers to exploration, description, and conceptualization of the content and structures of the subjective life: the particular lived world, for instance, what it is to be a person with schizophrenia (Stanghellini & Mancini, 2017; Parnas & Zandersen, 2021). Psychopathological phenomenology is not limited to a mere description of the subjective experience, but attempts to capture and define the core, configuration, structure, or center of gravity on which they gravitate and organize and disorganize the symptoms observed. Beyond the symptoms are individuals with their particular altered lifeworld. The patients do not have bunches of symptoms, but *disturbed* (backwards, confused) ways of being-in-the-world, which the symptoms reveal without themselves being the whole problem. The best help would not be, then, to eliminate the symptoms, but understand their meaning and change the relationship with them when a useless effort is involved, as is usually the case, such as struggling against the voices (Pérez-Álvarez et al., 2008).

Even though phenomenology uses a psychopathological language, it is far from the biomedical model, beginning with the notion of "symptom" sensibly, the meaning of which should be interpreted in the biographical context and circumstances of life. It would not be the first time that the symptoms understood as such open another way of having them without being *had* and dominated by them. By making them understandable in the context of life, the symptoms take on a new sense and enter in another narrative different from the biomedical one. In the end, the biomedical explanation is still a narrative, not *the* narrative, which because of its scientific foundation – which in fact it does not have – cancels out others. However, the biomedical narrative in terms of brain disease is more stigmatizing than any other and probably iatrogenic insofar as the medication it leads to is often worse than the disease. On the contrary, the hermeneutic phenomenological narrative reduces the stigma and opens other possibilities such as empathic comprehension and psychotherapy.

The phenomenological approach is different scientific conception from the natural positivist (statistical, cerebrocentric), based on qualitative methodology (without detriment to mixed methods), beginning with the phenomenologically informed semi-structured interview (Pérez-Álvarez & García-Montes, 2018). It also assumes another clinical procedure other than the nosological (in third person) based on the therapeutic relationship in which the interview (empathetic, understanding, exploratory, hermeneutic) continues to be the clinical method by antonomasia (Pérez-Álvarez, 2021, Chaps. 3 and 13).

For a phenomenological or for a psychodynamic approach (or one based on functional behavior or systemic analysis), the symptoms of schizophrenia are not aberrations, mere manifestations of breakdowns, or neurocognitive dysfunctions. The so-called "positive symptoms" of schizophrenia: Disorganized thinking, hallucinations, and delusions are not merely thinking without feeling, perceptions without object, and erroneous beliefs, as they are often dismissed. It is important to rethink positive symptoms.

1.3.2 *Starting Out by Rethinking "Positive Symptoms"*

Disorganized thinking still has its own internal organization and associative lines, even though they challenge common sense. Within its idiosyncrasy and strangeness, the thinking of people with schizophrenia can sometimes entail higher, more logical cognitive or perceptive functioning than the conventional thinking of "normal" people, although not necessarily in the general intelligence tests (Sass & Parnas, 2017). In particular, the way people with schizophrenia reason may be more logical than how "sane" people do, in tasks that require different types of reasoning (Cardella, 2020). The "paranoic-critical method" coined by Dalí enables links to be perceived between objects that are rationally or apparently unconnected. The unconventional attitude may often take precedence over conventionality. As one patient said, "My aversion to common sense is stronger than my instinct for survival" and thus the values of people with schizophrenia, including divergent forms of thought, could be beyond the banalities and common places of daily life (Stanghellini & Ballerini, 2007). Cases could always be put forward where their logic is impossible to grasp, but neither should the rationality of madness be minimized.

Hallucinations, far from being perceptions without object, have an object, more felt and experienced than "perceived" or heard sensorially, consisting of normal "objectivation" of processes and functionally tacit, silent like thought. It is interesting to recall that patients used to refer to "thoughts", and these were often subclinical, until the term "voices" was established and became prominent for clinicians – diagnosis, medication, and research (Katschnig, 2018; Yttri et al., 2020).

However, this may be that the experience of thoughts or voices is lived as inescapable interference: present-there and at the same time external. The truth is also that the experience occurs in an ontological space different from perceptive space. As strange as they may be for the patients and incomprehensible for the clinicians, the voices make sense in the biographical context, are related to real life situations, and often go on to form part of the person's life (McCarthy-Jones, 2012). Thus, the emergence of the voices has to do with real life situations, particularly, when one's position is threatened in matters that have to do with their very existence (Who am I?) and the intentions of others (Who are they?). They are very real experiences (*the real*, a Lacanian would say), which escape our understanding. It is not surprising that these vital questions are expressed in themes related with kinship and authority, sexuality, relations, gender identity, the meaning of life in the light of death and what the other wants, all existential themes (Moernaut et al., 2018).

Neither are delusions "erroneous beliefs" about the "outside world" according to the conceptions in use. Some delusions have the propositional structure of beliefs and are therefore disputable and are empirically tested. Unlike these empirical, epistemological, belief-type delusions, there are the ontological delusions that involve a whole transformation of awareness of the characteristic reality of schizophrenia. It is the distinction already established by Jaspers between primary or true delusions and secondary delusions arising from other factors, such as guilt in melancholia or a paranoid personality. Ontological delusions have an affective, experiential, immediate nature, revealed to the patient and imposed, not derived from reflection or inferential reasoning. The content of delusions in schizophrenia usually has a metaphysical, scatological, or charismatic sense, beyond worldly, empirical, ontic concerns. Thus, they are ontological delusions more than ontic, practical-worldly, empirical, paradoxically lived in a "double reality" with a subjective quality disconnected from the intersubjective world (Sass, 2014).

This double reality refers to the phenomenon described by Bleuler as "double bookkeeping", according to which two disjoint ways of being in the world, one delusional psychotic and the other worldly practical, coexist in patients with schizophrenia as kings, emperors, and popes, carrying out their daily tasks in the hospital without trying to exert their imaginary condition. Phillippe Pinel knew about this phenomenon well a century before when he recognized reasonability in madness which enabled dialogue with fools and moral treatment (Swain, 2009). Double bookkeeping is a paradoxical and enigmatic phenomenon. Patients refer to ontological convictions that seem mysterious to us, but are not problematic for them. They function like a sort of evidence from which we, as observers, are isolated. This aspect, which to clinicians seems enigmatic, is not a symptom like "pressure of thought" or "depressed affect". Rather it expresses a fundamental change in the structure of subjectivity which confers a particular quality to the many symptoms. An experienced clinician might notice an atmosphere (vital, experiential) of something paradoxical and strange in the patient's expression and the way he is. However, to go beyond this atmospheric stage, we need to conceptualize more clearly what is paradoxical and enigmatic about this impression (Parnas et al., 2021; Sass, 2014).

Schizophrenic delusions would not be, then, beliefs about mundane matters. Rather they refer to a different realm that transcends the shared social world. The "evidence" of the delusion does not refer to evidence in the shared world. The delusion is evident in itself, in a vital, experiential manner. The two attitudes or realities (delusional, practical), even in the case of an explicit contradiction, may coexist peacefully one next to the other (Parnas et al., 2021, p. 1516). More than a matter of erroneous beliefs about the world, delusions involve a qualitative change in how reality is experienced, including feelings of derealization and subjectivation combined with the intuition of a different type of transcendent reality (Feyaerts et al., 2021a, p. 243). Table 1.2 summarizes a qualitative study of delusional experience in schizophrenia showing the ontological transformation involved in delusions, beyond beliefs and the abovementioned double bookkeeping (Feyaerts et al., 2021b).

Beyond the symptoms, structural phenomenology finds that the structure or center of gravity of psychotic experiences would be in a certain alteration of the basic-self or minimal-self. The basic-self, minimal-self, or ipseity (from the Latin *ipse* = self or itself) refers to the tacit experience of one-self, implicit, pre-reflexive: the basic sense of existing as a vital subject of the experience and agent of action. It deals with, in any case, a sense of oneself anchored in one's own lived-body and in the implicit temporality (sense of permanence). This fundamental sense of self constitutes an organizing, and disorganizing, principle of experience, thoughts, and action. It is like a sort of infrastructure or "operating system" of tacit or implicit self-awareness of oneself, point of reference of the activity, and directionality toward the world and unthought of *doorway* to first-person experience. As such an "operating system", it functions even better to the extent that it is not noticed, as if it did not exist. Due to its own tacit functionality (implicit, prereflexive), the basic-self or ipseity consists of an experience hard to capture and realize, as intangible and ineffable as fundamental. Its strength is not in its patency. In fact, when it becomes patent, experience of the self and of the world is altered, which is what happens in schizophrenia. If we noted the presence of the eye, vision would be altered.

Table 1.2 Themes of delusional experience (Feyaerts et al., 2021b)

Psychosis as an ontological transformation
"In one single instance, everything was totally different. I found myself in an entirely different world."
The limits of language
"I am simply unable to formulate it. No, really, it's something I cannot formulate."
The detached observer of life
"I think that's the best description. You're on automatic pilot and you're an observer. You're doing all kinds of stuff, but it's like you're not really present, as if you're observing everything from your own perspective. When you're observing, you participate less."
Psychosis as a state of hyperreality
"I had a sort of heightened perception – I saw connections everywhere, connections which I alone saw, for example, on the doors of the psychiatric ward. The semantics of words revealed a hidden meaning."
Mystical unity
"I gained a new form of consciousness, discovered a new world which others couldn't follow."
The self in hyperreality
"I was convinced that others would consider me a figure of Jesus, that I had discovered heaven, and that I had proven the existence of the supernatural."
Double bookkeeping
I lived between two realities. Much of our time we are here on earth taking care of our daily business. But on the other hand, there is this question of the purpose of life, of god and the angles. I just couldn't get a grip on the situation."
Aftermath: The enduring impact and value of delusional experience
"Perhaps it's a dangerous thing to say that other people are more superficial and less profound. But still, there's something more fleeting or cursory in other people. They're more prone to pass over things more easily."
In search for a meaningful therapy
"I must admit I prefer rational thinking and philosophy over following therapy. I would be more inclined to read philosophical rather than psychological literature."

1.3.3 The Ipseity Disturbance Model

In their seminal article of 2003, the American psychologist Louis Sass and the Danish psychiatrist Josef Parnas proposed the ipseity disturbance model for conceptualizing schizophrenia based on a renewed long philosophical and clinical tradition (Sass & Parnas, 2003). The model now has growing research and semi-structured interviews for evaluating anomalous self-experience (EASE: Examination of Anomalous Self-Experience; Nordgaard et al., 2021) and anomalous world experience (EAWE: Examination of Anomalous World Experience; Sass et al., 2017). A phenomenological evaluation referring to these interviews may be found in Pérez-Álvarez and García-Montes (2018). The model is briefly described below.

The ipseity disturbance is described around three mutually interdependent points: hyperreflexivity, diminished sense of self, and hold or grip on the world. Hyperreflexivity refers to a heightened self-awareness (involuntary, nonintellectual) of normally and functionally unnoticed aspects (tacit, prereflexive) that form part of the infrastructure of the self ("operating system") as if the eye saw itself. Diminished sense of self refers to a decline in experience (passive and automatic), the self-identical subject of experience and action: the sense of belonging, that the experiences I am having are mine, and of the sense of agency as I am the one who performs the action. Diminished sense of self is understood to be a complementary aspect of hyperreflexivity as a compensatory effect. But hyperreflexivity could also be seen as a compensatory effect of the diminished sense of self (Sass & Parnas, 2007).

Loss of hold or grip on the world, on the other hand, refers to disturbance of the spatiotemporal structure of the experiential field, such that *familiar things* are decontextualized and become merely *strange objects*. The model assumes that distortion of the world experience involves previous anomalies of the basic self. However, since the self-and-the-world are mutually constructed (I am I and my circumstances), their disturbance may be conceived as mutual as well, without being able to say which came first. The model could begin with disturbed sense of the world, instead of the self (hyperreflexivity, diminished sense of self), as is usually done. In his day, Eugène Minkowski proposed "loss of *vital* contact with reality" as the "generative disturbance" of schizophrenia (Minkowski, 2001), renewed by Wolfgang Blankenburg as "loss of natural self-evidence" as expressed by a patient (Blankenburg, 2014) and by Giovanni Stanghellini as "common sense psychopathology" (Stanghellini, 2004). Table 1.3 presents the ipseity disturbance model with examples taken from patients.

The theory of ipseity disturbance provides an alternative to the problem of the diversity of symptoms characterizing schizophreni. The variety of aspects involved in schizophrenia, certainly disconcerting, is a problem for the biomedical conception, but not for a phenomenological conception. According to the ipseity theory, the apparent diversity of symptoms (positive, negative, affective withdrawal) would share a self-disturbance that involves the sense of self-identical subject of experience and action. The theory of ipseity disturbance relocates and reconceives schizophrenia in the perspective of self, of the subject, or the person. Thus, the ipseity theory and the phenomenological approach in general offer a new paradigm for understanding and treating schizophrenia. In reality, it is not new, but an old-new paradigm, renewed, from when psychopathology was done. Perhaps new for the new generations of clinicians trained on the biomedical model.

All in all, the phenomenological approach, including the ipseity theory, has its limitations, notably, negligence in the explanation: How is the ipseity disturbance, and in short, the psychotic disorder, generated. The strength of phenomenology is the description of the lived world – the psychotic experience, not so much the explanation of how it arose or where it is heading. According to the phenomenological approach, the psychotic experience (with its double bookkeeping) arises and comes from intersubjectivity in agreement with the self and the world, the person, and their circumstances, mutually constituting each other. In this sense, disorders are situated in the person's context and circumstances, derived from the vicissitudes of life, such as biographic events (Pérez-Álvarez et al., 2016). With respect to how culture and familiar circumstances can cause a person to go mad, the study by Louis Sass of the "Schreber case" (Sass, 1994) is exemplary. However, the explanation is not the strong point of phenomenology (as description is), so its alliance with clearly

Table 1.3 Components of ipseity disturbance model

Ipseity	Ipseity disturbance	Examples
Sense of oneself as existing as a vital and self-identical subject of experience and action.	Disturbance of sense of self: Global crisis of common sense or world taken-for-granted; loss of the natural self-evidence of things.	Elyn Sacks in *The Centre Cannot Hold*: "Consciousness gradually loses its coherence. The center cannot hold. The "me" becomes a haze, and the solid center from which one experiences reality breaks up like a bad radio signal. There is no longer a vantage point from which to look out, take things in, assess. No core holds things together, providing the lens through which we see the world"." (Sacks, 2007, p. 12). "[M]y sense of self is totally crushed when the "bubble" surrounding my self-consciousness is destroyed by this unstable permeability. […] until the entire self-experience disintegrates" (Kean, 2009).
	Hyper-reflexivity: Heightened self-awareness of normally unspoken aspects involving alienation.	One patient realized that he was someone "watching" his own receptivity to music, his own mind receiving or registering musical tones. He periodically experienced his own movements that he reflected upon and de-automated. His thought acquired acoustic qualities. (Sass & Parnas, 2003, p. 438).
	Diminished sense of self: Decline of one as a subject of experience and action.	Elyn Sacks: "Random moments of time follow one another. Sights, sounds, thoughts, and feelings don't go together. No organization principle takes successive moments in time and puts them together in a coherent way from which sense can be made. And it's all taking place in slow motion." (Sacks, 2007, p. 12).
	Loss of grip on the world of contact with the world: Loss of vital contact with reality, of natural self-evidence, or of common sense.	René in his *Diary of a schizophrenic*: "I looked at, for example, a chair or a jug, I no longer thought about its usefulness, about its function: for me it was no longer a jug for holding water or milk, or a chair made to sit down on. No! They had lost their names, their function, their meaning and had become 'things!' (p. 138). "People seemed to me as seen in a dream: I did not distinguish their particular character; they were 'human' and nothing else "(Sechehaye, 1947/2003, p. 156).

dialogic and contextual approaches is appreciated (Galbusera et al., 2021; Galbusera & Kyselo, 2019; Pérez-Álvarez et al., 2016; Seikkula, 2019), which in turn should appreciate a phenomenological "touch."

1.3.4 *What About Biology and Medication?*

The phenomenological approach does not exclude biology or medication. But neither does it put them in first place like the biomedical model. The biomedical model does not exclude the phenomenological approach either, in principle, but in the practice, it is marginalized as being secondary.

The phenomenological focus includes the biology forming part of the biography as lived-body and organism changed by the vicissitudes of life. The biography and lived-body are another (more pertinent) way of considering the body, not organic – cerebrocentric, mechanist – like the neurobiological approach. After all, genetic and neural mechanisms are not to be found anywhere, no matter how hard they are searched for. The more that is known about the genome and the brain, the more impoverished is the understanding of schizophrenia. In the end, schizophrenia is not a brain disease (*dementia praecox*) like Parkinson's or Alzheimer's. If it is still psychiatric, it is because of what it has of psyche. The abysm (vital, epistemological, and ontological) between the molecular levels (genetic, neurochemical, neural), and for example, "receive a mandate from God for a better way of life", will be acknowledged.

Medication is recognized as not properly a treatment correcting the supposed neurochemical imbalances causing the symptoms. Nor are they explained by chemistry, nor was antipsychotic medication developed based on knowledge of the cause of what is being treated.

This does not mean that medication is not useful as a *resource* in the context of psychotherapeutic and community benefits (alternatives to medication) such as Open Dialogue, Soteria Houses, and medication-free hospitalization by preference of patients (Pérez-Álvarez, 2021, Chap. 10; Standal et al., 2021; Stupak & Dobroczyński, 2021). What happens is that the way assistance services are "set up", medication becomes inevitable, not only because that is how it is established, but because, and for the same reason, there is no alternative, such as Open Dialogue for crisis help, psychotherapy, family, and community support, and not discarding medication as a resource for continued help. However, medication as the (last) resource that it should be is placed from the beginning as a first-line treatment, and that often begins a race toward chronification.

1.4 Implications of the Contextual Phenomenological "Turn"

Phenomenology restores lost psychopathological knowledge. Thus, psychopathology is reestablished beyond symptoms, and schizophrenia is relocated in the context of the person and their circumstances. This contextual phenomenological "turn" has five implications that should be highlighted here.

1.4.1 Qualitative Differences Between Psychotic Spectrum Disorders

Within sharing symptoms and forming part of the same spectrum, psychotic disorders – schizophrenias, melancholia, mania – have their own "centers of gravity" which make them basically different. The differences are revealed in a variety of

Table 1.4 Qualitative differences between psychotic spectrum disorders

	Schizophrenia	Melancholia	Mania
Qualitative differences	Loss of common sense and of conventionality. Need and fear of interpersonal contact. *Ontological* paranoia of centrality. Dissociation of the meaning of "words" converted into perceptive objects. *All* experience seems ineffable.	Conformism, "normopathy", and perfectionism. Hypersyntony with others. Paranoia *contingent* on feelings of guilt or shame. Language *only* seems limited for capturing their sorrow, sadness, or emptiness.	Hypersociability. Need for approval. "Sense of communion" with others. Paranoia *contingent* on feeling envied. Language as a torrent of associations changing from context to context.

ways. Thus, for example, while schizophrenia is characterized by loss of common sense ("natural self-evidence") and conventionality, melancholia is characterized by conformism and "normopathy" (conventionality), and mania by sociability and "sense of communion" with others. Table 1.4 presents some of these differences (Sass & Pienkos, 2013, 2015, 2016).

1.4.2 *New Life for Psychotherapy in Psychosis*

The biomedical model with medication in the fore does not exclude psychological help, but it does limit it. The phenomenological approach returns dialogue to psychosis and opens it to psychotherapy, without excluding medication as a resource. Medication-free treatment, beginning with personal treatment, listening to the person, not the drug, should be an option. As the psychotic disorder basically consists of disturbance of the experience of selfhood, of the world, and of others, psychotherapy would be the most logical help. To begin with, psychotherapy would be the help most in agreement with the nature of the problem and the person's needs, including listening, understanding, and open dialogue; all of this, in the context of an interpersonal, person-centered relationship, which psychotherapy provides like no other relationship (Fuchs, 2019; Galbusera et al., 2021; Nelson et al., 2021; Pérez-Álvarez, 2021, Chap. 13; Pérez-Álvarez et al., 2011; Škodlar & Henriksen, 2019; Stanghellini & Lysaker, 2007). Chemistry is much discussed, but as one patient said, "the "chemistry" with my psychotherapist was what helped me the most" (Pérez-Álvarez & García-Montes, 2012).

Psychotherapy in psychosis should not have the biomedical stamp of a treatment or intervention in order to repair mechanisms that have supposedly broken down and eliminate or reduce symptoms. More than reducing symptoms, it would be important to change the relationship with them (Pérez-Álvarez et al., 2008, 2011; Stanghellini & Rosfort, 2015). In this respect, a phenomenological approach would be skeptical of most common cognitive-behavioral interventions (Nelson et al., 2021; Sass, 2019). For example, psychotherapy of delusions would place less emphasis on how they could be refuted with empirical evidence or logical analysis, and more on alteration of the conditions that inspire and sustain them. And these, in turn, would deviate the focus of the treatment of delusions from themselves toward promotion of real participation in practical activity and in shared social forms of experience. It would also imply decreasing patient anxiety and excitation that feed the hypervigilance that seems to encourage delusions (Sass, 2019).

1.4.3 A Holistic Contextual Approach as a Scientific Framework

That the new paradigm is critical of the natural positivist scientific paradigm (biomedical, based-on-evidence) does not mean that it is outside of science. First rather, it revindicates a contextual holistic human science as the scientific framework most appropriate to the nature of psy disorders, including psychosis (Pérez-Álvarez, 2021; Pérez-Álvarez & García-Montes, 2019). A contextual holistic approach concentrates on the person and their circumstances. Only in the context of people's lived world can what happens to them be *understood* and *explained*. Understanding means both an open attitude – empathy and I-you relationship, as an aptitude for phenomenological exploration of people's lived world. This aptitude assumes phenomenological training (not a natural gift) with which to perform the exploration and qualitative descriptions of experiences in a variety of dimensions, such as bodily, the self (agency, intentionality), space and time lived in, and others. However, as already mentioned, the phenomenological exploration is not just the description of particular experiences, but attempts to capture and describe basic structures or existential dimensions, "centers of gravity", on which apparently heterogeneous phenomena are organized and disorganized (Stanghellini & Rossi, 2014).

In another vein, the explanation in human sciences, in this case, psy sciences, would not be found in the psychophysiological mechanisms involved in the subject being dealt with, but the history of learning, biographical experiences, and vicissitudes of life, in how the lived-world has been transformed and the disorder developed. It is not that psychophysiological mechanisms are not important, but that they form part of the same circuits, loops, and situations in which people are involved. Unfortunately, phenomenology has not bestowed as much biographical explanation as description, sometimes causing a slightly solipsist and individualist impression, which, however, does not correspond to its radically intersubjective nature. This is why phenomenology appreciates an alliance with dynamic and contextual approaches that precisely emphasize biographical history. It is in the context of the biographical history where the symptoms make sense: their comprehension and explanation (Stanghellini & Mancini, 2017; Vallina-Fernández et al., 2014).

1.4.4 *Qualitative Methodology for Research and Clinical Practice*

Scientific research and clinical practice according to a contextual holistic approach – focused on the person and their circumstances – require above all a qualitative methodology, without thereby renouncing the psychometric properties nor excluding quantitative methodology. Thus, the phenomenologically reported semi-structured interview is a method of particular significance in psychosis as yet unsurpassed (Pérez-Álvarez & García-Montes, 2018), without detracting from technological innovations such as outpatient evaluation (Fonseca-Pedrero et al., 2022). Interpretative phenomenological analysis, Grounded Theory, thematic analysis, discourse analysis, narrative analysis, and case studies are some of the qualitative methods to be considered. The study on delusional experience cited was done following the method known as "interpretative phenomenological analysis" (Feyaerts et al., 2021b). Recognition of the qualitative methodology as the clinical method of excellence and its dignification with the prestige and standards reached by quantitative methodology are pending tasks in research and clinical training. However, the interest in and presence of the qualitative methodology is growing. Thus, for example, the recent seventh edition of the *Manual of psychotherapy and behavior change* by Bergin and Garfield, considered the "polar star" and "bible" of psychotherapy, has two chapters on qualitative research indicative of its development and recognized importance (Levitt et al., 2021; McLeod et al., 2021). Qualitative methodology is not reduced to adding a few methods, but involves a contextual phenomenological approach focused on the person and their circumstances, as noted in this chapter. All in all, according to the diversity of psychology and methodological plurality, the most challenging task is the reasoned right use of qualitative and quantitative methods. Although the scientific method does not exist, nothing scientific exists without method (Pérez-Álvarez, 2018).

1.4.5 *The Contextual Phenomenological Approach as a General Framework*

Although a specific model of schizophrenia, the ipseity disturbance model, has been presented, the idea of this chapter was to show that there is life for psychosis beyond the biomedical model. The contextual holistic focus and qualitative methodology assume a pluralistic conception that may well include a variety of traditions, theories, and practices focusing on the person and their circumstances. Open Dialogue and Soteria Houses have been mentioned, and the Hearing Voices Movement, psychodynamic and systemic approaches and the Power, Threat Meaning Framework could also be cited as few examples of alternatives to the biomedical model really existing. Among these others, it is still worth highlighting the application of Acceptance and Commitment Therapy to psychosis that began in 2001 and is in continuous progress (Díaz Garrido et al., 2021; García-Montes & Pérez-Álvarez, 2001, 2005, 2010; García-Montes et al., 2004, 2021), including its integration into an existential perspective (Pérez-Álvarez et al., 2010).

More specifically, a contextual phenomenological approach (abbreviated from phenomenological, existential, behavioral, contextual) could group together a variety of alternatives otherwise dispersed, not without granting them a certain character. While the phenomenological aspect is interested in capturing and describing the particular lived world, the contextual aspect situates what happens to persons in the biographical context of present, past, and possible future circumstances. Both respects (phenomenological and contextual) represent an approach that is not reductionist, nor individualistic, dualistic, or biomedical, but precisely contextual phenomenological.

1.5 Conclusions

This chapter proposed reasoning a change of paradigm in psychosis from the dominant biomedical model to a contextual phenomenological approach. The introduction began by showing the unsustainability of the biomedical paradigm, as established as it may be, and the sustainability of a contextual phenomenological approach, although it may still be emerging. In continuation, the need for change in the biomedical paradigm is shown, taking schizophrenia as the reference. Although it may be its bastion, schizophrenia exposes the biomedical model. Two types of arguments have been used. On one hand, recent criticism of psychiatry in high impact journals indicates its drift with no way out. On the other, the fact that nobody goes mad for no reason (motives and sense) like reducing madness, or in this case schizophrenia, to supposed cerebral breakdowns. The biomedical model is not up to schizophrenia: it neither sympathizes *with* the psychotic experience that it does not understand nor *with* the persons reduced to symptoms to be treated. In the following section, the possibility of a new paradigm beyond symptoms, represented by the contextual phenomenological approach, is described. After reviewing the usual simplistic view of "positive symptoms", the ipseity disturbance model of schizophrenia is introduced. Thus, schizophrenia is situated in the context of the person and their circumstances. Finally, some scientific and clinical implications of the contextual phenomenological "turn" are arrived at. There is life beyond the biomedical model.

References

Blankenburg, W. (2014). *La pérdida de la evidencia natural. Una contribución a la psicopatologia de la esquizofrenia*. Ediciones Universidad Diego Portales (Original 1971).

Borsboom, D., Cramer, A. O. J., & Kalis, A. (2019). Brain disorders? Not really: Why network structures block reductionism in psychopathology research. *Behavioral and Brain Sciences, 42*(e2), 1–63. https://doi.org/10.1017/S0140525X17002266

Braslow, J. T., Brekke, J. S., & Levenson, J. (2021). Psychiatry's myopia – Reclaiming the social, cultural, and psychological in the psychiatric gaze. *JAMA Psychiatry, 78*(4), 349–350. https://doi.org/10.1001/jamapsychiatry.2020.2722

Cardella, V. (2020). Rationality in mental disorders: Too little or too much. *European Journal of Analytic Philosophy, 16*(2), 13–36. https://doi.org/10.31820/ejap.16.2.1

Cougle, J. R., Hom, M. A., & Matheny, N. L. (2017). Cognitive behavioral therapy: Empirically supported treatment and the movement to empirically supported practice. In D. McKay, J. S. Abramowitz, & E. A. Storch (Eds.), *Treatments for psychological problems and syndromes* (pp. 4–14). Wiley Blackwell. https://doi.org/10.1002/9781118877142.ch2

Díaz Garrido, J. A., Laffite Cabrera, H., & Zúñiga Costa, R. (Eds.). (2021). *Terapia de Aceptación y Compromiso en psicosis: Aceptación y Recuperación por niveles (ART)*. Pirámide.

Dumas-Mallet, E., & Gonon, F. (2020). Messaging in biological psychiatry: Misrepresentations, their causes, and potential consequences. *Harvard Review of Psychiatry, 28*(6), 395–403. https://doi.org/10.1097/HRP.0000000000000276

Fava, G. (2020). Psychiatry's intellectual crisis. Conversations in in critical psychiatry. Psychiatric. *Times, 37*(9), 38–40.

Feyaerts, J., Henriksen, M. G., Vanheule, S., Myin-Germeys, I., & Sass, L. A. (2021a). Delusions beyond beliefs: A critical overview of diagnostic, aetiological, and therapeutic schizophrenia research from a clinical-phenomenological perspective. *The Lancet Psychiatry, 8*(3), 237–249. https://doi.org/10.1016/S2215-0366(20)30460-0

Feyaerts, J., Kusters, W., Van Duppen, Z., Vanheule, S., Myin-Germeys, I., & Sass, L. (2021b). Uncovering the realities of delusional experience in schizophrenia: A qualitative phenomenological study in Belgium. *The Lancet Psychiatry, 8*(9), 784–796. https://doi.org/10.1016/S2215-0366(21)00196-6

Fonseca-Pedrero, E., Ródenas, G., Pérez-Albéniz, A., Al-Halabí, S., Pérez-Álvarez, M., & Muñiz, J. (2022). La hora de la evaluación ambulatoria. *Papeles del Psicólogo/Psychologist Papers, xx*. https://doi.org/10.23923/pap.psicol.2983

Fuchs, T. (2019). The interactive phenomenal field and the life space: A sketch of an ecological concept of psychotherapy. *Psychopathology, 52*(2), 67–74. https://doi.org/10.1159/000502098

Galbusera, L., & Kyselo, M. (2019). The importance of dialogue for schizophrenia treatment: Conceptual bridges between the open dialogue approach and enactive cognitive science. *HumanaMente, 12*, 261–291.

Galbusera, L., Fuchs, T., Holm-Hadulla, R. M., & Thoma, S. (2021). Person-centered psychiatry as dialogical psychiatry: The significance of the therapeutic stance. *Psychopathology*, 1–9. https://doi.org/10.1159/000519501

García-Montes, J. M., & Pérez-Álvarez, M. (2001). ACT como tratamiento de síntomas psicóticos. El caso de las alucinaciones auditivas. *Análisis y modificación de Conducta, 27*, 455–472.

García-Montes, J. M., & Pérez-Álvarez, M. (2005). Fundamentación experimental y primeras aplicaciones clínicas de la terapia de aceptación y compromiso en el campo de los síntomas psicóticos. *Revista Latinoamericana de Psicología, 37*(2), 379–393.

García-Montes, J. M., & Pérez-Álvarez, M. (2010). Exposition in existential terms of a case of "negative schizophrenia" approached by means of acceptance and commitment therapy. *International Journal of Existential Psychology and Psychotherapy, 3*(1), 1–18.

García-Montes, J. M., Luciano, C., Hernández, M., & Zaldívar, F. (2004). Aplicación de la terapia de aceptación y compromiso (ACT) a sintomatología delirante: un estudio de caso. *Psicothema, 16*(1), 117–124.

García-Montes, J. M., Pérez-Álvarez, M., López-Ríos, F., Sánchez-Sánchez, L. C., & Vallina-Fernández, O. (2021). Terapia de Aceptación y Compromiso aplicada a síntomas psicóticos positivos. In J. A. Díaz Garrido, H. Laffite Cabrera, & R. Z. Costa (Eds.), *Terapia de aceptación y compromiso en psicosis. Aceptación y recuperación por niveles (ART)* (pp. 349–375). Pirámide.

Gardner, C., & Kleinman, A. (2019). Medicine and the mind – The consequences of psychiatry's identity crisis. *New England Journal of Medicine, 381*, 1697–1699.

Haslam, N. (2016). Concept creep: Psychology's expanding concepts of harm and pathology. *Psychological Inquiry, 27*(1), 1–17. https://doi.org/10.1080/1047840X.2016.1082418

Ioannidis, J. P. A. (2019). Therapy and prevention for mental health: What if mental diseases are mostly not brain disorders? *Behavioral and Brain Sciences, 42*, e13. https://doi.org/10.1017/S0140525X1800105X

Irarrázaval, L. (2020). A phenomenological paradigm for empirical research in psychiatry and psychology: Open questions. *Frontiers in Psychology, 11*, 1399. https://doi.org/10.3389/fpsyg.2020.01399

Katschnig, H. (2018). Psychiatry's contribution to the public stereotype of schizophrenia: Historical considerations. *Journal of Evaluation in Clinical Practice, 24*(5), 1093–1100. https://doi.org/10.1111/jep.13011

Kean, C. (2009). Silencing the self: Schizophrenia as a self-disturbance. *Schizophrenia Bulletin, 35*(6), 1034–1036. https://doi.org/10.1093/schbul/sbp043

Klar, P., & Northoff, G. (2021). When the world breaks down: A 3-stage existential model of nihilism in schizophrenia. *Psychopathology, 54*(4), 169–192. https://doi.org/10.1159/000516814

Kusters, W. (2014). *A philosophy of madness: The experience of psychotic thinking*. The MIT Press.

Levitt, H., McLeod, J., & Stiles, W. B. (2021). The conceptualization, design, and evaluation of qualitative methods in research on psychotherapy. In M. Barkham, W. Lutz, & L. G. Castonguay (Eds.), *Bergin and Garfield's handbook of psychotherapy and behavior change* (pp. 51–86). Wiley.

McCarthy-Jones, S. (2012). *Hearing voices: The histories, causes and meanings of auditory verbal hallucinations*. Cambridge University Press.

McLeod, J., Stiles, W. B., & Levitt, H. (2021). Qualitative research: Contributions to psychotherapy practice, theory and policy. In M. Barkham, W. Lutz, & L. G. Castonguay (Eds.), *Bergin and Garfield's handbook of psychotherapy and behavior change* (pp. 351–384). Wiley.

Minkowski, E. (2001). *La esquizofrenia: psicopatología de los esquizoides y los esquizofrénicos*. FCE (original de 1927).

Moernaut, N., Vanheule, S., & Feyaerts, J. (2018). Content matters, a qualitative analysis of verbal hallucinations. *Frontiers in Psychology, 9*, 1958. https://doi.org/10.3389/fpsyg.2018.01958

Moncrieff, J. (2013). *Hablando claro. Una introducción a los fármacos psiquiátricos*. Herder.

Nelson, B., Torregrossa, L., Thompson, A., Sass, L. A., Park, S., Hartmann, J. A., & Alvarez-Jimenez, M. (2021). Improving treatments for psychotic disorders: Beyond cognitive behaviour therapy for psychosis. *Psychosis, 13*(1), 78–84.

Nordgaard, J., Henriksen, M. G., Jansson, L., Handest, P., Møller, P., Rasmussen, A. R., Sandsten, K. E., Nilsson, L. S., Zandersen, M., Zahavi, D., & Parnas, J. (2021). Disordered selfhood in schizophrenia and the examination of anomalous self-experience: Accumulated evidence and experience. *Psychopathology, 54*, 275–281. https://doi.org/10.1159/000517672

Paris, J. (2021). *El espectro bipolar. ¿Diagnóstico o moda?* NED.

Parnas, J., & Zandersen, M. (2021). Talking to patients and rediscovering disordered selfhood in schizophrenia. *Psychiatric Times, 38*(1), 23–25.

Parnas, J., Urfer-Parnas, A., & Stephensen, H. (2021). Double bookkeeping and schizophrenia spectrum: Divided unified phenomenal consciousness. *European Archives of Psychiatry and Clinical Neuroscience, 271*(8), 1513–1523. https://doi.org/10.1007/s00406-020-01185-0

Pérez-Álvarez, M. (2018). Psychology as a science of subject and comportment, beyond the mind and behavior. *Integrative Psychological & Behavioral Science, 52*(1), 25–51. https://doi.org/10.1007/s12124-017-9408-4

Pérez-Álvarez, M. (2021). *Ciencia y pseudociencia en psicología y psiquiatría: más allá de la corriente principal*. Alianza Editorial.

Pérez-Álvarez, M., & García-Montes, J. M. (2012). From neurochemistry to interpersonal chemistry: Towards a psychotherapy of schizophrenia. In A. J. Lancaster & O. Sharpe (Eds.), *Psychotherapy: New research* (pp. 1–21). Nova Science Publishers.

Pérez-Álvarez, M., & García-Montes, J. M. (2018). Evaluación fenomenológica más allá de los síntomas. In E. Fonseca-Pedrero (Ed.), *Evaluación de los trastornos del espectro psicótico* (pp. 331–363). Pirámide.

Pérez-Álvarez, M., & García-Montes, J. M. (2019). La filosofía de la ciencia aplicada a la psicología clínica: pensando en psicosis. In E. Fonseca-Pedrero (Ed.), *Tratamientos psicológicos para la psicosis* (pp. 123–144). Pirámide.

Pérez-Álvarez, M., García-Montes, J. M., Perona-Garcelán, S., & Vallina-Fernández, O. (2008). Changing relationship with voices: New therapeutic perspectives for treating hallucinations. *Clinical Psychology & Psychotherapy, 15*(2), 75–85. https://doi.org/10.1002/cpp.563

Pérez-Álvarez, M., García Montes, J. M., & Sass, L. (2010). La hora de la fenomenología en la esquizofrenia. *Clínica y Salud, 21*, 221–233.

Pérez-Álvarez, M., García-Montes, J. M., Vallina-Fernández, O., Perona-Garcelán, S., & Cuevas-Yust, C. (2011). New life for schizophrenia psychotherapy in the light of phenomenology. *Clinical Psychology & Psychotherapy, 18*(3), 187–201. https://doi.org/10.1002/cpp.716

Pérez-Álvarez, M., García-Montes, J. M., Vallina-Fernández, O., & Perona-Garcelán, S. (2016). Rethinking schizophrenia in the context of the person and their circumstances: Seven reasons. *Frontiers in Psychology, 7*, 1650. https://doi.org/10.3389/fpsyg.2016.01650

Sacks, E. (2007). *The centre cannot hold: A memoir of my schizophrenia*. Virago.

Salagre, E., & Vieta, E. (2021). Commentary on Kohne and van OS view on precision psychiatry. *Psychological Medicine, 51*, 1412–1414. https://doi.org/10.1017/S0033291720005309

Sass, L. A. (1994). Civilized madness: Schizophrenia, self-consciousness and the modern mind. *History of the Human Sciences, 7*(2), 83–120. https://doi.org/10.1177/095269519400700206

Sass, L. (2007). 'Schizophrenic person' or 'person with schizophrenia'?: An essay on illness and the self. *Theory & Psychology, 17*(3), 395–420. https://doi.org/10.1177/0959354307073152

Sass, L. (2014). Delusion and double book-keeping. In T. Fuchs, T. Breyer, & C. Mundt (Eds.), *Karl jaspers' philosophy and psychopathology* (pp. 125–147). Springer.

Sass, L. (2019). Three dangers: Phenomenological reflections on the psychotherapy of psychosis. *Psychopathology, 52*, 126–134. https://doi.org/10.1159/000500012

Sass, L. A., & Parnas, J. (2003). Schizophrenia, consciousness, and the self. *Schizophrenia Bulletin, 29*(3), 427–444. https://doi.org/10.1093/oxfordjournals.schbul.a007017

Sass, L. A., & Parnas, J. (2007). Explaining schizophrenia: The relevance of phenomenology. In M. C. Chung, B. Fulford, & G. Graham (Eds.), *Reconceiving schizophrenia* (pp. 63–95). Oxford University Press.

Sass, L., & Parnas, J. (2017). Thought disorder, subjectivity, and the self. *Schizophrenia Bulletin, 43*(3), 497–502. https://doi.org/10.1093/schbul/sbx032

Sass, L. A., & Pienkos, E. (2013). Space, time, and atmosphere: A comparative phenomenology of melancholia, mania, and schizophrenia, part II. *Journal of Consciousness Studies, 20*(7–8), 131–152.

Sass, L., & Pienkos, E. (2015). Faces of Intersubjectivity: A phenomenological study of interpersonal experience in melancholia, mania, and schizophrenia. *Journal of Phenomenological Psychology, 46*(1), 1–32. https://doi.org/10.1163/15691624-12341283

Sass, L., & Pienkos, E. (2016). Variedades de la experiencia de sí mismo: una fenomenología comparativa de la melancolía, la manía y la esquizofrenia. Parte I. *Revista Colombiana de Filosofía de la Ciencia, 14*(28). https://doi.org/10.18270/rcfc.v14i28.1655

Sass, L., Pienkos, E., Skodlar, B., Stanghellini, G., Fuchs, T., Parnas, J., & Jones, N. (2017). EAWE: Examination of anomalous world experience. *Psychopathology, 50*(1), 10–54. https://doi.org/10.1159/000454928

Sechehaye, M. A. (1947/2003). *La realización simbólica y Diario de una esquizofrénica*. FCE.

Seikkula, J. (2019). Psychosis is not illness but a survival strategy in severe stress: A proposal for an addition to a phenomenological point of view. *Psychopathology, 52*(2), 143–150. https://doi.org/10.1159/000500162

Škodlar, B., & Henriksen, M. G. (2019). Toward a phenomenological psychotherapy for schizophrenia. *Psychopathology, 52*(2), 117–125. https://doi.org/10.1159/000500163

Standal, K., Solbakken, O. A., Rugkåsa, J., Martinsen, A. R., Halvorsen, M. S., Abbass, A., & Heiervang, K. S. (2021). Why service users choose medication-free psychiatric treatment: A mixed-method study of user accounts. *Patient Preference and Adherence, 15*, 1647–1660. https://doi.org/10.2147/PPA.S308151

Stanghellini, G. (2004). *Disembodied spirits and Deanimated bodies: The psychopathology of common sense*. Oxford University Press.

Stanghellini, G., & Ballerini, M. (2007). Values in persons with schizophrenia. *Schizophrenia Bulletin, 33*(1), 131–141. https://doi.org/10.1093/schbul/sbl036

Stanghellini, G., & Lysaker, P. H. (2007). The psychotherapy of schizophrenia through the lens of phenomenology: Intersubjectivity and the search for the recovery of first- and second-person awareness. *American Journal of Psychotherapy, 61*(2), 163–179.

Stanghellini, G., & Mancini, M. (2017). *The therapeutic interview in mental health: A values-based and person-centered approach*. Cambridge University Press.

Stanghellini, G., & Rosfort, R. (2015). Disordered selves or persons with schizophrenia? *Current Opinion in Psychiatry, 28*(3), 256–263.

Stanghellini, G., & Rossi, R. (2014). Pheno-phenotypes: A holistic approach to the psychopathology of schizophrenia. *Current Opinion in Psychiatry, 27*(3), 236–241.

Stupak, R., & Dobroczyński, B. (2021). From mental health industry to humane care. Suggestions for an alternative systemic approach to distress. *International Journal of Environmental Research and Public Health, 18*(12), 6625. https://doi.org/10.3390/ijerph18126625

Swain, G. (2009). *Diálogo con el insensato*. Asociación Española de Neuropsiquiatría.

The Schizophrenia Commission. (2012). *The abandoned illness: A report from the schizophrenia commission*. Rethink Mental Illness.

Vallina-Fernández, Ó., Pérez-Álvarez, M., Fernández-Iglesias, P., Soto-Balbuena, C., Perona-Garcelán, S., & García-Montes, J. M. (2014). Person-based contextual therapy applied to a complex case of schizophrenia. *Psicothema, 26*(3), 299–307. https://doi.org/10.7334/psicothema2013.247

van Os, J., & Kohne, A. C. J. (2021). It is not enough to sing its praises: The very foundations of precision psychiatry may be scientifically unsound and require examination. *Psychological Medicine, 51*, 1415–1417. https://doi.org/10.1017/S0033291721000167

Whitaker, R. (2015). *Anatomía de una epidemia: medicamentos psiquiátricos andel asombroso aumento de las enfermedades mentales*. Capitán Swing.

World Health Organization. (2021). *Guidance on community mental health services: Promoting person-centred and rights-based approaches*. https://www.who.int/publications/i/item/9789240025707

Yang, C., Tang, J., Liu, N., Yao, L., Xu, M., Sun, H., Tao, B., Gong, Q., Cao, H., Zhang, W., & Lui, S. (2021). The effects of antipsychotic treatment on the brain of patients with first-episode schizophrenia: A selective review of longitudinal MRI studies. *Frontiers in Psychiatry, 12*, 593703. https://doi.org/10.3389/fpsyt.2021.593703

Yttri, J. E., Urfer-Parnas, A., & Parnas, J. (2020). Auditory verbal hallucinations in schizophrenia: Mode of onset and disclosure. *The Journal of Nervous and Mental Disease, 208*(9), 689–693. https://doi.org/10.1097/NMD.0000000000001179

Chapter 2
Eppur si mouve

**Juan Antonio Díaz-Garrido, Raquel Zúñiga, Horus Laffite,
and Eric Morris**

2.1 When Empiricism Faced the Challenge of Psychosis

In the 1950s, the introduction of neuroleptics, along with the discovery of chlorpromazine (synthesised by Charpentier, who was looking for an antimalarial compound and suggested to psychiatry by Laborit for its sedative properties and finally brought to the field of psychiatry, led to a new approach, and finally brought to the field of psychosis by Delay and Deniker), entailed a revolution in the treatment of psychosis that facilitated the deinstitutionalisation of the mentally ill patients, and with it the psychiatric reform, which has progressively spread globally.

Shorter (1997) noted that "chlorpromazine started a revolution in psychiatry, comparable to the introduction of penicillin in general medicine". The first neuroleptics were followed by numerous important empirical findings that pointed out the causality of psychosis in the functioning of the brain neurotransmitter systems. New generations of increasingly selective pharmacological molecules emerged, which seemed to presage that "Science" would be able to control "madness" once and for all.

However, more than 70 years have passed and the enormous expectations placed on antipsychotic drugs have not been fully fulfilled. In this regard, Thomas Insel

Eppursimouve ("and yet it moves"), a phrase attributed by Giuseppe Baretti to Galileo Galilei.

J. A. Díaz-Garrido (✉) · H. Laffite
Hospital Universitario de Gran Canaria Doctor Negrín, Las Palmas de Gran Canaria, Spain

R. Zúñiga
Hospital Universitario Canarias, Santa Cruz de Tenerife, Spain

E. Morris
La Trobe University, Melbourne, Australia
e-mail: Eric.Morris@latrobe.edu.au

J. A. Díaz-Garrido et al. (eds.), *Psychological Interventions for Psychosis*,
https://doi.org/10.1007/978-3-031-27003-1_2

(former president of the National Institute of Mental Health, NIMH) stated that "the long-term outcomes for people with "schizophrenia" remind us that 100 years after defining this disorder and 50 years after "breakthrough" medications, we still have much to learn" (Insel, 2013).

An increasing number of studies explicitly state the limitations of pharmacological treatment. Whitaker (2005) notes that since the introduction of chlorpromazine in the United States, the percentage of people with disabilities caused by mental disorders has increased fivefold, raising the question: Have we made any progress in the treatment of patients with severe mental illness?

Already in 1967, NIMH researchers found that at the one-year follow-up "patients who received placebo treatment in the drug study were less likely to be rehospitalised than those who received any of the three active phenothiazines" (Schooler et al., 1967). Three other studies (Carpenter et al., 1977; Rappaport et al., 1978; Mosher & Menn, 1978) were funded by the NIMH in an attempt to clarify this question. Their conclusion was disconcerting: the treatment with neuroleptics could increase the incidence of long-term relapse.

In the same vein, more recent studies (Kishimoto et al., 2014; Lepping et al., 2011; Stone et al., 2018; Leucht et al., 2009) demonstrate better long-term outcomes in those who did not receive neuroleptic medication or discontinued its use. These results seem to be related to other studies that link the long-term use of neuroleptic medication with impairment (Pillinger et al., 2020; Husa et al., 2014; Ibi et al., 2017; Pol, 2015; Furukawa et al., 2015; Lieberman et al., 2005), or with better functioning after its discontinuation (Albert et al., 2019), or even with negative symptomatology (Artaloytia et al., 2006).

This is in line with the model presented by the British psychiatrist Joanna Moncrieff in her work "A straight talking introduction to psychiatric drugs" (2013) where she postulates that taking psychiatric drugs merely serves to replace the original mental state of the problem with the drug-induced mental state; in other words, taking a drug does not bring an organism from an abnormal functioning system to a normal one, as an illness-centred model assumes; on the contrary, it keeps the organism in an abnormal and biologically stressed state.

The main empirical theories about the (organic) cause of psychosis and the mechanisms of drugs in psychosis have also been strongly questioned. A recent meta-analysis rejects the dopaminergic and glutamatergic hypotheses as to the origin of psychosis (McCutcheon et al., 2021), which would leave the pharmacological explanation and approach to psychosis without an "efficient cause". Other studies report that there is no discernible difference in effectiveness between first- and second-generation antipsychotics, as well as negative effects associated with both (Saucedo-Uribe et al., 2020; Stone et al., 2018; Leucht et al., 2009). Or that, at best, their efficacy has been overestimated (Morrison et al., 2012).

With all of this and in line with Whitaker (2008), "the evidence calls for selective, cautious use of the drugs…" because, while the benefit of medication in reducing distress and unwanted phenomena is undeniable, there is also evidence of a subgroup of people who have had a psychotic episode and do not require neuroleptic medication (Wils et al., 2016; Stephens, 1978). Moncrieff herself points out that, if the disturbance is very severe, the drug-induced abnormal state may be preferred by the patient or by the people who are trying to help him or her.

2.2 Myths and Legends

Eugen Bleuler (1911/1993) built on Kraepelin's concept by coining the term schizophrenia, although he pointed out that with this term he was referring to a group that includes several diseases, the schizophrenia group. According to Bleuler, the term "dementia praecox" was inappropriate, since in many cases the deterioration either does not appear early or does not occur at all (Jablensky, 2010; Bleuler, 1911/1993). He distinguished between fundamental symptoms and accessory symptoms. The fundamental symptoms are those that are "present in all cases and in all periods of illness" (Bleuler, 1911/1993, p. 20) and, therefore, characteristic of schizophrenia, represented by the four "A's": impaired associations, disturbance of affectivity, ambivalence, and autism; Bleulerian fundamental symptoms correspond to a large extent to what we currently consider symptomatology of a negative character, while those that he called accessory symptoms correspond to the positive phenomenology. This approach emphasises the dynamic and positive character of the process, which allowed an approach to the psychodynamic perspective and thus to therapy.

Kurt Schneider's psychopathological contributions produced a turning point for the conceptualisation of schizophrenia when his work was belatedly rediscovered by anglophone psychiatry, where due to "misunderstandings or ignorance" of the author's context, definitions of the first-rank symptoms were reworked (Hoenig, 1982) and dogmatised with increasing interest, as these coincided with the positive symptomatology for which antipsychotic drugs were working. This position has been incorporated by the main diagnostic criteria manuals until their most recent versions (ICD-11 and DSM-5), since in their previous versions these positive symptoms (mainly delusions and hallucinations) were prioritised over the rest symptoms for the diagnosis of schizophrenia. However, Schneider (1997) pointed out the following:

> Among the many abnormal modes of experience that occur in schizophrenia, there are some that we call first-rank symptoms, not because we consider them "fundamental disorders", but because they have a completely special weight for the diagnosis. This assessment... refers only to the diagnosis. But it says nothing about the theory of schizophrenia.... In order to establish the diagnosis of schizophrenia, it is not necessary that the first-rank symptoms are present. (pp. 170–172)

The theoretical misrepresentation reflected in the nosological manuals about the importance of positive symptomatology in schizophrenia relegated to residual consideration phenomenon such as negative symptomatology and cognitive impairment, which have been shown to be central to people's distress and lack of adaptation to their environment.

2.3 Brave New World[1]

The critical and crude exposition of the alternative data that question the efficacy and adverse effects of neuroleptics has often been interpreted as an anti-psychiatric stance. Van Os and Kohne (2021) report that the commitment to a vision of schizophrenia that does not take a reductionist, brain pathology causes is often understood and labelled as "anti-psychiatry". On the contrary, the proposal put forward is for a reconceptualisation of psychosis, beyond the consideration of it as a biologically determined deteriorating illness with the associated reductionist search for univocal explanatory biomarkers. It can be argued that this reductionist, biological framing of prychosis has had limited impact in improving care and supporting personal recovery: additionally, it may contribute culturally to maintenance of the usual clinical practice in psychosis, centred almost exclusively on the use of medication. This focus on medication (and limited consideration of other treatment approaches) may bring with it unfortunate consequences. It can reinforce a mercantilist perspective of health, promoted by the pharmaceutical industry, and maintained and reinforced by a cultural system that encourages the imperious need to obtain "fast food" happiness, as well as the possibility of resolving any discomfort by pharmacological (magical) means. This system, which may promote the avoidance of unwanted experiences at almost any cost, and therefore of life itself, also makes use of another devastating tool to mould and homogenise its consumers: the stigma.

Dainius Pûras (2017), United Nations' (2017, 2018) Special Rapporteur on health rights, during the Human Rights Council in Geneva in 2017, stated that "...mental health systems... are based on outdated practices that violate human rights". During that intervention, he denounced that the decision-making is in the hands of "biomedical gatekeepers" supported by the pharmaceutical industry who advocate that people with mental disorders are dangerous and that biomedical interventions are necessary in most cases, concepts that perpetuate stigma and discrimination, as well as the coercive practices that are still widely accepted in mental health systems nowadays.

Pûras advocates overcoming the over-reliance on medication and the biased use of "evidence" that "was contaminating knowledge about mental health", encouraging a "paradigm shift to ensure compliance with the UN Convention on the Rights of Persons with Disabilities". According to Pûras, paternalistic and over-medicalised concepts must give way to participatory, psychosocial care and support in the community. Cost-effective and inclusive options with successful outcomes exist and are being used all over the world today; they just need to be enlarged and sustained (Pūras, 2017).

[1] Brave New World is the title of the novel published by the British writer Aldous Huxley in 1932. It refers to a utopian world where malaise and sadness were eliminated with the use of a single drug (soma) and without side effects.

The field of mental health professionals is also compromised, as research, scientific literature, and training are dominated with the medical-biological and pharmaco-centric perspective, promoting "mainstream psychiatry" (Pérez-Álvarez, 2021), through semiological straitjacketing and thus the conceptualisation and understanding of psychosis as a "disease", something that in many cases prevents the development of studies and non-pharmacological therapeutic applications (despite their evidence).

"Reviews and guidelines serve to consolidate the psychopharmacological dominance and unidimensional treatments rather than to guide the implementation of much more complex (but not more costly) multi- and inter-professional systems" (Tizón, 2016, p. 22).

As Lisa Cosgrove and Emili Wheeler (2013) state

> …prohibiting industry relationships is a necessary but insufficient solution; the disease model with its reductionism and de-politicised approach also must be challenged… until this epistemic shift is made, industry will continue to enjoy its colonisation of psychiatry.

Although there are comparative studies that support drug-free psychotherapy (Francey et al., 2020; Morrison et al., 2018; Bergstöm et al., 2018), the number of these is ridiculous compared to studies on the efficacy of pharmacotherapy, which is also financially supported and institutionalised. Furthermore, the comparison between psychopharmacological treatment and psychotherapy within the framework of evidence-based medicine is not adequate, given that the purpose of the interventions is not the same, since the first one seeks the reduction of the symptomatology, while psychotherapy does not have this as its ultimate goal (Pérez-Álvarez, 2014).

The psychotherapeutic approach to psychosis is not exempt from criticism. On the one hand, there is a significant shortage of qualified professionals for this type of human problem. On the other hand, the "expert perspective" can dominate the intervention, giving priority to the authority of the professional, their psychotherapeutic model, and their preconceived ideas about psychosis, instead of giving voice to the person and their experience, leaving the person invalidated and disempowered, restricting and limiting their freedom to decide, and therefore incurring epistemic injustice (Fricker, 2017).

Studies such as Stovel et al. (2016) and Wang et al. (2018) have shown how people with psychosis perceive themselves as disempowered by biomedical perspectives, having this and effect on the loss of power in their decision-making.

Other difficulties seen in the approach to psychosis are found at the structural level, such as the fragmentation of services, contradictory interests and priorities, difficulties in the funding and provision of resources, as well as the complex relationships between the administrations with social and health competences, which generate a significant lack of definition on the responsibilities, duplication of efforts, and a break in the continuity of care (Hadley et al., 1996; cited by Vallina, 2003).

2.4 The Right to Decide

In 2013, the British Psychological Society's Division of Clinical Psychology contemplated the need for a paradigm shift in relation to functional psychiatric diagnoses, advocating a multifactorial approach, which contextualises distress and behaviour, and which recognises the complexity of the interactions involved in all the human experience (Awenat et al., 2013).

From this position emerges an alternative model to traditional diagnostic systems, "The Power Threat Meaning Framework" (Johnstone & Boyle, 2018a, b). Cooke (2014) proposes as directions: a commitment to integral and team work, the replacement of paternalism with collaboration, free choice for the person to choose the treatment and to be able to express themselves freely about their experiences in a non-punitive framework, as well as an approach aimed at the prevention and working against discrimination and stigma. Recently, Valery and Prouteau (2020) pointed out that beliefs about biological causality in mental health problems constitute one of the variables most closely related to professional stigma.

Morrison et al. (2012) in their famous article "Antipsychotics: Is it time to introduce patient choice?", ask whether antipsychotics should always be the first line of choice. Van Os stated that "in the short-term antipsychotics work very well, but in the long-term people have to make their own choices", and puts the focus on "a model that increases resilience rather than suppressing symptoms and helps people to live with them" adding that "what works is the care that provides hope and where everyone works towards their life goals" (quoted in Barnés, 2018). Moreover, when people with psychosis are asked about their needs and preferences (e.g. Freeman et al., 2019), they identify challenges that are treatable with social and psychological approaches. For the types of care that meets these needs to be possible, a global change in the conceptualisation of psychosis is necessary, as well as the development of institutional and legislative policies aimed at modifying the support systems for people, working in a top-down process to dismantle and modify the current stigma, without forgetting the "bottom-up" process, such as the associative movements of people with psychotic experiences, families, and professionals who advocate for an appropriate change to the twenty-first century, such as the recently established drug-free hospital unit at the Åsgård Psychiatric Hospital in Tromso, UNN Åsgård (Norway).

The right to decide on treatment and life course for a person with psychosis is a controversial issue. Refusal or criticism of medication has been typically seen as a lack of awareness or insight that is part of the illness itself. However, there is evidence that most people with a diagnosis of severe mental disorder are actually capable of making decisions about treatment (Cairns et al., 2005), as well as making accurate assessments of the effects of medication (Day et al., 1995), and yet they are ignored or their opinion is not given the same consideration as that of other people (Bindman et al., 2003; Szmukler, 2004).

Nevertheless, the right to decide is an area in which progressive advances are taking place, driven by non-hospitalisation focused positions and forms of intervention and care such as: the Soteria houses initiated by Mosher (Calton et al., 2008; Mosher, 1999), the treatment adapted to needs (Alanen, 2011), or the approach in Switzerland by Emmenegger (2016), among others. See the Guidance on Community Mental Health services: Promoting person-centred and rights-based approaches, published by WHO in 2021. (Guidance on community mental health services Promoting person-centred and rights-based approaches.) (WHO, 2021).

It has been described that the use of coercive measures and physical restraint in mental health or social services is not only experienced as humiliating, but in many cases, it also produces a traumatic effect, increased by unclear and contradictory explanations about these measures, the imperative or paternalistic treatment, and the use of confusing and critical comments that do not take into consideration the emotional and cognitive situation of the person, giving rise to the experience that has been called "sanctuary trauma" (Anthony, 1993) or "welfare trauma" (Díaz-Garrido et al., 2021), especially when these services and professionals should be the guarantors of the person's safety and care, and from them one would expect understanding, patience, and comfort.

A paradoxical effect occurs, where interventions focus on the containment of suffering and not on establishing a dialogue about the personal experience of psychosis. It is significant that the admitted patients report insufficient access to psychotherapy, which is considered a high priority for them (Jones et al., 2010; Lelliott & Quirk, 2004).

Therefore, the experience of being admitted into a psychiatric unit can be a traumatic experience with detrimental implications, in the form of longer hospital stays (Calkins & Corso, 2007; LeBel & Goldstein, 2005), difficulty in establishing therapeutic alliance and adherence to treatment (NASMHPD, 2009; Frueh et al., 2005; Robins et al., 2005), as well as the increase on the relapses and readmission (LeBel & Goldstein, 2005).

Perhaps, a non-institutional, non-medicalising, and admission-avoidance approach should be the priority; an approach that encourages a networking perspective, providing a contextual and relational understanding and getting closer to the proposal of contemporary human rights approaches (von Peter et al., 2019).

Stigma is a complex concept in which multiple effects and influences occur at different levels, which we try to represent through the following concepts: social stigma, self-stigma, and iatro-stigma (Fig. 2.1) (Díaz-Garrido et al., 2021).

Some studies suggest that an alternative system to the usual one (Open Dialogue, Soteria-Berne houses and models based on mutual support) would be effective and more economical. Following these studies, Stupak and Dobroczyński (2021) propose the possibility of reducing expenditure on medication and hospital stays, allocating these resources to better care, which would have an impact on better social and occupational functioning of these people. However, the implementation of such a system "currently seems unlikely because of the influence of parties interested in maintaining the status quo, that is to a large degree associated with the neoliberal cultural and economic order".

From our point of view, the free decision of the individual becomes the backbone that has to guide the whole process of intervention and recovery, as well as being the

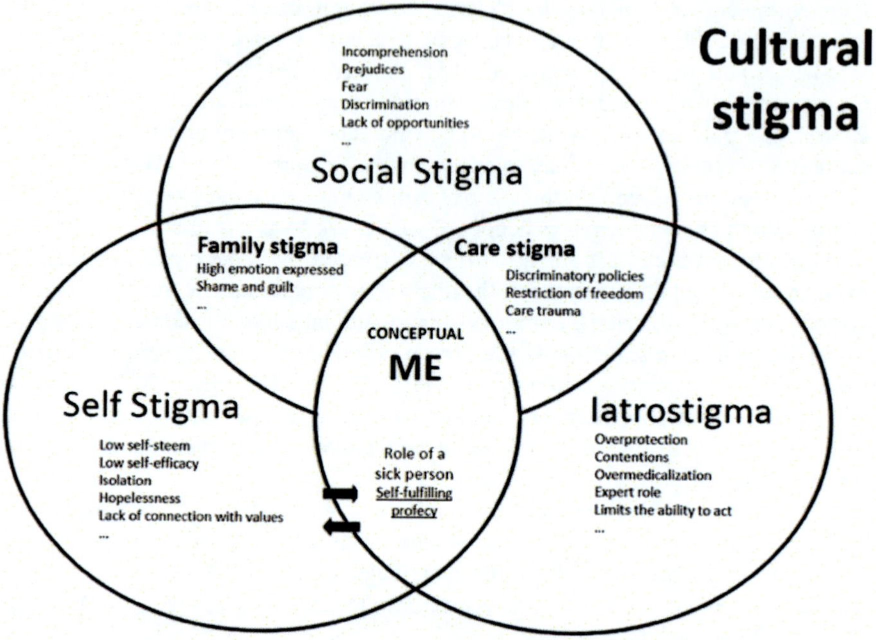

Fig. 2.1 Social stigma, self-stigma and iatro-stigma (Retrieved from Díaz-Garrido et al., 2021). Stigma conditions and hinders people's free decision making. From the conceptualisation and labelling "schizophrenic", "psychotic", to the very understanding influenced by different factors about what psychosis is, it hinders the development of a purposeful life, with its capacity for self-development and self-fulfilment. Social prejudices deeply mark the person with psychosis and label them as "strange", "violent", "unpredictable", facilitating segregation, isolation, and lack of opportunities for personal, social, and professional development. (Penn & Martin, 1998)

fundamental principle of the paradigm shift, minimising the use of punitive resources such as involuntary admission, forced treatment, and restraints; respecting the type of treatment that the person wishes to receive, be it exclusively pharmacological, psychological, or of mixed nature, knowing the risks or consequences of not adopting one or the other.

This stance would be congruent with recovery-oriented practices, for example, the CHIME model (Leamy et al., 2011): connectedness, hope, and optimism about the future, identity, meaning in life, and empowerment.

2.5 Towards a Paradigm Shift

In 2017, Thomas Insel said, "I spent 13 years at NIMH really pushing on the neuroscience and genetics of mental disorders, and when I look back on that I realise that while I think I succeeded at getting lots of really cool papers published by cool scientists at fairly large costs –I think $20 billion– I don't think we've moved the needle in reducing suicide, reducing hospitalisations, improving the recovery for the tens of millions of people who have mental illness" (Cited in Rogers, 2017).

Currently, a global movement is taking place from different theoretical-practical conceptions, philosophical approaches, non-governmental organisations, associations of people with psychotic experiences and family members, authors of recognised prestige, and a paradigm shift in the approach and conceptualisation of psychosis; a change that goes from the name itself ("integration disorder" in Japan, "attunement disorder" in Korea, "Salience Syndrome" or "Psychotic Spectrum Syndrome" among other proposals), to more contextualised and person-centred work orientations.

The fundamental principle of this paradigm shift is the person-centred approach and the development of transdiagnostic models, rejecting classical nosological labels. In addition, interventions linked to the person's context, the establishment of a more symmetrical therapeutic relationship, and the introduction of the person's choice are considered essential.

Many of the perspectives involved in the paradigm shift are based on principles such as: empowerment, radical acceptance, non-control, validation, etc., and therefore on changing the relationship with symptoms rather than eliminating them, which take on a new dimension in the way of understanding the approach to psychosis.

New conceptions of the severe mental disorder must take into consideration the person holistically, with his or her interests, goals, and values as the centre and direction of the treatment. They must also take into consideration that psychotic phenomena and experiences are multi-causal in nature, with strong involvement of the attachment, the trauma, and the dissociation components (Bloomfield et al., 2021).

The progress towards recovery-based treatments involves a reworking of the concept of functionality, understood as the choice of relevant and valuable directions and actions for the person experiencing psychotic phenomenology.

The paradigm shift requires the involvement of all professionals, starting from the withdrawal of the role of expert, to adopt a position of respect and trust in the person's capacity for growth, accompanying him or her and giving structure and support in the freely chosen valuable direction.

Examples of this paradigm shift are: the Power Framework, Threat and Meaning, Open Dialogue, Hearing Voices, contextual models such as Acceptance and Commitment Therapy (ACT), Leveled Acceptance and Recovery Therapy (ART), Compassion Focused Therapy (CFT), Person-Based Cognitive Therapy, Functional Analytic Therapy (FAP), Dialectical Behavioural Therapy (DBT), mindfulness-based therapies, Metacognitive Therapy, person-centred attention, the "Icarus" project, and the post-psychiatric movement, among others.

2.6 Conclusions

From the proposals for the reconceptualisation of psychosis, through the recognition of the right to the free decision of the person in the duly informed choice of treatment, the new types of treatments and approaches, to the consideration of attachment, trauma and stigma as an experience strongly associated with people with psychotic phenomena, changes are taking place in all areas related to psychosis, which seem to lead us towards a (r)evolution in the way of understanding and supporting people who live with this reality.

Although there is still a long way to go, a lot of resistance to overcome, providing discourses and arguments empirically sound to convince, we are participating in and witnessing the beginning of a paradigm shift, which, although it is in doubt, and takes some time, "and yet it moves".

References

Alanen, Y. (2011). *Schizophrenie – Erscheinungsformen und die bedürfnisangepassteBehandlung*. Klett-Cotta.

Albert, N., Randers, L., Allott, K., Jensen, H. D., Melau, M., Hjorthøj, C., & Nordentoft, M. (2019). Cognitive functioning following discontinuation of antipsychotic medication. A naturalistic sub-group analysis from the OPUS II trial. *Psychological Medicine, 49*(7), 1138–1147. https://doi.org/10.1017/S0033291718001836

Anthony, W. A. (1993). Recovery from mental illness: The guiding vision of the mental health service system in the 1990s. *Psychosocial Rehabilitation Journal, 16*(4), 11–23. https://doi.org/10.1037/h0095655

Artaloytia, J. F., Arango, C., Lahti, A., Sanz, J., Pascual, A., Cubero, P., Prieto, D., & Palomo, T. (2006). Negative signs and symptoms secondary to antipsychotics: A double-blind, randomized trial of a single dose of placebo, haloperidol, and risperidone in healthy volunteers. *The American Journal of Psychiatry, 163*(3), 488–493. https://doi.org/10.1176/appi.ajp.163.3.488

Awenat, F., Berger, M., Coles, S., Dooley, C., Foster, S., Hanna, J., Hemmingfields, J., Johnstone, L., Nadirshaw, Z., Wainwright, T., & Whomsley, S. (2013). *Classification of behaviour and experience in relation to functional psychiatric diagnoses: Time for a paradigm shift DCP Position Statement*. The British Psychological Society. Puedeleerseen https://cutt.ly/rUzrlTc

Barnés, H. (2018). *El holandés que quiere revolucionar la salud mental: "Es mucho más que tratar síntomas"*. El confidencial (25 de abril). Disponible en https://bit.ly/3faWVeU

Bergström, T., Seikkula, J., Alakare, B., Mäki, P., Köngäs-Saviaro, P., Taskila, J. J., Tolvanen, A., & Aaltonen, J. (2018). The family-oriented open dialogue approach in the treatment of first-episode psychosis: Nineteen–year outcomes. *Psychiatry Research, 270*, 168–175. https://doi.org/10.1016/j.psychres.2018.09.039

Bindman, J., Maingay, S., & Szmukler, G. (2003). The Human Rights Act and mental health legislation. *The British Journal of Psychiatry, 182*, 91–94. https://doi.org/10.1192/bjp.182.2.91

Bleuler, E. (1911/1993). *Demencia Precoz. El grupo de las esquizofrenias* (2ª ed.). [Dementia Praecox: The schizophrenia group]. Lumen.

Bloomfield, M., Chang, T., Woodl, M. J., Lyons, L. M., Cheng, Z., Bauer-Staeb, C., Hobbs, C., Bracke, S., Kennerley, H., Isham, L., Brewin, C., Billings, J., Greene, T., & Lewis, G. (2021). Psychological processes mediating the association between developmental trauma and spe-

cific psychotic symptoms in adults: A systematic review and meta-analysis. *World Psychiatry, 20*(1), 107–123. https://doi.org/10.1002/wps.20841
Cairns, R., Maddock, C., Buchanan, A., David, A. S., Hayward, P., Richardson, G., Szmukler, G., & Hotopf, M. (2005). Prevalence and predictors of mental incapacity in psychiatric in-patients. *The British Journal of Psychiatry, 187*, 379–385. https://doi.org/10.1192/bjp.187.4.379
Calkins, L., & Corso, A. S. (2007). Patient variables associated with the therapeutic use of seclusion and restraint in inpatient psychiatry. *New York Medical Journal, 2*(2).
Calton, T., Ferriter, M., Huband, N., & Spandler, H. (2008). A systematic review of the Soteria paradigm for the treatment of people diagnosed with schizophrenia. *Schizophrenia Bulletin, 34*(1), 181–192. https://doi.org/10.1093/schbul/sbm047
Carpenter, W., McGlashan, T., & Strauss, J. (1977). The treatment of acute schizophrenia without drugs: An investigation of some current assumptions. *The American Journal of Psychiatry, 134*, 14–20.
Convención sobre los derechos de las personas con discapacidad. Disponible en https://www.un.org/esa/socdev/enable/documents/tccconvs.pdf
Cooke, A. (Ed.). (2014). *Understanding psychosis and schizophrenia*. Division of Clinical Psychology/The British Psychological Society. Disponible en https://www.bps.org.uk/system/files/user-files/DivisionofClinicalPsychology/public/understanding_psychosis_-_final_19th_nov_2014.pdf
Cosgrove, L., & Wheeler, E. E. (2013). Industry's colonization of psychiatry: Ethical and practical implications of financial conflicts of interest in the DSM-5. *Feminism & Psychology, 23*(1), 93–106. https://doi.org/10.1177/0959353512467972
Day, J. C., Wood, G., Dewey, M., & Bentall, R. P. (1995). A self-rating scale for measuring neuroleptic side-effects. Validation in a group of schizophrenic patients. *The British Journal of Psychiatry, 166*(5), 650–653. https://doi.org/10.1192/bjp.166.5.650
Díaz Garrido, J. A., Laffite, H., & Zúñiga, R. (2021). Terapia de Aceptación y Recuperación por niveles (ART). En J. A. Díaz Garrido, H. Laffite, & R. Zúñiga (Eds.), *Terapia de Aceptación y Compromiso en psicosis: Aceptación y Recuperación por niveles (ART)*. Pirámide.
Emmenegger, T. (2016). *Freedom is a daily exercise. Psychiatry without coercion? A Swiss experience*. Ticino. Recuperado a partir de. http://www.salutmental.org/wpcontent/uploads/2016/11/Emmenegger-2016.pdf. FEAFES. (2009).
Francey, S., O'Donoghue, B., Nelson, B., Graham, J., Baldwin, L., Pan Yuen, H., Kerr, M., Ratheesh, A., Allott, K., Alvarez-Jimenez, M., Fornito, A., Harrigan, S., Thompson, A., Wood, S., Berk, M., & McGorry, P. (2020). Psychosocial intervention with or without antipsychotic medication for first-episode psychosis: A randomized noninferiority clinical trial. *Schizophrenia Bulletin Open, 1*(1), sgaa015. https://doi.org/10.1093/schizbullopen/sgaa015
Freeman, D., Taylor, K. M., Molodynski, A., & Waite, F. (2019). Treatable clinical intervention targets for patients with schizophrenia. *Schizophrenia Research, 211*, 44–50. https://doi.org/10.1016/j.schres.2019.07.016
Fricker, M. (2017). *Injusticia epistémica*. Herder.
Frueh, B. C., Knapp, R. G., Cusack, K. J., Grubaugh, A. L., Sauvageot, J. A., Cousins, V. C., Yim, E., Robins, C. S., Monnier, J., & Hiers, T. G. (2005). Patients' reports of traumatic or harmful experiences within the psychiatric setting. *Psychiatric Services (Washington, DC), 56*(9), 1123–1133. https://doi.org/10.1176/appi.ps.56.9.1123
Furukawa, T. A., Levine, S. Z., Tanaka, S., Goldberg, Y., Samara, M., Davis, J. M., Cipriani, A., & Leucht, S. (2015). Initial severity of schizophrenia and efficacy of antipsychotics: Participant-level meta-analysis of 6 placebo-controlled studies. *JAMA Psychiatry, 72*(1), 14–21. https://doi.org/10.1001/jamapsychiatry.2014.2127
Hoenig, J. (1982). Kurt Schneider and Anglophone psychiatry. *Comprehensive Psychiatry, 23*(5), 391–400. https://doi.org/10.1016/0010-440x(82)90152-3
Husa, A. P., Rannikko, I., Moilanen, J., Haapea, M., Murray, G. K., Barnett, J., Jones, P. B., Isohanni, M., Koponen, H., Miettunen, J., & Jääskeläinen, E. (2014). Lifetime use of antipsychotic medication and its relation to change of verbal learning and memory in midlife

schizophrenia – An observational 9-year follow-up study. *Schizophrenia Research, 158*(1–3), 134–141. https://doi.org/10.1016/j.schres.2014.06.035
Ibi, D., de la Fuente Revenga, M., Kezunovic, N., Muguruza, C., Saunders, J. M., Gaitonde, S. A., Moreno, J. L., Ijaz, M. K., Santosh, V., Kozlenkov, A., Holloway, T., Seto, J., García-Bea, A., Kurita, M., Mosley, G. E., Jiang, Y., Christoffel, D. J., Callado, L. F., Russo, S. J., Dracheva, S., et al. (2017). Antipsychotic-induced Hdac2 transcription via NF-κB leads to synaptic and cognitive side effects. *Nature Neuroscience, 20*(9), 1247–1259. https://doi.org/10.1038/nn.4616
Insel, T. (2013). *Antipsychotics: Taking he long view* (Blog). Disponible en http://bit.ly/3d6Cgpq
Jablensky, A. (2010). The diagnostic concept of schizophrenia: Its history, evolution, and future prospects. *Dialogues in Clinical Neuroscience, 12*(3), 271–287. https://doi.org/10.31887/DCNS.2010.12.3/ajablensky
Johnstone, L., Boyle, M., Cromby, J., Dillon, J., Harper, D., Kinderman, P., Longden, E., Pilgrim, D., & Read, J. (2018a). *The Power Threat Meaning Framework: Overview*. British Psychological Society. Available from www.bps.org.uk/PTM-Overview
Johnstone, L., Boyle, M., Cromby, J., Dillon, J., Harper, D., Kinderman, P., Longden, E., Pilgrim, D., & Read, J. (2018b). *The Power Threat Meaning Framework: Towards the identification of patterns in emotional distress, unusual experiences and troubled or troubling behaviour, as an alternative to functional psychiatric diagnosis*. British Psychological Society. Available from www.bps.org.uk/PTM-Main
Jones, J., Nolan, P., Bowers, L., Simpson, A., Whittington, R., Hackney, D., & Bhui, K. (2010). Psychiatric wards: Places of safety? *Journal of Psychiatric and Mental Health Nursing, 17*(2), 124–130. https://doi.org/10.1111/j.1365-2850.2009.01482.x
Kishimoto, T., Robenzadeh, A., Leucht, C., Leucht, S., Watanabe, K., Mimura, M., Borenstein, M., Kane, J. M., & Correll, C. U. (2014). Long-acting injectable vs oral antipsychotics for relapse prevention in schizophrenia: A meta-analysis of randomized trials. *Schizophrenia Bulletin, 40*(1), 192–213. https://doi.org/10.1093/schbul/sbs150
Leamy, M., Bird, V., Le Boutillier, C., Williams, J., & Slade, M. (2011). Conceptual framework for personal recovery in mental health: Systematic review and narrative synthesis. *The British Journal of Psychiatry, 199*(6), 445–452. https://doi.org/10.1192/bjp.bp.110.083733
Lebel, J., & Goldstein, R. (2005). The economic cost of using restraint and the value added by restraint reduction or elimination. *Psychiatric services (Washington, DC), 56*(9), 1109–1114. https://doi.org/10.1176/appi.ps.56.9.1109
Lelliott, P., & Quirk, A. (2004). What is life like on acute psychiatric wards? *Current Opinion in Psychiatry, 17*(4), 297–301.
Lepping, P., Sambhi, R., Whittington, R., Lane, S., & Poole, R. (2011). Clinical relevance of findings in trials of antipsychotics: Systematic review. *British Journal of Psychiatry, 198*(5), 341–345. https://doi.org/10.1192/bjp.bp.109.075366
Leucht, S., Corves, C., Arbter, D., Engel, R. R., Li, C., & Davis, J. M. (2009). Second-generation versus first-generation antipsychotic drugs for schizophrenia: A meta-analysis. *Lancet, 373*(9657), 31–41. https://doi.org/10.1016/S0140-6736(08)61764-X
Lieberman, J. A., Stroup, T. S., McEvoy, J. P., Swartz, M. S., Rosenheck, R. A., Perkins, D. O., Keefe, R. S., Davis, S. M., Davis, C. E., Lebowitz, B. D., Severe, J., Hsiao, J. K., & Clinical Antipsychotic Trials of Intervention Effectiveness (CATIE) Investigators. (2005). Effectiveness of antipsychotic drugs in patients with chronic schizophrenia. *The New England Journal of Medicine, 353*(12), 1209–1223. https://doi.org/10.1056/NEJMoa051688
McCutcheon, R. A., Merritt, K., & Howes, O. D. (2021). Dopamine and glutamate in individuals at high risk for psychosis: A meta-analysis of in vivo imaging findings and their variability compared to controls. *World Psychiatry, 20*(3), 405–416. https://doi.org/10.1002/wps.20893
Moncrieff, J. (2013). *Hablando claro. Una introducción a los fármacos psiquiátricos*. Herder.
Morrison, A., Hutton, P., Shiers, D., & Turkington, D. (2012). Antipsychotics: Is it time to introduce patient choice? *British Journal of Psychiatry, 201*(2), 83–84. https://doi.org/10.1192/bjp.bp.112.112110
Morrison, A. P., Law, H., Carter, L., Sellers, R., Emsley, R., Pyle, M., French, P., Shiers, D., Yung, A. R., Murphy, E. K., Holden, N., Steele, A., Bowe, S. E., Palmier-Claus, J., Brooks, V., Byrne, R., Davies, L., & Haddad, P. M. (2018). Antipsychotic drugs versus cognitive behav-

ioural therapy versus a combination of both in people with psychosis: A randomised controlled pilot and feasibility study. *The Lancet. Psychiatry, 5*(5), 411–423. https://doi.org/10.1016/S2215-0366(18)30096-8

Mosher, L. (1999). Soteria and other alternatives to acute psychiatric hospitalization: A personal and professional review. *The Journal of Nervous and Mental Disease, 187*(3), 142–149. https://doi.org/10.1097/00005053-199903000-00003

Mosher, L. R., & Menn, A. Z. (1978). Community residential treatment for schizophrenia: Two-year follow-up. *Hospital & Community Psychiatry, 29*(11), 715–723. https://doi.org/10.1176/ps.29.11.715

National Association of State Mental Health Program Directors [NASMHPD]. (2009). *Training curriculum for creation of violence-free, coercion-free treatment settings and the reduction of seclusion and restraint* (7.a ed.). National Association of State Mental Health Program Directors, Office of Technical Assistance.

Penn, D. L., & Martin, J. (1998). The stigma of severe mental illness: Some potential solutions for a recalcitrant problem. *The Psychiatric Quarterly, 69*(3), 235–247. https://doi.org/10.1023/a:1022153327316

Pérez-Álvarez, M. (2014). *Las terapias de tercera generación como terapias contextuales*. Síntesis.

Pérez-Álvarez, M. (2021). *Ciencia y Pseudociencia en psicología y psiquiatría*. Alianza Editorial.

Pillinger, T., McCutcheon, R. A., Vano, L., Mizuno, Y., Arumuham, A., Hindley, G., Beck, K., Natesan, S., Efthimiou, O., Cipriani, A., & Howes, O. D. (2020). Comparative effects of 18 antipsychotics on metabolic function in patients with schizophrenia, predictors of metabolic dysregulation, and association with psychopathology: A systematic review and network meta-analysis. *The Lancet. Psychiatry, 7*(1), 64–77. https://doi.org/10.1016/S2215-0366(19)30416-X

Pol, Y. E. (2015). Antipsicóticos para la esquizofrenia: paradigma de los medicamentos psiquiátricos [Antipsychoticsforschizophrenia: theparadigmofpsychiatricdrugs]. *Saludcolectiva, 11*(1), 115–128. https://doi.org/10.1590/S1851-82652015000100009

Pūras, D. (2017). *OHCHR | World needs "revolution" in mental health care – UN rights expert*. Ohchr.org. Retrieved January 5, 2022, from https://www.ohchr.org/EN/NewsEvents/Pages/DisplayNews.aspx?NewsID=21689

Rappaport, M., Hopkins, H. K., Hall, K., Belleza, T., & Silverman, J. (1978). Are there schizophrenics for whom drugs may be unnecessary or contraindicated? *International Pharmacopsychiatry, 13*(2), 100–111. https://doi.org/10.1159/000468327

Robins, C. S., Sauvageot, J. A., Cusack, K. J., Suffoletta-Maierle, S., & Frueh, B. C. (2005). Consumers' perceptions of negative experiences and "sanctuary harm" in psychiatric settings. *Psychiatric Services (Washington, DC), 56*(9), 1134–1138. https://doi.org/10.1176/appi.ps.56.9.1134

Rogers, A. (2017). *Star neuroscientist Tom Insel leaves the google-spawned verily for … a startup?* Wired. Retrieved January 11, 2022, from https://www.wired.com/2017/05/star-neuroscientist-tom-insel-leaves-google-spawned-verily-startup/

Saucedo Uribe, E., Carranza Navarro, F., Guerrero Medrano, A. F., García Cervantes, K. I., Álvarez Villalobos, N. A., Acuña Rocha, V. D., Méndez Hernández, M., Millán Alanís, J. M., Hinojosa Cavada, C. M., Zúñiga Hernández, J. A., & Fernández Zambrano, S. M. (2020). Preliminary efficacy and tolerability profiles of first versus second-generation Long-Acting Injectable Antipsychotics in schizophrenia: A systematic review and meta-analysis. *Journal of Psychiatric Research, 129*, 222–233. https://doi.org/10.1016/j.jpsychires.2020.06.013

Schneider, K. (1997). *Psicopatología clínica* (1ª ed.). Fundación de Archivos de Neurobiología (Ed. Original: Schneider, K. (1946). KlinischePsychopathologie).

Schooler, N., Goldbertg, S., Boothe, H., & Cole, J. (1967). One year after discharge: Comnunity adjustment of schizopherenic patients. *American Journal of Psychiatry, 123*, 986–995.

Shorter, E. (1997). *A history of psychiatry*. Wiley.

Stephens, J. H. (1978). Long-term prognosis and followup in schizophrenia. *Schizophrenia Bulletin, 4*, 25–47.

Stone, J. M., Roux, S., Taylor, D., & Morrison, P. D. (2018). First-generation versus second-generation long-acting injectable antipsychotic drugs and time to relapse. *Therapeutic Advances in Psychopharmacology, 8*(12), 333–336. https://doi.org/10.1177/2045125318795130

Stovell, D., Wearden, A., Morrison, A. P., & Hutton, P. (2016). Service users' experiences of the treatment decision-making process in psychosis: A phenomenological analysis. *Psychosis*. https://doi.org/10.1080/17522439.2016.1145730

Stupak, R., & Dobroczyński, B. (2021). From mental health industry to humane care. Suggestions for an alternative systemic approach to distress. *International Journal of Environmental Research and Public Health, 18*(12), 6625. https://doi.org/10.3390/ijerph18126625

Szmukler, G. (2004). Mental health legislation in the era of community psychiatry. *Psychiatry, 3*(3), 16–19. https://doi.org/10.1383/psyt.3.3.16.30678

Tizón, J. (2016). La importancia del diálogo democrático para la integración social, familiar y personal. En J. Seikkula & T. Arnkill (Eds.), *Diálogos terapéuticos en la red social*. Herder.

United Nations General Assembly. (2017). *Human Rights Council*. Thirsty-fourth session. Disponible en a_hrc_34_32_mental_health_and_human_rights_2017.docx

United Nations General Assembly. (2018). *Human Rights Council*. Thirsty-fourth session. Disponible en https://www.ohchr.org/Documents/Issues/MentalHealth/A_HRC_39_36_EN.pdf

Valery, K. M., & Prouteau, A. (2020). Schizophrenia stigma in mental health professionals and associated factors: A systematic review. *Psychiatry, 290*, 113068. https://doi.org/10.1016/j.psychres.2020.113068

Vallina, O. (2003). Los orígenes de la cronicidad: intervenciones iniciales en psicosis. *Boletín de la Asociación Madrileña de Rehabilitación Psicosocial, 15-16*, 15–27.

van Os, J., & Kohne, A. C. J. (2021). It is not enough to sing its praises: The very foundations of precision psychiatry may be scientifically unsound and require examination. *Psychological Medicine, 51*, 1415–1417. https://doi.org/10.1017/S0033291721000167

von Peter, S., Aderhold, V., Cubellis, L., Bergström, T., Stastny, P., Seikkula, J., & Puras, D. (2019). Open dialogue as a human rights-aligned approach. *Frontiers in Psychiatry, 10*, 387. https://doi.org/10.3389/fpsyt.2019.00387

Wang, K., Link, B. G., Corrigan, P. W., Davidson, L., & Flanagan, E. (2018). Perceived provider stigma as a predictor of mental health service users' internalized stigma and disempowerment. *Psychiatry Research, 259*, 526–531. https://doi.org/10.1016/j.psychres.2017.11.036

Whitaker, R. (2005). Anatomy of an epidemic. *Ethical Human Psychology and Psychiatry, 7*, 23–35.

Whitaker, R. (2008). Deinstitutionalization and neuroleptics: The myth and reality. In Y. In Alanen, M. González de Chávez, A. S. Silver, & B. Martindale (Eds.), *Psychotherapeutic approaches to schizophrenic psychoses: Past, present and future*. Routledge.

Wils, R. S., Gotfredsen, D. R., Hjorthøj, C., Austin, S. F., Albert, N., Secher, R. G., Thorup, A. A. E., Mors, O., & Nordentoft, M. (2016). Antipsychotic medication and remission of psychotic symptoms 10years after a first-episode psychosis. *Schizophrenia Research, 182*, 42–48. https://doi.org/10.1016/j.schres.2016.10.030

World Health Organization, WHO. (2021). *Guidance on community mental health services: Promoting person-centred and rights-based approaches*. Who.int. (2022). Retrieved January 11, 2022, from https://www.who.int/publications/i/item/9789240025707

Chapter 3
Rethinking Antipsychotics: Evidence-Based Medicine Calls for a Dramatic Change in Their Use

Robert Whitaker

3.1 Introduction

In conventional histories of psychiatry, the arrival of antipsychotics into asylum medicine in the 1950s is characterized as a great advance in care. In *A History of Psychiatry*, Edward Shorter puts it this way: "Chlorpromazine initiated a revolution in psychiatry, comparative to the introduction of penicillin in general medicine." Thanks to this new drug, schizophrenia patients "could lead relatively normal lives and not be confined to institutions" (Shorter, 1998).

Ever since, antipsychotics have been a first-line treatment for treating acute episodes of psychosis, and by the 1980s, the drugs were regularly prescribed for "maintenance" purposes. Randomized clinical trials have found that they reduce the risk of relapse, which is cited as evidence they provide a long-term benefit. Today, there is increased use of injectables to improve "medication adherence," with antipsychotics now said to protect against early death.

However, there is an evidence-based history that can be dug out from the scientific literature that tells of how long-term use of antipsychotics increases the chronicity of psychotic symptoms, lowers recovery rates, and increases the risk of early death. Indeed, recovery rates for schizophrenia patients have declined since the introduction of antipsychotics (and notably so since the introduction of atypical antipsychotics in the mid 1990s). The "standard mortality rate" for schizophrenia patients has worsened in the past decades too.

As a guild, psychiatry boasts that its practices are "evidence-based," and yet it turns a blind eye to the abundant evidence that tells of a drug-based paradigm of care that does great harm. The latter tells of a medical specialty that needs to rethink its prescribing practices, which, unfortunately, it resists doing.

R. Whitaker (✉)
President of Mad in America Foundation, Cambridge, MA, USA

J. A. Díaz-Garrido et al. (eds.), *Psychological Interventions for Psychosis*,
https://doi.org/10.1007/978-3-031-27003-1_3

3.2 The Case for Antipsychotics

The evidence that is cited for the use of antipsychotics is composed of two parts. The evidence for their short-term use comes from trials that have this design: patients with psychotic symptoms are withdrawn from antipsychotic medication and then randomized to placebo or to an antipsychotic, with their symptoms then assessed at the end of 4–6 weeks. A meta-analysis of 167 such studies conducted over the past 60 years found that 51% of those treated with an antipsychotic had at least a "minimal" response compared to 30% of the placebo group (Leucht et al., 2017).

Evidence for the long-term use of antipsychotics comes from "relapse" studies. Patients that have stabilized fairly well on an antipsychotic are randomized either to continued drug treatment or to placebo, and in a 2012 Cochrane review of 65 such studies conducted from 1959 to 2011, the 12-month relapse rate for the drug-withdrawn group was 64%, versus 27% for the drug-maintained cohort. "The results clearly demonstrate the superiority of antipsychotics compared to placebo in preventing relapse," the researchers concluded (Leucht et al., 2012).

In the past two decades, several teams of researchers have pored through mortality data and concluded that although antipsychotics increase mortality risks for non-psychiatric patients, they are protective against early death when prescribed to patients with a psychotic diagnosis.

3.3 Critiques of the RCT Evidence

Leucht's 2017 meta-analysis of the short-term trials revealed that the short-term "effectiveness" of antipsychotics is of a minimal sort. The median difference in reduction of symptoms between the medicated and placebo patients on the 210-point Positive and Negative Symptoms Scale (PANSS) is only 9.6 points, which is less than the 15-point difference on PANSS necessary for a treatment to provide a clinical benefit of at least minimal importance (Hermes et al., 2012).

It appears that second-generation antipsychotics may be even less effective than the first-generation drugs. A meta-analysis of 38 RCTs of second-generation antipsychotics found that the only 41% of the patients "responded" to the antipsychotic, compared to a 24% response rate for placebo. This is an NNT of 6: six patients must be treated with an atypical antipsychotic to provide one additional response beyond placebo, which means that five of every six patients are exposed to the adverse effects of the drugs without receiving any benefit (Leucht et al., 2009).

The other problem with the short-term trials of antipsychotics is that the placebo group is in fact a drug-withdrawal cohort, and this confounds response rates that might occur in medication-naïve patients. Indeed, there has never been a good-quality trial in medication-naïve patients, an absence in the evidence base that led Cochrane investigators to conclude that "data are too sparse to assess the effects of antipsychotic medication on outcomes in early-episode schizophrenia" (Bola &

Soydan, 2007). In other words, after 60 years of the use of antipsychotics to curb acute episodes of psychosis, there is no evidence that they provide a benefit in medication-naïve patients.

The relapse literature is similarly compromised by a biased trial design. The studies are conducted in a subgroup of patients that have stabilized on the drugs, and the placebo group is once again a drug-withdrawal group. As such, all these studies show that there is an increased risk of relapse for some period after an antipsychotic is withdrawn from a subgroup of good-responders to the drugs—those that have been stable on the medication. They do not provide an assessment of how medicated patients are faring over longer periods of time and in domains that measure their functioning and quality of life.

3.4 The Case Against Antipsychotics

There is a counter-narrative that exists in the research literature. In broad terms, it tells of a medical profession that is deluded about its own history and the merits of its drugs, with such delusion born of a refusal to confront findings, spanning across seven decades of research, that tell of medications that worsen long-term outcomes.

3.4.1 Outcomes of Psychotic Patients From 1945 to 1955

The conventional narrative in psychiatry tells how patients diagnosed with schizophrenia, prior to the 1955 arrival of chlorpromazine in asylum medicine, were destined to become chronically ill and confined to a life inside a mental hospital. However, a review of discharge rates for first-episode schizophrenia patients from 1945 to 1955 reveals a very different understanding.

- At Warren State Hospital in Pennsylvania, 62% of first-episode psychotic patients admitted between 1946 and 1950 were discharged within 12 months. At the end of 3 years, 73% were living outside the hospital (Cole, 1959).
- At Delaware State Hospital, 85% of first-episode schizophrenia patients admitted from 1948 to 1950 were discharged within 5 years, and on January 1, 1956—6 years or more after initial hospitalization—70% were successfully living in the community (Cole, 1959).
- At Hillside Hospital in Queens, New York, more than half of the 87 schizophrenia patients discharged in 1950 never relapsed during the next 4 years (Lehrman, 1961).

A review of discharge rates in Norway during this period revealed a similar outcome. Of 6315 patients hospitalized for "functional psychoses" from 1948 to 1952, 63% had been discharged and never readmitted by the end of 1953; another 9% had been discharged and readmitted at some point during that period (Odegard, 1964).

The same was true for first-episode patients at a mental hospital in Scotland. From 1949 to 1953, 63% were discharged and never relapsed during the follow-up period; 21% were discharged but relapsed at some point; and only 16% became chronically ill (McWalter et al., 2006).

The conventional history of psychiatry, which tells of how antipsychotics made it possible to treat the seriously mentally ill in the community, is belied by these data. From 1945 to 1955, roughly two-thirds of first-episode patients were discharged and living in the community at the end of follow-up periods that ranged from 1 to 5 years.

It's also noteworthy that the California Department of Mental Health, in a study of first-episode patients admitted to mental hospitals in 1956, found that 88% of those treated without neuroleptics were discharged within 18 months, compared to 74% of those treated with the drugs (Epstein et al., 1962).

3.4.2 *The Revolving Door Appears*

After antipsychotics were introduced, discharge rates for first-episode patients didn't change much. However, within a few years, a worry arose that discharged patients might be returning to the hospital more frequently than before, a pattern dubbed the "revolving door syndrome." At least four retrospective studies assessed whether this was the case.

- In the United States., a retrospective study that compared 5-year outcomes for psychotic patients admitted to Boston Psychopathic Hospital in 1947 to a similar group of patients admitted in 1967 found that the relapse rate was higher for the latter group (69% versus 55%). The 1967 group was also much more likely to be "socially dependent"—on welfare and other forms of social support (Bockoven & Solomon, 1975).
- A British study of 100 schizophrenia patients found that those treated in 1956/1957 had a "higher rate of readmission" in the 3 years following discharge than those treated in 1952/1953 (Pritchard, 1967).
- A Norwegian study that compared outcomes for first-episode patients admitted in 1948–1952 with those admitted in 1955–1959 found that while there may have been a slight improvement in discharge rates after the arrival of chlorpromazine, the total number of readmissions increased 41.6%, which the researchers described as "characteristic of the drug period" (Odegard, 1964).
- A study of 221 first-episode schizophrenia patients admitted into Scottish hospitals from 1949 to 1957, with patients followed for 3 years, found that while there was no significant difference in the percentage that suffered a single "attack" (63% in the predrug era; 69% in the postdrug era), there was an "increased relapse frequency" in males following the introduction of chlorpromazine (McWalter et al., 2006).

These retrospective studies all hinted at a disconcerting possibility: The use of antipsychotics with first-episode patients didn't improve discharge rates, at least not to any significant degree, yet increased the likelihood that discharged patients would relapse and return to the hospital. This concern led the National Institute of Mental

Health in the United States to conduct three clinical trials in the 1970s to assess the longer-term impact of antipsychotics.

The first such study, known as the Soteria Project, was led by the head of schizophrenia research at the NIMH, Loren Mosher. The study was quasi-randomized, with schizophrenia patients treated conventionally in a hospital or in a residential setting (Soteria) staffed by ordinary people. At Soteria, patients were not immediately treated with antipsychotics. The drugs would be prescribed only if the patients failed to improve after a few weeks. Eventually, Mosher opened two such houses, with a total of 82 patients treated during the 10-year experiment. At the end of 2 years, the Soteria patients, in comparison to those treated conventionally in the hospital, "had lower psychopathology scores, fewer [hospital] readmissions, and better global adjustment" (Matthews et al., 1979; Bola & Mosher, 2003). In terms of antipsychotic use, 42% of the Soteria patients had never been exposed to the drugs, 39% had used them on a temporary basis, and 19% had come to use them on a constant basis. Bola and Mosher concluded that "contrary to popular views, minimal use of antipsychotic medications combined with specially designed psychosocial intervention for patients newly identified with schizophrenia spectrum disorder is not harmful but appears to be advantageous."

In a second study at Agnews State Hospital in California, led by Maurice Rappaport, 80 young males newly diagnosed with schizophrenia were randomized into drug and placebo cohorts. Both groups stayed in the hospital for 6 weeks on average, and then were followed for 3 years, during which time they could choose to take an antipsychotic or stop taking the medication. At the end of 3 years, it was the never exposed group—24 of the 41 randomized to placebo in the hospital—that had, by far, the best outcomes. The worst outcome was seen in the group randomized to an antipsychotic who stayed on the medication throughout the 3 years (see Fig. 3.1). "Our findings suggest that antipsychotic medication is not the treatment of choice, at least for certain patients, if one is interested in long-term clinical improvement," Rappaport and colleagues wrote. "Many unmedicated-while-in-hospital patients showed greater long-term improvement, less pathology at follow-up, fewer rehospitalizations, and better overall functioning in the community than patients who were given chlorpromazine while in the hospital" (Rappaport et al., 1978).

The third study, led by William Carpenter, was conducted at NIHM's own research facility, and at the end of 1 year, the unmedicated patients, who had been treated with psychotherapy, had relapsed at a lower rate. They also suffered less from depression, blunted emotions, and retarded movements. Carpenter concluded that "antipsychotic medication may make some schizophrenia patients more vulnerable to future relapse than would be the case in the natural course of the illness" (Carpenter et al., 1977).

3.4.3 Antipsychotic-Induced Dopamine Supersensitivity

In the late 1970s and early 1980s, two Canadian physicians, Guy Chouinard and Barry Jones, put forth an explanation of why antipsychotics could make psychotic patients more vulnerable to relapse and worsen long-term outcomes. Chlorpromazine

Rappaport's Study: Three-Year Outcomes

Medication use (in hospital/after discharge)	Number of Patients	Severity of Illness (1= best outcome; 7 = worst outcome)	Rehospitalization
No meds/off	24	1.7	8%
Antipsychotic/off	17	2.79	47%
No meds/on	17	3.54	53%
Antipsychotic/on	22	3.51	73%

Fig. 3.1 Rappaport's study: Three-year outcomes. (Source: Rappaport et al., 1978)

and other antipsychotics blocked dopamine receptors in the brain, and in response to this blockade, the brain increased its density of dopamine receptors. This drug-induced "dopamine supersensitivity," they wrote, could lead "to both dyskinetic symptoms and psychotic symptoms … an implication is that the tendency toward psychotic relapse in a patient who has developed such a supersensitivity is determined by more than just the normal course of the illness" (Chouinard et al., 1978).

Drug-induced dopamine supersensitivity told of how neuroleptics, over time, acted as a trap. This change in brain physiology made patients particularly vulnerable to relapse when the drugs were withdrawn, and yet, if they stayed on the drugs indefinitely, it increased the risk that they would become chronically psychotic. In 1982, Chouinard and Jones reported that 30% of 216 schizophrenia outpatients they studied showed signs of drug-induced tardive psychosis. When this sets in, they wrote, "new schizophrenic symptoms or original symptoms of greater severity will appear" (Chouinard & Jones, 1982).

3.4.4 Cross-Cultural Studies

In two cross-cultural studies conducted in the 1970s and 1980s, one 5 years in length and the other 2 years in length, the World Health Organization (WHO) twice found that schizophrenia patients in three "developing" countries—India, Nigeria, and Colombia—had much better outcomes than patients in the United States and other "developed" countries. In the poor countries, only 16% of schizophrenia patients were regularly maintained on antipsychotic drugs, versus 61% of the patients in the rich countries. The outcomes were the best in India and Nigeria, where usage of antipsychotic medication was the lowest, and the worst in the Soviet Union, which had the highest medication use and highest percentage of patients who became chronically ill (Leff et al., 1992; Jablensky et al., 1992).

In 1997, the WHO investigators interviewed the patients in the two studies once more. After 15 years, the "outcome differential" held up for "general clinical state, symptomatology, disability, and social functioning." In the developing countries, where only a small percentage of patients had been maintained on antipsychotics, 53% were "never psychotic" anymore, and 73% were employed (Hopper & Wanderling, 2000).

3.4.5 MRI Studies

The advent of MRI technology in the 1990s enabled researchers to measure brain volumes in schizophrenia patients. In a series of reports from 1994 to 1998, researchers found that antipsychotics caused basal ganglion structures and the thalamus to swell, and the frontal lobes to shrink, with these changes in volumes "dose related" (Chakos et al., 1994; Madsen et al., 1998, Gur et al., 1998a). In 1998, Raquel Gur concluded that the swelling of the basal ganglia and thalamus was "associated with greater severity of both negative and positive symptoms" (Gur et al., 1998b).

Next, Beng-Choon Ho and Nancy Andreasen, long-time editor-in-chief of the *American Journal of Psychiatry*, reported that schizophrenia patients suffered from a shrinkage of the frontal lobes over the long term, and that this shrinkage was associated with a worsening of negative symptoms and functional impairment, and after 5 years, a decline in cognitive function. Initially, they attributed this shrinkage to the disease, but subsequently concluded that the "more drugs you've been given, the more brain tissue you lose" (Ho et al., 2003; Andreasen, 2005; Dreifus, 2008, Ho et al., 2011).

Numerous other studies have concluded that antipsychotic use is associated with shrinkage of brain volumes. In a summary review of this literature, German investigators concluded that these "changes in brain structure" could "exert adverse effects on neurocognition, negative and positive symptoms and psychosocial functioning" (Aderhold et al., 2014).

In sum, the MRI studies tell of an iatrogenic process: Antipsychotics cause changes in brain volumes that are associated with a worsening of symptoms and functional impairment.

3.4.6 Longitudinal Studies

In the late 1970s, Martin Harrow and Thomas Jobe began a long-term study of 200 patients diagnosed with schizophrenia and other psychotic disorders at two Chicago-area hospitals. Forty-six percent were first-episode patients, and the median age of the cohort was 22.9 years, which meant that Harrow and Jobe would track the course of their lives starting from the onset of their illness, or shortly thereafter. All patients were treated conventionally in the hospital and discharged. Over the next 20 years, Harrow and Jobe periodically assessed how well they were doing and whether they were taking antipsychotic medication.

At the end of year two, there was little difference between the schizophrenia patients on medication and those who had stopped taking an antipsychotic. But over the next two and a half years, the outcomes for the two groups diverged in dramatic ways. The medicated group, overall, did not get better during this period. At the end of 4.5 years, only 6% were in recovery and few were working. In contrast, as a group, those off medication improved markedly, and by the end of 4.5 years, 39% were in recovery and more than 60% were working (Harrow & Jobe, 2007) (see Fig. 3.2).

This stark difference in outcomes remained throughout the study. At year 15, outcomes for the off-medication group were as follows: 40% had "recovered," 44% had a "fair outcome," and 16% had a "uniformly poor" outcome. In contrast, the 15-year outcomes for those on antipsychotics were dramatically worse: 5% had "recovered," 46% had a "fair outcome," and 49% had a "uniformly poor" outcome (Harrow & Jobe, 2007). The medicated patients had worse outcomes in every domain: anxiety symptoms, psychotic symptoms, cognitive function, and work history (Harrow et al., 2012, 2014; Harrow & Jobe, 2013).

The same was true for patients with milder psychotic disorders at baseline: those who stopped taking antipsychotic medication had better long-term outcomes. Most notably, schizophrenia patients off medication had better long-term

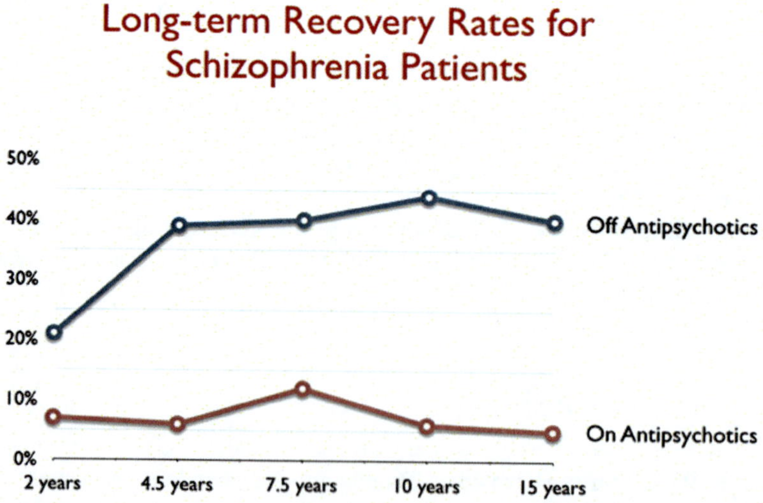

Fig. 3.2 Long-term recovery rates for schizophrenia patients. (Source: Harrow & Jobe, 2007)

outcomes than those with milder psychotic disorders who stayed on antipsychotics throughout the study.

As Harrow and Jobe discussed their results, they stated that drug-induced dopamine supersensitivity could be the reason that medicated patients had such poor long-term outcomes. "How unique among medical treatments is it that the apparent efficacy of antipsychotics could diminish over time or become ineffective or harmful?" they wrote. "There are many examples for other medications of similar long-term effects, with this often occurring as the body readjusts, biologically, to the medications" (Harrow & Jobe, 2013).

Other longitudinal studies also have found higher recovery rates for psychotic patients that don't take antipsychotic medication. To wit:

- In a randomized study conducted in the Netherlands, psychotic patients who had stabilized on an antipsychotic were either maintained on the drug or withdrawn from it (or tapered down to a low dose). At the end of 7 years, the withdrawn/low-dose group had a much higher recovery rate, 40% versus 18% (Wunderink et al., 2013).
- In an Australian study, 81 first-episode patients stabilized on antipsychotic medication were randomized to treatment as usual or to a specialized therapy designed to increased medication adherence. Although the specialized therapy did increase compliance over a 30-month period, the increased use of medication was associated with "decreases in psychosocial functioning and increases in negative symptoms" (Gleeson et al., 2009).
- A Finnish study of 70 schizophrenia patients born in 1966 found that, in an assessment of how they were doing in 2000, the 24 off antipsychotic medication were more likely to be working, more likely to be in remission, and had better clinical outcomes (Moilanen et al., 2013).
- A Danish study of 486 first-episode schizophrenia spectrum patients diagnosed from 1998 to 2000 found that at the end of 10 years, when 303 patients were still in the study, the 121 who were off antipsychotic medication were more likely than the medicated group to be in remission (74% vs. 49%), and more likely to be employed (37% vs. 16%) (Wils et al., 2017) (see Fig. 3.3).

3.4.7 *Summary of 60 Years of Research*

This "case against antipsychotics" is comprised of research of different types that together tell a coherent story. Here are the various pieces of the research puzzle:

- A majority of first-episode psychotic patients in the decade prior to the arrival of chlorpromazine recovered in the hospital and stayed well after being discharged into the community. They had an episode of schizophrenia.
- Once antipsychotics were introduced, Bockoven's retrospective study told of an increase in relapse rates and a decline in functional outcomes for psychotic patients.

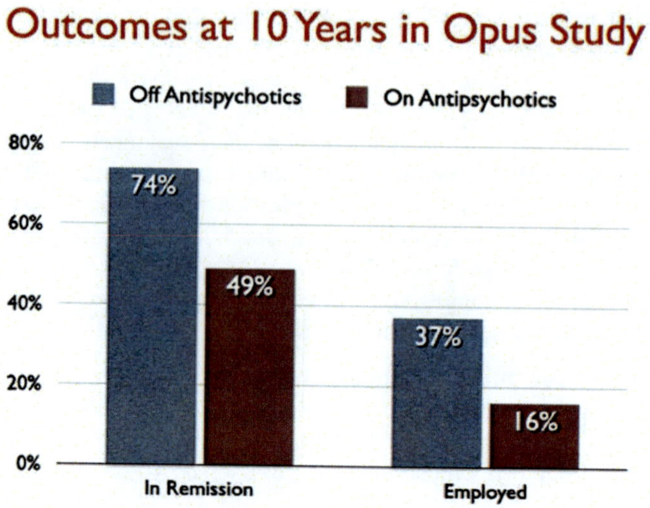

Fig. 3.3 Outcomes at 10 years in Opus study. (Wils et al., 2017)

- In the 1970s, three NIMH-funded studies found that regular antipsychotic use was associated with worse long-term outcomes, including a greater chronicity of psychotic symptoms.
- An explanation for this long-term worsening was then put forward: The drugs induce a dopamine supersensitivity that makes patients more biologically vulnerable to psychosis.
- Two cross-cultural studies by the WHO found that longer term schizophrenia outcomes were much better in developing countries where most patients weren't maintained on antipsychotics.
- MRI technology enabled researchers to study drug-induced changes in brain volumes, and they reported that such changes were associated with a worsening of symptoms and functional outcomes.
- Longitudinal studies of various types, including the Harrow and Jobe study funded by the NIMH, told of better longer outcomes for schizophrenia-spectrum patients who stopped taking antipsychotic medication.

3.5 Proof of Principle

This research tells of drugs that, on the whole, worsen long-term outcomes. However, some individuals do respond fairly well to the drugs, even over the longer term, and thus benefit from their use. As such, this review provides evidence for selective use of antipsychotics, based on two principles: no immediate use of the drugs (to see if patients can improve without their use), and if the drugs need to be prescribed to help stabilize patients, to try to limit their long-term use.

The developers of Open Dialogue Therapy in northern Finland adopted this selective-use model in the early 1990s. Here are their 5-years results: At the end of 5 years, 67% of their patients have never been exposed to an antipsychotic; 23% have used them for a time; and 20% use them on a continual basis. Two-thirds had recovered and never relapsed, 80% were asymptomatic, and 73% were working or in school (Seikkula et al., 2006).

These 5-year results are markedly superior to longer-term outcomes in the U.S. and other developed countries where patients are regularly maintained on antipsychotics. They serve as "proof of principle" that adopting a selective-use model can markedly improve outcomes for those diagnosed with psychotic disorders.

3.6 Psychiatry's Cognitive Dissonance

During the past 10 years, I have written about this history in various forums, including in a book titled *Anatomy of an Epidemic* (Whitaker, 2010, 2016). Others have done so as well, most notably Peter Breggin, Joanna Moncrieff, and Peter Gotzsche.

However, for the most part, prescribing practices in the United States and other "developed" countries remain the same, and if anything, there is now a push to use injectable antipsychotics in order to ensure "medication compliance." The field, by doing so, is doubling down on its belief that antipsychotics provide a long-term benefit.

The history of medicine is replete with accounts of physicians being resistant to change. Physicians that have adopted a prescribing practice loath to admit that their drug treatment may do more harm than good, and even though they may proclaim that their practices are "evidence-based," they are primed to sort through the evidence in a way that will support their current practices. The modern explanation for this behavior is that the physicians suffer from a "cognitive dissonance" that prevents them from reviewing the evidence with an open mind, although the words of the journalist Upton Sinclair are worth recalling too: "It is difficult to get a man to understand something when his salary depends upon his not understanding it."

Sinclair's aphorism certainly applies to American psychiatrists. In 1980, the American Psychiatric Association (APA) adopted a "disease model" when it published the third edition of its *Diagnostic and Statistical Manual,* and the profession made the prescribing of psychiatric drugs the central feature of its medical practice, with many psychiatrists describing themselves as "psychopharmacologists."

Moreover, the APA, together with pharmaceutical companies, successfully exported this disease model to psychiatrists in developed countries around the world, all of which has produced an international guild that resists reviewing the evidence presented here, or else eager to discount it as flawed.

An example of this resistance can be found in a 2017 article published in the *American Journal of Psychiatry* titled "The Long-term Effects of Antipsychotic Medication on Clinical Course in Schizophrenia" (Goff et al., 2017). The article was authored by Jeffrey Lieberman, a former president of the American Psychiatric

Association, and seven other psychiatrists who described themselves, in an accompanying press release, as an "an international panel of experts in antipsychotic pharmacology, neuroimaging, and neuropathology." They said they had undertaken this effort to respond to critics of neuroleptics, naming in particular Gotzsche, Moncrieff, and myself.

Their article revisited much of the research that has been presented here. Although it isn't possible in the space of this article to fully deconstruct their paper, a brief review reveals much about how they sorted through the evidence.

Discharge Rates Before and After the Arrival of Chlorpromazine The studies of discharge rates prior to 1955 and immediately afterwards belief the conventional narrative that antipsychotics represented a great leap forward in the treatment of psychotic disorders and enabled deinstitutionalization. However, Lieberman and colleagues didn't write anything about the discharge rates from 1945 to 1955. Instead, when discussing this issue, they wrote that the Norwegian and Scottish studies had found "that increased rates of discharge" were "associated with initial antipsychotic treatment." They had cherry-picked the one finding that seemed to support the belief that chlorpromazine had made it possible to treat schizophrenia patients in the community; they didn't mention, however, that the discharge rates in those two studies increased from around 63% to 69%, a minimal increase at best.

Retrospective Studies of Rehospitalization Rates Lieberman and colleagues didn't review any of the four studies that told of higher rehospitalization rates following the introduction of antipsychotics. They ignored the retrospective study of patients treated at Boston Psychopathic Hospital in 1947 and 1967, which found an increase in the relapse rate and a decline in functioning for patients treated with antipsychotics—the principal study in the U.S. that assessed this rehospitalization question.

The Three NIMH-Funded Studies in the 1970s Rappaport, Mosher, and Carpenter found superior long-term outcomes for those off antipsychotics (or for those treated with psychosocial care that minimized use of the drugs). Lieberman and colleagues dismissed all three as flawed in some way or as inconsequential. Rappaport's study was said to have had an excess of dropouts in the placebo arm that confounded the result (a criticism belied by the fact that there were more patients randomized to placebo than to drug that were still in the study at the end of 3 years.) As for Mosher's and Carpenter's experiments, these studies, Lieberman and colleagues wrote, were "difficult to interpret due to highly selective patient samples, diagnostic heterogeneity, and high attrition rates."

Drug-Induced Dopamine Supersensitivity While acknowledging that antipsychotics may induce a dopamine supersensitivity, Lieberman and colleagues—rather than exploring whether this biological change could account for the findings in the retrospective studies and the longitudinal studies—simply declared that there was no evidence that was detrimental to psychotic patients. "Clinical studies have not provided compelling evidence that treatment with antipsychotics worsens the course of illness, increases risk of relapse, or causes cognitive deficits," they wrote. They also did not mention the study by Chouinard and Jones that found that 30% of the schizophrenia patients showed signs of drug-induced tardive psychosis.

MRI Studies of Brain Volumes Even though Gur, Andreasen, and others had told of how antipsychotics cause changes in brain volumes that are associated with a worsening of symptoms and functional decline, Lieberman and colleagues disputed their conclusions. They argued that it wasn't possible to disentangle drug effects from disease effects, and thus maybe it was the disease that was causing the brain shrinkage. Even if the changes were drug caused, they wrote, "it is possible that antipsychotics may have deleterious effects on normal brain but protective effects in the presence of schizophrenia-related neuropathology." (In other words, the brain shrinkage is good for schizophrenia patients, and bad for everyone else.)

Harrow's Longitudinal Study The NIMH funded Harrow's study with the expectation that it would provide a picture of the long-term course of schizophrenia, with medication use a variable to be assessed. It is the most important and thorough study of long-term outcomes ever conducted during the pharmacological era. However, Lieberman and colleagues dismissed it with a couple of quick sentences and cited no outcomes data, simply stating that the superior outcomes for the unmedicated patients were likely due to their being less ill at baseline. They wrote this even though, having reviewed critical writings on this topic, they knew that in fact the opposite was true, and that those who were diagnosed with milder disorders at baseline who stayed on the drugs had worse outcomes than those with more severe diagnoses who stopped taking the medication. They would have seen the graphic shown in Fig. 3.4.

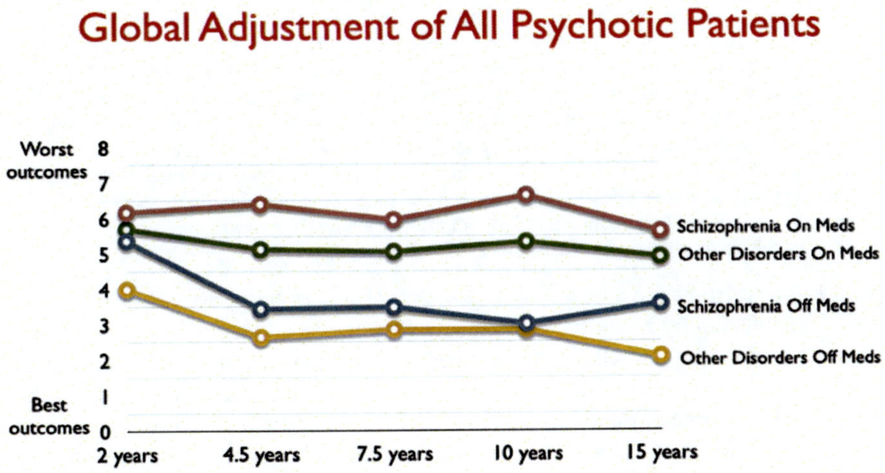

Fig. 3.4 Global adjustment of all psychotic patients. (Source: Harrow & Jobe, 2007)

What this brief review reveals is that Lieberman and colleagues had no interest in exploring the evidence that tells of possible harm done by antipsychotics over the long term. Instead, they were bent on reasserting belief in the efficacy of antipsychotics and dismissing evidence of harm done. They did so by ignoring critical studies; dismissing clinical studies as flawed; never presenting any of the quantitative data that told of harm; never citing conclusions drawn by the authors of these papers; waving away concerns related to dopamine supersensitivity and drug-induced brain shrinkage; and spending so little time on Harrow's study that readers could only conclude it was of little consequence.

And, of course, having reviewed the "case against antipsychotics" in this way, they then pointed to the RCTs of antipsychotics as good evidence that these drugs provide a short-term benefit and reduce relapse rates over the long term.

Remarkably, Lieberman and colleagues revealed their real intent—and their animosity towards anyone who would dare challenge the merits of antipsychotics—by issuing a press release to accompany the publication of the article, with Lieberman also appearing in a Medscape video to declare victory and to disparage the critics.

The press release by the Columbia University Department of Psychiatry stated that critics had raised concerns with the potential to "mislead some patients (and their families) to refuse or discontinue antipsychotic treatment." However, after conducting a "comprehensive examination" of all possible evidence, experts in the field—Lieberman and the other seven authors—had come to a definitive conclusion about the merits of antipsychotics. "For patients with schizophrenia and related psychotic disorders, antipsychotic medications do not have negative long-term effects on patients' outcomes or the brain. In addition, the benefits of these medications are much greater than their potential side effects" (Columbia University Department of Psychiatry, 2017).

In his video, Lieberman went even further in his denunciation of critics.

> The critics who gave rise to this notion that antipsychotic treatment adversely affects long-term outcomes were sowing seeds of untruth and, in their pursuit of some ideological goal or need for self-serving acclamations, were ignoring entirely the harm that they were causing many people who unwittingly would accept these as credible statements and follow their guidance. As I film this video, the contents of the new article are embargoed, so I cannot reveal the contents just yet. But let me just say that this is an extremely well-composed paper that provides a scholarly and rigorous review of relevant lines of evidence. It comes to a very clear and definitive conclusion that we all should take note of the findings, apply them in our clinical practices, and use them where need be in the education of patients and against the reputation of individuals who are really trying to create mischief for their own nefarious purposes (Lieberman, 2017).

Such is the resistance to a history of research that tells of harm done. It is resistance most likely fueled by a mixture of cognitive dissonance and a desire to protect psychiatry's guild interests. All eight of the authors were psychiatrists. Five of the eight also disclosed financial ties to drug companies, with at least three serving on speaker bureaus for multiple companies. Lieberman disclosed no current conflicts of interest, but he had a past filled with such conflicts: In 2009, he disclosed having had financial ties to 15 drug companies in the previous 2 years.

3.7 Early Death

The defenders of antipsychotics now regularly cite findings, mostly coming from researchers in Finland and Sweden, that these drugs lower mortality rates in psychotic patients. Lieberman and colleagues cited several of these studies as well, which are now being touted as evidence supporting long-term use of the drugs.

Even at first glance, this is a finding that seems to defy logic.

Antipsychotics are well known to cause adverse effects that raise the risk of dying from cardiac, respiratory, and endocrine diseases (Corell et al., 2015). Studies of antipsychotics prescribed to nonpsychiatric patients have found that this treatment consistently ups mortality rates (Ralph & Espinet, 2018; Weintraub et al., 2016; Ray et al., 2009; Basciotta et al., 2020; Calsolaro et al., 2019; Harrison et al., 2021; Hoang et al., 2011; Jayatilleke et al., 2018; Maust et al., 2015; Jennum et al., 2015). Australian investigators concluded that this was true for psychiatric patients too (Ralph & Espinet, 2018). UK investigators, utilizing a database of 11 million people treated in primary care settings from 1995 to 2010, concluded that those with a psychiatric diagnosis of depression, bipolar disorder, and schizophrenia who used antipsychotics were 1.75 times more likely to die than patients with a similar diagnosis who did not use the drugs (Murray-Thomas et al., 2013).

Studies of schizophrenia cohorts have also found that mortality rates among schizophrenia patients increased in lockstep with dosage and number of antipsychotics prescribed. In a study of 88 chronic patients in Ireland, the researchers concluded that "the greater the number of antipsychotics given concurrently, the shorter was patient survival" (Waddington et al., 1998). Finnish investigators, after studying a cohort of 99 patients, similarly found that there was "a graded relationship between the number of neuroleptic drugs prescribed and mortality of those with schizophrenia. This relationship and the excess mortality among people with schizophrenia could not be explained by coexistent somatic diseases or other known risk factors for premature death" (Joukamaa et al., 2006).

The research that has led to an opposite conclusion that these drugs when given to psychotic patients protect against early death is of a different type. It comes from a mining of prescription databases and death records for patients diagnosed with schizophrenia or some other serious psychotic disorder, and then calculating deaths per patient year of exposure to the drugs versus deaths per patient year when they are off medication (Tiihonen et al., 2009; Taipale et al., 2020). Given the regular use of antipsychotics to treat psychotic disorders, the death-per-patient-year methodology is bound to find a positive outcome for the drug.

For instance, imagine the data from four patients who suffer a first episode at age 20. One patient takes an antipsychotic for 30 years and dies at age 50 while on the drug. A second patient takes an antipsychotic for 29 years, develops tardive dyskinesia and diabetes, stops taking the drug at age 49, and dies a year later. A third patient takes an antipsychotic for 6 months, stops taking it, and then commits suicide during the first month off the drug. A fourth patient stops taking the drugs immediately after discharge from the hospital and is alive 30 years later.

In this scenario, the only patient still alive at age 50 is the one who stopped drug treatment immediately after discharge. All the other three, treated within a drug-based paradigm of care, are dead by age 50. Yet, if you calculate death rates by years of exposure to drug or no medication, the death rate is four times as high for the "unmedicated" group.

Here's the math: The first patient counts for one death per 30 years of drug exposure. The person who dies after 29 years on the drug is counted as *surviving* 29 years on medication and *dying* in 1 year while off medication—the death is chalked up to being off medication. The person who commits suicide in the first month after withdrawing from the drug is counted as surviving 6 months on the drug and dying in 1 month off medication, even though abrupt withdrawal is known to increase the risk of suicide (Herings & Erkins, 2003). The fourth patient counts for 30 years of survival off medication. The four patients together have a total of 59 years and 1 month on medication, and 31 years and 1 month off medication. Two of the three deaths are attributed to being off medication. Thus, calculating deaths-per-patient years produces this mortality rate for the four patients: one death for every 59.5 years on drug and one death for every 15.5 years off medication.

Thus, you have a paradigm of care which leads to patients treated with antipsychotics dying 15–25 years early, and yet, with this methodology, you have a finding that antipsychotics markedly reduce the risk of death in this population (Parks, et al., 2006).

Indeed, even as many in psychiatry are embracing this belief, standard mortality rates for patients diagnosed with schizophrenia and bipolar disorder are *worsening.*

In 2007, Australian researchers conducted a systematic review of published reports of mortality rates of schizophrenia patients in 25 nations. They found that the standard mortality rates (SMRs) for "all-cause mortality" rose from 1.84 in the 1970s to 2.98 in the 1980s to 3.20 in the 1990s (Saha et al., 2007).

The standard mortality rate measures how much more likely the schizophrenia patients are to die than the general population, and thus by the 1990s, according to the Australian researchers, schizophrenia patients were three times more likely to die in any 1 year than those without the diagnosis. In Finland and Sweden, where researchers have mined databases to conclude that antipsychotics protect against early, studies of actual cohorts of schizophrenia patients since the 1990s produced an SMR of 4.5 for the Finnish patients and 4.8 for the Swedish patients (Kiviniemi, 2014; Torniainen et al., 2015).

Meanwhile, in the UK, investigators reported that the SMR for bipolar patients had risen steadily from 2000 to 2014, increasing by 0.14 per year, while the SMR for schizophrenia patients had increased gradually from 2000 to 2010 (0.11 per year) and then more rapidly from 2010 to 2014 (0.34 per year.) "The mortality gap between individuals with bipolar disorders and schizophrenia, and the general population, is widening," they wrote (Hayes et al., 2017).

Even as early death for psychiatric patients treated with second-generation antipsychotics worsens, the guild celebrates their pills for "lengthening lives."

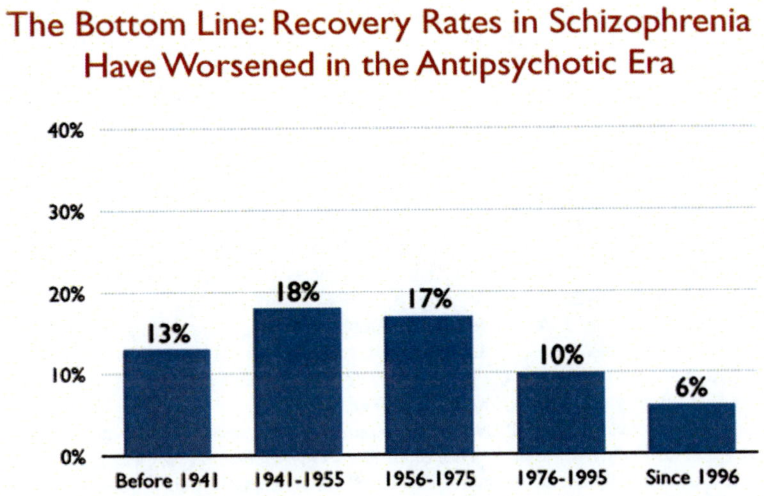

Fig. 3.5 The bottom line: Recovery rates in schizophrenia have worsened in the antipsychotic era. (Source: Jaaskelainen et al., 2013)

3.8 Conclusion

The World Health Organization cross-culture studies conducted in the 1970s and 1980s told of a failed paradigm of care in the United States and other developed countries. It is now 2021, and the latest study of recovery rates in the United States and other developed countries tells of a continued worsening of outcomes. The recovery rate for schizophrenia patients in the atypicals era has declined to 6%, which is the worst outcome that has been recorded in the last 100 years (Jaaskelainen et al., 2013) (see Fig. 3.5).

Such is the state of psychiatric care for psychotic patients in the current era. Worsening outcomes, worsening mortality rates, and increased use of long-acting injectable antipsychotics to ensure that patients remain "medication compliant." The evidence reviewed here cries out for a rethinking of the use of these drugs.

References

Aderhold, V., Weinmann, S., Hagele, C., & Heinz, A. (2014, May). Heinzfrontale Hirnvolumenminderung durch Antipsycotika? *Der Nervenarzt.*

Andreasen, N. (2005). Longitudinal changes in neurocognition during the first decade of schizophrenia illness. *International Congress on Schizophrenia Research, 2005*, 348.

Basciotta, M., Zhou, W., Ngo, L., Donnino, M., Marcantonio, E. R., & Herzig, S. J. (2020). Antipsychotics and the risk of mortality or cardiopulmonary arrest in hospitalized adults. *Journal of the American Geriatrics Society, 68*(3), 544–550. https://doi.org/10.1111/jgs.16246

Bockoven, J. S., & Solomon, H. C. (1975). Comparison of two five-year follow-up studies: 1948 to 1952 and 1967 to 1972. *The American Journal of Psychiatry, 132*(8), 796–801. https://doi.org/10.1176/ajp.132.8.796

Bola, J. R., & Mosher, L. R. (2003). Treatment of acute psychosis without neuroleptics: Two-year outcomes from the Soteria project. *The Journal of Nervous and Mental Disease, 191*(4), 219–229. https://doi.org/10.1097/01.NMD.0000061148.84257.F9

Bola, J., & Soydan, H. (2007). Antipsychotic medication for early episode schizophrenia. In The Cochrane Collaboration (Ed.), *Cochrane database of systematic reviews* (p. CD006374). Wiley. https://doi.org/10.1002/14651858.CD006374

Calsolaro, V., Antognoli, R., Okoye, C., & Monzani, F. (2019). The use of antipsychotic drugs for treating behavioral symptoms in Alzheimer's disease. *Frontiers in Pharmacology, 10*, 1465. https://doi.org/10.3389/fphar.2019.01465

Carpenter, W. T., McGlashan, T. H., & Strauss, J. S. (1977). The treatment of acute schizophrenia without drugs: An investigation of some current assumptions. *The American Journal of Psychiatry, 134*(1), 14–20. https://doi.org/10.1176/ajp.134.1.14

Chakos, M. H., Lieberman, J. A., Bilder, R. M., Borenstein, M., Lerner, G., Bogerts, B., Wu, H., Kinon, B., & Ashtari, M. (1994). Increase in caudate nuclei volumes of first-episode schizophrenic patients taking antipsychotic drugs. *The American Journal of Psychiatry, 151*(10), 1430–1436. https://doi.org/10.1176/ajp.151.10.1430

Chouinard, G., & Jones, B. (1982). Neuroleptic-induced supersensitivity psychosis, the "hump course," and tardive dyskinesia. *Journal of Clinical Psychopharmacology, 2*(2), 143–144.

Chouinard, G., Jones, B. D., & Annable, L. (1978). Neuroleptic-induced supersensitivity psychosis. *The American Journal of Psychiatry, 135*(11), 1409–1410. https://doi.org/10.1176/ajp.135.11.1409

Cole, J. O. (Ed.). (1959). *Psychopharnmacology*. National Academy of Science.

Columbia University Department of Psychiatry. (2017, May 12). *Benefits of antipsychotics outweigh risks, experts find.* Press release. https://www.columbiapsychiatry.org/news/benefits-antipsychotics-outweigh-risks-find-experts?utm_source=redirect&utm_campaign=Lieberman_antipsychotics-longterm. Accessed 30 Dec 2021.

Correll, C. U., Detraux, J., De Lepeleire, J., & De Hert, M. (2015). Effects of antipsychotics, antidepressants and mood stabilizers on risk for physical diseases in people with schizophrenia, depression and bipolar disorder. *World Psychiatry, 14*(2), 119–136. https://doi.org/10.1002/wps.20204

Dreifus, C. (2008). Using imaging to look at changes in the brain. *New York Times*, September 16.

Epstein, L. J., Morgan, R. D., & Reynolds, L. (1962). An approach to the effect of ataraxic drugs on hospital release rates. *American Journal of Psychiatry, 119*(1), 36–47. https://doi.org/10.1176/ajp.119.1.36

Gleeson, J. F. M., Cotton, S. M., Alvarez-Jimenez, M., Wade, D., Gee, D., Crisp, K., Pearce, T., Newman, B., Spiliotacopoulos, D., Castle, D., & McGorry, P. D. (2009). A randomized controlled trial of relapse prevention therapy for first-episode psychosis patients. *The Journal of Clinical Psychiatry, 70*(4), 477–486. https://doi.org/10.4088/JCP.08m04407

Goff, D. C., Falkai, P., Fleischhacker, W. W., Girgis, R. R., Kahn, R. M., Uchida, H., Zhao, J., & Lieberman, J. A. (2017). The long-term effects of antipsychotic medication on clinical course in schizophrenia. *American Journal of Psychiatry, 174*(9), 840–849. https://doi.org/10.1176/appi.ajp.2017.16091016

Gur, R. E., Cowell, P., Turetsky, B. I., Gallacher, F., Cannon, T., Bilker, W., & Gur, R. C. (1998a). A follow-up magnetic resonance imaging study of schizophrenia. Relationship of neuroanatomical changes to clinical and neurobehavioral measures. *Archives of General Psychiatry, 55*(2), 145–152. https://doi.org/10.1001/archpsyc.55.2.145

Gur, R. E., Maany, V., Mozley, P. D., Swanson, C., Bilker, W., & Gur, R. C. (1998b). Subcortical MRI volumes in neuroleptic-naive and treated patients with schizophrenia. *The American Journal of Psychiatry, 155*(12), 1711–1717. https://doi.org/10.1176/ajp.155.12.1711

Harrison, S. L., Sluggett, J. K., Lang, C., Whitehead, C., Crotty, M., Corlis, M., Wesselingh, S., & Inacio, M. C. (2021). Initiation of antipsychotics after moving to residential aged care facilities and mortality: A national cohort study. *Aging Clinical and Experimental Research, 33*(1), 95–104. https://doi.org/10.1007/s40520-020-01518-y

Harrow, M., & Jobe, T. H. (2007). Factors involved in outcome and recovery in schizophrenia patients not on antipsychotic medications: A 15-year multifollow-up study. *The Journal of Nervous and Mental Disease, 195*(5), 406–414. https://doi.org/10.1097/01.nmd.0000253783.32338.6e

Harrow, M., & Jobe, T. H. (2013). Does long-term treatment of schizophrenia with antipsychotic medications facilitate recovery? *Schizophrenia Bulletin, 39*(5), 962–965. https://doi.org/10.1093/schbul/sbt034

Harrow, M., Jobe, T. H., & Faull, R. N. (2012). Do all schizophrenia patients need antipsychotic treatment continuously throughout their lifetime? A 20-year longitudinal study. *Psychological Medicine, 42*(10), 2145–2155. https://doi.org/10.1017/S0033291712000220

Harrow, M., Jobe, T. H., & Faull, R. N. (2014). Does treatment of schizophrenia with antipsychotic medications eliminate or reduce psychosis? A 20-year multi-follow-up study. *Psychological Medicine, 44*(14), 3007–3016. https://doi.org/10.1017/S0033291714000610

Hayes, J. F., Marston, L., Walters, K., King, M. B., & Osborn, D. P. J. (2017). Mortality gap for people with bipolar disorder and schizophrenia: UK-based cohort study 2000–2014. *British Journal of Psychiatry, 211*(3), 175–181. https://doi.org/10.1192/bjp.bp.117.202606

Herings, R. M. C., & Erkens, J. A. (2003). Increased suicide attempt rate among patients interrupting use of atypical antipsychotics. *Pharmacoepidemiology and Drug Safety, 12*(5), 423–424. https://doi.org/10.1002/pds.837

Hermes, E. D. A., Sokoloff, D., Stroup, T. S., & Rosenheck, R. A. (2012). Minimum clinically important difference in the positive and negative syndrome scale with data from the clinical antipsychotic trials of intervention effectiveness (CATIE). *The Journal of Clinical Psychiatry, 73*(4), 526–532. https://doi.org/10.4088/JCP.11m07162

Ho, B.-C., Andreasen, N. C., Nopoulos, P., Arndt, S., Magnotta, V., & Flaum, M. (2003). Progressive structural brain abnormalities and their relationship to clinical outcome: A longitudinal magnetic resonance imaging study early in schizophrenia. *Archives of General Psychiatry, 60*(6), 585–594. https://doi.org/10.1001/archpsyc.60.6.585

Ho, B.-C., Andreasen, N. C., Ziebell, S., Pierson, R., & Magnotta, V. (2011). Long-term antipsychotic treatment and brain volumes: A longitudinal study of first-episode schizophrenia. *Archives of General Psychiatry, 68*(2), 128–137. https://doi.org/10.1001/archgenpsychiatry.2010.199

Hoang, U., Stewart, R., & Goldacre, M. J. (2011). Mortality after hospital discharge for people with schizophrenia or bipolar disorder: Retrospective study of linked English hospital episode statistics, 1999-2006. *BMJ, 343*(sep13 1), d5422–d5422. https://doi.org/10.1136/bmj.d5422

Hopper, K., & Wanderling, J. (2000). Revisiting the developed versus developing country distinction in course and outcome in schizophrenia: Results from ISoS, the WHO collaborative followup project. International Study of Schizophrenia. *Schizophrenia Bulletin, 26*(4), 835–846. https://doi.org/10.1093/oxfordjournals.schbul.a033498

Jaaskelainen, E., Juola, P., Hirvonen, N., McGrath, J. J., Saha, S., Isohanni, M., Veijola, J., & Miettunen, J. (2013). A systematic review and meta-analysis of recovery in schizophrenia. *Schizophrenia Bulletin, 39*(6), 1296–1306. https://doi.org/10.1093/schbul/sbs130

Jablensky, A., Sartorius, N., Ernberg, G., Anker, M., Korten, A., Cooper, J. E., Day, R., & Bertelsen, A. (1992). Schizophrenia: Manifestations, incidence and course in different cultures. A World Health Organization ten-country study. *Psychological Medicine. Monograph Supplement, 20*, 1–97. https://doi.org/10.1017/s0264180100000904

Jayatilleke, N., Hayes, R. D., Chang, C.-K., & Stewart, R. (2018). Acute general hospital admissions in people with serious mental illness. *Psychological Medicine, 48*(16), 2676–2683. https://doi.org/10.1017/S0033291718000284

Jennum, P., Baandrup, L., Ibsen, R., & Kjellberg, J. (2015). Increased all-cause mortality with use of psychotropic medication in dementia patients and controls: A population-based register study. *European Neuropsychopharmacology, 25*(11), 1906–1913. https://doi.org/10.1016/j.euroneuro.2015.08.014

Joukamaa, M., Heliövaara, M., Knekt, P., Aromaa, A., Raitasalo, R., & Lehtinen, V. (2006). Schizophrenia, neuroleptic medication and mortality. *British Journal of Psychiatry, 188*(2), 122–127. https://doi.org/10.1192/bjp.188.2.122

Kiviniemi, M. (2014). *Mortality, disability, psychiatric treatment and medication in first-onset schizophrenia in Finland: The register linkage study*. Doctoral dissertation, University of Oulo, Finland. http://jultika.oulu.fi/files/isbn9789526206325.pdf. Accessed 28 May 2020.

Leff, J., Sartorius, N., Jablensky, A., Korten, A., & Ernberg, G. (1992). The International Pilot Study of Schizophrenia: Five-year follow-up findings. *Psychological Medicine, 22*(1), 131–145. https://doi.org/10.1017/s0033291700032797

Lehrman, N. S. (1961). Follow-up of brief and prolonged psychiatric hospitalization. *Comprehensive Psychiatry, 2*, 227–240. https://doi.org/10.1016/s0010-440x(61)80015-1

Leucht, S., Corves, C., Arbter, D., Engel, R. R., Li, C., & Davis, J. M. (2009). Second-generation versus first-generation antipsychotic drugs for schizophrenia: A meta-analysis. *The Lancet, 373*(9657), 31–41. https://doi.org/10.1016/S0140-6736(08)61764-X

Leucht, S., Tardy, M., Komossa, K., Heres, S., Kissling, W., & Davis, J. M. (2012). Maintenance treatment with antipsychotic drugs for schizophrenia. *Cochrane Database of Systematic Reviews*. https://doi.org/10.1002/14651858.CD008016.pub2

Leucht, S., Leucht, C., Huhn, M., Chaimani, A., Mavridis, D., Helfer, B., Samara, M., Rabaioli, M., Bächer, S., Cipriani, A., Geddes, J. R., Salanti, G., & Davis, J. M. (2017). Sixty years of placebo-controlled antipsychotic drug trials in acute schizophrenia: Systematic review, Bayesian meta-analysis, and meta-regression of efficacy predictors. *American Journal of Psychiatry, 174*(10), 927–942. https://doi.org/10.1176/appi.ajp.2017.16121358

Lieberman, J. (2017, May 12). *Two major developments in psychiatry*. Medscape video. https://medscape.com/viewarticle/879623. Accessed 30 Dec 2021.

Madsen, A. L., Keidling, N., Karle, A., Esbjerg, S., & Hemmingsen, R. (1998). Neuroleptics in progressive structural brain abnormalities in psychiatric illness. *Lancet (London, England), 352*(9130), 784–785. https://doi.org/10.1016/s0140-6736(05)60678-2

Matthews, S. M., Roper, M. T., Mosher, L. R., & Menn, A. Z. (1979). A non-neuroleptic treatment for schizophrenia: Analysis of the two-year postdischarge risk of relapse. *Schizophrenia Bulletin, 5*(2), 322–333. https://doi.org/10.1093/schbul/5.2.322

Maust, D. T., Kim, H. M., Seyfried, L. S., Chiang, C., Kavanagh, J., Schneider, L. S., & Kales, H. C. (2015). Antipsychotics, other psychotropics, and the risk of death in patients with dementia: Number needed to harm. *JAMA Psychiatry, 72*(5), 438. https://doi.org/10.1001/jamapsychiatry.2014.3018

Mcwalter, H. S., Mercer, R., Sutherland, M., & Watt, A. (2006). Outcomes of treatment of schizophrenia in a North-East Scottish mental hospital. *The American Journal of Psychiatry*. https://doi.org/10.1176/ajp.118.6.529

Moilanen, J., Haapea, M., Miettunen, J., Jääskeläinen, E., Veijola, J., Isohanni, M., & Koponen, H. (2013). Characteristics of subjects with schizophrenia spectrum disorder with and without antipsychotic medication—A 10-year follow-up of the Northern Finland 1966 Birth Cohort study. *European Psychiatry: The Journal of the Association of European Psychiatrists, 28*(1), 53–58. https://doi.org/10.1016/j.eurpsy.2011.06.009

Murray-Thomas, T., Jones, M. E., Patel, D., Brunner, E., Shatapathy, C. C., Motsko, S., & Van Staa, T. P. (2013). Risk of mortality (including sudden cardiac death) and major cardiovascular events in atypical and typical antipsychotic users: A study with the general practice research database. *Cardiovascular Psychiatry and Neurology, 2013*, 1–15. https://doi.org/10.1155/2013/247486

Odegard, O. (1964). Pattern of discharge from Norwegian psychiatric hospitals before and after the introduction of the psychotropic drugs. *American Journal of Psychiatry, 120*(8), 772–778. https://doi.org/10.1176/ajp.120.8.772

Parks, J., Svendsen, D., Singer, P., & Foti, M. E. (2006). *Morbidity and mortality in people with serious mental illness*. National Association of State Mental Health Program Directors. Retrieved from https://www.nasmhpd.org/sites/default/files/Mortality%20and%20Morbidity%20Final%20Report%208.18.08_0.pdf

Pritchard, M. (1967). Prognosis of schizophrenia before and after pharmacotherapy: II. Three-year follow-up. *The British Journal of Psychiatry: The Journal of Mental Science, 113*(505), 1353–1359. https://doi.org/10.1192/bjp.113.505.1353

Ralph, S. J., & Espinet, A. J. (2018). Increased all-cause mortality by antipsychotic drugs: Updated review and meta-analysis in dementia and general mental health care. *Journal of Alzheimer's Disease Reports, 2*(1), 1–26. https://doi.org/10.3233/ADR-170042

Rappaport, M., Hopkins, H. K., Hall, K., Belleza, T., & Silverman, J. (1978). Are there schizophrenics for whom drugs may be unnecessary or contraindicated? *International Pharmacopsychiatry, 13*(2), 100–111. https://doi.org/10.1159/000468327

Ray, W. A., Chung, C. P., Murray, K. T., Hall, K., & Stein, C. M. (2009). Atypical antipsychotic drugs and the risk of sudden cardiac death. *New England Journal of Medicine, 360*(3), 225–235. https://doi.org/10.1056/NEJMoa0806994

Saha, S., Chant, D., & McGrath, J. (2007). A systematic review of mortality in schizophrenia: Is the differential mortality gap worsening over time? *Archives of General Psychiatry, 64*(10), 1123. https://doi.org/10.1001/archpsyc.64.10.1123

Seikkula, J., Aaltonen, J., Alakare, B., Haarakangas, K., Keränen, J., & Lehtinen, K. (2006). Five-year experience of first-episode nonaffective psychosis in open-dialogue approach: Treatment principles, follow-up outcomes, and two case studies. *Psychotherapy Research, 16*(2), 214–228. https://doi.org/10.1080/10503300500268490

Shorter, E. (1998). *A history of psychiatry: From the era of the asylum to the age of Prozac*. Wiley.

Taipale, H., Tanskanen, A., Mehtälä, J., Vattulainen, P., Correll, C. U., & Tiihonen, J. (2020). 20-year follow-up study of physical morbidity and mortality in relationship to antipsychotic treatment in a nationwide cohort of 62,250 patients with schizophrenia (FIN20). *World Psychiatry, 19*(1), 61–68. https://doi.org/10.1002/wps.20699

Tiihonen, J., Lönnqvist, J., Wahlbeck, K., Klaukka, T., Niskanen, L., Tanskanen, A., & Haukka, J. (2009). 11-year follow-up of mortality in patients with schizophrenia: A population-based cohort study (FIN11 study). *The Lancet, 374*(9690), 620–627. https://doi.org/10.1016/S0140-6736(09)60742-X

Torniainen, M., Mittendorfer-Rutz, E., Tanskanen, A., Björkenstam, C., Suvisaari, J., Alexanderson, K., & Tiihonen, J. (2015). Antipsychotic treatment and mortality in schizophrenia. *Schizophrenia Bulletin, 41*(3), 656–663. https://doi.org/10.1093/schbul/sbu164

Waddington, J. L., Youssef, H. A., & Kinsella, A. (1998). Mortality in schizophrenia: Antipsychotic polypharmacy and absence of adjunctive anticholinergics over the course of a 10-year prospective study. *British Journal of Psychiatry, 173*(4), 325–329. https://doi.org/10.1192/bjp.173.4.325

Weintraub, D., Chiang, C., Kim, H. M., Wilkinson, J., Marras, C., Stanislawski, B., Mamikonyan, E., & Kales, H. C. (2016). Association of antipsychotic use with mortality risk in patients with Parkinson disease. *JAMA Neurology, 73*(5), 535. https://doi.org/10.1001/jamaneurol.2016.0031

Whitaker, R. (2010). *Anatomy of an epidemic*. Crown.

Whitaker, R. (2016). *The case against psychiatric drugs: A review of their long-term effects*. Mad in America Foundation. Google Scholar.

Wils, R. S., Gotfredsen, D. R., Hjorthøj, C., Austin, S. F., Albert, N., Secher, R. G., Thorup, A. A. E., Mors, O., & Nordentoft, M. (2017). Antipsychotic medication and remission of psychotic symptoms 10 years after a first-episode psychosis. *Schizophrenia Research, 182*, 42–48. https://doi.org/10.1016/j.schres.2016.10.030

Wunderink, L., Nieboer, R. M., Wiersma, D., Sytema, S., & Nienhuis, F. J. (2013). Recovery in remitted first-episode psychosis at 7 years of follow-up of an early dose reduction/discontinuation or maintenance treatment strategy: Long-term follow-up of a 2-year randomized clinical trial. *JAMA Psychiatry, 70*(9), 913–920. https://doi.org/10.1001/jamapsychiatry.2013.19

Chapter 4
Neuroleptics Do Much More Harm Than Good and Should Not Be Used

Peter C. Gøtzsche

4.1 Introduction

When you see a patient with a psychosis, the first thing important to realise is that neuroleptics are *not* the solution. Yet, the current paradigm in psychiatry is that psychosis should be treated with neuroleptics as first-line therapy.

I have stopped calling these drugs by their official name, antipsychotics, because it is a misnomer. Neuroleptics do not have any specific antipsychotic effect. They work by impairing important brain functions, and they do this in the same way, whether given to patients with psychosis, to healthy volunteers, or to animals (Breggin, 2008; Gøtzsche, 2015). They cannot cure people, only dampen their symptoms, which come with a lot of harmful effects. For example, they do not just dampen psychotic thoughts but all thoughts, which tend to render the patients inactive and passive. Two physicians have described how a single dose of haloperidol knocked them down (Belmaker & Wald, 1977). They experienced a marked slowing of thinking and movement, profound inner restlessness, a paralysis of volition and a lack of physical and psychic energy, and being unable to read or work. David Healy found the same in 20 staff from his hospital who received droperidol (Moncrieff, 2013). Everyone felt anxious, restless, disengaged, and demotivated to do anything; a psychologist volunteer found it too complicated just to obtain a sandwich from a sandwich machine.

By contrast, antibiotics do not make false promises. They work as intended, and the best of them kill bacteria and save lives, with virtually no harms, e.g. penicillin for meningitis or sepsis with streptococci.

P. C. Gøtzsche (✉)
Institute for Scientific Freedom, Copenhagen, Denmark
e-mail: pcg@scientificfreedom.dk

J. A. Díaz-Garrido et al. (eds.), *Psychological Interventions for Psychosis*,
https://doi.org/10.1007/978-3-031-27003-1_4

Neuroleptics do the opposite. They kill many patients, and they make it difficult for those who survive to come back to a more normal life. This is true for all psychiatric drugs. They change brain functions and bring the patient to an unknown territory where the patient has not been before. This is problematic because you cannot bring the patient from a chemically induced new condition back to a more normal state unless you taper off the drugs, and even then, it will not always be possible, as the patient might have developed irreversible brain damage (Gøtzsche, 2022a). In contrast, the aim of psychological treatments is to change a brain that is not functioning well back towards a more normal state.

It is therefore not surprising that in all countries where this has been investigated, the increased use of psychiatric drugs has been accompanied by an increase in disability pensions (Whitaker, 2015). If they had worked like insulin for diabetes, which psychiatrists sometimes say to convince the patients to take drugs they don't like, we would have seen *fewer* disability pensions.

4.2 What Is the Effect of Neuroleptics on Psychosis?

The effect in the placebo-controlled trials is less than the minimal clinically relevant effect, which corresponds to about 15 points on the Positive and Negative Syndrome Scale (PANSS) (Leucht et al., 2006), commonly used in the trials. Yet, what was reported in placebo-controlled trials of newer drugs submitted to the FDA was only 6 points (Khin et al., 2012), even though scores easily improve when someone is knocked down by a tranquillizer and expresses abnormal ideas less frequently (Moncrieff, 2013).

It should also be considered that these trials were seriously flawed and exaggerated the effect. There are at least four reasons for this (Gøtzsche, 2022a).

4.2.1 Cold Turkey in the Placebo Group

In every single trial but two, the patients were already on a drug similar to the one being tested against placebo. After a short wash-out period without this drug, the patients were randomised to the new drug or placebo. There are three main problems with this design.

First, the patients who are recruited for the trials are those who have not reacted too negatively on getting such a drug before (Moncrieff & Cohen, 2006). They will likely therefore not react negatively to the new drug, which means that the trials will underestimate the harms of the drugs.

Second, when patients who have tolerated a drug are randomised to placebo, they will likely react more negatively to this than if they had not been in treatment before. This is because all psychiatric drugs have a range of effects, some of which can be perceived as positive, e.g. emotional numbing.

Third, the cold turkey that some patients in the placebo group go through harms them. It is therefore not surprising that the new drug seems to be better than placebo. Introducing longer wash-out periods does not remove this problem. If people have been permanently brain-damaged before entering the trials, wash-out periods cannot compensate, and even if that is not the case, they could suffer from withdrawal symptoms for months or years (Breggin, 2008, 2012).

When my research group searched for placebo-controlled trials in psychosis that only included patients who had not received such a drug earlier, we found only one trial (Wang et al., 2013). It was from China and appeared to be unreliable (Danborg & Gøtzsche, 2019).

The first trial that was not flawed was published in March 2020 (Francey et al., 2020), 70 years after the discovery of the first neuroleptic, chlorpromazine.

However, even 70 years wasn't enough for the psychiatrists to come to their senses. They were not yet ready to draw the consequences of their results, which their abstract demonstrates:

"Group differences were small and clinically trivial, indicating that treatment with placebo medication was no less effective than conventional antipsychotic treatment (Mean Difference = −0.2, 2-sided 95% confidence interval −7.5 to 7.0, t = 0.060, p = 0.95). Within the context of a specialised early intervention service, and with a short duration of untreated psychosis, the immediate introduction of antipsychotic medication may not be required for all cases of first episode psychosis in order to see functional improvement. However, this finding can only be generalised to a very small proportion of FEP [first episode psychosis] cases at this stage, and a larger trial is required to clarify whether antipsychotic-free treatment can be recommended for specific subgroups of those with FEP."

What this means for people who are willing to interpret the evidence clearly is:

Our study was small, but it is unique because it only included patients who had not been treated with a neuroleptic before. We found that neuroleptics are not needed for patients with untreated psychosis. This is great progress for patients, as these drugs are highly toxic and make it difficult for them to come back to a normal life. Based on the totality of the evidence we have, the use of neuroleptics in psychosis cannot be justified. Such pills should only be used in placebo-controlled randomised trials of drug-naïve patients.

The authors of a 2011 systematic review of neuroleptics for early episode schizophrenia pointed out that the available evidence doesn't support a conclusion that neuroleptic treatment in an acute early episode of schizophrenia is effective (Bola et al., 2011). This is one of the very few Cochrane reviews of psychiatric drugs that can be trusted (Gøtzsche, 2015, 2022a). There are huge problems with most Cochrane reviews, e.g. Cochrane reviews in schizophrenia routinely include trials in a meta-analysis where half of the data are missing.

To find out for how long patients should be advised to continue taking their drugs, so-called maintenance studies, also called withdrawal studies, have been carried out. These studies are also highly misleading because of cold turkey effects. A large meta-analysis of 65 placebo-controlled trials found that only three patients needed to be treated with neuroleptics to prevent one relapse after 1 year (Leucht et al., 2012), which looks very impressive, but the result is totally unreliable. The apparent benefit of continued treatment with neuroleptics decreased over time and was close to zero after 3 years. Thus, what was seen after 1 year was iatrogenic harm, which was described as a benefit.

When follow-up is longer than 3 years, it turns out that discontinuing neuroleptics is the best option. There is only one appropriately planned and conducted maintenance trial, from Holland. It has 7 years of follow-up, and patients who had their dosages decreased or discontinued fared much better than those who were randomised to continue taking their pills: 21 of 52 (40%) versus 9 of 51 (18%) had recovered from their first episode of schizophrenia (Wunderink et al., 2013).

Leading psychiatrists interpret the maintenance studies to mean that the drugs are highly effective at preventing new episodes of psychosis (Gøtzsche, 2015, 2022b) and that the patients should therefore continue taking the drugs for years or even for life. But why would drugs that have almost no effect in the acute situation, apart from knocking patients down, be expected to be highly effective for preventing relapse? Using a little common sense tells us that this can hardly be correct.

Danish researchers tried to repeat the Dutch study, but their trial was abandoned because the patients were scared about what would happen if they did not continue taking their drugs (Gøtzsche, 2022a). They have learned – heavily assisted by their psychiatrists – to identify themselves with pill takers and have forgotten what life was about before they came on the pills.

A psychiatrist involved with the failed trial told me about another, recent withdrawal trial, carried out in Hong Kong (Hui et al., 2018). The researchers treated first-episode patients with quetiapine for 2 years; discontinued the treatment in half of the patients by introducing placebo; and reported the results at 10 years. A poor clinical outcome occurred in 35 (39%) of 89 patients in the discontinuation group and in only 19 (21%) of 89 patients in the maintenance treatment group.

I immediately suspected that the trial was flawed – as this result was the exact opposite of the Dutch result – and that they had tapered off the neuroleptic far too quickly and had caused a cold turkey. As there was nothing about their tapering scheme in the article, I looked up an earlier publication, of the results at 3 years (Chen et al., 2010). They didn't taper at all; all patients randomised to placebo were exposed to a cold turkey.

The 10-year report was highly revealing: "A post-hoc analysis suggested that the adverse consequences of early discontinuation were mediated in part through early relapse during the 1-year period following medication discontinuation." The manufacturer of quetiapine funded the trial in Hong Kong, which was seriously flawed in favour of their drug.

The investigators defined a poor outcome as a composite of persistent psychotic symptoms, a requirement for clozapine treatment, or death by suicide. They called their trial double-blind, but it is impossible to maintain the blind in a trial with cold turkey symptoms, and it is highly subjective whether there are any psychotic symptoms and whether clozapine should be given. I'm much more interested in whether the patients return to a normal life, and a table showed that after 10 years, 69% of those who continued taking their drug were employed versus 71% in the cold turkey group, a quite remarkable result considering the iatrogenic harms inflicted on the latter group.

I consider this trial highly unethical because some patients commit suicide when they experience cold turkey effects. Robert Whitaker has demonstrated that this trial design is lethal (Whitaker, 2002). One in every 145 patients who entered the trials for risperidone, olanzapine, quetiapine, and sertindole died, but none of these deaths were mentioned in the scientific literature, and the FDA didn't require them to be mentioned. The suicide rate in these clinical trials was 2–5 times higher than the norm.

The Hong Kong investigators' attempt at explaining away what they found is breathtaking. They wrote that their result in the third year raised the suggestion that "there might be a time window or critical period during which a relapse might be course-modifying." The plausibility of the existence of such a time window between year two and three is zero. As it is highly variable when or if a patient relapses, there cannot exist any such time window. The psychiatrists deliberately harmed half of their patients, but they concluded they did nothing wrong and that their patients, or their disease, or a "time window" were to blame.

4.2.2 *Lack of Blinding*

Because of the conspicuous harms of psychiatric drugs, trials labelled double-blind are not double-blind. Quite a few patients – and their doctors – know who is on drug and who is on placebo (Gøtzsche, 2015). It takes very little unblinding in a trial before the small differences recorded can be explained purely by bias in the outcome assessment on a subjective rating scale (Moncrieff et al., 2004; Hróbjartsson et al., 2013).

In trials supposed to be double-blind, investigators may report positive effects that only exist in their imagination. This occurred in a famous trial funded by the US National Institute of Mental Health in 1964, which is still highly cited as evidence that neuroleptics are effective. It was a trial of 344 newly admitted patients with schizophrenia who were randomised to phenothiazines such as chlorpromazine, or to placebo (Cole, 1964). The investigators reported, without offering any numerical data, that the drugs reduced apathy and made movements less retarded, the exact opposite of what these drugs do to people, which the psychiatrists had admitted a decade earlier (Whitaker, 2015). The investigators claimed a huge benefit for social participation (effect size of 1.02) and that the drugs make the patients less indifferent to the environment (effect size 0.50). The drugs do the opposite. They also claimed, with no data, that 75% versus 23% were markedly or moderately improved and suggested that the drugs should no longer be called tranquillizers but antischizophrenic drugs. Their study contributed to shaping the erroneous beliefs that schizophrenia can be cured with drugs and that neuroleptics should be taken indefinitely (Whitaker, 2002).

4.2.3 *Irrelevant Outcomes*

A score on a rating scale doesn't tell us whether the patient is well. Hundreds of placebo-controlled trials of neuroleptics have been carried out, but I have not seen any that measured whether the patients came back to a normal productive life. If such trials existed, I would have known about them because the drug companies and many psychiatrists would have used the results incessantly in their marketing of the benefit of these drugs. Unless, of course, they showed that the drugs made the situation worse and were therefore buried in company archives.

The situation is the same for other psychiatric drugs. According to the American Psychiatric Association's disease manual, DSM-5, major depression is present when the patient exhibits 5 or more of 9 symptoms that "cause clinically significant distress or impairment in social, occupational, or other important areas of functioning." Given how the disorder is defined, it makes no sense that drug trials don't use these outcomes (Gøtzsche, 2015).

4.2.4 *Industry Sponsored Trials*

Almost all placebo-controlled trials are planned, conducted, and analysed by the drug industry. A Cochrane review that included 48 papers that in total comprised thousands of individual trials found that industry-sponsored studies more often had favourable efficacy results, favourable harms results, and favourable conclusions for the drug or medical device of interest, compared with non-industry-sponsored studies (Gøtzsche, 2013).

4.3 What Is the Effect of Neuroleptics on Mortality?

Eight years ago, I tried to find out how many people are killed by psychotropic drugs (Gøtzsche, 2015). My results were shocking. Based on the most reliable studies I could find, randomised trials and good comparative cohort studies, I estimated that psychiatric drugs are the third leading cause of death, after heart disease and cancer. Perhaps they are not quite that harmful, but there is no doubt that they kill hundreds of thousands of people every year. I have estimated that just one neuroleptic drug, olanzapine, had killed 200,000 patients up to 2007 (Gøtzsche, 2013).

If we want to find out how many people psychiatric drugs kill, we might think that placebo-controlled randomised trials would be ideal, but that's not the case, and schizophrenia is a prime example. As just noted, the cold-turkey design of these trials has caused some patients to commit suicide in the placebo group.

We would therefore need to find patients who were not already in treatment with neuroleptics before they were randomised. In trials in dementia, pre-treatment is not so likely. A meta-analysis of such trials showed that neuroleptics kill people

(Schneider et al., 2005). The meta-analysis included trials of newer drugs, aripiprazole, olanzapine, quetiapine, and risperidone, in patients with Alzheimer's disease or dementia, and deaths were recorded up till 30 days after discontinuing the double-blind treatment. For every 100 patients treated, there was one additional death on the drug (3.5% versus 2.3% died, $p = 0.02$).

This is bad enough, but it is actually worse than this. The trials generally ran for only 10–12 weeks, although most patients in real life are treated for years. Moreover, in published psychiatric drug trials, half of the deaths are missing, on average (Hughes et al., 2014). I therefore looked up the corresponding FDA data based on the same drugs and trials (FDA, 2022).

As expected, some deaths had been omitted from the publications, and the death rates were now 4.5% versus 2.6%, which means that neuroleptics kill two patients in a hundred in less than 3 months.

I also found a Finnish study of 70,718 community-dwellers newly diagnosed with Alzheimer's disease, which reported that neuroleptics killed 4–5 people per year compared to patients who were not treated (Koponen et al., 2017). If the patients received more than one neuroleptic, the risk of death was increased by 57%. As this was not a randomised trial, the results are not fully reliable, but taken together, these data show a death rate so high that I cannot recall having seen any other drug the patients don't need that is so deadly.

Elderly patients are often treated with several drugs and are more vulnerable to their harmful effects, which means that the increase in the death rate is likely higher than in young patients. Yet, I still think we will need to extrapolate these results to young people with schizophrenia, as they are the best we have. In evidence-based healthcare, we base our decisions on the best available evidence. This means the most reliable evidence, which are the data just above. Thus, absent other reliable evidence, we will need to assume that neuroleptics are also highly lethal for young people. We should therefore not use these drugs for anyone; also because a clinically relevant effect on psychosis has never been demonstrated in reliable trials (see above).

According to the FDA, most of the deaths in the demented patients appeared to be either cardiovascular (e.g. heart failure, sudden death) or infectious (e.g. pneumonia). Young people on neuroleptics also often die suddenly from cardiovascular causes. And I would expect some of them to die from pneumonia. Neuroleptics and forced admission to a closed ward make people inactive. When they lie still in their bed, they can get pneumonia, which the psychiatrists might not detect, as they have not had much training in internal medicine, and as their focus is on the patients' mental state.

The psychiatrists are fully aware – and have often written about it – that the lifespan for patients with schizophrenia is 15 years shorter than for other people (Hjorthøj et al., 2017), but they don't blame their drugs or themselves, but the patients. It is true that these people have unhealthy lifestyles and may abuse other substances, in particular tobacco. But it is also true that some of this is a consequence of the drugs they receive. Some patients say they smoke because it counteracts some of the harms of neuroleptics, which is correct because tobacco increases dopamine while the drugs decrease dopamine.

It is also indisputable that neuroleptics kill some patients with schizophrenia because they can cause huge weight gains, hypertension, and diabetes, but how common is it?

When I tried to find out why young people with schizophrenia die, I faced a roadblock, carefully guarded by the psychiatric guild. It is one of the best kept secrets about psychiatry that the psychiatrists kill many of their patients with neuroleptics (Gøtzsche, 2015, 2022a).

In 2012, Wenche ten Velden Hegelstad and 16 colleagues published 10-year follow-up data for 281 patients with a first-episode psychosis (the TIPS study) (Hegelstad et al., 2012). Although their average age at entry into the study was only 29 years, 31 patients (12%) died in less than 10 years. However, the authors' detailed article was about recovery and symptom scores. They took no interest in all these deaths, which appeared in a flowchart of patients lost to follow-up and were not commented upon anywhere in their paper.

This was remarkable but not uncommon for psychiatry. I wrote to Hegelstad and asked for details about the deaths, and she replied that they were preparing a manuscript detailing the information I asked for. The paper came out the next month, in *World Psychiatry* (Melle et al., 2017), but the number of deaths was now different from their first paper, and the information I had requested wasn't anywhere.

Robert Whitaker and I therefore wrote to the editor of this journal, professor Mario Maj, asking for his help in getting a unique insight into why so many patients had died so young. We hoped he would ensure that the knowledge the investigators had in their files became public by publishing our short letter to the editor and by asking them to respond: "That would be a great service to psychiatry, the patients, and everyone else with an interest in this vitally important issue."

We explained in our letter that the authors had reported that 16 patients died by suicide, 7 by accidental overdoses or other accidents, and 8 from physical illnesses, including 3 from cardiovascular illness. But it was not clarified, for example, if the psychiatrists had overdosed the patients, which is not uncommon, or if "accidental overdoses" meant something else.

Eight days later, we were told by Maj, "Unfortunately, although it is an interesting piece, it does not compete successfully for one of the slots we have available in the journal for letters."

So, there was no space in the journal for our letter of 346 words, no longer than a journal abstract, and no interest in helping young people survive by finding out what kills them at such a young age. This was psychiatry at its worst, protecting itself while literally killing the patients.

I appealed Maj's decision explaining that people I had talked to in several countries about deaths in young people with schizophrenia – psychiatrists, forensic experts, and patients – had all agreed that we desperately need the kind of information we asked Maj to ensure we got from the very valuable cohort of patients Melle et al. reported in his journal (Gøtzsche, 2022a). I ended my letter this way:

"What Melle et al. have published in your journal is not an adequate account of why these young people died. Therefore, we call on you to ensure these data get out in the open, for the benefit of the patients. We believe it is your professional and ethical duty – both as a journal editor and as a doctor – to make this happen. This is not a matter about the slots you have available in the journal for letters. It is a matter of prioritization."

We did not hear from Maj again.

TIPS was supported by grants from 15 funders, including the Norwegian Research Council, the US National Institute of Mental Health, three drug companies (Janssen-Cilag, Eli Lilly and Lundbeck), and other funders in Norway, Denmark, and USA. I asked all the funders for detailed information on the deaths, emphasizing that funders have an ethical obligation to ensure that information of great importance for public health, which has been collected in a funded study, gets published.

The silence was daunting.

Janssen-Cilag replied: "We find the data on mortality published by Melle et al., 2017 in *World Psychiatry* fully satisfactory." Both they and Eli Lilly encouraged us to contact the authors, which was absurd, as I had written to the companies that the authors had refused to share their data with us.

Lundbeck did not reply.

In December 2017, the Norwegian Research Council published its policy about making research data accessible for other researchers, which left no doubt that this should happen, without delay, and not later than when the researchers published their research. Five months after I had written to the Norwegian Research Council, I received a letter from Ingrid Melle, who had been asked by the council to respond to me. This led to some clarification, e.g. Melle explained that accidental drug overdose means taking too much of an illegal substance, or substance, or too strong a substance by accident, and that it does not refer to prescription drugs. If information about overdoses was ambiguous, it was defined as probable suicide.

The really interesting question was why 16 young people (6%) committed suicide in just 10 years? And why this vitally important information was not explored by the researchers? We cannot conclude it was their schizophrenia that led to suicide. It is more likely the drugs enforced upon them, other forced treatments, involuntary admissions to psychiatric wards, humiliation, stigmatisation, and loss of hope, e.g. when patients are told that their disease is genetic, or can be seen in a brain scan, or is lifelong, or requires lifelong treatment with neuroleptics. I am not making this up (Gøtzsche, 2015, 2022b). Some textbooks recommend lifelong treatment for some or even most patients (Gøtzsche, 2022b). It is no wonder they might kill themselves when there is no hope.

There are countless unreliable studies that purport to show that neuroleptics decrease mortality. You should not pay any attention to these studies, which are all fatally flawed. I have done post-mortem dissections on some of them (Gøtzsche, 2015). The main problem is that the patients that are being compared – those on drugs and those not – are not comparable to begin with. Whitaker once wrote to me that it requires extraordinary mental gymnastics by the psychiatrists to conclude that these drugs, which cause obesity, metabolic dysfunction, diabetes, tardive dyskinesia, lethal cardiac arrhythmias, and so on, protect against death.

4.4 Are Patients' Rights Being Respected?

Apart from cancer chemotherapy, neuroleptics are some of the most toxic drugs ever invented. It therefore makes no sense that many patients are forced to take them against their will. This is unethical and a huge violation of basic human rights.

Virtually all psychiatrists claim that they cannot practice without coercion, but this isn't true (Gøtzsche, 2015). Examples from several countries have shown that coercion is not needed. According to Italy's Mental Health Law, the danger criterion is not a legal justification for forced treatment; it is a case for the police, just as in Iceland, where no chains, belts, or other physical constraints have been used since 1932. Physical restraint is an enormous assault on patients who have experienced sexual abuse, which many patients have, some even while they were locked up.

At Akershus University Hospital in Norway, they don't have a regime for rapid tranquillisation and have never needed one (Gøtzsche, 2015). At a psychosis ward in London, they waited on average about 2 weeks before starting neuroleptics on newly admitted people. In the end, most patients chose to take some medication, often in very small doses, so it is very well possible that it was respect, time, and shelter that helped them, not the "sub-treatment threshold doses." Germany has also shown how it can be done (Zinkler & von Peter, 2019).

With good management and training of staff in de-escalation techniques, it is possible to practice psychiatry without coercion (Fiorillo et al., 2011; Scanlan, 2010).

There must be 24-h support facilities without any compulsion, so that the hospital is no longer the only place you can go to when you are in acute crisis (Zinkler & von Peter, 2019). For example, there could be refuges with the possibility of accommodation and where the money follows the patient and not the treatment. We also need social and worthy services for people who are on their way back into society after having been in contact with psychiatry.

Psychiatry seems to be the only area in society where the law is systematically being violated all over the world - even Supreme Court and Ombudsman decisions are being ignored and psychiatrists lie routinely in court to obtain what they want (Gøtzsche, 2015, 2022a). In my research group, we studied 30 consecutive cases from the Psychiatric Appeals Board in Denmark and found that the law had been violated in every single case (Gøtzsche et al., 2019; Gøtzsche & Sørensen, 2020).

All 30 patients were forced to take neuroleptics they didn't want, even though less dangerous alternatives could be used, e.g. benzodiazepines. The psychiatrists had no respect for the patients' views and experiences. In all 21 cases where there was information about the effect of previous drugs, the psychiatrists stated that neuroleptics had had a good effect, whereas none of the patients shared this view (Gøtzsche & Sørensen, 2020).

The harms of prior medication played no role either in the psychiatrist's decision making, not even when they were serious, e.g. we suspected or found akathisia or tardive dyskinesia in seven patients, and five patients expressed fear of dying because of the forced treatment. An expert confirmed our suspicion that a patient had developed akathisia on aripiprazole, but on the same page, the expert – a high-ranking member of the board of the Danish Psychiatric Association – recommended forced treatment with this drug even though it was stopped because of the akathisia.

The power imbalance was extreme. We had reservations about the psychiatrists' diagnoses of delusions in nine cases. There is an element of catch-22 when a psychiatrist decides on a diagnosis and the patient disagrees. According to the psychiatrist, the disagreement shows that the patient has a lack of insight into the disease, which is a proof of mental illness. The abuse involved psychiatrists using diagnoses or derogatory terms for things they didn't like or didn't understand; the patients felt misunderstood and overlooked; their legal protection was a sham; and the harm done was immense (Gøtzsche & Sørensen, 2020).

The patients or their disease were blamed for virtually everything untoward that happened. The psychiatrists didn't seem to have any interest in trauma, neither previous ones nor those caused by themselves. Withdrawal reactions were not taken seriously – we didn't even see this, or a similar term, being used although many patients suffered from them.

It is a very serious transgression of the law and of professional ethics when psychiatrists exaggerate the patients' symptoms and trivialise the harms of the drugs to maintain coercion, but this often happens, and the patient files can be very misleading or outright wrong, too. In this way, the psychiatrists can be said to operate a kangaroo court, where they are both investigators and judges and lie in court about the evidence, where after they sentence the patients to a treatment that is deadly for some of them and harmful for everyone.

When the patients complain about this unfair treatment, which isn't allowed in any other sector of society, it is the same judges (or their friends that won't disagree with them) whose evidence and judgments provide the basis for the verdicts at the two appeal boards, first the Psychiatric Patients' Complaints Board, and next, the Psychiatric Appeals Board. It doesn't matter the slightest bit what the patients say. As they have been declared insane, no one finds it necessary to listen to them. This is a system so abominable that it looks surreal, but this is the reality, not only in Denmark, but all over the world. When we assessed the records for 30 consecutive petitions for mental health commitment in which an involuntary medication order was requested from Anchorage, Alaska, we found that the legal procedures can best be characterized as a sham where the patients are defenseless (Tasch & Gøtzsche, 2023).

When anyone proposes to abolish coercion, psychiatrists often mention rare cases, such as severe mania where the patients may be busily spending their entire wealth. But this can be handled without forced hospitalisation and treatment. For example, an emergency clause could be introduced that removes the patients' financial decision-making rights at short notice.

Furthermore, a few difficult cases cannot justify that massive harm is inflicted on the patients, which also makes it difficult to recruit good people to psychiatry. No one likes coercion, and it destroys the patient's trust in the staff, which is so important for healing and for the working environment in the department.

In many countries, a person considered insane can be committed to a psychiatric ward involuntarily if the prospect of cure or substantial and significant improvement of the condition would be significantly impaired otherwise. No drugs can accomplish that.

The other lawful reason for forcing drugs on people is if they present an obvious and substantial danger to themselves or others. This is also an invalid argument. Psychiatric drugs cause violence (Gøtzsche, 2015), and they cannot protect against violence unless the patients are drugged to such an extent that they have become zombies.

Treatment with neuroleptics kill many patients, also young people, and many more become permanently brain damaged. There are videos of children and adults with akathisia and tardive dyskinesia that show how horrible these brain damages can be (What does akathisia and tardive dyskinesia look like? Undated). It took psychiatry 20 years to recognise tardive dyskinesia as a iatrogenic illness (Breggin, 2008), even though it is one of the worst harms of neuroleptics and affects about 4–5% of the patients per year (Moncrieff, 2015), which means that most patients in long-term treatment will develop it. In 1984, Poul Leber from the FDA extrapolated the data and indicated that, over a lifetime, all patients might develop tardive dyskinesia (Breggin, 2008). Three years later, the president of the American Psychiatric Association said at an Oprah Winfrey show that tardive dyskinesia was not a serious or frequent problem (Karon, 2009).

Coercion should be abolished. This is our duty, according to the United Nations Convention on the Rights of Persons with Disabilities, which virtually all countries have ratified (Gøtzsche, 2015). The Psychiatry Act is not necessary, as the Emergency Guardian Act provides the opportunity to intervene when it is imperative, and the science shows that it is not rational or evidence-based to argue that forced treatment is in the best interests of patients (Gøtzsche, 2019).

If you are not convinced, you should read *The Zyprexa Papers* by lawyer Jim Gottstein (Gottstein, 2020). It is a book about illegal, forced drugging that destroyed patients. Gottstein needed to go to the Supreme Court in Alaska before he got any justice, and he ran a great personal risk by exposing documents that were supposed to be secret.

4.5 What Should Doctors Do Instead of Using Neuroleptics?

Neuroleptics are not needed and should be taken off the market. Their availability is immensely harmful because doctors cannot handle them, but use them far too much, in far too high doses, and for far too long, with devastating consequences.

I cannot imagine any situation in psychiatry where these drugs are needed, apart from the very tragic situation where they have changed the patients' brain so much that it is too painful for the patients to taper off them even if done very slowly. Some of the brain damage these pills cause is permanent and dose-related, i.e. tardive dyskinesia (Ho et al., 2011).

If acutely disturbed patients need something to calm them down, benzodiazepines are far less dangerous and even seem to work better (Dold et al., 2012). When I have asked patients if they would prefer a benzodiazepine or a neuroleptic next time, they developed a psychosis and felt they needed a drug, all of them have said they preferred a benzodiazepine. Why don't they get it then?

I know psychiatrists in several countries that don't use psychiatric drugs or electroshock. They handle even the most severely disturbed patients with empathy, psychotherapy, and patience (Gøtzsche, 2015).

The aim of psychological treatments is to change a brain that is not functioning well back towards a more normal state. Psychiatric drugs also change the brain, but they create an artificial third state – an unknown territory – that is neither normal nor the malfunctioning state the patient came from.

This is problematic because you cannot go from the chemically induced third state back to normal unless you taper off the drugs, and even then, it will not always be possible, as the patient might have developed irreversible brain damage.

A human approach to emotional pain is very important, and treatment outcomes depend more on therapeutic alliances than on whether psychotherapy or pharmacotherapy is used (Krupnick et al., 1996).

Most of the problems patients face are caused by maladaptive emotion regulation, and psychiatric drugs make matters worse, as their effects constitute maladaptive emotion regulation. In contrast, psychotherapy aims at teaching patients to handle their feelings, thoughts and behaviour in better ways. This is called adaptive emotion regulation. It may permanently change patients for the better and make them stronger when facing life's challenges.

There are substantial issues to consider when reading reports about trials that have compared psychotherapy with drugs. The trials are not effectively blinded, neither for psychotherapy nor for drugs, and the prevailing belief in the biomedical model would be expected to influence the psychiatrists' behaviour during the trial and to bias their outcome assessments in favour of drugs over psychotherapy. Trials that show that the effects of a drug and psychotherapy combined are better than either treatment alone should also be interpreted cautiously, and short-term results are misleading. We should only take long-term results into consideration, e.g. results obtained after a year or more.

I will not advocate combination therapy. Doing effective psychotherapy can be difficult when the patients' brains are numbed by psychoactive substances, which may render them unable to think clearly or to evaluate themselves. The lack of insight into feelings, thoughts, and behaviours is called medication spellbinding (Breggin, 2006, 2008). The main biasing effect of medication spellbinding is that the patients underestimate the harms of psychiatric drugs.

For psychotherapy, there are many competing schools and methods, and it is not so important which method you use. It is far more important that you are a good listener and meet your fellow human being where that person is, as Danish philosopher Søren Kierkegaard advised us to do two centuries ago.

Psychotherapy seems to be useful for the whole range of psychiatric disorders, also psychoses (Morrison et al., 2014). A comparison between Lappland and

Stockholm illustrates the difference between an empathic approach and immediately enforcing drugs upon patients with a first-episode psychosis (Seikkula et al., 2006; Svedberg et al., 2001). The Open Dialogue Family and Network Approach in Lappland aims at treating psychotic patients in their homes, and the treatment involves the patient's social network and starts within 24 h after contact. The patients were closely comparable to those in Stockholm, but in Stockholm, 93% were treated with neuroleptics against only 33% in Lappland, and 5 years later, ongoing use was 75% versus 17%. After 5 years, 62% in Stockholm versus 19% in Lappland were on disability allowance or sick leave, and the use of hospital beds had also been much higher in Stockholm, 110 versus only 31 days, on average. It was not a randomised comparison, but the results are so strikingly different that it would be irresponsible to dismiss them. There are many other results supporting the non-drug approach (Gøtzsche, 2015), and the Open Dialogue model is now gaining momentum in several countries.

Psychotherapy does not work for everyone. We need to accept that some people cannot be helped no matter what we do, which is true also in other areas of healthcare. Some therapists are not so competent or do not work well with some patients; it may therefore be necessary to try more than one therapist.

Physical and emotional pain have similarities. Just like we need physical pain in order to avoid dangers, we need emotional pain to guide us in life (Nilsonne, 2017). An acute condition like psychosis is often related to trauma and tend to self-heal if we are a little patient. Through the process of healing – whether assisted by psychotherapy or not – we learn something important that can be useful if we get in trouble again. Such experiences can also boost our self-confidence, whereas pills may prevent us from learning anything because they numb our feelings and thoughts. Pills can also provide a false sense of security and deprive the patient of real therapy and other healing human interactions – doctors may think they need not engage themselves as much when a patient is taking drugs.

Being treated humanely is difficult in today's psychiatry. If you panic and go to a psychiatric emergency ward, you will probably be told you need a drug, and if you decline and say you just need rest to collect yourself, you might be told that the ward is not a hotel (Nilsonne, 2017).

4.6 Conclusions

Neuroleptics should not be used for psychosis, indeed for anything. They are far too harmful compared to the unspecific dampening of symptoms they may accomplish, which can be obtained with other methods, e.g. with a short-term course of benzodiazepines. If we break a leg, we would not be satisfied with a treatment that reduces the pain so little that we cannot feel the difference, while the leg is still broken. But this is where we are with neuroleptics and most other psychiatric drugs (Gøtzsche, 2015, 2022a, b).

What is most important is to take an interest in the patients and listen to them, going many years back in time, which will often reveal that traumas have played an important role for the patients' current condition.

A paper that analysed the 41 most rigorous studies found that people who had suffered childhood adversity were 2.8 times more likely to develop psychosis than those who had not ($p < 0.001$) (Varese et al., 2012). Nine of the 10 studies that tested for a dose-response relationship found it. Another study found that people who had experienced three types of trauma (e.g. sexual abuse, physical abuse, and bullying) were 18 times more likely to be psychotic than non-abused people, and if they had experienced five types of trauma, they were 193 times more likely to be psychotic (95% confidence interval 51–736 times) (Shevlin et al., 2008).

Patients with severe traumas in their past can sometimes be cured by psychotherapy. Drugs have never cured anyone.

It is of course much more challenging for psychiatrists to take a keen interest in their patients and their uniqueness, which also makes themselves vulnerable, but it is also much more rewarding. Sometimes, patients the system had given up upon and put on disability pension were brought back to life this way. Nothing can be more rewarding for a psychiatrist than this.

We clearly need a revolution in psychiatry, nothing less. The current paradigm, with a focus on biological psychiatry with all its hundreds of receptors and genes, each of which predisposes just a little bit to the condition (Gøtzsche, 2022b), has been a disaster. It is time to realise this. We cannot change people's genes anyway, so why this obsession with heredity? Its only purpose is that it makes psychiatry look more "scientific," but this is not the way to go in research if we want to help our patients.

References

Belmaker, R. H., & Wald, D. (1977). Haloperidol in normals. *The British Journal of Psychiatry, 131*, 222–223.

Bola, J., Kao, D., & Soydan, H. (2011). Antipsychotic medication for early episode schizophrenia. *Cochrane Database of Systematic Reviews, 6*, CD006374.

Breggin, P. R. (2006). Intoxication anosognosia: The spellbinding effect of psychiatric drugs. *Ethical Human Psychology and Psychiatry, 8*, 201–215.

Breggin, P. R. (2008). *Brain-disabling treatments in psychiatry: Drugs, electroshock, and the psychopharmaceutical complex*. Springer.

Breggin, P. (2012). *Psychiatric drug withdrawal: A guide for prescribers, therapists, patients and their families*. Springer.

Chen, E. Y., Hui, C. L., Lam, M. M., Chiu, C. P., Law, C. W., Chung, D. W., et al. (2010). Maintenance treatment with quetiapine versus discontinuation after one year of treatment in patients with remitted first episode psychosis: Randomised controlled trial. *The BMJ, 341*, c4024.

Cole, J. O. (1964). Phenothiazine treatment in acute schizophrenia; effectiveness: The National Institute of Mental Health Psychopharmacology Service Center Collaborative Study Group. *Archives of General Psychiatry, 10*, 246–261.

Danborg, P. B., & Gøtzsche, P. C. (2019). Benefits and harms of antipsychotic drugs in drug-naïve patients with psychosis: A systematic review. *International Journal of Risk & Safety in Medicine, 30*, 193–201. Free access.

Dold, M., Li, C., Tardy, M., Khorsand, V., Gillies, D., & Leucht, S. (2012). Benzodiazepines for schizophrenia. *Cochrane Database of Systematic Reviews, 11*, CD006391.

FDA package insert for risperidone (Risperdal). https://www.accessdata.fda.gov/drugsatfda_docs/label/2009/020272s056,020588s044,021346s033,021444s03lbl.pdf. Accessed 30 May 2022.

Fiorillo, A., De Rosa, C., Del Vecchio, V., Jurjanz, L., Schnall, K., Onchev, G., et al. (2011). How to improve clinical practice on involuntary hospital admissions of psychiatric patients: Suggestions from the EUNOMIA study. *European Psychiatry, 26*, 201–207.

Francey, S. M., O'Donoghue, B., Nelson, B., Graham, J., Baldwin, L., Yuen, H. P., et al. (2020). Psychosocial intervention with or without antipsychotic medication for first episode psychosis: A randomized noninferiority clinical trial. *Schizophrenia Bulletin Open*. https://doi.org/10.1093/schizbullopen/sgaa015

Gottstein, J. (2020). *The Zyprexa papers*. Jim Gottstein.

Gøtzsche, P. C. (2013). *Deadly medicines and organised crime: How big pharma has corrupted health care*. London: Radcliffe Publishing.

Gøtzsche, P. C. (2015). *Deadly psychiatry and organised denial*. People's Press.

Gøtzsche, P. C. (2019). Forced drugging with antipsychotics is against the law: Decision in Norway. *Mad in America* (May 4). https://www.madinamerica.com/2019/05/forced-drugging-antipsychotics-against-law/

Gøtzsche, P. C. (2022a). *Mental health survival kit and withdrawal from psychiatric drugs*. L H Press.

Gøtzsche, P. C. (2022b). *Critical psychiatry textbook*. Institute for Scientific Freedom.

Gøtzsche, P. C., & Sørensen, A. (2020). Systematic violations of patients' rights and lack of safety: Cohort of 30 patients forced to receive antipsychotics. *Indian Journal of Medical Ethics, 5*(4), 312–318. Free access.

Gøtzsche, P. C., Vinther, S., & Sørensen, A. (2019). Forced medication in psychiatry: Patients' rights and the law not respected by Appeals Board in Denmark. *Clinical Neuropsychiatry, 16*, 229–233. Free access.

Hegelstad, W. T., Larsen, T. K., Auestad, B., Evensen, J., Haahr, U., Joa, I., et al. (2012). Long-term follow-up of the TIPS early detection in psychosis study: Effects on 10-year outcome. *The American Journal of Psychiatry, 169*, 374–380.

Hjorthøj, C., Stürup, A. E., McGrath, J. J., & Nordentoft, M. (2017). Years of potential life lost and life expectancy in schizophrenia: A systematic review and meta-analysis. *Lancet Psychiatry, 4*, 295–301.

Ho, B. C., Andreasen, N. C., Ziebell, S., Pierson, R., & Magnotta, V. (2011). Long-term antipsychotic treatment and brain volumes: A longitudinal study of first-episode schizophrenia. *Archives of General Psychiatry, 68*, 128–137.

Hróbjartsson, A., Thomsen, A. S., Emanuelsson, F., Tendal, B., Hilden, J., Boutron, I., et al. (2013). Observer bias in randomized clinical trials with measurement scale outcomes: A systematic review of trials with both blinded and nonblinded assessors. *CMAJ, 185*, E201–E211.

Hughes, S., Cohen, D., & Jaggi, R. (2014). Differences in reporting serious adverse events in industry sponsored clinical trial registries and journal articles on antidepressant and antipsychotic drugs: A cross-sectional study. *BMJ Open, 4*, e005535.

Hui, C. L. M., Honer, W. G., Lee, E. H. M., Chang, W. C., Chan, S. K. W., Chen, E. S. M., et al. (2018). Long-term effects of discontinuation from antipsychotic maintenance following first-episode schizophrenia and related disorders: A 10 year follow-up of a randomised, double-blind trial. *Lancet Psychiatry, 5*, 432–442.

Karon, B. P. (2009). All I know about Peter Breggin. In C. B. Pert et al. (Eds.), *The Conscience of Psychiatry. The reform work of Peter R. Breggin, MD*. Lake Edge Press.

Khin, N. A., Chen, Y. F., Yang, Y., Yang, P., & Laughren, T. P. (2012). Exploratory analyses of efficacy data from schizophrenia trials in support of new drug applications submitted to the US Food and Drug Administration. *The Journal of Clinical Psychiatry, 73*, 856–864.

Koponen, M., Taipale, H., Lavikainen, P., Tanskanen, A., Tiihonen, J., Tolppanen, A. M., et al. (2017). Risk of mortality associated with antipsychotic monotherapy and polypharmacy among community-dwelling persons with Alzheimer's disease. *Journal of Alzheimer's Disease, 56*, 107–118.

Krupnick, J. L., Sotsky, S. M., Simmens, S., Moyer, J., Elkin, I., Watkins, J., et al. (1996). The role of the therapeutic alliance in psychotherapy and pharmacotherapy outcome: Findings in the National Institute of Mental Health Treatment of Depression Collaborative Research Program. *Journal of Consulting and Clinical Psychology, 64*, 532–539.

Leucht, S., Kane, J. M., Etschel, E., Kissling, W., Hamann, J., & Engel, R. R. (2006). Linking the PANSS, BPRS, and CGI: Clinical implications. *Neuropsychopharmacology, 31*, 2318–2325.

Leucht, S., Tardy, M., Komossa, K., Heres, S., Kissling, W., Salanti, G., et al. (2012). Antipsychotic drugs versus placebo for relapse prevention in schizophrenia: A systematic review and meta-analysis. *Lancet, 379*, 2063–2071.

Melle, I., Olav Johannesen, J., Haahr, U. H., Ten Velden, H. W., Joa, I., Langeveld, J., et al. (2017). Causes and predictors of premature death in first-episode schizophrenia spectrum disorders. *World Psychiatry, 16*, 217–218.

Moncrieff, J. (2013). *The bitterest pills*. Palgrave Macmillan.

Moncrieff, J. (2015). Antipsychotic maintenance treatment: Time to rethink? *PLoS Medicine, 12*, e1001861.

Moncrieff, J., & Cohen, D. (2006). Do antidepressants cure or create abnormal brain states? *PLoS Medicine, 3*, e240.

Moncrieff, J., Wessely, S., & Hardy, R. (2004). Active placebos versus antidepressants for depression. *Cochrane Database of Systematic Reviews, 1*, CD003012.

Morrison, A. P., Turkington, D., Pyle, M., et al. (2014). Cognitive therapy for people with schizophrenia spectrum disorders not taking antipsychotic drugs: A single-blind randomised controlled trial. *Lancet, 383*, 1395–1403.

Nilsonne, Å. (2017). *Processen: möten, mediciner, beslut*. Stockholm.

Scanlan, J. N. (2010). Interventions to reduce the use of seclusion and restraint in inpatient psychiatric settings: What we know so far, a review of the literature. *International Journal of Social Psychiatry, 56*, 412–423.

Schneider, L. S., Dagerman, K. S., & Insel, P. (2005). Risk of death with atypical antipsychotic drug treatment for dementia: Meta-analysis of randomized placebo-controlled trials. *JAMA, 294*, 1934–1943.

Seikkula, J., Aaltonen, J., Alakare, B., Haarakangas, K., Keränen, J., & Lehtinen, K. (2006). Five-year experience of first-episode nonaffective psychosis in open-dialogue approach: Treatment principles, follow-up outcomes, and two case studies. *Psychotherapy Research, 16*, 214–228.

Shevlin, M., Houston, J. E., Dorahy, M. J., & Adamson, G. (2008). Cumulative traumas and psychosis: An analysis of the national comorbidity survey and the British Psychiatric Morbidity Survey. *Schizophrenia Bulletin, 34*, 193–199.

Svedberg, B., Mesterton, A., & Cullberg, J. (2001). First-episode non-affective psychosis in a total urban population: A 5-year follow-up. *Social Psychiatry and Psychiatric Epidemiology, 36*, 332–337.

Tasch, G., & Gøtzsche, P. C. (2023). Systematic violations of patients' rights and safety: Forced medication of a cohort of 30 patients in Alaska. Psychosis (in press).

Varese, F., Smeets, F., Drukker, M., Lieverse, R., Lataster, T., Viechtbauer, W., et al. (2012). Childhood adversities increase the risk of psychosis: A meta-analysis of patientcontrol, prospective- and cross-sectional cohort studies. *Schizophrenia Bulletin, 38*, 661–671.

Wang, C. H., Li, Y., Yang, J., Su, L. Y., Geng, Y. G., Li, H., et al. (2013). A randomized controlled trial of olanzapine improving memory deficits in Han Chinese patients with first-episode schizophrenia. *Schizophrenia Research, 144*, 129–135.

What does akathisia and tardive dyskinesia look like? (Undated). *Videos of children and adults who have been permanently brain damaged by neuroleptics*. https://www.deadlymedicines.dk/lectures/

Whitaker, R. (2002). *Mad in America: Bad science, bad medicine, and the enduring mistreatment of the mentally ill*. Perseus Books Group.

Whitaker, R. (2015). *Anatomy of an epidemic* (2nd ed.). Broadway Paperbacks.

Wunderink, L., Nieboer, R. M., Wiersma, D., Sytema, S., & Nienhuis, F. J. (2013). Recovery in remitted first-episode psychosis at 7 years of follow-up of an early dose reduction/discontinuation or maintenance treatment strategy: Long-term follow-up of a 2-year randomized clinical trial. *JAMA Psychiatry, 70*, 913–920.

Zinkler, M., & von Peter, S. (2019). End coercion in mental health services – Toward a system based on support only. *Laws, 8*, 19.

Chapter 5
Advocating for Integrated Therapy in the Social Environment to Treat Schizophrenia Problems

Luis Valero-Aguayo, Miguel Valenzuela-Hernández, Sara Oneca de Miguel, Juan José Ruiz-Sánchez, and Juan Antonio Díaz-Garrido

Psychological therapy, in its various forms, has been effective improving the lives of people diagnosed with schizophrenia or severe mental disorders. However, the historical tradition treats these problems from a psychiatric and almost exclusively medical, neurological, or pharmacological approach. These pharmacological treatments have eliminated lifelong institutionalisation of these people, but have not really addressed either the causes or the consequences of these problems. Psychology, as a science of behaviour and human relationship, has addressed some of the causes of family and social stress, and it has provided effective treatment systems to address the personal and social consequences of this problem; it has reduced many of the behaviours associated with this category called "psychosis"; and it has improved living conditions, autonomy, and personal life similar to those of other people. In this chapter, we will address some of these solutions, in defence of a psychological and social approach to the problems of schizophrenia. We are not only trying to prevent some of the variables that cause these problems to arise, but also trying to change the professional approach, the family, social, economic, and even political environment that would allow us to improve the resolution of these problems.

L. Valero-Aguayo (✉)
Faculty of Psychology, University of Málaga, Málaga, Spain
e-mail: lvalero@uma.es

M. Valenzuela-Hernández
Ítaca Formation, Córdoba, Spain
e-mail: miguel@itacaformacion.es

S. Oneca de Miguel
Psychology Center Oneca, Pamplona, Navarra, Spain

J. J. Ruiz-Sánchez
Andalusian Health Service, Úbeda District Mental Health Unit, Jaén, Spain

J. A. Díaz-Garrido
Universitary Hospital of Gran Canaria Doctor Negrín, Las Palmas de Gran Canaria, Spain

J. A. Díaz-Garrido et al. (eds.), *Psychological Interventions for Psychosis*,
https://doi.org/10.1007/978-3-031-27003-1_5

5.1 Problem Definition

The high variability of psychotic spectrum disorders, both in their possible aetiopathogenesis, their course and prognosis, and even their different response to different types of intervention, leads us to believe that there are as many psychoses and psychotic experiences as there are diagnosed individuals. This aspect was already anticipated by Bleuler himself (1911/1993) when he spoke of the "group of schizophrenias". It could be stated, paraphrasing Van Os (2016), that "schizophrenia does not exist", highlighting the need to redefine and reconceptualise what we call psychosis.

The approach to problems that are included under the category of "schizophrenia", "psychosis", or "severe mental disorder" is based on a medical and biological definition of the problem. A "mental illness" is assumed to underlie everything that the person displays to family members or professionals. From this conception, a person who shows several of the symptoms at a given moment (in a "break") will already have that illness permanently and chronically.

Thus, we must start by defining what the personal, psychological, or relational problems that are grouped under the category of "schizophrenia" consist of. We will start from a basis that does not assume a "disease" or "psychopathological disorder" common to all these problems. Giving them a name does not mean that we know what they are, let alone what causes them. Only the scientific method allows us to know the causes of these problems and to be able to predict and change them. But we cannot do this based on names, but only on the basis of variables that are measured and are independent of the phenomenon itself. Thus, explaining that a person tells us that he/she hears voices in his/her head because of schizophrenia is not a scientific explanation. It is circular, tautological reasoning, because we have already defined schizophrenia by a strange behaviour such as hearing voices.

What we may therefore consider common to this diagnostic category are certain behaviours that appear strange, inappropriate, and even dangerous to the social context. However, none of the behaviours ("symptoms") of schizophrenia are different from other behaviours that we consider "normal", which are accepted by the social context. Many people have experiences of "hearing voices"and have beliefs about their environment that they perceive as strange (an estimated 10%), yet they do not find them distressing and do not contact mental health services. In any case, it is parameters such as frequency, intensity, duration, or history of these behaviours that differ from the rest of the population. They are like others, only stronger, more intense, or longer lasting.

This already leads us to a relativistic and external position (social, environmental, contextual), since the definition of schizophrenia problems must start not only from the description of the behaviours included in that set, but also from their parameters and why they are considered abnormal. None of these behaviours can be analysed without the context in which they happen, without the family, work, social, economic, etc., environment that determines that they are strange or unusual. For example, that some of these behaviours arise with massive cannabis ingestion suggests biological or neurological factors. However, in Jamaican and Rastafarian culture, this practice is considered part of the religious context, they are considered normal, and for them there are no mental health problem issues involved. Similarly, in Maori culture (New Zealand), people with these strange experiences are considered special, they would be a gift to that person, and would have a value in the social and religious reality of their culture.

We are not going to go into the classic definitions of psychopathology, nor how they have been formed and modified historically. We will start from the descriptions made by the DSM-5 (APA, 2013) and ICD-11 (WHO, 2019) diagnostic system itself, to show the characteristic behaviours we are referring to, which would be the following:

1. *Delusions*, defined as "fixed beliefs that are not susceptible to change even if there is evidence to the contrary". That is, cognitive-verbal behaviour about oneself or others that the social context considers to be unrealistic, exaggerated, or bizarre. How is this psychopathological behaviour different from believing in aliens, abductions, ghosts, telepathy, conspiracy theories, intelligence surveillance, the rejection of vaccines, or animal food? If we are objective, none. The difference is in the context that determines what is accepted and what is not, in each historical and social moment, and some of them are even applauded by that same social environment.
2. *Hallucinations*, defined as "visual or auditory perceptions that occur without the presence of an external stimulus". That is, also cognitive-verbal behaviours of reporting events that are not seen, heard, or perceived by others. This type of behaviour can be common in any person. Even the DSM makes the distinction that hypnagogic images around sleep would not be considered hallucinations and would even be normal in religious cultural contexts. How are these hallucinations different from the "flying flies" we see if we had an eye problem, or the tinnitus we continually hear as background noise? Nobody sees or hears them from the outside, but they are there. In any case, it could be the way these hallucinations are told, which would be different from other similar behaviours that are socially accepted.
3. *Disorganised speech*, also defined as disorganised thinking, describes the individual's verbal behaviour in a format not understandable to the audience of that speech. Again, how is such language different from the thoughtless and loquacious speech of our neighbour, or the hundreds of pages of some post-modern philosophers that only they understand? In any case, it could be the absence of referential content in such speech that makes the difference, but again it is the audience (social and verbal context) that determines that such speech is unacceptable and strange.
4. *Disorganised motor behaviour*, defined as various types of motor responses that are aimless, repetitive, stereotyped, unpredictable, inappropriate, or bizarre, including "catatonia" such as a near total decrease in movement. There is no need to define much more here, what is the difference with respect to the hyperactivity of many children and young people, or the extravagant behaviours of

many youtubers? Precisely, the difference lies in the context in which these responses are given, because now we are not on the dance floor, or recording a video, but in the everyday context with other family members, who are the ones who will consider these movements to be strange and extravagant, and therefore will have to be changed.

5. *Low probability behaviours*, considered as "negative symptoms", all defined as diminished habitual behaviour, ranging from low expression of emotions, reduced daily activities, reduced speech, reduced social contacts, or lack of experiencing pleasure in activities. The definition here is also very clear, as these are the usual behaviours of daily life that would be characterised by a very low frequency and intensity. Again, how are these behaviours different from the ones we all have on weekends, the many hours a day sitting on the sofa in front of the TV, or the routine and boredom of an unemployed person? In any case, it would be the parameter of intensity that would define them, in addition to the family environment that would consider that "you can't just lie around all day doing nothing".

With these definitions, at least we now know what to focus, what to look for, what to study, and what parameters to measure to know if we are able to change these problems. Thus, with this category we are basically referring to those five behaviours, which are also common to most people, but when applied to a specific individual, they are considered to have an illness called "psychosis"or "schizophrenia". However, they are just behaviours like any others, but with altered parameters in their frequency, intensity or duration, and the social environment determines that they are strange, rare, inappropriate, etc., so they must be changed or suppressed. If the social environment does not manage to do so, professional help is sought to do so, or even to do so by force, against the individual's own will.

5.2 Searching for Causes

There are no innocent questions and answers in the contexts of so-called mental health problems. All questions and answers have *implications and consequences*, not only for the people treated in these systems, but also for the professionals who apply them. Moreover, any questions and answers about the problems of psychosis and how to treat them are connected to certain *scientific, theoretical, and philosophical conceptions*, and also within historical and socio-cultural frameworks. Any interpretation that is made will always be within supposedly scientific frameworks, although these criteria are in turn determined by a cultural and historical context.

Interestingly, Coll-Florit et al. (2019) used discourse analysis to record the opinions and statements that both professionals and affected people made about schizophrenia and their situation. Broadly speaking, they found that psychiatrists were the ones who presented more metaphors about illness, separating the individual from the illness and presenting it as a battle or a fight against something independent from the person; on the other hand, both the users themselves and psychologists and other professionals used more metaphors about mental experiences, the mind and emotions, as well as their fears; and only psychologists also considered social life, the family environment, communication, as metaphors for this problem. The use of one type of metaphor or another implies a lot about how these problems are seen from different points of view, and how that also determines the way of approaching and treating them.

As professionals, we propose that it is not the same to place ourselves in a *closed knowledge*, with rigid rules and norms of categorisation and treatment, which is supposed to be independent of the time, moment, and place in which both clinicians and those who have these psychotic experiences live, as it is to place ourselves in an *open, evolutionary, adaptive knowledge*, integrated in the cultural, social, economic, and historical context that each person with these experiences and also professionals live in. It is not the same to consider *the psychotic experience as an illness* (whether neurological, genetic, psychological, or mental), as it is to consider it *as a subjective phenomenological experience* (also with its personal and historical causes). The latter would be interpreted according to the cultural narrative of the moment, and the mission of professionals would be to help the person to be the protagonist of his/her own life.

Thus, it is not the same to consider these experiences as *a failure that springs from within the person*, from their brain or their mental activity, as it is to consider it as *the result of multiple dysfunctional exchanges* throughout their lives, including the biological changes that this entail. It is not the same to conceive of psychosis problems as *a disorder of the brain*, which is the usual psychiatric conception, as it is to conceive of it alternatively as *a socially acquired identity disorder*.

5.2.1 Searching for Biological Causes

In the history of psychotic spectrum disorders, many biologically based alterations have been proposed as possible causes of these problems. This suggests that we know nothing certain about the necessary and sufficient biological causes for these disorders to appear. As Díaz-Garrido et al. (2021) and Fonseca-Pedrero and Lemos-Giráldez (2019) state, today we cannot affirm that there are etiopathogenic markers of functional and/or structural alterations of a cerebral or genetic nature that are the cause of psychosis problems. At most, we can consider them as working hypotheses that many researchers continue to explore every day. The fact that so many biological causes are found may imply that these causes are not being looked for where they may actually be. They are looking inside the brain, but the brain is only a necessary element for behaviour to occur, it is not the cause of behaviour. To find the causes of any psychological phenomenon, as in other sciences, we have to find the *necessary-and-sufficient variable* for that phenomenon to happen. The brain is a necessary variable: without neurons, without neurotransmitters, without the prefrontal cortex, etc., we could hardly behave; but *the sufficient variable* is the interaction of the organism with its environment (physical and social). Without that interaction, no behaviour would develop. Even some people with severe neuronal deterioration manage to have certain interactions with their environment (e.g. moving their fingers or gazing), but without these minimal interactions we would say that they are in a coma or clinically dead.

The above does not imply that we deny that some kind of brain damage, neural function, or brain structure may underlie, as *a necessary but not the only cause* of the various psychotic problems. *The social context would also be a necessary cause* for the development of psychotic problems. Early models already spoke of an integration of factors, such as that of Zubin and Spring (1977), on the confluence of genetic factors, life events, and interpersonal conflicts in a person's life, together with a certain susceptibility or vulnerability as personality characteristics. This integration theory has sought explanations in specific aetiological factors for each type of behaviour (Gleeson et al., 2007) and is the basis of the traumatogenic model (Read et al., 2001) and other approaches that integrate genetic and environmental variables (Freeman and Garety, 2003; Petrones, 2004).

We could consider these interactions and experiences as *necessary causes* (certain contexts and crises must be present for the characteristic behaviours to appear), but *they are not sufficient causes either*. There are people who go through similar traumatic or stressful interactions and do not necessarily develop these problems, although they may develop different mental health problems.

In this logic, then, we are arguing for a multi-causal origin of psychosis problems, where *the brain and its malfunctioning may be a necessary cause*, but also *interaction with the social environment would be another necessary cause*. The latter is usually not considered in research, as it tends to always follow the medical model of physical illness, thus discarding a large part of the "causality" of these problems. It remains to be found *which would be sufficient causes*, i.e. those which, if they appear in the individual's history, can be proven to produce these problems with certainty.

5.2.2 Covariations and Biological Correlates

A large part of the difficulty in finding these causes lies in the research methodology, as correlational and epidemiological studies are mainly used, which allow us to glimpse hundreds of "causes" (as many correlations as we wish to obtain), or *post-hoc* studies that draw conclusions *a posteriori*, when the problem has already been created and causes are assumed, and that sometimes the treatments themselves have contributed to create.

Unfortunately, all studies on possible causes of psychosis problems are correlational, and correlation does not imply finding causation. Many biomedical studies are based on studying some neural variable, including the coloured pixels of the *functional magnetic resonance images (fMRI)* and their correlation with some characteristics of people diagnosed with schizophrenia, in any case comparing with normative populations without such a diagnosis. But these illuminated pixels only indicate the activation of certain neuronal groups or areas, which are previously indicated by the experimenter, and how they relate to the motor or cognitive activity that the individual is doing precisely at that moment. We see that, even in this type of highly technological research, interaction is essential as *a necessary variable*, the *f* of *f*RMI precisely indicates *the functionality* of the behaviour.

On the other hand, psychological studies attempting to find personality traits or specific characteristics in their history, life episodes, family characteristics, susceptibility to stress, etc., are always correlational. They are generally based only on questionnaires, on verbal information given by the individual and/or his/her family, to which are added the diagnoses and assessments of clinical professionals. They cannot really offer many efficient causes for schizophrenia problems either, and they are always based on *post-hoc* studies, when the problem has already presented itself in clinics or health centres. From the very first moment, it is usual that people start to be medicated, and from then on their whole life. It is quite difficult to separate "causes" when medical treatment becomes exclusive and compulsory, with its own iatrogenic effects, and therefore indistinguishable from the very problems it is trying to solve. The toxic effect of the antipsychotics (or neuroleptics) themselves in the long term, producing cognitive impairment, structural alterations, shorter life expectancy, or lower recovery rate, is not without criticism (Harrow et al., 2012; Omachi & Sumiyoski, 2018; Wunderink et al., 2013).

5.3 Rethinking the Causes

In this knowledge open to other alternatives in the search for causes, we can start from the approach of Pérez-Álvarez (2003), and Pérez-Álvarez and García-Montes (2006), on the causes of psychological disorders in general. These authors speak of the four causes of psychological disorders, which in this case we could also extend to the four causes of psychotic disorders.

1. *The efficient cause.* It tries to answer the question of what, who or whose causes psychotic experiences to appear. In this sense, the efficient cause would be found in the relationships between people and the circumstances of life, generally bad or adverse for the person. The individual has these experiences that he or she does not know how to interpret, which makes him or her confront his/her immediate family and social environment, and to which he/she reacts in an exaggerated or inadequate manner. Further to this reasoning, Guerin (2020a, b) proposes that psychotic experiences are an adaptive resource that people use in the face of bad life experiences, after having tried other alternative resources and having failed. For example, Ordoñez et al. (2012) found that, among those admitted to psychiatric units, at least 75% of people reported traumatic experiences, and 69% of women and 59% of men had suffered sexual or physical abuse in childhood. Clearly, there are multiple efficient causes, ranging from childhood abuse

and neglect, poor prenatal health, maternal stress, experiences in war situations, poverty, cannabis use, etc. (Cantor-Graae, 2007).

2. *The material cause.* It tries to find the entity or matter of these psychotic experiences. From a contextual and phenomenological perspective, the contents of these experiences would be based on intense suffering, so that the individual gives answers to cope with this suffering, which changes the experience of the self as an entity from which one acts (the voices heard are those of others) and as the director of one's own life (and these others order what to do). The person does not manage to verbally relate their subjective experiences in an adequate and articulate way to others, with expressions or discourse that others understand. His experiences are his/her own, no one else has them, and no one else has taught him how to name them, how to integrate them into his/her personal self, or how to describe them in words that others understand. From this perspective, then, psychosis problems are presented as disorders of personal identity, where hyperreflexibility (Pérez-Álvarez, 2008), depersonalisation of one's own experiences, and the loss of common sense with the social environment, would be the matter or entities that compose them, regardless of the symptoms or forms that appear in each person thus diagnosed.
3. *The formal cause.* This responds to the form, configuration, or topography of the different behaviours ("symptoms") of these psychotic experiences. In this case, the DSM and the ICD diagnostic systems capture these forms very descriptively. The experiences are lived subjectively by the individual with their personal history and current interactions, but when they describe them, or are described by family members, they begin to be classified, ordered, and categorised. It would be a "secondary elaboration" (Pérez-Álvarez, 2003, 2019) where professionals ask questions and obtain information, based on questionnaires that are confirmed with themselves, so as to delimit the different behaviours presented by that person, always within the categories and parameters defined by those same systems. However, we must not limit ourselves to these categories or "symptoms", because we must also consider the culture and the historical and social moment in which the problem arises. Historical studies have already shown how these "symptoms" can change throughout history, and how they are closely related to the social and cultural environment (religion, political system, technology, media). Possibly, the fact that more importance is given to the so-called "positive symptoms" than to the "negative symptoms" is due to the fact that the drug is listened to more than the individual (González-Pardo and Pérez-Álvarez, 2007). But what we have in our hands, and what we have to treat, is not an illness, nor a disorder, nor a set of symptoms, but *a person with alterations in their way of being in the world.* Alterations involve suffering for these people (and their relatives in many cases), and which would be the formal causes that the professional has to find out and remedy.
4. *The final cause.* This responds to the function, the results, the purpose, or what the psychotic experiences are for, both for the individual and for those close to them and the professionals who care for them. It is about finding out what these psychotic behaviours are for, what consequences they have, what happens to the

individual when he/she suffers, and what actions the social environment takes with regard to them. As we will see below, the social and contextual perspectives that are emerging look for these whys and wherefores in the individual's need to adapt to the social environment that exerts its power and stress; in short, the social function of the dominant power to eliminate any source of dissidence or alteration of the established order. We could even analyse a function of maintaining the problem as a chronic illness that obtains a high economic return and a justification for the social power to have "something" to deal with.

In this situation, professionals trained in contextual and social analysis should approach psychotic experiences in a functional way, addressing these final causes. Their clinical exchanges should aim at shifting the focus of people with these experiences from fighting against these experiences (their thoughts, voices, hallucinations, hyper-reflexivity), to fighting to open up a horizon towards a valuable life. The aim is for the person to direct his/her life and to be the protagonist of positive social interactions, valuable for his/her life, even if and in spite of these psychotic experiences are still present. In each person, it will be necessary to look for the "causes", which will not always be the same in those who receive this diagnosis, to try to change them or in any case to offer alternative ways, to confront this environment that is hostile to them.

In addition, a professional who deals with mental health problems must question his/her own work in depth, must have a broad knowledge of the social relations and movements, both in their history and in their economy, which condition many of the problems classified as "disorders". If professionals do not take a critical look, detached in time and space from the present problem, it is difficult to even realise those four ultimate causes that could account for the emergence and maintenance of mental health problems. However, if this more relativistic, more philosophical, and phenomenological perspective is adopted, perhaps professionals will find other ways of approaching and helping people suffering from psychotic problems.

5.4 The Medical and Pharmacological Approach

The emergence of medications, and especially the appearance of chlorpromazine in 1952, developed a biological model according to which "something is wrong in the psychotic brain", be it neurotransmitters, structural changes, or any other issue. Symptoms associated with these malfunctions emerge and are organised into different disorders. As new drugs emerged, new pathologies were created to be treated with these drugs. All with four fundamental objectives in the case of schizophrenia: symptom control, reducing the frequency and severity of psychotic episodes, improving quality of life, and facilitating the social, occupational and family integration of the person with this diagnosis (SEP, 2000).

What was happening a few years before this "psychopharmacological revolution"? It is interesting to remember that the DSM was developed in the midst of a real battle with the democratic intention (but the science is not democratic) of reaching consensus. With the support of the pharmacological industry, what was really intended was to restore psychiatric prestige in the medical world, which was at a low ebb after the criticisms of the 1970s. Suffice it to recall Hobson's (2003) "... the development of drugs that interact with brain chemical systems is the most important advance in the history of modern psychiatry". No doubt it is, but the psychiatry is among the most powerful sections in the medical world, and it is thanks to the enormous amounts that the psychopharmaceutical industries pour into this section of medicine. The reality at this point in the twenty-first century is that the supposed biological cause of any *mental disorder* has not been found. One of the reasons for this is that we would need to know the brain model of "normal functioning", and this does not exist either, so it is difficult to compare to find the differences. Indeed, a recent meta-analysis of 40 studies (McCutheon et al., 2021) comparing neuronal activity in people at high risk of schizophrenia and others without problems has shown the absence of such differences.

It all seems relatively simple and even consistent with the accepted social model. We attribute the origin of so-called "psychotic" behaviours to a place in a "damaged brain", a problem with neurotransmitters, genes, or some other cause over which we seem to have no choice. We then look for substances that appear to be able to repair these "defects". So, once we have the "symptoms" and the chemical treatments to compensate for them, we act medically. No one is responsible, it is a "chemical condemnation" and as such we can only accept it and live to reduce the symptoms that are considered the problem, and not so much the situations that are experienced in the context. Thus, the family already knows that the cause is a brain problem, and the only thing to do is to pity and treat the person "as if he/she were mad". The individual, for his/her part, does not have much to decide either, only to take the pharmacological treatment even if the short, medium, and long-term side effects make him feel worse and worse, with less and less energy, with movements that he/she does not seem to be able to control, with his/her attention completely scattered, without energy. This is what he/she has to do, to "stabilise" him/herself, and not to be a nuisance.

The professionals of the *Rethinking* project (Crespo-Facorro et al., 2016) produced a consensus document on the efficacy, effectiveness, and efficiency of treatments applied to the problem of schizophrenia. In these conclusions, they state that first- and second-generation antipsychotics are effective, provided there is good compliance, for the so-called "positive symptoms", while cognitive-behavioural interventions have also been shown to be useful, albeit with a moderate effect size. However, they state that there are no drugs that have shown efficacy for "negative symptoms" (primary or secondary), and some of them may even produce negative symptomatology in people who do not have problems (Arango et al., 2013). It also appears that injectable, long-acting, second-generation antipsychotics have advantages in reducing problems and facilitating the coexistence of the individual and his/her family. However, there are also studies that do not show improvements over traditional treatments in symptom reduction, cognitive and social functioning, or relapse prevention (Kishimoto et al., 2014; Lemos et al., 2010). On the other hand, other types of drugs (antidepressants, benzodiazepines, anticonvulsants) that have also been used seem to show little efficacy (Buchanan et al., 2010).

The great shortcoming of this type of pharmacological studies, however, is that they fail to evaluate the social functioning and quality of life of these people, since efficacy studies generally only evaluate the "symptoms" and their changes. They do not consider the individual as a whole, as a human being in his/her social context, so the social functioning of that person, his/her family, social and work interactions, etc., are not assessed. Nor is the person's own opinion taken into account. If we consider the importance of the subjective experience of schizophrenia, and how the individual is able to adapt to it, the assessment of that experience and the person's own opinion about his/her recovery, inclusion in the social environment, or quality of life, are also fundamental aspects to consider in the effectiveness of a treatment. In this sense, recent research has been incorporating more subjective element of the concept of "recovery" (Disky et al., 2015), where the person expresses their satisfaction, their feelings about their current situation, and evaluates both the service received, and their progress and quality of life in the present.

The difficulties in carrying out this type of studies and assessments undoubtedly result from the pressure of care, the scarcity of resources, and medicalisation as an exclusive health resource. If it is an *illness*, as it is socially understood, then it must be *cured* with drugs. In this way, the patient is stripped of his or her own ability to cope.

A further reason for the necessary change in the field of mental health is the iatrogenic nature of the treatments. "Antipsychotic"drugs have had a geometric increase, so that it seems hardly credible that they have solved anything beyond the profit results of the pharmaceutical companies, and all the "contracted" science that has moved in around them. The more drugs patented, the more everyday realities become illnesses, resulting in an increasing number of supposed illnesses that are coupled with the emergence of new psychotropic drugs (Goldarcre, 2019; Gotzsche, 2020).

In short, the biocommercial paradigm has not proved useful for treating mental illness, although we must recognise that the use of drugs can contribute at specific times to allowing the person to be in a better position to solve the problems that lead to suffering. However, a sensible, controlled, and time-limited consumption that alters the person's coping conditions as little as possible; and that is also explained as what it is for: to reduce physical discomfort, but not to treat a problem that has its social roots. It is precisely at this level, the way the person relates to and is in his/her various social contexts, that will be the key to intervention.

5.5 The Psychological Treatments

Traditionally, psychological treatments for schizophrenia problems have really been seen as adjuncts or complements to pharmacological therapy. Since the latter does not achieve optimal results, especially not in the long term, and has high side effects and poor adherence to treatment, there has been a need to include other forms of intervention to help improve the situation. In this case, the psychological treatments with the greatest experimental support that appear in the NICE guidelines (2014), those of the APA (2019), the RANZ-CP of Australia (2016), the CPA of Canada (2017), of other professional associations on the subject, and also in Spain the *Guide of the Ministry of Health and Consumer Affairs* (GPC, 2009) are usually the following: cognitive-behavioural therapy, social skills training, cognitive-social training, assertive-community treatment and employment support, family intervention, and psychoeducation.

These are being incorporated with other forms of intervention based on metacognitive rehabilitation, or therapies based on acceptance and mindfulness. Although they differ from one guide to another, they tend to have common elements, albeit with varying degrees of effectiveness. An extensive description of these reviews can be found in these same international guidelines and in various writings (Fonseca-Pedrero, 2019; Fonseca-Pedrero et al., 2021; McDonagh et al., 2018; Ridenour et al., 2019; Shirivastava, 2020).

5.5.1 Psychological Treatment with Empirical Support

Cognitive-Behavioural Therapy In general, this type of therapy is an extension of cognitive-behavioural techniques applied to other problems, but now adapted to the specific characteristics of these people. In this case, a diversity of behavioural techniques include not only contingency management (e.g. token economy in institutions), but also teaching self-management and self-control, coping skills training, controlling anxiety dealing with others, changing depressive and ruminative thoughts, etc. Particular emphasis is placed on reducing the distress and disability associated with psychotic behaviours, reducing emotional disturbance and achieving greater involvement of the individual in relapse prevention and social adaptation. The review and meta-analysis by Wood et al. (2020), based on 23 randomised cognitive studies, showed positive effects after therapy and at follow-up, not on "positive" behaviours but on "negative" behaviours, daily functioning, and readmissions.

Fundamentally, cognitive-behavioural strategies focus on people's beliefs, trying to change these schemas, to confront reality, or to modify automatic thoughts. In our view, however, what they can achieve is the strengthening of these delusions. Focusing on the content by insisting on it is a form of positive reinforcement, which paradoxically increases them by trying to change them. Hence, from the most recent therapies, the central objective is changed towards the acceptance of these thoughts, the description, and vision of these hallucinations as true, although in the background, giving priority to vital objectives, personal values, and relations with the environment, in spite of continuing to have these strange experiences that the individual does not know how to handle.

Social Skills Training This type of intervention, which is common to the previous one, focuses on improving social competences, adequate processing of social information, and social cognition about their environment. In addition, interactive skills, emotional skills, instrumental roles, and social norms are taught to facilitate the individual's social inclusion. On this basis, neuropsychological rehabilitation therapies ("cognitive rehabilitation techniques") have also been proposed that focus on cognitive skills training, learning new supervised skills for managing the everyday or work environment. A meta-analysis of 27 studies (Turner et al., 2018) of randomised group comparisons has shown that social skills training has better results than controls and standardised treatment groups on "negative symptoms", and also on other problem behaviours, especially on measures of social integration and functioning. This effectiveness was also maintained in long-term follow-ups.

Cognitive-Social Training This perspective that adds the word "social" to the cognitive refers to the degree to which people integrate that social information or have social and emotional processing skills, empathy, knowledge of social norms, involvement in social settings, etc. (Baez et al., 2013). This theory goes so far as to determine its components in emotional processing, social perception, theory of mind and attributional style and even ventures to identify in which brain areas these "social mental processes" could be located (Pinkham, 2014). From our perspective, this psychological and cognitive theory has little "social" element. It implies looking again for causes *within* the individual, rather than in the interactions he/she makes with his/her environment. Problems of social relations, social malfunctioning, or maladjustment are attributed to a certain "social cognition". From this cognitive approach, we are back to having to deal with the "mind" and something supposedly altered within the individual.

Assertive-Community Treatment This is an intervention model aimed at organising the health system around the problem, rather than a treatment technique. It consists of a multidisciplinary team that tries to implement most of the available services (treatment, rehabilitation, health, social and economic support). The aim is to maintain a comprehensive service for people with severe and complex mental disorders, of a chronic nature, and with severe effects on their daily functioning. In many cases, these people have only received uncoordinated, piecemeal treatment, wandering from professional to professional, without receiving comprehensive care in all the aspects. The ultimate goals of this form of intervention are not so much to refer problems, but to keep the individual in contact with health and care services, reduce the incidence and duration of hospitalisations, improve adherence to treatment and therapeutic guidelines, and thereby improve the social functioning and quality of life of these individuals (Vanderlip et al., 2017). In fact, it is the programme recommended as public health policy by the WHO (2008) and has been implemented in many European countries.

Family Intervention Since the deinstitutionalisation of people with psychosis in the last century, families have been at the forefront of all forms of intervention. They are important not only as a possible source of conflicts and stress (remember the "expressed emotion"), which have to be addressed in joint sessions and therapeutic indications for day-to-day life, but also as a "family burden" since they are the ones who have to face all the episodes, conflicts, discomfort, stigma, and difficulties of all kinds. Thus, professional support for the family, attending to their emotional and relational needs, avoiding blaming, and the creation of a good therapeutic alliance are crucial for the maximum benefit of any programme. Systematic reviews (McFarlane, 2016; Sin et al., 2017) indicate a 50–60% reduction in problems compared to treatment as usual, especially when such family intervention is applied in the first episodes or early phase of the psychosis problem and is also combined with some of the other evidence-based therapies.

Whatever the theoretical basis for intervention in the family, it is also combined with "psychoeducation" and problem solving that arise throughout the therapeutic process. However, from our point of view, these interventions are very much influenced by the medical-psychiatric model, where family members are usually asked to help with pharmacological adherence, monitoring of the person, or day-to-day care. In addition, if the basis of an "illness" model is assumed by the relatives, then they adopt more roles of "caregivers" than "problem-solvers". Generally, these programmes increase the information available to family members, and they improve interactions within the family, as well as adherence to treatment, and overall family satisfaction, but do not show improvements in behaviours characteristic of "psychosis".

Psychoeducation This is practically a type of intervention that is present in all other forms of treatment, since an element of information and education is always included in all programmes, especially for the family. The aim is to provide relevant information about the problem and the planned form of treatment, as well as strategies for the management of their environment regarding the difficulties that arise in day-to-day life, medication intake, reactions to episodes, emotional treatment, etc. In many cases, this information is also included in the form of readings and even online support programmes. The inclusion of this element aimed at family members and caregivers within rehabilitation programmes has shown better final results (Sin et al., 2017). A meta-analysis study (Alhadidi et al., 2020) of 11 randomised studies shows that adding psychoeducation to the programme results in fewer relapses and lower readmission rates, while increasing the sense of well-being and control by the family environment, than groups that did not include this component in the intervention.

5.5.2 Psychological Treatment as Support

One of the arguments most often put forward for the need for psychology to collaborate in interventions on psychosis is the need for adherence to pharmacological treatment. It is preached that the individual must be "aware of the illness", i.e. he/

she must accept and assume the role he/she is forced to play, recognise that he/she has an "illness", and that the only possible treatment that will benefit him/her is pharmacological treatment. This "recognition" is an essential factor for the initiation of pharmacological or psychological therapy. Without it, the success of any voluntary intervention by the individual is difficult, and it is a predictor of subsequent pharmacological success (Ayesa-Arriola et al., 2011). However, it focuses the entire problem on the individual and not on the relationship with the social context. It is logical that if the person accepts that he/she "has" an illness and that there is nothing he/she can do to change but take medication, then he/she will adjust to this demand. In this way, psychologists also contribute to the psychopathologisation of problems, making the individual the only one to be blamed, and the person's life is decontextualised.

This insistence on "illness awareness" also has another side which is called "self-stigmatisation". That is, as soon as the diagnosis is received, the individual himself assumes the possible discrimination of his/her family, friends, and relatives. This leads to self-isolation and reluctance to seek help, support, or alternative ways to improve their situation. Thus, the person with a diagnosis of schizophrenia is not only confronted with the real fact of stigmatisation by the social environment, which isolates him/her, sees him/her as strange, and does not want to be around him/her, but also a self-assumed role believed to be true by the individual himself/herself, which leads to more isolation and fewer possibilities of interactions with others.

We believe that psychology is in urgent need of a critical revision to question this profoundly iatrogenic model, which views human distress in terms of the "ghost in the machine", a ghost that also seems to have a broken mechanism. Thus, psychological intervention should not focus on decreasing hallucinatory behaviours (e.g. "focusing" or "reality testing"), since focusing on them may increase them, or at least increase their evocation and verbalisation. The aim would be that the individual would interpret these experiences differently, adapt to them, and that they do not determine his/her actions in everyday life. It is also useful to try to find out their functionality, what triggers them, what behaviours follow, and what happens after these episodes, always trying to focus on the functionality, rather than on the form or content of these experiences.

However, official psychology also plays the role of a social loudspeaker for the biocommercial model, as it accepts without nuance the biological discourse of alterations that need a chemical solution, instead of understanding the profound social and relational component that leads to situations of personal suffering. A change in health policies is needed, with a more social and community orientation in health services, which prioritise this reality of social functioning and quality of life in the success of the treatments that are implemented.

5.6 The Contextual and Social Perspective

It is important to establish from the outset what this contextual and social perspective implies, as they are polysemous terms, and are used with multiple other theoretical conceptions. It is not only psychology that uses the word "social", but also community psychiatry interventions, and even social services. We will consider here as fundamental, both as causes and as objects of change, the immediate context, and the wider social context in which the individual with these problems lives. Context, then, will be the whole set of variables and factors that directly (and also indirectly) affect psychosis problems (van Os, 2010). In other words, we consider variables that are external to the problems to be more important and more addressable. By changing immediate family interactions, social interactions with friends and acquaintances, work environment, personal autonomy, economic independence, living conditions, opportunities, and accessibility to resources, etc., it is more likely that many of the psychotic behaviours, which until now have been addressed from an individual perspective, can be solved.

Programmes Focused on "Community Intervention" They have a behavioural and cognitive-behavioural basis, as they integrate various strategies already endorsed for intervention in other types of clinical problems. In this case, training in daily living skills, social skills, assertiveness, coping, social emotional management, work integration, etc., are used. Controlled studies of this type show the efficacy of such training and employment support to be very effective for the individual's daily life, decreasing substance use, hospitalisations, and decreasing the risk of social exclusion (Liberman and Kopelowicz, 2005; Killackey, 2009). Among the social approaches, experiences started already in the 1980s with the so-called "case management programmes". Here a tutor or manager acts as a guide and coordinator between the different mental health devices and the individual, facilitating different types of programmes, support, social options, etc. In Spain, this type of experience has not been very successful due to a lack of funding and training for the professionals on the team. On the contrary, models of individual intervention and psychosocial reintegration have been devised and implemented, such as the previously mentioned "assertive community treatment", combining individual, psychological, pharmacological, and social approaches (Mesa-Velasco et al., 2021), which have reduced hospitalisations and the severity of the problems (Wilkinson et al., 1995). Although they are minor, self-help groups and social clubs have also other strategies to use the social context to improve the interaction problems of these people. Such services can create a non-clinical context that can benefit communication and the learning of appropriate social skills, as well as providing support and social reinforcement, breaking isolation, and improving the social network for these individuals.

Psychological and Social Interventions Without Drugs Pharmacological management and the "deactivation" of the individual that this involves means that experiences or interventions that do not include pharmacological treatment are rare. Recent research has begun to compare the efficacy of different interventions with and without pharmacological treatment (or with the lowest possible doses). The review by Cooper et al. (2020) has identified 17 non-drug studies, but of these only 9 randomised studies comparing drug and non-drug groups, and mostly with small samples. In these results, interventions with the psychological treatments described above, but without adjunctive medication, achieve the same overall results as those using only medication as the exclusive treatment. Psychotic behaviours decrease at a medium level, but social functioning improves greatly.

Interventions Focused on the Social Function We have already mentioned the social function of the medical-psychiatric model that tries to impose a single form of treatment based on drugs and unique biologistic causes. Actually, from a more contextual and social perspective, we can consider that the dominant powers (from the family to the state) try to impose their social narrative, and the control of social behaviours in established frameworks, so that those who escape (or try to avoid) these frameworks, showing alternative narratives and stories, are forced into a form of treatment that renders them useless for their daily lives and prevents them from coping with these functions of power and social control. This social analysis also emerges from the British mental health movement on the *Power, Threat, and Meaning Framework* (Johnstone et al., 2018), which views mental health experiences as an individual's reaction to a social and political framework of power, which exerts pressure and stress, and to which they rebel, flee, try to adapt, or fight back. In this sense, psychotic behaviours would have a reason as an adaptation and reaction to the suffering of this power, and where the individual reacts and tries to cope as best he/she can with these threats from the social environment. This framework is finally understood from the "meaning" that the individual gives to that power and that threat, that is, from the perception and subjectivity that the person gives to that situation, which makes him/her suffer, react, or remain paralysed in the face of all those interactions that oppress him/her.

Interventions from the Functional Context The maintenance of psychotic problems can also be analysed from the functional analysis of behaviour (Ramnerö and Törneke, 2008) based on the principles of learning, where the direct consequences of a behaviour on the environment are studied. When a behaviour occurs, usually strange to its context, it receives consequences from the social environment, which usually reacts by being surprised, altered, attacked, immobilised, or by moving away, isolating the individual, avoiding his or her social presence, etc. From what we know about the laws of learning, this strange behaviour will be repeated if it receives contingencies. In these cases of "bizarre" or "psychotic" behaviours, they are considered as an attempt at dysfunctional adaptation to adverse life situations (Pankey and Hayes, 2003; García-Montes et al., 2006; Pérez-Álvarez, 2019) and would have a function or purpose of avoiding the aversive emotional experience derived from these situations (e.g. direct escape, avoidance of the aversive situation, experiential avoidance). But in attempting to do so, they encounter new social contingencies that chronically maintain them. If that context does not change (family, lifestyle, and social relationships usually remain stable), then they become chronic, long-lasting behaviours. They would have a maintenance function through their immediate effects, by eliminating responsibilities, confrontations, problems with others, etc., and even maintaining socially reinforced behaviours by attracting a great deal of attention and care. In many cases, the set of variables that follow psychotic behaviours says a lot about their chronic maintenance, including the reactions of professionals, who tend to strengthen these formal causes (by insisting on the "symptoms") and also the final causes (by reinforcing their maintenance). In these cases, the intervention must seek to change these contingencies, not only by teaching family members and relatives, but also by trying to change the moment-to-moment interactions that the individual has in his/her daily life. This also involves social and economic changes, of a more global nature, but which form part of the macro-contingencies that maintain social behaviour, so that they would also be the object of change in these psychotic problems. Interdisciplinary work is therefore essential, not only with the medical professionals that already exist, but also with social workers, employment counsellors, support tutors, etc., who can really do a great deal of work to avoid the chronicity of the problems.

Acceptance-Based and Life-Based Interventions These are the new approaches that have emerged from the so-called "third-generation therapies" or also "contextual therapies" (such as *Acceptance and Commitment Therapy*; Hayes et al., 2012) in which the emphasis is on the individual's relationship to his/her environment, including here his/her verbal context. The fundamental idea is that the more the individual struggles with his/her private events (hallucinations, recurrent ideas, and thoughts), the more he/she is increasing them, so that this struggle is the centre of his/her life and becomes the source of all other problems. The therapy, then, basically consists of accepting these events as true, observing them, describing them, and "letting them go", in order to focus on the present life here and now. Psychological flexibility is sought, so that extraneous thoughts and experiences do not become the centre of everything, but rather the personal values, the life goals that a person has.

This view is also shared by phenomenological and experiential theories, which attribute a deficient construction of the self, the way of living intersubjectivity with others, and the lack of relationship with the world (Ayesa-Arriola et al., 2011; Martín-Murcia & Cangas, 2021; Parnas and Handest, 2003). This type of interventions can also include "open dialogue" and "hearing voices" approaches that emphasise personal experience and help to understand them within the social and family context (Ruddle et al., 2011; Valtanen, 2019). The review of Ventura-Martins et al. (2017) and Louise et al. (2018) about these therapies have shown their effectiveness in reducing psychological behaviours, anxiety, and depression, as well as functioning in daily life. More details of these therapies and their effectiveness can be found in other chapters of this book, and in manuals such as Díaz-Garrido et al. (2021) and Fonseca-Pedrero (2019).

Social-Contextual Approach Essentially, here, we advocate the search for causes and solutions to the problems of schizophrenia in the individual's social and experiential environment. Focusing on the "brain" or the "mind" has not led very far to effective long-term solutions. It is necessary to focus on the outside, on the interactions that occurred in that person's life, and those that are happening at the moment. It would be by changing those interactions and that context that better long-term solutions could be found. When the individual has an autonomous, socially positive life, economic independence, and life goals, these problems of "psychosis"can be considered solved.

Our approach is: **contextual, social, and external,** since we assume that the causal variables of the problems are outside the individual, in the interactions that happened in his/her history and in the present. At the moment the first "psychotic break" appears, history can no longer be changed, but the person's future can be changed. Thus, the therapeutic goal should be not so much to change the individual, but to change his/her environment or social context, and the way he/she interacts with these contexts, including the verbal interactions and the explanation of the experiences he/she suffers. If we assume a causality or triggering of psychotic problems from difficult and stressful situations, then we must also look for the remedy in those situations, starting with the family. New crises and readmissions are much more likely if the person lives with very critical family members.

From this social-contextual approach, we also follow the ideas of Guerin (2016, 2017, 2020a, b), the individual's living conditions from childhood and adolescence shape the various behaviours, and some of them will be strangers to their environment. They will not emerge suddenly, but increase or exaggerate from weaker ones, which are socially "spoiled" or "punished", and the individual tends to adapt or try to escape from these new conditions, sometimes exaggerating even more, reacting in an emotional and strong way, which often leads to institutionalisation and medication. In this way, both negative environments and bizarre behaviours feedback, becoming entrenched and chronically maintained.

Therefore, our analysis is that the intervention should not focus on an inner self, but **on the concrete interactions that happen in everyday life** between that person and his/her family. Direct observation in real context is what can indicate the aversive situation that the individual is experiencing. The family should be taught how to interact without punishing, because if the family members do so, it is because they do not know any other repertoire, nor do they know how to deal with the problems. The so-called "psychoeducation" described above, we believe, is not enough; it is only information about the problem from a medical-illness point of view, rather than information about the daily reality of these social interactions. Information has little power to modify behaviours, it has to be a direct training, and if possible in the family environment, to observe and start modifying these interactions in situ. Therapy should be brought into the home, not in an "artificial" or "professional" context, which is not functional to produce the same negative interactions that usually occur in daily life, but should take place at mealtimes, chats, discussions, etc. Family intervention is missing this great opportunity for action. In these cases, social interventions through living with others outside the family, "protected homes", or supervised living may be valid options, although so far there is little research on their effectiveness.

On the other hand, life today pivots around work and money. This is the context that determines a large part of new social behaviours as well. Thus, in a person with these "psychotic" problems, the fact of **being employed and financially independent** are the fundamental factors for a *full functional recovery*. This should be the ultimate goal of therapeutic interventions, where the individual moves from a sufferer's sick role to a normalised role as an autonomous person. However, discrimination and stigma towards these people greatly hinder these goals. Sheltered workshops and associations of "sheltered work" or "special employment centres" are some options, as long as they do not become a refuge isolated from the real social and working environment and do not become yet another form of abuse of unprotected workers by employers.

The aim should be to ensure that integration into the labour market is real, in a normalised job, alongside other workers without problems, and not to persist in the tendency to "ghettoise" or "overprotect" when trying to deal with employment issues. Logically, the initial difficulties are based on deficits in social and professional skills to develop some work, but experiences with so-called "artistic" jobs show the usefulness of this approach. A person with such problems may not be able to be in construction or in an office, working rigorous hours and under the stress of abusive bosses, and may quickly give up because he/she does not know how to cope with the circumstances. However, he/she may be able to develop a job writing articles, being a blogger, radio scriptwriter, theatre actor, artistic painter, or studio musician (El País, 2004; La Colifata, 2021). As we argued above, psychotic-type behaviours can be presented by anyone, and it is a matter of degree whether they are considered pathological or not. In fact, the line between psychotic and creative behaviour in many artists is a fine one (see the examples of van Gogh, Munch, Martín-Ramírez, Wölfli, Nijinsky, John Nash, Joyce, Hemingway, Virginia Woolf, Philip K. Dick, Kafka, Jack Kerouac, Syd Barret, Peter Green, and a long etcetera).

5.7 What Do We Want to Achieve with the Therapy?

Studies of empirically validated therapies and practices always base their conclusions on quantitative changes that are assumed to be the effect of the treatment. Depending on the design used, these changes will be more or less reliable in terms of their conclusions, but always quantitative and based on changes in scores on questionnaires or structured interviews with scales of the "clinical" opinion of professionals. Very few studies base their conclusions on direct observation of the behaviours of the persons to whom these diagnoses are given; at most family members are asked, again with a standardised questionnaire and opinion scales. Even studies on pharmacological efficacy only measure the information that the individual or the professional gives on the frequency and type of drug prescribed; very few studies measure the amount of metabolites of these drugs in the blood, in order to have something objective to go by. Obviously, all these scales and opinions are then converted into numbers, and from there they are used as if continuous variables had been measured. Nothing could be further from the truth, because in essence our studies on therapies are always based on language, on the opinion of the family, the professional, or the individual. Does anyone measure the frequency or duration of clinically relevant behaviours (even if they are called "symptoms")?

Not only that, but what studies measure the real changes in that person's life? Certainly, very few. Only a small number measure so-called "quality of life" (again, an opinion), frequency of readmissions, time between visits, months in employment, or some socio-economic variables that might be somewhat more objective. But efficacy studies, and subsequent meta-analysis studies, do not usually capture these variables, but only quantitative changes in the questionnaires.

Obviously, these are necessary data, but it also leads us to a reflection on what is the change (objective) we want to achieve with any therapy, and with any intervention programme, whether in an institution or in the public health system. The objective, we believe, would not only be a quantitative change, but several changes that may reflect the real performance of the intervention on the individual's daily life. In this sense, **we advocate the use of more direct measures of behaviour, measures in the daily life of the individual** (or within an institution, if that is the case). This would involve measuring the so-called "clinically relevant behaviours", i.e. those behaviours that mostly lead to a diagnosis. Some of these were described at the beginning of this chapter. This implies focusing on and trying to change specific behaviours rather than "psychopathologies". But it would not be a matter of "clinically opining", for example, that hallucinations or delusions have decreased, but of observing and directly measuring the number of such statements a person gives per unit of time; or the amount of time they can remain silent or static in an interview; or recording the frequency of irrational speech; or the speed at which they talk about how their week has gone. That kind of data would be more objective and direct than the opinion of a professional who will, at most, do an interview and a general observation for a few minutes.

Hence, it is necessary to incorporate other data on daily life, social contacts and relationships, time and types of work, habits of independence and personal autonomy, pro-social behaviour in their environment, leisure, and entertainment behaviour, etc., into efficacy research. But, observed directly and not from questionnaires, since they would only represent the opinion (again) of professionals, relatives, or the individual him/herself.

In addition, **any intervention must seek the maximum autonomy and independence of the individual** to function in his/her social environment, in all aspects of family, relationships, friends, work, finances, leisure, etc. We believe that what should be sought is that social functioning, appropriate to the environment, even with (despite having) "symptoms". If a pharmacological treatment reduces these symptoms but prevents this social functioning, because it cancels out the individual, we are not really on the best path to effective intervention. Many psychological, social, and contextual treatments have shown that such functioning is possible even if the individual continues to maintain some of these behaviours. Precisely, as we said earlier, contextual therapies seek functioning in the here and now life of the individual, even if hallucinatory behaviours are still present. As we said at the beginning, we all hallucinate and we all have our delusions and paranoias, it is a question of degree. It is a continuum, and it is in this balance that we can seek the autonomy and freedom of the individual to develop his/her life as a person.

5.8 Towards the Future

We are not trying to reissue an old confrontation, more mythological than real, between psychiatry and psychology. We are dealing with the urgent need to replace a biocommercial paradigm (García-Valdecasas and Vispe, 2011) dominant in mental health care in general, with one that, without denying the importance of biology, focuses on psychological and social aspects, not by whim but by seeking a real benefit for people.

Tailoring to the needs of the individual involves the use of social, psychological, and biological treatments in a coherent package for each particular person. Experiences from Finland with support systems and community, in team-based treatment units called "open dialogue" (Lakerman, 2014), and prevention experience in Melbourne (Phillips et al., 2007; RANZ-CP, 2016) have been significant. Social interventions seek to reduce the impact of social exclusion. The labelling of the individual and their isolation from the social environment results in significant disadvantage and loss of opportunity and entitlement in relation to others. People so diagnosed tend to have less money, be lonely, very socially disconnected, unemployed, and are possible victims of any abuse or neglect. Also the Norwegian experience (Johannessen et al., 2005; Ulland et al., 2014) integrates pharmacological interventions with psychological ones, where the prevalence of patients with schizophrenia problems is among the lowest in Europe, where they consider that homeless people (usually with this type of problems) are entitled to housing, social support, and psychological and/or social treatment; in addition to a system of care from the first episode, where they receive immediate support and individualised treatment to adapt their situation to the family and social environment.

Rethinking's multidisciplinary team (Crespo-Facorro et al., 2016) includes a series of recommendations, which we endorse as our own, for the improvement of comprehensive care for people with schizophrenia:

- Provide an integrated, evidence-based package of care that meets physical and mental health needs.
- Provide support for people with schizophrenia to live in their usual environment.
- Develop mechanisms to help them navigate complex employment and social benefit systems.
- Provide specific support, information, and educational programmes for family members and careers.
- Regularly review and improve care procedures.
- Involve all stakeholders: users, professionals, relatives, and organisations.

- Provide support for research and search for new treatments in proportion to their social impact.
- Establish well-funded awareness-raising campaigns as part of ongoing action plans.

Many factors remain to be addressed in this brief proposal for change. There is certainly room for a more social and contextual (political?) analysis of why the factors that contribute to the production of problems of psychological discomfort (poverty undoubtedly has a prominent place here) disappear from the variables taken into account, and we only focus on organic factors. Behind this we consider that there is a whole socio-political construction of reality, where the term illness is something "politically constructed" and for the benefit of the system.

We are undoubtedly advocating those treatments should not be placed in the hands of "pharmaceutical" psychiatry, but in the hands of multidisciplinary teams where factors such as social integration, work, confrontation of discomfort, etc., are also objectives and actors in the treatment formats. In short, therefore, to improve care for people with these problems, the new forms of treatment must include ecological, contextual, and relevant assessments for the quality of life of people with schizophrenia, not only quantitative statistical data, but also the real repercussions that the programmes have on the lives of people, families, and the social environment in general.

References

Alhadidi, M. M. B., Abdullah, K. L., Yoong, T. L., Hadid, L. A., & Danaee, M. (2020). A systematic review or randomized controlled trial of psychoeducation interventions for patients diagnosed with schizophrenia. *International Journal of Social Psychiatry, 66*(6), 542–552. https://doi.org/10.1177/0020764020919475

American Psychiatric Association. (2013). *Diagnostic and statistical manual of mental disorders* (5th ed.). APA.

American Psychiatric Association. (2019). *The American Psychiatric Association practice guideline for the treatment of patients with schizophrenia*. APA.

Arango, C., Garibaldi, G., & Marder, S. R. (2013). Pharmacological approaches to treating negative symptoms: A review of clinical trials. *Schizophrenia Research, 150*(1–2), 346–352. https://doi.org/10.1016/j.scheres.2013.07.026

Ayesa-Arriola, R., Rodríguez-Sánchez, J. M., Morelli, C., Pelayo- Terán, J. M., Pérez-Iglesias, R., Mata, I., Martínez-García, O., Pardo-García, G., & Vázquez-Barquero, J. L. (2011). Insight dimensions in first-episode psychosis patients: Clinical, cognitive, pre- morbid and socio-demographic correlates. *Early Intervention in Psychiatry, 5*, 140–149. https://doi.org/10.1111/j.1751-7893.2010.00249.x

Baez, S., Herrera, E., Villarin, L., Theil, D., González-Gadea, M. L., Gomez, P., Mosquera, M., Huepe, D., Strejilevich, S., Vigliecca, N. S., Malthaus, F., Decty, J., Manes, F., & Ibañez, A. M. (2013). Contextual social cognition impartments in schizophrenia and bipolar disorder. *PLoS One, 8*(3), e57664. https://doi.org/10.1371/journal.pone.0057664

Bleuler, E. (1911/1993). *Demencia Precoz. El grupo de las esquizofrenias* (2ª ed.). [Dementia Praecox: The schizophrenia group]. Lumen.

Buchanan, R. W., Kreyenbuhl, J., Kelly, D. L., Noel, J. M., Boggs, D. L., Fischer, B. A., Himelhoch, S., Fang, B., Peterson, E., Aquino, P. R., & Keller, W. (2010). The 2009 schizophrenia PORT psychopharmacological treatment recommendations and summary statements. *Schizophrenia Bulletin, 36*(1), 71–93. https://doi.org/10.1093/schbul/sbp116

Cantor-Graae, E. (2007). The contribution of social factors to the development of schizophrenia: A review of recent findings. *The Canadian Journal of Psychiatry, 52*(5), 277–286. https://doi.org/10.1177/070674370705200502

Coll-Florit, M., Miranda, X., & Climent, S. (2019). Metáforas de la esquizofrenia: Un estudio sobre el discurso de afectados y profesionales [Metaphors of schizophrenia: A study of the discourse of sufferers and professionals]. *Revista Española de Lingüística Aplicada, 32*(1), 1–31. https://doi.org/10.1075/resla.16003.col

Cooper, R. E., Laxhman, N., Crellin, N., Moncrieff, J., & Priebe, S. (2020). Psicosocial interventions for people with schizophrenia or psychosis on minimal or non-antipsychotic medication: A systematic review. *Schizophrenia Research, 225*, 15–30. https://doi.org/10.1016/j.schres.2019.05.020

CPA. (2017). *Canadian treatment guidelines on psychosocial treatment of schizophrenia in adults.* Canadian Psychiatric Association. https://capa-apc.org

Crespo-Facorro, B., Bernardo, M., Argimon, J. M., Arrojo, M., Bravo-Ortiz, M. F., Cabrera-Cifuentes, A., Carretero-Roman, J., Franco-Martin, M. A., García-Portilla, P., Haro, J. M., Olivares, J. M., Panadés, R., Pino-Montes, J., Sanjuán, J., & Arango, C. (2016). Eficacia, eficiencia y efectividad en el tratamiento multidimensional de la esquizofrenia: Proyecto Rethinking [Rethinking Project: Efficacy, efficiency, and effectiveness in the multidimensional treatment of schizophrenia]. *Revista de Psiquiatría y Salud Mental, 10*(1), 4–10. https://doi.org/10.1016/j.rpsm.2016.09.001

Díaz-Garrido, J. A., Laffite, H., & Zúñiga, R. (2021). *Terapia de aceptación y compromiso en psicosis: Aceptación y recuperación por niveles (ART)* [Acceptance and Commitment Therapy in psychosis: Accepcance and Recovery by Levels]. Pirámide.

Disky, J., Lalitha, K., Gandhi, S., Desai, G., & Nagarajaiah, P. (2015). Consumer perspectives on the concept of recovery in schizophrenia: A systematic review. *Asian Journal of Psychiatry, 14*, 13–18. https://doi.org/10.1016/j.ajp.2015.01.006

El Pais. (2004, 24 November). *Terapia en directo: Un programa radiofónico elaborado por personas con enfermedad mental cumple cuatro años en Málaga* [Live therapy: A radio programme produced by people with mental illness in four years old in Malaga]. (Newspaper report 24-11-2004). https://elpais.com/diario/2004/11/24/andalucia/1101252160_850215.html. Programa de radio disponible en http://www.canalmalaga.es/romper-barreras

Fonseca-Pedrero, E. (coord.) (2019). *Tratamientos psicológicos para la psicosis* [Psychological treatments for psychosis]. Pirámide.

Fonseca-Pedrero, E., & Lemos-Giráldez, S. (2019). El síndrome psicótico: Pasado, presente y futuro [The psychotic syndrome: Past, present and future]. In E. Fonseca-Pedrero (Ed.), *Tratamientos psicológicos para la psicosis* (pp. 25–78). [Psychological treatments for psychosis]. Pirámide.

Fonseca-Pedrero, E., Paíno, M., Perona-Garcelán, S., Rodríguez-Testal, J. F., & Vallina, O. (2021). Tratamientos psicológicos para la psicosis [Psychological treatments for psychosis]. In E. Fonseca-Pedrero (Ed.), *Manual de tratamientos psicológicos. Adultos* (pp. 251–304). [Psychological treatment manual: Adults]. Pirámide.

Freeman, D., & Garety, P. A. (2003). Connecting neurosis and psychosis: The direct influence of emotion on delusions and hallucinations. *Behaviour Research and Therapy, 41*, 923–947. https://doi.org/10.1016/S0005-7967(02)00104-3

García-Montes, J. M., Pérez-Álvarez, M., & Cangas, A. J. (2006). Aproximación al abordaje clínico de los síntomas psicóticos desde la aceptación [Acceptance-based approach to the clinical management of psychotic symptoms]. *Apuntes de Psicología, 24*(1–3), 293–230. https://www.apuntesdepsicologia.es/index.php/revista/article/view/107/109

García-Valdecasas, J., & Vispe, A. (2011). Mercaderes en el templo: Hegemonía del paradigma biocomercial en psiquiatría [Merchants in the temple: Hegemony of the biocommercial paradigm in psychiatry]. *Revista de la Asociación Española de Neuropsiquiatría, 110*, 321–341. https://doi.org/10.4321/S0211-57352011000200010

Gleeson, J. F. M., Krstev, H., & Killackey, E. (2007). Integration and the psychotherapies for schizophrenia and psychosis. In J. F. M. Gleeson, E. Killackey, & H. Krstev (Eds.), *Psychotherapy for psychoses: Theoretical, cultural, and clinical integration* (pp. 1–14). Routledge. https://doi.org/10.4324/9780203937976

Goldarcre, B. (2019). *Mala farma* [Bad pharma]. Paidós Contextos.

González-Pardo, H., & Pérez-Álvarez, M. (2007). *La invención de los trastornos mentales. ¿Escuchando al fármaco o al paciente?* [The invention of mental disorders: Listening the drug or the patient?]. Alianza Editorial.

Gotzsche, P. (2020). *Psicofármacos que matan y denegación organizada* [Killing psychotropic drugs and organised denial]. Los Libros del Lince.

GPC. (2009). *Guía práctica clínica sobre la esquizofrenia y el trastorno psicótico incipiente* [Clinical practice guideline on schizophrenia and incipient psychotic disorder]. Plan de Calidad para el Sistema Nacional de Salud del Ministerio de Sanidad y Consumo. https://portal.guiasalud.es

Guerin, B. (2016). *How to rethink psychology: New metaphors for understanding people and their behavior*. Routledge. [Spanish translation in Editorial Tsara].

Guerin, B. (2017). *How to rethink mental illness: The human contexts behind the labels*. Routledge. [Spanish translation in Editorial Tsara].

Guerin, B. (2020a). *Turning psychology into social contextual analysis*. Routledge.

Guerin, B. (2020b). *Turning mental health into social action*. Routledge.

Harrow, M., Jobe, T. H., & Faull, R. N. (2012). Do all schizophrenia patients need antipsychotic treatment continuously throughout their lifetime? A 20-year longitudinal study. *Psychological Medicine, 42*(10), 2145–2155. https://doi.org/10.1017/S0033291712000220

Hayes, S. C., Strosahl, K. D., & Wilson, K. G. (2012). *Acceptance and commitment therapy: The process and practice of mindful change* (2nd ed.). Guilford Press.

Hobson, J. A. (2003). *La farmacia de los sueños* [The pharmacy of dreams]. Ariel Neurociencia.

Johannesen, J., Stubhaug, B., & Skandsen, J. (2005). Mental health services in Norway. *International Psychiatry, 2*(9), 13–15. https://doi.org/10.1192/S1749367600007347

Johnstone, L., Boyle, M., Cromby, J., Dillon, J., Harper, D., Kinderman, P., Longden, E., Pilgrim, D., & Read, J. (2018). *The power threat meaning framework: Overview*. British Psychological Society. (Spanish translation in Asociación Española de Neuropsiquiaría). https://focusmadrid.com/files/2020/02/El-Marco-de-Poder-Amenaza-y-Significado.pdf

Killackey, E. (2009). Psychosocial and psychological interventions in early psychosis: Essential elements for recovery. *Early Interventions in Psychiatry, 3*, 17–21. https://doi.org/10.1111/j.1751-7893.2009.00126x

Kishimoto, T., Robenzadeh, A., Leucht, C., Leucht, S., Watanabe, K., Mimura, M., Borenstein, M., Kane, J. M., & Correll, C. U. (2014). Long-acting injectable vs oral antipsychotics for relapse prevention in schizophrenia: A meta-analysis of randomized trials. *Schizophrenia Bulletin, 40*(1), 192–213. https://doi.org/10.1093/schbul/sbs150

La Colifata. (2021). *Programa de radio de FM e Internet* [FM and Internet radio programme] (Radio broadcast). https://lacolifata.com.ar

Lakerman, R. (2014). The Finnish open dialogue approach to crisis intervention in psychosis: A review. *Psychotherapy in Australia, 20*(3), 28–35. https://doi.org/10.3316/informit.267467486046068

Lemos, S., Vallina, O., Fernández, P., Fonseca, E., & Paino, M. (2010). Bases clínicas para un nuevo modelo de atención a las psicosis [Clinical bases for a new model of care for psychosis]. *Clínica y Salud, 21*(3), 299–318. https://doi.org/10.5093/cl2010v21n3a7

Liberman, R. P., & Kopelowicz, A. (2005). *Psychiatric rehabilitation Kaplan and Sadock's comprehensive textbook of Psychiatry*. Lippincott Williams and Wilkins.

Louise, S., Fitzpatrick, M., Strauss, C., Rossell, S. L., & Thomas, N. (2018). Mindfulness-and acceptance-based interventions for psychosis: Our current understanding and a meta-analysis. *Schizophrenia Research, 192*, 57–63. https://doi.org/10.1016/j.schres.2017.05.023

Martín-Murcia, F., & Cangas, A. J. (2021). The axiological structure in psychosis. En K. Fukao (eds). P*sychosis, phenomenology, psychopathology, and pathophysiology* (pp. 1–10). IntechOpen. https://www.interchopen.com/chapters/77050

McCutcheon, R. A., Merritt, K., & y Howes, O.D. (2021). Dopamine and glutamate in individuals at high risk for psychosis: A meta-analysis of in vivo imaging findings and their variability compared to controls. *World Psychiatry, 20*(3), 405–416. https://doi.org/10.1002/wps.20893

McDonagh, M. S., Dana, T., Selph, D. T., Devine, E. B., Cantor, A., Bougatsos, C., Blanzina, I., Crusing, S., Fu, R., Kopelovich, S. L., Monroe-DeVita, M., & Haupt, D. W. (2018). Treatment for schizophrenia in adults: A systematic review. *Agency for Healthcare Research and Quality. Report Nº 17*(18)EHC031-EF. https://www.ncbi.nlm.nih.gov/books/NBK487628/

McFarlane, W. R. (2016). Family interventions for schizophrenia and the psychoses: A review. *Family Process, 55*(3), 460–482. https://doi.org/10.1111/famp.12235

Mesa-Velasco, R., García-Navarro, B., Nieto-Campos, A., & San Román-Mata, S. (2021). El tratamiento asertivo comunitario en pacientes de salud mental en España: Características y situación actual [Assertive community treatment in mental health patients in Spain: Characteristics and current situation]. *Journal of Sport and Health Research, 13*(3), 347–362. https://doi.org/10.58727/jshr.91213

NICE. (2014). *Psychosis and schizophrenia in adults: Treatment and management. National Clinical Guideline N° 178*. National Collaborating Center for Mental Health/National Institute for Health and Care Excellence.

Omachi, Y., & Sumiyoshi, T. (2018). Dose reduction/discontinuation of antipsychotic drugs in psychosis; Effect on cognition and functional outcomes. *Frontiers in Psychiatry, 9*, 447. https://doi.org/10.3389/fpsyt.218.00447

Ordoñez, N., Lemos, S., Paino, M., Fonseca, E., García, L., & Pizarro, J. P. (2012). Relación entre psicosis y experiencias traumáticas tempranas [Relationship between psychosis and early traumatic experiences]. *Anuario de Psicología, 44*(3), 283–294. https://revistes.ub.edu/index.php/Anuario-psicologia/article/download/11105/13854/0

Pankey, J., & Hayes, S. (2003). Acceptance and Commitment Therapy for psychosis. *International Journal of Psychology and Psychological Therapy, 3*(2), 331–328. https://www.redalyc.org/pdf/560/56030212.pdf

Parnas, J., & Handest, P. (2003). Phenomenology of anomalous self- experience in early schizophrenia. *Comprehensive Psychiatry, 44*(2), 121–134. https://doi.org/10.1053/comp.2003.50017

Pérez-Álvarez, M. (2003). *Las cuatro causas de los trastornos psicológicos* [The four causes of psychological disorders]. Editorial Universitas.

Pérez-Álvarez, M. (2008). Hiperreflexivility as a condition of mental disorder: A clinical and historical perspective. *Psicothema, 20*(2), 181–187. https://www.psicothema.com/pdf/3445.pdf

Pérez-Álvarez, M. (2019). Diagnóstico más allá de los síntomas: Un enfoque centrado en el mundo de la vida de las personas [Diagnosis beyond symptoms: An approach centred on the world of people's lives]. *Cuadernos de Psiquiatría Comunitaria, 16*(1), 22–38.

Pérez-Álvarez, M., & García-Montes, J. M. (2006). Entendimiento filosófico de la esquizofrenia [Philosophical understanding of schizophrenia]. *Apuntes de Psicología, 24*(1–3), 11–29. https://www.apuntesdepsicologia.es/index.php/revista/article/view/69/71

Petronis, A. (2004). Schizophrenia, neurodevelopment, and epigenetics. In M. S. Keshavan, J. L. Kennedy, & R. M. Murray (Eds.), *Neurodevelopment and schizophrenia* (pp. 174–190). Cambridge University Press.

Phillips, L. J., Francey, S. M., Leicester, S. B., Bechdolf, A., & Morrison, A. P. (2007). Development of psychotherapy in the pre-psychosis phase: Comparison of three approaches Australia, Germany, and UK. In J. F. M. Gleeson, E. Killackey, & H. Krstev (Eds.), *Psychotherapy for psychoses: Theoretical, cultural, and clinical integration* (pp. 117–134). Routledge. https://doi.org/10.4324/9780203937976

Pinkham, A. E. (2014). Social cognition in schizophrenia. *Journal of Clinical Psychiatry, 75*(2), 14–19. https://doi.org/10.4088/JCP.13065su1.04

Ramnerö, J., & Törneke, N. (2008). *The ABCs of human behavior: Behavioral principles for the practicing clinician*. Context Press.

RANZ-CP. (2016). *Clinical practice guidelines for the management of schizophrenia and related disorders*. Royal Australian and new Zeeland College of Psychiatrist. https://www.ranzep.org/home

Read, J., Perry, B. D., Moskowitz, A., & Connolly, J. (2001). The contribution of early traumatic events to schizophrenia in some patients: A traumagenic neurodevelopmental model. *Psychiatry: Interpersonal and Biological Processes, 64*, 319–345. https://doi.org/10.1521/psyc.64.4.319.18602

Ridenour, J. M., Hamm, J. A., & Czaja, M. (2019). A review of psychotherapeutic models and treatments for psychosis. *Psychosis, 11*(3), 248–260. https://doi.org/10.1080/17522439.2019.1615111

Ruddle, A., Mason, O., & Wykes, T. (2011). A review of hearing voices groups: Evidence and mechanisms of change. *Clinical Psychology Review, 31*(5), 757–766. https://doi.org/10.1016/j.cpr.2011.03.010

SEP. (2000). *Consenso español de expertos para recomendaciones de actuación en el tratamiento de la esquizofrenia* [Spanish expert consensus for recommendations for action in the treatment of schizophrenia]. Sociedad Española de Psiquiatría. http://www.p3-info.es/PDF/SEP.pdf

Shrivastava, A. (2020). *Schizophrenia treatment outcomes: An evidence-based approach to recovery*. Springer.

Sin, J., Guillard, S., Spain, D., Cornelius, V., Chen, T., & Henderson, C. (2017). Effectiveness of psychoeducational interventions for family cares of people with psychosis: A systematic review and meta-analysis. *Clinical Psychology Review, 56*, 13–24. https://doi.org/10.1016/j.cpr.2017.05.002

Turner, D. T., McGlanaghy, E., Cuijpers, P., van der Gaag, M., Karyotaki, E., & MacBeth, A. (2018). A meta-analysis of social skills training and related interventions for psychosis. *Schizophrenia Bulletin, 44*(3), 475–491. https://doi.org/10.1093/schbul/sbx146

Ulland, D., Andersen, A. J. W., Larsen, I. B., & Seikkyla, J. (2014). Generating dialogical practices in mental health: Experiences from Southern Norway, 1998–2008. *Administration and Policy in Mental Health and Mental Health Services Research, 41*, 410–419. https://doi.org/10.1007/s10488-013-0479-3

Valtanen, K. (2019). The psychiatrist's role in implementing open dialogue model of care. *Australian and New Zealand Journal of Family Therapy, 40*(3), 319–329. https://doi.org/10.1002/anzf.1382

van Os, J. (2010). The environment and schizophrenia. *Nature, 468*, 203–212. https://doi.org/10.1038/nature09563

van Os, J. (2016). "Schizophrenia" does not exist. *British Medical Journal, 352*, i375. https://doi.org/10.1136/bmj.i375

Vanderlip, E. R., Henwood, B. F., Hrouda, D. R., Meyer, P. S., Monroe-DeVita, M., Studer, L. M., Schweikhard, A. J., & Moser, L. (2017). Systematic literature review of general health care intervention within programs of assertive community treatment. *Psychiatric Services, 68*(3), 218–224. https://doi.org/10.1176/appl.ps.201600100

Ventura-Martins, M. J. R., Castilho, P., Barreto-Carvalho, C., Pereira, A. T., Santos, V., Gumley, A., & Ferreria, A. (2017). Contextual cognitive-behavioral therapies across the psychosis continuum. *European Psychologist, 22*(2), 83–100. https://doi.org/10.1027/1016-9040/a000283

WHO. (2019). *International coding of deseases*. World Health Organization. https://icd.who.int/es

Wilkinson, G., Piccinelli, M., Falloon, I. A., & Kreakorian, H. (1995). An evaluation of community-based psychiatric care for people with treated long-term mental illness. *British Journal of Psychiatry, 167*, 26–37. https://doi.org/10.1192/bjp.167.1.26

Wood, L., Williams, C., Billings, J., & Johnson, S. (2020). A systematic review and meta-analysis of cognitive behavioural informed psychological interventions for psychiatric inpatients with psychosis. *Schizophrenia Research, 220*, 133–144. https://doi.org/10.1016/j.schres.2020.03.041

World Health Organization. (2008). *WHO Europe: Policies and practices for mental health in Europe. Meet the challenges*. http:/www.euro.who.int/_data/assets/pdf_file/0006/96450E91732.pdf

Wunderink, L., Roeline, M., Nieboer, M., Wiersma, D., Sytema, S., & Nienhuis, F. J. (2013). Recovery in emitted first-episode psychosis at 7 years of follow-up of an early dose reduction/discontinuation or maintenance treatment strategy. Long-term follow-up of a 2-year randomized clinical trial. *JAMA Psychiatry, 70*(9), 913–920. https://doi.org/10.1001/jamapsychiatry.2013.19

Zubin, J., & Spring, B. (1977). Vulnerability: A new view of schizophrenia. *Journal of Abnormal Psychology, 86*(2), 103.126. https://doi.org/10.1037/0021-843X.86.2.103

Chapter 6
Contextualizing 'Psychosis' Behaviors and What to Do About Them

Bernard Guerin

6.1 Basic Analyses

6.1.1 Behaviors

The psychoses and schizophrenia have long been one of the most contentious of the groupings of 'mental health' issues (Bleuler, 1911; Jung, 1907/1960; Luhrmann & Marrow, 2016; Schilder, 1976; Sullivan, 1974). Furthermore, there are also several international groups, many even including psychiatrists and clinical psychologists, requesting that this category be dismantled since it makes little sense (Bentall, 2006; International Society for Psychological and Social Approaches to Psychosis, ISPS, 2017). Here I will ignore the DSM labels anyway since they are fictions, but the *behaviors* which have been observed and documented in the DSM are clearly not. The people who have had these behaviors shaped are usually suffering and in great pain and confusion.

The current DSM-5 clustering of 'psychosis' contains five main groups of very disparate behaviors:

- *Grossly disorganized or abnormal motor behavior (including catatonia).*
- *Negative symptoms (especially diminished emotional expression and avolition—a decrease in motivated self-initiated purposeful activities).*
- *Delusions.*
- *Disordered thinking (speech)—frequent derailment or incoherence.*
- *Hallucinations.*

It is also often associated with *traumatic* and *dissociative* behaviors, and sometimes concurrent with major mood changes of depression, mania, or both (but

B. Guerin (✉)
University of South Australia, Magill, Australia
e-mail: Bernard.Guerin@unisa.edu.au

J. A. Díaz-Garrido et al. (eds.), *Psychological Interventions for Psychosis*,
https://doi.org/10.1007/978-3-031-27003-1_6

labelled '*schizoaffective*' by the DSM). Thus, even without any form of diagnosis, we can still observe the sorts of behaviors that were previously labeled by this arbitrary category and observe them and the contexts which shape them. We should no longer be guided by the DSM category system, but if they must be categorized, this can be done more functionally (Guerin, 2017, 2020a). There is more in (3) below.

6.1.2 Contexts for 'Mental Health' Behaviors

Many people have now proposed that 'mental health' behaviors are shaped when people are trying to deal with extremely bad life situations, such as living with traumatic events, abuse, poverty, threats of all sorts, violence, etc. (Boyle & Johnstone, 2020; Frankl, 2006; Guerin, 2020a; Johnstone et al., 2018) and not because of any brain disease, chemical imbalance, or 'cognitive dysfunction' (Johnstone, 2014). People are adapting to their bad worlds to get along and survive, but this is not working out well. As we will see below, they are in life situations in which *none of their normal behaviors have any real effect to change anything*. Behaviors that would normally bring about some change in the world, mostly in the 'social world', no longer work. Of particular importance for the group of behaviors listed as 'psychosis', *language use* no longer has the effects it normally has. Language is 'broken,' meaning that it no longer gets the outcomes that it normally has through the person's discursive communities and social relationships. Or to put this better, the person still has all their language skills, but they have no discursive communities that support their talking without punishment or neglect.

However, we must be clear that such bad life situations shape *many* different behavioral patterns to cope with, deal with, put up with, or escape from these bad contexts. Figure 6.1 illustrates this broader idea of the bad life situations of many people and some of the diverse behaviors shaped from these. The broadest question for analysis is this: *For someone (though no fault of their own) who is trying to live in these bad life conditions, what behaviors are shaped and which more specific life environments shape the more specific different behaviors?*

However, when looking at those outcomes of bad life situations which are called 'mental health' issues rather than criminal, escapist, exiting, or 'putting up with' responses, there are indeed some specific conditions which seem to predict that the 'mental health' behaviors will be shaped when trying to deal with such bad life situations. In particular, the following extra conditions are suggested for any contextual analyses of 'mental health' behaviors, as opposed to just criminal activities, bullying or exiting:

- Having weak, bad, or contradictory social relationships and few opportunities for resources.
- Therefore, being *trapped* in a bad situation so the other options are not available (such as simple exiting, talking your way out, or bullying your way out).

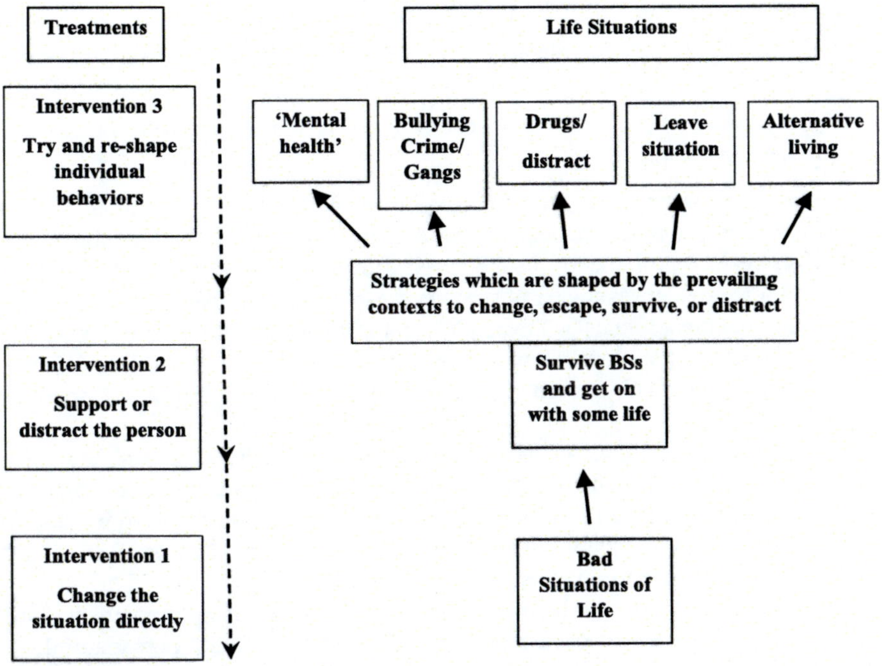

Fig. 6.1 Various behaviors shaped by living in bad life situations

- Any alternative behaviors which *might* be done are blocked, usually by other people.
- The source or origin of your bad situations cannot easily be *seen* or *observed* (so we can further specify which life contexts these are most likely to be; Guerin, 2020a).
- As a result, some ordinary behaviors which still *seem* to have *some* effect on *some* people *some* of the time in your life are shaped to become exaggerated or altered; but these are just those behaviors remaining possible with such restrictive worlds.

So, the profile of contexts shaping the 'mental health' behaviors is one of very restrictive life contexts with few behavioral options possible and so few effective consequences possible. This is not only just in situations of poverty or abuse, since restrictive life environments with few alternative behaviors can occur in any place in society. In fact, the more wealth a family has, the more they might act to 'protect' those family members by restricting their life options, although the wealth can be used to purchase alternative options for the person being restricted so that the 'mental health' behaviors do not become shaped.

This means that what have been called the 'mental health' behaviors are really *behaviors that have been shaped by living in restrictive bad life situations*. It turns out (Guerin, 2021) that those behaviors listed under the DSM categories of 'schizophrenia' and 'psychosis' have been shaped in some of the worst and most restrictive life situations (Bloomfield et al., 2021). But added to this, is that most of these listed behaviors have also been shaped by extremely punishing or neglectful *discursive* environments.

Analyzing the contexts of 'psychotic' behaviors as primarily shaped by broken discursive communities.

Before moving on to the more specific behaviors labelled as 'psychotic', I will make a few quick points about contextualizing talking and thinking, since such behaviors feature prominently in the 'psychotic' behaviors: 'If we ask ourselves what is it that gives the character of strangeness to the substitutive formation and the symptom in schizophrenia, we eventually come to realize that it is the predominance of what has to do with words over what has to do with things' (Freud, 1915/1984, p. 206). This is even now clear for the 'negative symptoms' (Moernaut et al., 2021).

For a social contextual analysis, language use is just a behavior like any other, although it has some special properties. But the key thing for language use analysis is that *language is only shaped and maintained by people*, not by anything else in the world. Cats do not shape saying "cat", only people can do that (even if they sometimes occasion the social behaviors).

So, *using words is always about doing things to people*. Using language is just a fancy way of doing all of our social behaviors which we could potentially do in other ways, without words. Basically, when we talk about language use, we are talking about managing our social relationships and the outcomes of those relationships. *Using language and managing social relationships become synonymous.*

The point to take from this is that *if there are 'dysfunctions' of speech, talking or thinking, then these are really 'dysfunctions' of social relationships and getting resources (effects) through social relationships*. Typically, this means that "your words are broken": that is, your words are no longer doing what they should do or have done in the past—*there are only punishing consequences or no consequences anymore*. Your language is no longer working to do anything, and this is because of social relationship problems. Under these conditions, we *see ordinary language uses become exaggerated and distorted*, such as occur with the label of 'psychosis' but also elsewhere in the DSM.

In this analysis, it is analytically and functionally important that the social relationship problems are *occurring over many situations and social relationships*. So, it is not that there is a 'withdrawal' from one or two people (who might be directly punishing), but a more widespread withdrawal from most social relationships. This could occur in environments in which (1) the larger societal systems are not working for the person (e. g., poverty or patriarchy), (2) many or most of their known social relationships are bad (e. g., abusive and violent families), or (3) they have a very restricted range of social contacts anyway and these are all bad (e. g., highly oppressive or restrictive families). Clearly, the first clinical step for repairing broken language use must be to build some sort of social relationship with such people in which the therapist can be trusted. Trying to focus solely on a quick and language-led recovery (talking therapies) is unlikely to work.

Contextualizing 'thinking' is a bit trickier because it is even harder to see the social origins of shaping than for spoken or written language uses. I have suggested that a good way to envisage and contextualize thinking is that it is made of the same language events which occur for talking—all the ways we have been shaped to speak in specific contexts—but our 'thoughts' are those which do not get said out loud (Guerin, 2020b, Chapter 4; cf. Skinner 1957). We 'have' the language responses in any specific context regardless of whether we say them out loud or not (they have already been shaped in context), and *those which are not said out loud comprise what we call our 'thinking'*.

To analyze thinking, therefore, needs additional special forms of observation, analysis, and 'therapy'. We need to (1) first find out the social contexts in which those discourses have been said out loud in the past, might be said, and with which audiences or social relationships these would be said. Second, (2) we must analyze the contexts under which those discourses are now *not* said out loud and which constitute thinking. Sometimes this is innocuous, as when we are interrupted, or no one is present. But in other cases, more clinically relevant, language use is not said out loud because there are audiences or social relationships in which some of the talking out loud has been *punished* or *ignored*. These cases of being shaped to think language responses instead of saying them out loud include those called 'repressed thoughts' by Freud and others.

6.1.3 Analysis of 'Psychosis' Behaviors Shaped in Context

What we need to do for analysis, therefore, is to find out how the behaviors of 'psychosis' have been shaped by bad life contexts and bad discursive contexts especially. When people are trapped in restrictive and bad life situations, there are numerous everyday behaviors that can get shaped to exaggeration—the whole realm of 'mental health' behaviors in fact. Many are done because they are opportunistic, others because there are few alternative behaviors which make any difference at all. People over time usually show many of these different 'mental health' behaviors, as well as behaviors to escape, bully or fight their way out, get distracted, or ignore the bad life situation and 'put up with it' (Guerin, 2020c). People do not get one 'disease' and that is all, as fictionized by the DSM. They are shaped to different and various behaviors over time.

Since the use of language is our primary way of dealing with people and social relationships, we therefore see distortions and exaggeration in the uses of language under restrictive and bad life situations. For example, we observe silence, exaggeration of stories and comments, fantasy stories, etc. With language use messed up, we also therefore can observe reductions in thinking things through, concentration, memory, planning, etc. We can observe exaggerated and 'strange' ways of talking about 'self'. We can also observe people trying to find new audiences for their language use, and in many cases this is seen through such people frequently approaching strangers and trying to talk and tell stories (often catchy exaggerated stories).

Talking to strangers might be the only reasonable conversation such a person has all day, even if the stranger soon finds an excuse to leave. But strangers are usually polite for a short time, and there is no responsibility since they will not be encountered again most likely.

It can be seen, then, that having defective discursive communities can lead to a wide range of multiple problems which do not initially seem to bear on the 'psychotic' behaviors, including concentration, thinking abilities, coherence of storytelling, coherence of a 'self', and selection of audiences. This occurs after years of any use of language being punished, ignored, or constantly opposed.

I will now try to spell this out briefly with each of the five major groups of 'symptoms'.

6.1.3.1 Grossly Disorganized or Abnormal Motor Behavior

This group of behaviors which is lumped together by the DSM encompasses ordinary behaviors which have been shaped out of the ordinary or exaggerated because they at least have some consequences (albeit dysfunctional usually). Taken directly from the DSM, I mix in here the following DSM listed 'behaviors': appear dramatic, emotional, or erratic; appear odd or eccentric, eccentricities of behavior; disorganized or abnormal motor behavior; motor control disrupted from normal; being reckless, impulsivity; increased energy; increased spending; overactivity; repetitive behaviors applied rigidly (Guerin, 2017).

These seem clearly, as a group, to be ordinary behaviors shaped into exaggeration. The general analysis would be that the bad life situations have restricted all possible 'normal' behaviors to change it or to exit in some way. These 'unusual actions' will certainly have effects, especially in the social contexts, but will not necessarily lead to the bad situation changing. In the case of living in bad societal contexts (poverty, male dominance), they are also not likely to change much. Some of these actions will provide distraction from the person's bad life contexts, but probably not change much. Some might inadvertently lead to making new social contacts which could eventually help. Strong and weak forms of 'catatonia' are also a form of exiting, but also not ones which are likely to help change the bad situations.

6.1.3.2 Negative Symptoms

Negative symptoms are a curious mixture of behaviors which have been disputed over the history of psychiatry (Bleuler, 1912; Jung, 1907/1960). The main 'behavior' is the absence of a 'normal' behavior. The behaviors include: blunting of affect; poverty of speech and thought; apathy; anhedonia; reduced social drive; loss of motivation; lack of social interest; and inattention to social or cognitive input. The DSM writes:

> *Negative symptoms* account for a substantial portion of the morbidity associated with schizophrenia but are less prominent in other psychotic disorders. Two negative symptoms

> are particularly prominent in schizophrenia: diminished emotional expression and avolition. *Diminished emotional expression* includes reductions in the expression of emotions in the face, eye contact, intonation of speech (prosody), and movements of the hand, head, and face that normally give an emotional emphasis to speech. *Avolition* is a decrease in motivated self-initiated purposeful activities. The individual may sit for long periods of time and show little interest in participating in work or social activities. Other negative symptoms include alogia, anhedonia, and asociality. *Alogia* is manifested by diminished speech output. *Anhedonia* is the decreased ability to experience pleasure from positive stimuli or a degradation in the recollection of pleasure previously experienced. *Asociality* refers to the apparent lack of interest in social interactions and may be associated with avolition, but it can also be a manifestation of limited opportunities for social interactions. (APA, 2013, p. 88)

From a social contextual point of view, keeping in mind the strong functional links given earlier between social relationships and the observed behaviors of thinking, they are all *withdrawal* or *exiting* strategies from 'normal' social relationships. In this sense, they will be functionally related to depression and catatonia, since they both are similar strategies shaped differently (but using the DSM does not encourage making these links).

Some recent research talking to people who had been labelled as having 'negative symptoms' also found that, when put in context, these behaviors were primarily issues of *language use* rather than problems of the brain (Moernaut et al., 2021). The main behaviors of 'negative symptoms' were due to the people *not being able to put into words* their unusual experiences: '…a failure of narratives to account for perplexing experiences participants are confronted with in psychosis' (p. 1). If still questioned (by a therapist) about their experiences, they tended to employ 'meta-narratives', that is, talking about the fact that they could not talk about their experiences and spurious explanations as to why. These authors concluded: "The standard characterization of negative symptoms as a loss of normal functioning should be revised, as this does not match participants' subjective experiences. Negative symptoms rather represent hard to verbalize experiences. This difficulty of linguistic expression is not a shortcoming of the person experiencing them, but characteristic of the experiences themselves." Once again, then, what looks like failure of functioning (reduced speech, lack of concentration and planning, etc.) is really about the person's language no longer working in a normal way because of the bad social relationships they have been subjected to, usually over long periods.

The 'negative symptoms' are also common as everyday behaviors, and mostly non-problematic, but in bad environments we see the exaggeration of these otherwise normal 'withdrawal' behaviors. If you are in a meeting and get severely criticized, it is likely your language use will also shut down (while you plan revenge; cf. 'dissociachotic', Ball, 2020). But 'negative symptoms' are 'generalized' behaviors which will function in different ways across *many* different life contexts as ways of (originally, at least) attempting to cope with bad or threatening situations—they are not a response to a specific bad situation such as being punished in one meeting. It is important to note for these behaviors, therefore, that the actual functioning cannot be gleaned by the form or topography of the behaviors, they always need contextualizing. And they could change at any time to another form.

Other behaviors likely to be found with the same people are: crying spells; desperation; feeling overwhelmed; unable to adjust a particular stressor; being awake throughout the night; decreased sleep; sleeping troubles; disturbance of eating, or eating-related behavior; somatic changes that affect the individual's capacity to function; spending less time with friends and family; staying home from work or school; attention seeking; increased sex drive; increased alcohol and drug use (Guerin, 2017).

There are almost certainly exceptions but in general, time should not be spent on interpreting the 'meaning' or 'sign' of the particular behaviors in this group, but focus more on:

- what the person's overwhelming, general, or bad situation is about and what other responses might help change their environment ("What has happened to you?")
- what social relationships do they still have which are present and what the person's discourses say about these social relationships,
- the possible *generalized audiences* for these behaviors ('generalized other', 'social norms', media, 'someone', 'everyone', 'men', strangers),
- who is requiring some sort of response be made at all; where is that pressure coming from (it could be from therapists, in fact, demanding that the person put everything into words, "express your feelings", when they cannot do this; Moernaut et al., 2021).

6.1.3.3 Disorganized Thinking

For the 'schizophrenic' behaviors listed by the DSM as 'disorganized thinking', I include: slowing down of thoughts and actions; concentration difficulties; consciousness disrupted from normal; memory disrupted from normal; perception disrupted from normal; racing thoughts; rapid speech; disorganized thinking; cognitive or perceptual distortions; preoccupation;

intolerance of uncertainty; repetitive mental acts applied rigidly.

As outlined earlier, for social contextual analysis, *any issues with talking or thinking are issues with social relationships*. When social relationships are messed up, then our language also get messed up because language only does anything to people. People in bad situations can have their language stop working or functioning because they can no longer get any effects or consequences from talking, or else only punishing effects. Any features of language can then be shaped to become exaggerated or transformed, if this gets at least some effect or change. There are many variations in the DSM, but there are also probably many others with nuanced differences that are worth exploring.

So, the important analysis here is to remember that language use is only shaped through the effects on people, so that when social relationships get bad and other alternatives are not possible, then language ceases to function, at least in the normal ways. With language being perhaps the most frequent behavior through which we all have effects in our worlds, all the functionings of language become undone. This includes most of what are currently called 'cognitive' functions such as memory, concentration, 'processing', self, beliefs, etc. (Guerin, 2020b). If we think of memory as storytelling in language, then memory will be disrupted in bad life situations in which language is not having any effect on the people around (Janet, 1925/1919). Talking and thinking will be slowed down, and hence 'concentration' slowed.

Some forms of 'disorganized thinking' in the DSM, but which are functionally related in the above way, in addition to the one labelled 'disorganized thinking', are 'slowing down of thoughts and actions', 'concentration difficulties', 'consciousness disrupted from normal', and 'memory disrupted from normal'. It is suggested that all are *shaped from trying to deal with punishing, restricted or negligent social relationships*, which means that the language no longer works as it normally would in getting people to do things (help, laugh, bond, entertain, etc.). With heavily punishing audiences for any talk, as seems to be implicated for those who have received labels of 'schizophrenia' and 'psychoses', we would perhaps expect more of 'slowing down of thoughts and actions' and 'concentration difficulties'. We would also expect that in such socially punishing contexts a lot of talking would be replaced with thinking (Guerin, 2020b, Chapter 3).

To put this all together, when social relationships are massively broken and no longer get any effects, then language will also be broken since that is the main way we get effects in life. This can be replaced by violent or bullying behaviors to have effects, but it also means that language functioning is messed up. Of importance is that if language is heavily or generally punished or no longer gets the common effects, then this will also 'break' parts of behavior which are considered important in social life:

- Self-talk and what this can get us in our social worlds.
- Memory.
- Planning and future talk.
- Increased frequency of engaging strangers in conversation since they are polite for a period in most cases and will not be seen again, so there are no further obligations or responsibly.
- A strong form of cynicism and noticing of hypocrisy in people's behavior and talk.
- Lack of concentration and what looks like 'slowing down' of language use.

6.1.3.4 Delusions

It is proposed that similar social relationship issues have shaped the behaviors under theDSM label of 'delusions' (Guerin, 2023). This group can also include: dysfunctional beliefs; intrusive and unwanted thoughts; grandiose ideas, grandiosity; hallucinations; recurrent and persistent thoughts. As for before, there will almost inevitably be cross-overs found between all these behaviors as people are shaped into different behaviors by similar and recurring bad life situations.

For social contextual analysis, people's beliefs are just language use and not something stored or possessed 'inside' them (Guerin, 2020c). Our beliefs are shaped by our social relationships and we *use* our beliefs to do all our regular social behaviors (Guerin, 2020c, Table 4.1). Beliefs are like tools we can use to strategize our social worlds. These strategies are not just to agree with what your significant others believe. For example, you can state your 'beliefs' to build a self-identity by using *differences* to those around you; you can also use beliefs to compete with others around you (Guerin, 2020c, Chapter 4).

For the cases of 'delusional beliefs', the person has been shaped into at least one very common way of engaging in social relationships—through the common and ubiquitous use of storytelling (Frank, 2010; Guerin, 2023). However, since this has not worked or been functional in changing anything in the person's world, it once again becomes exaggerated into certain types of *stories with social properties which get attention and which make it difficult to refute*. Such stories include rumors, gossip, conspiracy stories, and urban legends (Guerin & Miyazaki, 2006).

The social properties include telling *abstract* stories, so they are difficult for people to challenge despite any objections by listeners (even therapists report this). They also provide somewhat interesting, engaging, and even entertaining discourses for the person in all parts of life, although this becomes more difficult as they get more exaggerated and extreme. However, with delusional stories to tell, the person can at least engage in *some* social interactions which potentially could help change their bad life situations. However, these probably work best for new audiences and those who are strangers, rather than the same delusions being told over to the same known people. It must also be remembered that any aversiveness from poor stories being told repeatedly can also function as yet another type of exiting or withdrawal strategy—a way of getting away from people or having them back off.

6.1.3.5 Hallucinations (Auditory)

Both visual hallucinations and auditory hallucinations (voice hearing) are related to delusions, dysfunctional beliefs, intrusive and unwanted thoughts, grandiose ideas, grandiosity, and recurrent and persistent thoughts. They all pertain to language and imagery responses, including thinking, becoming exaggerated under very bad life situations. I would also include panic attacks in this functional group even though they are remote from the others within the DSM.

For the case of auditory hallucinations, which includes voice hearing, it is easier to see the analysis. I have proposed earlier already that thinking is the same as talking but is under further external contexts (usually punishing) such that they are not said out loud. It is also clear that hearing music, voices, and other sounds are 'normal' behaviors, but wrongly talked about as originating from inside the head. We 'normally' have a dominant, command or 'me' voice, but this is shaped by all the discourses, conversations, dialogues, media, television, etc. around us constantly in everyday life for all our life. Our talking and arguing with those commonly around us also figures prominently in all this.

So, it is no wonder that under extreme bad life situations when a person's language is not working to have any effect and get things done, these other behaviors will also be exaggerated. And what is then heard as an 'auditory hallucination' (hearing voices or noises) will originate from the many discourses around us as responses which are not said out loud. If we normally have a conflict with someone, and cannot say out loud all the things we are shaped to, then we will ruminate over this for a time afterwards until it is resolved (Kheng & Guerin, 2020)

An anthropological study by Luhrmann et al. (2015) and Luhmann (1912) shows this clearly. They talked to people who hear voices in India, Ghana, and the United States and interviewed for some of the social relationship contexts for the voices.

> Broadly speaking the voice-hearing experience was similar in all three settings. Many of those interviewed reported good and bad voices; many reported conversations with their voices, and many reported whispering, hissing or voices they could not quite hear. In all settings there were people who reported that God had spoken to them and in all settings there were people who hated their voices and experienced them as an assault. Nevertheless, there were striking differences in the quality of the voice-hearing experience, and particularly in the quality of relationship with the speaker of the voice. Many participants in the Chennai and Accra samples insisted that their predominant or even only experience of the voices was positive – a report supported by chart review and clinical observation. Not one American did so. Many in the Chennai and Accra samples seemed to experience their voices as people: the voice was that of a human the participant knew, such as a brother or a neighbor, or a human-like spirit whom the participant also knew. These respondents seemed to have real human relationships with the voices – sometimes even when they did not like them. This was less typical of the San Mateo sample, whose reported experiences were markedly more violent, harsher and more hated… In general the American sample experienced voices as bombardment and as symptoms of a brain disease caused by genes or trauma... Five people even described their voice-hearing experience as a battle or war, as in 'the warfare of everyone just yelling'. (p. 42)

> More than half of the Chennai sample (n = 11) heard voices of kin, such as parents, mother-in-law, sister-in-law or sisters. Another two experienced a voice as husband or wife, and yet another reported that the voice said he should listen to his father. These voices behaved as relatives do: they gave guidance, but they also scolded. They often gave commands to do domestic tasks. Although people did not always like them, they spoke about them as relationships. One man explained, 'They talk as if elder people advising younger people'. A woman heard seven or eight of her female relatives scold her constantly. They told her that she should die; but they also told her to bathe, to shop, and to go into the kitchen and prepare food. Another woman explained that her voice took on the form of different family members – it 'talks like all the familiar persons in my house'. Although the voice frightened her and sometimes, she claimed, even beat her, she insisted that the voice was good: 'It teaches me what I don't know'. (p. 43)

6.1.3.6 Hallucinations (Visual)

Visual hallucinations are likely to co-occur with delusions, dysfunctional beliefs; intrusive and unwanted thoughts; auditory hallucinations; grandiose ideas, grandiosity; recurrent and persistent thoughts.

People in everyday life report imagery, some more than others, and it is usually very persuasive, direct, and impactful. More so than hearing or talking. The same analyses therefore apply that when trapped in very bad life situations, strong visual hallucination imagery can appear, shaped by the change it usually incurs.

In this way the shaping and effects of visual hallucinations are like those of hearing voices and panic attacks. They are all normal behaviors shaped by bad life situations. They do not contain a message, as is sometimes claimed, but do signal that the life situation is out of control. In earlier times (premodern, imagery was probably more frequently used, since language has become the dominant behaviors in modernity. Seeing visions was also more common, therefore, and likewise signaled that something was wrong with the *community's* life situation that needed changing. So indirectly they probably contained another sort of message as they do now.

6.2 How to Support People Who Have Been Shaped into the 'Psychosis' Behaviors?

Having looked at the behaviors shaped when trying to live in bad life situations, and the specific behaviors shaped by the extra 'mental health' conditions, we can finally look at what might be done to change such shaped behaviors. I want to separate out two parts of this: how to respond to someone with these behaviors, and how to attempt to change or lessen such behaviors.

6.2.1 How to Respond Within a Social Relationship or 'Therapeutic Alliance'

What is typically done with these 'disorders' is to support the person by distraction, forced removal, or capacity-reducing drugs, and hope that over time their bad situations will change (which they can do, of course). Often, they have bureaucratic forms to deal with as well. None of these are helpful for people in such situations.

From the analysis here, the support person must remember that the person is used to non-effectual social behavior and language use, so the best strategy is finding ways to show that what the person is saying does indeed have some effects on the listener (typically the therapist to start). This is not done through asking a lot of questions ("When did these delusions first occur?"), nor just reflecting back what they tell you ("You seem to be feeling very confused"). Better is to be clear that their words are beginning to get some of the usual effects of people using language. Even for those of us outside of these life bad situations, being interrogated or being asked a lot of questions about our own conduct, history, and the like is an unusual discourse in everyday life and is at least mildly punishing.

So, one better strategy is to just listen and then be clear about what effect the person's words are having on you (Guerin et al., 2021). In doing this, one must be 'authentic' or honest, since the people will easily know if it is being made up—they have had a lifetime of observing fake responding. Getting them to talk about their experiences or history, or anything they wish, is the best way to proceed. [But one must also beware of the neoliberal shaping of modern therapy to be quick and efficient when doing this.] Once the person has talked and you have listened and shown you have been affected, then other things can be done, but often that by itself is enough.

6.2.2 *How to Change the Behaviors*

The ideal task of therapy from the social contextual approach is to analyze the person's bad life situations and *try to change those life situations or find a different strategy for the person which actually works to have some life effects*. Just changing the actual behaviors alone as they appear, as typically done in CBT, will not be enough if the person will remain in their same bad environments. Moving the person to a completely new life world might even be necessary (e.g., Haley, 1973). Also, of importance is finding activities and especially new social connections *in which they can have an effect on people or make a difference*, since this has not been possible for some time in their lives.

To put this succinctly, the message is to: *fix the person's bad life situations, don't try and fix the person*. And to do this by responding that is sensitive to their long histories of poor outcomes from any use of language.

If we look back to Fig. 6.1, it suggests that there are at least three 'layers' of treatment for life issues arising from trying to live in bad situations.

Level 3 For Level 3, there are attempts made to directly change the *behaviors* shaped by the bad life situations in partnership with the person (always), without changing the life situation itself. If the person is doing 'delinquent' behaviors, then try and stop or change those behaviors. If the person is having anxious thoughts, then try and stop, block, or replace those thoughts. Typical procedures here are done through clinical psychology (CBT), behavior modification, coaching into alterative behaviors, educational programs, and many more methods going back a long time (Janet, 1925/1919).

Level 2 The interventions or treatments called Level 2 are attempts to just help people cope with their bad life situations; that is, put up with it or cushion the bad effects. Counselling, therapy, and clinical psychology all do this, as does social work for people with 'mental health' behaviors and other behaviors listed in Fig. 6.1 (violence, drugs, bullying, crime). Psychiatric medications are the same in that they placate people and make it easier for them to put up with their 'symptoms', but psychiatric drugs do not 'cure' anything and have more troublesome side effects including difficulties with eventual withdrawal. Recreational drugs can have the same Level 2 outcomes as well.

Level 1 These are attempts to directly change the person's bad life world. That is, go into the person's world and work with them to change their bad life situations. This rarely happens in psychiatry and clinical psychology (with a few exceptions), and such clinicians are usually *not* allowed to do this professionally. Some social workers do most of this, as do other 'care workers' and community helpers.

For many of those with 'mental health' behaviors, that is, who have had behaviors shaped through bad life situations, the above is sufficient. However, when dealing with those who have been shaped into behaviors in the 'psychosis' label, often it is nearly impossible to go in and change the 'home' life situation. There is often crime, abuse, drug use, etc., for which many others are involved, making this difficult or impossible to change. In such cases, it becomes necessary to work with the person *to create new life contexts* and reduce the impact of the person's original life situation. This is easier for discursive communities than the more physical problems of normal life (abuse, poverty, etc.). I will deal with creating new discursive communities in more detail below.

In reality all three levels are needed. Regardless of whether Levels 1 or 3 are implemented, people need to be socially and materially supported and cared for throughout (Level 2). Many bad life situations are extremely difficult to change, so supporting the person to put up with their predicaments until the bad situations resolve themselves 'naturally' is probably what a large number of purported 'cures' are really doing. If you have some form of therapy or treatment over 1–2 years, frequently the bad life situation will change during that period anyway.

A curious feature of contextual approaches is that when a context changes, the behaviors which have been shaped do not become 'cured' or 'stopped,' but they simply disappear and do not occur. When you are seated in front of a piano, then your playing behaviors occur. When the piano is absent then the behaviors simply disappear (unless there is another context for piano playing present). Your piano playing does not get 'wiped out', 'erased', or 'cured'.

Table 6.1 shows some of the therapy discourses used with the medial model of the outcomes being sought. Table 6.1 also shows some of the terms that are used for contextual approaches when changes occur. It is important to note that you often do not wish for the behavior to completely be erased in any case, since there will likely be contexts in life when those behaviors are functional. We do not want people in therapy to have crying erased, just attuned to new contexts.

6.2.3 *Dealing with Language Use Issues*

The general treatment of 'psychosis' behaviors we have seen follows along the same lines. But those who have such behaviors shaped are usually in *extreme* bad life situations, so Level 2 is necessary throughout. Level 1 and 3 treatments often are difficult to do even in partnership with the person. But we have seen that a lot of the

Table 6.1 Therapy is said to be successful when the behaviours

Medical models of 'mental health'	Contextual models of 'mental health'
Stop	Disappear
Are 'cured'	Become irrelevant
Are blocked	Become unnecessary
Are corrected	Go into the background
Are erased	Fade away
	Do not show up anymore
	Can still be used in appropriate contexts

symptoms are language-based, which really means they are social relationship-based. We have also seen that the specific behaviors are not so important and should not be overinterpreted. So the main thrust is to work on Level 1 and change the bad *discursive* life worlds such people are living in.

The main part of interventions, therefore, from a social contextual approach is to find some activities, probably not related to their 'symptoms', *which allow the person to act in the world and have some effects through using their language*. These do not have to be positive or pleasurable effects, as we have seen from their symptoms. Having effects on other *people* is probably the best, but initially this can be difficult to manage. Music and art therapy can function in this way (Guerin, 2019a, b; Killick, 2017). Similar events occur in newer treatments for voice hearers (Romme & Escher, 2000). So instead of focusing on the 'delusions' or trying to refute them (CBT), find ways with the person for them to engage with new listeners in *other* types of storytelling that have 'normal' effects. Many of the newer 'social' treatments for 'psychosis' are probably doing this inadvertently (Haddock & Slade, 1996; Meaden & Fox, 2015; Mullen, 2021; Putman & Martindale, 2022; Ruiz, 2021a, b).

So, because the behaviors labelled as 'psychosis' are commonly language-based, finding ways to allow the people with 'psychosis' behaviors *to have effects on people using their language* would be the best step. Devise activities in which the person can talk, so that this talking actually has consequences on another person, agreeing, obeying, bonding, etc. Talking about things unrelated to their shaped language behaviors is probably the best. That is, do not discuss their delusions, etc. but other things in life, and other forms of storytelling (Frank, 2010).

Basically, their social relationships and the consequences which can be gained from social relationships need to be repaired (*fix the person's bad* ***discursive*** *situations, don't try and fix the person*). Some therapists probably do this incidentally from talking to people, but it could be done in much better ways with real trust. *The therapist needs to let the person with 'psychosis' behaviors have real effects with consequences(effects) through other people*, this is what has been missing in their lives. But ironically, *clinical training frequently requires the clinician to not show any signs that the person has affected them in any way*.

Finding ways to support a person into developing such language-use-with-effects can occur *within therapy* in many ways. It is usually done inadvertently by most therapists, but a lot more could be done by not just asking questions and listening to answers but by arranging so that the person can achieve outcomes with their language use. Asking questions and getting answers in therapy is usually *only* for the benefit (effect) of the therapist. This might be as simple as the person asking the therapist a question and getting an answer, which is often not allowed in therapy. Many therapies almost certainly do some of these without it being explicit (Haddock & Slade, 1996; Meaden & Fox, 2015; Mullen, 2021; Putman & Martindale, 2022; Ruiz, 2021a, b).

If one looks through the sociolinguistic research, one can find a myriad of potential methods for this. As one example, 'adjacency pairs' is a sociolinguistic term for common pairs of statements in everyday conversation where the first has a reliable or common outcome or effect: questions have the effect of getting an answer; thanking gets "you're welcome"; a greeting gets a return greeting effect; a request gets a fulfilment; etc. The point of these is not to learn what people commonly do but to begin using language, possibly with new audiences than those who have shaped the 'psychosis' behaviors, and get some effects occurring. This is what has been missing. Therapists need to become much more sensitive or attuned to what effects language has, and how that applies *within therapy* to those they are supporting (Guerin et al., 2021).

We can go beyond the 'therapeutic alliance' as a potential breeding ground for getting effects or outcomes for language use and begin to involve other people outside of the therapy situation. Those shaped into 'psychosis' behaviors typically do not need communication training or language instruction—they have presumably learned all that before. What they lack are supportive discursive communities. This can be done by helping the person to find new groups and social relationships where their talking is more effective. The outcomes of talk do not have to be all kindness, positive and understanding; rather, *the talk needs to let the person have effects on other people, to get things done with their language in the way we all do*. Self-help groups are important, but there is a myriad of other groups who could provide this basic resource, community, and special-interest groups. If your talk always receives only positive and affirming replies, such as in some self-groups, this can wear thin, as it does in everyday conversations. There is much sociolinguistic research on other forms of language use which can have effects, such as politeness, and directives (Guerin, 1997).

But the other main sensitivity is about what is said out loud and what is 'thought'. From a long time of being punished, thinking (talking but not out loud) is prevalent, and so another goal is to increase out loud talking. Again, this does not just mean to get the person saying anything out loud or trying to talk about 'feelings' or difficult topics, but just to have their discourses receive outcomes or effects when out loud, rather than merely being thought when they get no outcomes. So, what is talked about in this way is almost irrelevant, and if nonsensitive topics were done more, this would likely increase more rapidly. Forcing someone to talk about what is difficult or impossible to say out loud (Guerin, 2020a, Chapter 7; Moernaut et al., 2021) is counterproductive to having them learn to talk and get reasonable or useful outcomes. Again, ironically, therapists are taught to only talk about and address serious personal issues, and things that are difficult to even say, when conducting therapy.

Eventually, then, the person with new audiences and getting effects other than punishment and neglect when they talk will begin reestablishing their talking about plans, memories, 'self', and improve their concentration and remembering.

6.2.4 Building a Discursive Life History

Finally, if the person is willing to talk about their history and context, we can now add another type of finding out their contextual history. This is to ask directly about the *discourses and outcomes of those discourses* in their lives. Table 6.2 gives some ideas of what can be asked. Remember that this is really about the person's social relationships, and what they have been able to do with those audiences in the past.

Table 6.2 Contextualizing delusions as beliefs and stories and the sorts of questions which can elicit something of a person's current and historical discursive practices

Person's current and historical discursive practices
Who do you talk with normally in life? (current and historical)
What do you talk about? (current and historical)
Do have a lot of people to talk to or only few? (current and historical)
Do the people around you pay attention when you talk? (current and historical)
Do they do things you might ask them to do? (current and historical)
Do they enjoy your what you say? (current and historical)
Who listens to your stories?
How do they each typically respond?
Have the stories increased in length over time?
Have new parts to the story been added?
How do you keep people's attention when talking to them?
Do you have responses ready if someone challengers what you say?
Do you tell exactly the same stories to everyone?
Do you change the stories slightly for different people?
What happens when you tell other stories (what you did during the day, etc.)?
Do people pay attention or not?
Example of contextual questions for a delusion
When did the delusional stories begin?
Who were the listeners? Friends? Family? Strangers?
Do the delusional stories get people listening? Who?
What does this discourse do to people who are told?
What can it be used for in conversation?
What are its consequences in conversation?
What are the social properties of saying something like this?
What can it do to listeners?
Who are the audiences it is currently told to?
Who were the past audiences for this delusion and what effects did it have on them?

References

Ball, M. (2020). *Dissociachotic: Seeing non psychosis*. Paper presented at A disorder for everyone! Challenging the culture of psychiatric diagnosis and exploring trauma informed alternatives. Cornwall, UK.

Bentall, R. P. (2006). Madness explained: Why we must reject the Kraepelinian paradigm and replace it with a 'complaint-orientated' approach to understanding mental illness. *Medical Hypotheses, 66*, 220–233.

Bleuler, E. (1911). *Dementia praecox or the group of schizophrenias*. International Universities Press.

Bleuler, E. (1912). *The theory of schizophrenic negativism*. NY: The Journal of Nervous and Mental Disease Publishing Company. (Nervous and mental disease monographs series, Number 11).

Bloomfield, M. A. P., Chang, T., Wood, M. J., et al. (2021). Psychological processes mediating the association between developmental trauma and specific psychotic symptoms in adults: A systematic review and meta-analysis. *World Psychiatry, 20*, 107–123.

Boyle, M., & Johnstone, L. (2020). *A straight talking introduction to the power threat meaning framework: An alternative to psychiatric diagnosis*. PCCS Books.
Frank, A. W. (2010). *Letting stories breathe: A socio-narratology*. University of Chicago Press.
Frankl, V. E. (2006). *Man's search for meaning*. Beacon Press.
Freud, S. (1915/1984). The unconscious. (In the Penguin freud library volume 11) : Penguin Books.
Guerin, B. (1997). Social contexts for communication: Communicative power as past and present social consequences. In J. Owen (Ed.), *Context and communication behavior* (pp. 133–179). Context Press.
Guerin, B. (2017). *How to rethink mental illness: The human contexts behind the labels*. Routledge.
Guerin, B. (2019a). What does poetry do to readers and listeners, and how does it do this? Language use as social activity and its clinical relevance. *Revista Brasileira de Análise do Comportamento, 15*, 100–114.
Guerin, B. (2019b). Contextualizing music to enhance music therapy. *Revista Perspectivas em Análise Comportamento, 10*, 222–242.
Guerin, B. (2020a). *Turning mental health into social action*. Routledge.
Guerin, B. (2020b). *Turning psychology into social contextual analysis*. Routledge.
Guerin, B. (2020c). *Turning psychology into a social science*. Routledge.
Guerin, B. (2021). Contextualizing the 'psychotic' behaviors: A social contextual approach. In J. A. Díaz-Garrido, H. Laffite Cabrera, & R. Zúñiga Costa (Eds.), *Terapia de aceptación y compromiso en psicosis: Aceptación y recuperación por niveles (ART)* (Acceptance and commitment therapy for psychosis: Acceptance and Recovery by Levels (ART)) (pp. 533–550). Ediciones Pirámide (Spanish translation).
Guerin, B. (2023). *Delusions as storytelling gone wrong in bad life situations: Exploring a discursive contextual analysis of delusions with clinical implications*. University of South Australia: Unpublished paper.
Guerin, B., & Miyazaki, Y. (2006). Analyzing rumors, gossip, and urban legends through their conversational properties. *The Psychological Record, 56*, 23–34. [Translated into Spanish in: *Revista Latinoamericana de Psicología, 35*, 257–272].
Guerin, B., Ball, M., & Ritchie, R. (2021). *Therapy in the absence of psychopathology and neoliberalism*. University of South Australia: Unpublished paper.
Haddock, G., & Slade, P. D. (Eds.). (1996). *Cognitive-behavioural interventions with psychotic disorders*. Routledge.
Haley, J. (1973). *Uncommon therapy: The psychiatric techniques of Milton H. Erickson, M.D.* Norton.
ISPS. (2017, July). *ISPS Liverpool declaration*. http://www.isps2017uk.org/making-real-change-happen
Janet, P. (1925/1919). *Psychological healing: A historical and clinical study*. George Allen & Unwin.
Johnstone, L. (2014). *A straight talking introduction to psychiatric diagnosis*. PCCS Books.
Johnstone, L., Boyle, M., Cromby, J., Dillon, J., Harper, D., Kinderman, P., et al. (2018). *The power threat meaning framework: Towards the identification of patterns in emotional distress, unusual experiences and troubled or troubling behaviour, as an alternative to functional psychiatric diagnosis*. British Psychological Society.
Jung, C. G. (1907/1960). *The psychogenesis of mental disease*. Princeton University Press.
Kheng, C., & Guerin, B. (2020). *"I just can't get that thought out of my head": Contextualizing rumination as an everyday discursive-social phenomenon and its clinical significance*. University of South Australia: Unpublished paper.
Killick, K. (Ed.). (2017). *Art therapy for psychosis: Theory and practice*. Routledge.
Luhrmann, T. M. (1912). *When God talks back: Understanding the American evangelical relationships with God*. Vintage Books.
Luhrmann, T. M., & Marrow, J. (Eds.). (2016). *Our most troubling madness: Case studies in schizophrenia across cultures*. University of California Press.

Luhrmann, T. M., Padmavati, R., Tharoor, H., & Osei, A. (2015). Differences in voice-hearing experiences of people psychosis in the USA, India and Ghana: Interview-based study. *British Journal of Psychiatry, 206*(1), 41–44.
Meaden, A., & Fox, A. (2015). *Innovations in psychosocial interventions for psychosis: Working with the hard to reach.* Routledge.
Moernaut, N., Krivzov, J., Lizon, M., Feyaerts, J., & Vanheule, S. (2021). Negative symptoms in psychosis: Failure and construction of narratives. *Psychosis, 14*, 1–10.
Mullen, M. (2021). *The dialectical behavior therapy skills workbook: Manage your emotions, reduce symptoms and get back your life*. New Harbinger.
Putman, N., & Martindale, B. (2022). *Open dialogue for psychosis: Organising mental health services to prioritise dialogue, relationship and meaning*. Routledge.
Romme, M., & Escher, S. (2000). *Making sense of voices: A guide for mental health for professionals working with voice-hearers*. Mind Publications.
Ruiz, J. J. (2021a). ACT de grupo para personas con experiencias psicóticas. In J. A. Díaz-Garrido, H. Laffite Cabrera, & R. Zúñiga Costa (Eds.), *Terapia de aceptación y compromiso en psicosis: Aceptación y recuperación por niveles (ART)* (Acceptance and commitment therapy for psychosis: Acceptance and Recovery by Levels (ART)) (pp. 261–288). Ediciones Pirámide (Spanish translation).
Ruiz, J. J. (Ed.). (2021b). *FACT de Grupo. Integrando ACT y FAP de Grupo*. Ediciones Psara.
Schilder, P. (1976). *On psychoses*. International Universities Press.
Skinner, B. F. (1957). *Verbal behavior*. Prentice Hall.
Sullivan, H. S. (1974). *Schizophrenia as a human process*. Norton.

Chapter 7
Culturally Adapted CBT for Psychosis

Farooq Naeem, Saiqa Naz, and Peter Phiri

7.1 Culture and Psychosis

Culture shapes the presentation, subjective phenomenology, and coping with psychotic symptoms (Luhrmann et al., 2015). Elevated rates of schizophrenia have been reported for clients from "cultural minority" populations in studies from England, with the highest rates for the Black Caribbean, followed by Black African and then Asian groups (Fearon et al., 2006). Overall, it has been reported that the migrant and ethnic minority populations have approximately a three-fold increased incidence of schizophrenia (Cantor-Graae & Selten, 2005). Vast differences exist in treatment access, experiences, and outcomes of schizophrenia, with disadvantages consistently reported for minority populations in Western countries (Degnan et al., 2016). Such inequalities for ethnic minorities include poorer engagement with services and professionals, more coercive care pathways, compulsory hospital admissions and involvement in the criminal justice system, higher doses of medication, and inferior access to psychological therapies (Bhui et al., 2003).

Cognitive behavioural therapy for psychosis (CBTp) is an evidence-based adjunct to medication in treating schizophrenia (Wykes et al., 2008) and is

F. Naeem (✉)
Centre for Addiction and Mental health, University of Toronto, Toronto, ON, Canada

S. Naz
Sheffield Specialist Psychotherapy Service, Sheffield Health and Social Care NHS Foundation Trust, Sheffield, UK

P. Phiri
Southern Health NHS Foundation Trust, Research & Innovation Department, Southampton, UK

Psychology Department, Faculty of Environmental and Life Sciences, University of Southampton, Southampton, UK
e-mail: peter.phiri@southernhealth.nhs.uk

J. A. Díaz-Garrido et al. (eds.), *Psychological Interventions for Psychosis*,
https://doi.org/10.1007/978-3-031-27003-1_7

recommended by National Treatment Guidelines in High-Income Countries (APA, 2006; NICE, 2014). However, like other modern therapies, cognitive behaviour therapy was developed in the West and is therefore underpinned by Western explanatory models of illness. The explanatory models of illness are often rooted in local cultural and religious beliefs and values, which need to be addressed in any psychosocial intervention as these play a very important role in help-seeking and health-related behaviours (Joel et al., 2003; Lloyd et al., 1998). There is evidence suggesting that people from some of the cultures in the Global South can attribute spiritual causes to psychotic symptoms (Zafar et al., 2008) and are more likely to consider seeking help from faith healers or spiritual leaders compared to other people with their western counterparts. Therefore, it has been recommended that CBTp needs cultural adaptation before its application in Non-Western culture (Naeem et al., 2014, 2015c). Our work to culturally adapt CBT for psychosis has shown that numerous adjustments need to be made for CBT to be acceptable, accessible, and effective (Naeem et al., 2014; Rathod et al., 2010).

7.2 Need for Ethno-Psychotherapy and Ethno-CBT

As the countries in the Global North are becoming culturally diverse, governments are under considerable pressure to address health disparities by providing equitable, culturally sensitive, appropriate, and effective clinical services relevant to the different population's cultural backgrounds. At the same time, countries in the Global South, due to the improved economic condition and access to online knowledge, have led to an awareness of modern psychotherapies. As a result of these critical considerations, there is a huge drive towards the delivery of culturally adapted psychological therapies. The study of psychotherapy across cultures and subcultures is known as ethno-psychotherapy (Naeem et al., 2015b). It, therefore, implies that ethno-CBT (Cognitive Behaviour Therapy) will be the branch of ethno-psychotherapy concerned with culture and CBT.

7.3 The Ethno-CBT

Cultural adaptation of CBT was initially defined as "making adaptations in how therapy is delivered, through the acquisition of awareness, information, and skills appropriate to a given culture, without compromising the theoretical underpinnings of CBT." (Naeem, 2012). It, therefore, can be said that the primary goal of cultural adaptation is to "improve engagement with a client who does not share the therapist's cultural background."

7.4 Cultural Adaptation: Historical Background

Some therapists in the United States have created recommendations for adapting psychosocial interventions based on their work with non-Western cultures, assuming that individuals from non-Western cultures may have distinct sets of beliefs, values, and perceptions. There are a few known guides or models of cultural adaptation: Ecological Validity Model (Bernal et al., 1995; Bernal & Sáez-Santiago, 2006); Cultural Accommodation Model (Leong & Lee, 2006); model of essential elements (Podorefsky et al., 2001); Cultural Adaptation Process Model (Domenech-Rodríguez & Wieling, 2005); data-driven adaptation; heuristic framework (Barrera Jr. & Castro, 2006); Psychotherapy Adaptation and Modification model (Hwang, 2006); and adaptation model for American Indians (Whitbeck, 2006). However, none of the previous adaptation frameworks has been tested through RCTs.

On the other hand, these first recommendations explain therapists' own experiences dealing with patients from racialized populations, provide therapy suggestions in general, and address broader philosophical, theoretical, and clinical concerns. Furthermore, none of the frameworks focused solely on CBT, and the guidelines did not directly derive from research addressing cultural variables.

7.5 Current Evidence

7.5.1 *Culturally Adapted Psychotherapies*

A recent review of current literature revealed that more than 10 review articles and meta-analyses of culturally adapted psychosocial interventions had been published (Rathod et al., 2018). The reviews reported effect sizes ranging from 0.23 to 0.75, with the majority reporting moderate to large effect sizes. Most of the evaluations looked at a wide range of mental health conditions and populations. One focused on schizophrenia (Degnan et al., 2016), while five focused on depressive symptoms (Anik et al., 2021; Chowdhary et al., 2014; Rojas-García et al., 2014, 2015; van Loon et al., 2013). One review focused on online and internet-based interventions (Spanhel et al., 2021). One review focused on Latinos (Sutton, 2015). The rest of the reviews included studies of different ethnic and cultural groups. Two reviews focused on youth (≤18 years) (Hodge et al., 2010; Huey Jr. & Polo, 2008). One study focused on postnatal depression among women (Rojas-García et al., 2014). While most reviews attempted to characterize cultural adaptation, only two used a systematic method to define the nature and process in-depth (Chowdhary et al., 2014; Degnan et al., 2016). Two meta-analyses (Rojas-García et al., 2014, 2015) focused on culturally adapted interventions for depressed persons from low socioeconomic status (Rojas-García et al., 2014, 2015).

7.5.2 *Culturally Adapted CBT for Psychosis*

So far, only two pilot trials and one fully powered RCT of CBTp have been published (Habib et al., 2014; Naeem et al., 2015c; Rathod et al., 2013). In their review and meta-analysis of culturally adapted psychosocial interventions for schizophrenia. Degnan et al. (2016) used qualitative methodology to evaluate the nature of cultural adaptations. First, they assessed the process and components of adaption using sound methodology. The authors evaluated the nature of cultural adaptations reported in the included research using a qualitative approach. The authors' nine themes after the adaptations were thematically examined were language, concepts, family, communication, content, cultural norms and practices, setting and delivery, therapeutic partnership, and treatment goals. However, both researches took data from RCTs, which may have hampered the identification of themes because authors did not always record adaptations or characterize the adaptation process separately. This could have made it impossible to create a full picture.

Degnan et al. (2016) reported minimal variation in symptomatic effect depending on the type of intervention. However, interventions were more successful when patients attended with relatives rather than alone. They also reported that interventions adapted for Chinese and majority populations are less effective for schizophrenia than non-Chinese and minority populations.

7.6 Southampton Adaptation Framework for CBTp

We developed the Southampton Adaptation Framework for CBT (Naeem, Ayub, et al., 2009) to culturally adapt CBT in 2009. Over the years, the framework evolved and has been described in detail in our recent publications in its current form (Naeem et al., 2015b, 2016, 2019). This framework has also been used to adapt CBT for depression and anxiety in Saudi Arabia (Algahtani et al., 2019) and Morocco (Rhermoul et al., 2017) and psychosis in China (Li et al., 2017) and for emotional dysregulation in learning disability in Canada (McQueen et al., 2018). Currently, the framework is being used in Canada to adapt CBT for depression and anxiety for the South Asian population (Naeem et al., 2021). We have used the framework to adapt and test CBT using an RCT design in various areas, such as depression (Naeem, Gul, et al., 2015a), schizophrenia (Naeem et al., 2015c), OCD (Aslam et al., 2015), and self-harm (Husain et al., 2014).

7.6.1 *Methodology for Adaptation*

We used a mixed-methods approach (see Fig. 7.1). We started with qualitative studies using open-ended interviews (Naeem et al., 2009b, 2010, 2012) to gather the information that can be used to develop more or less precise guidelines for

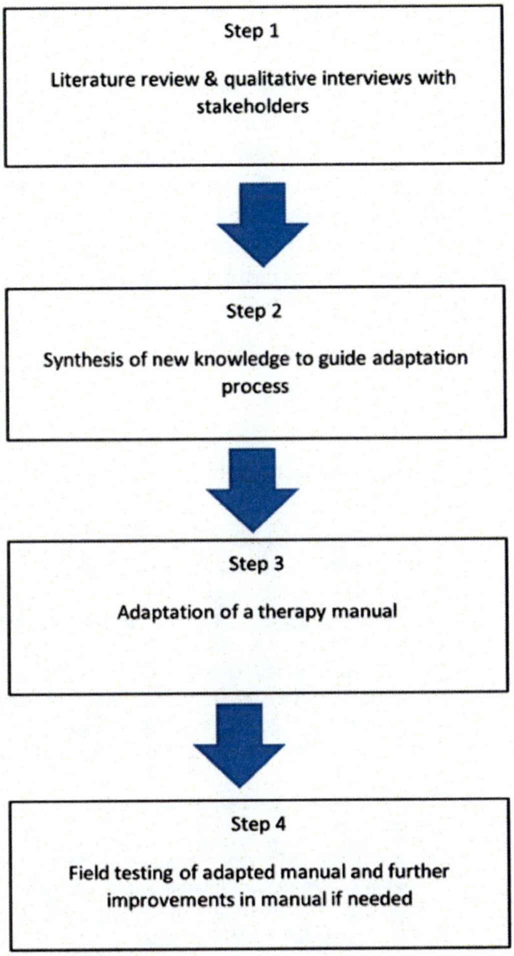

Fig. 7.1 Steps in adapting psychotherapy

adaptation. Through time, these interviews have evolved into semi-structured interviews that can be carried out by less experienced researchers with supervision (Li et al., 2017). Patients, their caregivers' therapists or mental health experts, and community leaders have all been involved in the past. The qualitative research looked into issues such as patients', carers', and community leaders' beliefs about a condition, its origins, and treatment, particularly non-medical therapies, as well as patients' experiences with any non-pharmacological assistance they received. Professionals were interviewed about their experiences, obstacles, and, if any, solutions. A name-the-title technique (Naeem et al., 2009b) was used to find equivalent terminology rather than using literal translations. Following the adaptation of CBT in each area, a feasibility pilot study was often done to see if the modified therapy was acceptable. Finally, to determine the therapy's efficacy, a larger RCT was done.

7.7 The Fundamental Areas of Cultural Competence in CBT

According to our findings, the following areas of cultural competency termed the "triple-A principle" must be covered to effectively adapt CBT for a specific culture: (1) awareness of important cultural issues and treatment preparation; (2) assessment and engagement; and (3) adjustments and modifications (see Table 7.1). Cultural awareness, in turn, refers to three important areas: (a) Culture – culture, religion, and spirituality; (b) context – evaluation of the healthcare system's capabilities and features; (c) the cultural context of cognitions and dysfunctional beliefs.

Table 7.1 Components of Southampton adaptation framework

Major areas	Minor areas
Awareness of culture and religion	1. Cause and effect model of mental illness used by the population in focus (Bio-Psycho-Socio-Spiritual Model) 2. Language and terminology (literal translations don't work) 3. Communication styles, idioms of distress, and personal boundaries 4. Family and caregivers' involvement 5. Health system-related issues (for future implementation-number of therapists, resources, distance from the treatment facility) 6. Considerations of gender, sex-related issues 7. Pathways to care (traditional healers, faith healers, religious leaders, elders) 8. Coping strategies and cultural strengths- religion, spirituality, cultural practices
Assessment and engagement	1. Self-awareness in therapists about their own belief system 2. Common presenting complaints and concerns 3. Assessment of acculturation and immigration status 4. Racism and racial or other trauma 5. Stigma, shame, and guilt 6. Barriers to seeking therapy and engagement with therapy 7. Awareness of illness, its causes, and its treatment 8. Beliefs about illness, its causes, and its treatment
Adjustments in therapy	1. Culturally acceptable patient-therapist relationship (attitude towards authority in a given culture) 2. Psycho–education and access to therapy 3. Cultural variations in dysfunctional beliefs 4. Acceptable therapy settings and style 5. Adjustments or modifications are required in therapy settings 6. Use of culturally favourable communication strategies such as stories or images 7. Understanding barriers in therapy such as how to ensure homework assignments are completed 8. Adjustments in therapy techniques

7.7.1 *Awareness of Cultural and Spiritual Knowledge*

A. Religion and spirituality play a vital role in many non-Western European societies. A biopsychosocial–spiritual paradigm of illness is used by patients from many non-Western cultures (Naeem et al., 2015b). This model impacts their beliefs, particularly regarding health, well-being, disease, and seeking help when they are in trouble. Views on the cause-effect link are influenced by culture and religion (Cinnirella & Loewenthal, 1999). For example, a mishap could be attributed to the 'evil eye' or 'God's will.' When faced with adversity, people frequently turn to religious coping mechanisms (Bhugra & Rosemarie, 1999). On the other hand, many beliefs and stigmas around mental illness may be rooted in religion and spirituality. Understanding ideas about the causes of mental illness is critical because they can influence therapy and help-seeking options and pathways (Lloyd et al., 1998). A culturally adapted intervention should consider the spiritual or religious components of the cause and effect model of a person with schizophrenia and their carers.

Historically, the connection between religiousness and psychosis has been studied (Menezes & Moreira-Almeida, 2010). However, religion may be present in the psychotic patients' lives as part of the problem as well as part of the solution (Mohr & Huguelet, 2004). One study from the United States reported that one in seven psychotic patients was very worried about ideas and religious practices (Sylvia & Pfeifer, 2009). A Nigerian study of schizophrenic patients who sought help from local healers before looking for psychiatric help reported that a substantial number of the patients from all educational levels sought care from either native healers or syncretic churches: this was true for both Christians and Moslems (Erinosho, 1977). The utilization of traditional healers before psychiatric contact suggests that psychiatric disorder is well placed within the belief system despite modernizing influences. One study from India reported that good outcomes among 323 patients observed for 2 years were associated with an increase in patients' religious activities (Verghese et al., 1989). de Dantas et al. (1999) conducted an analysis of 200 psychiatric admissions in Brazil and found that religious symptoms with moderate to very strong intensity were present in 15.7% of the cases. Another study reported a prevalence rate of 21.3% of religious deliria among German inpatients of only 6.8% among Japanese inpatients, demonstrating that different cultures produce different effects regarding religious delusions (Tateyama et al., 1993). Another study from the USA reported that of 1136 psychiatric inpatients, 328 had deliria and 93 had deliria of religious content (Appelbaum et al., 1999). Therefore, it can be seen that although religion cannot be considered an etiologic factor in schizophrenia, it influences the content of patients' thoughts and their behaviour and probably the outcome.

Language, gender, and family-related factors play a major role in providing culturally adapted CBT for psychosis and should all be taken into account. Language obstacles are a major concern in this regard and must be taken into account as a priority. Literal translations are ineffective when translating from a European language to a non-European language. Cultures have a wide variety of communication styles. The idea of assertiveness, for example, is absent in many non-Western European cultures. When speaking to an elder in a non-European culture, assertiveness may be unacceptable in some instances. As a result, assertiveness strategies should be applied with culturally sensitivity, such as learning the "apologies technique," which involves using phrases like "With a big apology, before a person disagrees," etc. (Farooq Naeem, 2013; Hays & Iwamasa, 2006). You are dealing with the family in communal societies, not simply the individual. Involving family members can boost treatment involvement, ensure that homework assignments are completed, and improve follow-up.

B. It is critical to evaluate the context and the healthcare system's capacity. For example, distance from the treatment facility may be a problem for patients in many low- and middle-income nations where psychiatric clinics are limited to larger cities (Li et al., 2017; Naeem et al., 2010). On the other hand, many patients in the Global South, as well as some from racialized and immigrant communities in the Global North, may be unaware of the healthcare system, mental health problems, available psychiatric treatments, and their likely outcomes, which can lead to underutilization of culturally adapted interventions if due consideration is not paid to these factors.

Women from some cultures are less likely to attend therapy as they might need permission from a man and might be dependent on men to be brought to the clinic (Shaikh & Hatcher, 2005). When working with female patients, it would help to engage the accompanying man or the family during the assessment and psychoeducation them. In many low- and middle-income countries where psychiatric facilities are limited to bigger cities, distance from the treatment facility might be a barrier for all patients (Li et al., 2017; Naeem et al., 2010; Naeem et al., 2009a). The availability of culturally sensitive therapists can be a further systemic barrier. Patients' knowledge of the healthcare system, available treatments, and their likely outcomes are key factors influencing service utilization and engagement.

C. The content of Cognitive errors and dysfunctional beliefs vary from culture to culture. There is at least some evidence from research from Turkey and Hong Kong, for example, provides evidence of such variations (Sahin & Sahin, 1992; Tam et al., 2007). Typical beliefs that a Western European therapist could deem dysfunctional include the belief that one must rely on others, please others, submit to the demands of those in authority, and sacrifice one's own needs for the benefit of family; however, these beliefs are normal and in some instances even admirable in persons from the communal societies (Chen & Davenport, 2005; Farooq Naeem, 2013; Laungani, 2004).

7.7.2 Assessment and Engagement

Being aware of the aforementioned cultural and religious challenges can aid in conducting a culturally sensitive evaluation and engaging customers from other cultures. The therapist can begin by starting with the patient's ideas about mental illness, healing, and healers. "What do you think is the cause of the illness?" "Who can treat these symptoms?" and "What is the optimal treatment for these symptoms?" are some of the questions that might help the therapist get understanding. Next, the therapist should inquire about the patient's spiritual and religious basis of symptoms. The therapist can then ask about the patient's experience and expectations of the healthcare system and their interactions with any healers (e.g. faith healers, religious healers, magicians, and herbalists). Because some patients with psychosis have religious or spiritual concerns, assessing these carefully and in a non-judgmental way is critical. In case of any doubts, it is highly recommended that a spiritual or religious leader is consulted. The initial examination should explore the shame, guilt, and stigma attached to mental illness within the clients' context. Finally, structured assessments using validated tools can be used to assess the patient's beliefs about disease and its treatment (Lloyd et al., 1998) and their level of acculturation (Frey & Roysircar, 2004; Wallace et al., 2010). Therapists should make themselves familiar with the biopsychosocial (Kinderman, 2014) and the spiritual models of illness (Verghese, 2008) to formulate clients' problems. Finally, teaching the patient and their family on the biopsychosocial causes of illness is an important aspect of the evaluation process.

Patients from non-Western cultures have been found to drop out of therapy at high rates (Rathod & Kingdon, 2014). Therefore, the initial few sessions are always crucial. Because some patients expect instant relief from bothersome symptoms, emphasizing symptom management at the start of therapy can increase participation and raise the patient's trust in the therapist.

7.7.3 Adjustments to the Therapy

CBT techniques, in our opinion, do not require large modifications to function for people from non-western European cultures. Minor changes, however, will be required. Problem solving, activity scheduling, and behavioural experiments are examples of procedures that require just minor alterations. Non-Western patients prefer muscle relaxation and breathing techniques. Breathing exercises are popular in non-Western cultures and are part of many religious and spiritual traditions. Because most clients with depression and anxiety focus on physical symptoms, thought diaries can be employed with a column for physical symptoms. It takes a lot of effort to assist clients in recognizing their thoughts and emotions. Thus, the therapist should take the time to explain these to them.

To begin, a more directive counselling style might be beneficial. A collaborative approach might be adopted as therapy progresses. A saint or guru who provides sermons is the non-Western form of spiritual and emotional healing, instead of professional teaching through "Socratic dialogue," valued in individualistic Western countries. If Socratic discussion is employed without adequate preparation, patients from non-Western cultures often feel uncomfortable. This is an important consideration since Socratic dialogue is of great significance when dealing with delusions.

In non-western cultures, stories to explain a point are frequent. Experienced healers use stories from non-Western cultural backgrounds to communicate their messages. When combined with visuals in handouts, stories can be quite engaging. Similarly, due to low literacy levels, homework compliance is low in many non-western societies. The patient could be provided audio cassettes or bibliographic materials from the session and encouraged to count negative thoughts with beads or counters, commonly used in Asia and Africa, instead of pen and paper. Family members can also play an important part in assisting their homework and ensuring that they attend therapy sessions.

7.8 Future Directions

Current evidence suggests that culturally adapted CBT for psychosis is effective. However, this is an emerging field, and therefore a lot of work needs to be done. There needs to be further research into adaptation to find out what works. There is also a need for further studies evaluating the effectiveness of adapted interventions compared with non-adapted interventions instead of usual care. Most importantly, there is a need to conduct economic evaluation studies to determine how beneficial culturally adapted interventions are compared with standard therapies. Future studies should also focus on potential moderators of cultural adaptation on the outcome. It might be worth considering adding a checklist for culturally adapted interventions in consort guidelines.

References

Algahtani, H. M. S., Almulhim, A., AlNajjar, F. A., Ali, M. K., Irfan, M., Ayub, M., & Naeem, F. (2019). Cultural adaptation of cognitive behavioural therapy (CBT) for patients with depression and anxiety in Saudi Arabia and Bahrain: A qualitative study exploring views of patients, carers, and mental health professionals. *The Cognitive Behaviour Therapist, 12*. https://doi.org/10.1017/S1754470X1900028X

Anik, E., West, R. M., Cardno, A. G., & Mir, G. (2021). Culturally adapted psychotherapies for depressed adults: A systematic review and meta-analysis. *Journal of Affective Disorders, 278*, 296–310. https://doi.org/10.1016/j.jad.2020.09.051

APA. (2006). *Practice guidelines for the treatment of psychiatric disorders*. American Psychiatric Pub.

Appelbaum, P. S., Robbins, P. C., & Roth, L. H. (1999). Dimensional approach to delusions: Comparison across types and diagnoses. *The American Journal of Psychiatry, 156*(12), 1938–1943. https://doi.org/10.1176/ajp.156.12.1938

Aslam, M., Irfan, M., & Naeem, F. (2015). Brief culturally adapted cognitive behaviour therapy for obsessive compulsive disorder: A pilot study. *Pakistan Journal of Medical Sciences, 31*(4), 874–879. https://doi.org/10.12669/pjms.314.7385

Barrera, M., Jr., & Castro, F. G. (2006). A heuristic framework for the cultural adaptation of interventions. *Clinical Psychology: Science and Practice, 13*(4), 311–316. https://doi.org/10.1111/j.1468-2850.2006.00043.x

Bernal, G., & Sáez-Santiago, E. (2006). Culturally centered psychosocial interventions. *Journal of Community Psychology, 34*(2), 121–132. https://doi.org/10.1002/jcop.20096

Bernal, G., Bonilla, J., & Bellido, C. (1995). Ecological validity and cultural sensitivity for outcome research: Issues for the cultural adaptation and development of psychosocial treatments with Hispanics. *Journal of Abnormal Child Psychology, 23*(1), 67–82. https://doi.org/10.1007/BF01447045

Bhugra, K. B., & Rosemarie, M. D. (1999). Cultural identity and its measurement: A questionnaire for Asians. *International Review of Psychiatry, 11*(2–3), 244–249. https://doi.org/10.1080/09540269974438

Bhui, K., Stansfeld, S., Hull, S., Priebe, S., Mole, F., & Feder, G. (2003). Ethnic variations in pathways to and use of specialist mental health services in the UK. Systematic review. *The British Journal of Psychiatry: the Journal of Mental Science, 182*, 105–116. https://doi.org/10.1192/bjp.182.2.105

Cantor-Graae, E., & Selten, J.-P. (2005). Schizophrenia and migration: A meta-analysis and review. *The American Journal of Psychiatry, 162*(1), 12–24. https://doi.org/10.1176/appi.ajp.162.1.12

Chen, S. W.-H., & Davenport, D. S. (2005). Cognitive-behavioral therapy with Chinese American clients: Cautions and modifications. *Psychotherapy: Theory, Research, Practice, Training, 42*(1), 101–110. https://doi.org/10.1037/0033-3204.42.1.101

Chowdhary, N., Jotheeswaran, A. T., Nadkarni, A., Hollon, S. D., King, M., Jordans, M. J. D., Rahman, A., Verdeli, H., Araya, R., & Patel, V. (2014). The methods and outcomes of cultural adaptations of psychological treatments for depressive disorders: A systematic review. *Psychological Medicine, 44*(06), 1131–1146. https://doi.org/10.1017/S0033291713001785

Cinnirella, M., & Loewenthal, K. M. (1999). Religious and ethnic group influences on beliefs about mental illness: A qualitative interview study. *British Journal of Medical Psychology, 72*(4), 505–524. https://doi.org/10.1348/000711299160202

de Dantas, C. R., Pavarin, L. B., & Dalgalarrondo, P. (1999). Symptoms of religious content on psychiatric patients. *Brazilian Journal of Psychiatry, 21*, 158–164. https://doi.org/10.1590/S1516-44461999000300007

Degnan, A., Baker, S., Edge, D., & Drake, R. (2016). The nature and efficacy of culturally-adapted psychosocial interventions for schizophrenia: A systematic review and meta-analysis.

Domenech-Rodríguez, M., & Wieling, E. (2005). Developing culturally appropriate, evidence-based treatments for interventions with ethnic minority populations. In *Voices of color: First-person accounts of ethnic minority therapists* (pp. 313–333). Sage Publications, Inc. https://doi.org/10.4135/9781452231662.n18

Erinosho, O. A. (1977). Social background and pre-admission sources of care among Yoruba psychiatric patients. *Social Psychiatry, 12*(2), 71–74. https://doi.org/10.1007/BF00579114

Farooq Naeem, M. A. (2013). *Culturally adapted CBT (CaCBT) for depression, therapy manual for use with South Asian Muslims* [Kindle Edition].

Fearon, P., Kirkbride, J. B., Morgan, C., Dazzan, P., Morgan, K., Lloyd, T., Hutchinson, G., Tarrant, J., Fung, W. L. A., Holloway, J., Mallett, R., Harrison, G., Leff, J., Jones, P. B., & Murray, R. M. (2006). Incidence of schizophrenia and other psychoses in ethnic minority groups: Results from the MRC AESOP Study. *Psychological Medicine, 36*(11), 1541–1550. https://doi.org/10.1017/S0033291706008774

Frey, L. L., & Roysircar, G. (2004). Effects of acculturation and worldview for white American, South American, South Asian, and Southeast Asian students. *International Journal for the Advancement of Counselling, 26*(3), 229–248. https://doi.org/10.1023/B:ADCO.0000035527.46652.d2

Habib, N., Dawood, S., Kingdon, D., & Naeem, F. (2014). Preliminary evaluation of Culturally Adapted CBT for Psychosis (CA-CBTp): Findings from developing culturally-sensitive CBT project (DCCP). *Behavioural and Cognitive Psychotherapy, FirstView*, 1–9. https://doi.org/10.1017/S1352465813000829

Hays, P. A., & Iwamasa, G. Y. (Eds.). (2006). *Culturally responsive cognitive-behavioral therapy: Assessment, practice, and supervision*. American Psychological Association.

Hodge, D. R., PhD, K. F. J., & PhD, M. G. V. (2010). Culturally sensitive interventions and health and Behavioral health youth outcomes: A meta-analytic review. *Social Work in Health Care, 49*(5), 401–423. https://doi.org/10.1080/00981381003648398

Huey, S., Jr., & Polo, A. J. (2008). Evidence-based psychosocial treatments for ethnic minority youth. *Journal of Clinical Child & Adolescent Psychology, 37*(1), 262–301. https://doi.org/10.1080/15374410701820174

Husain, N., Afsar, S., Ara, J., Fayyaz, H., Rahman, R. u., Tomenson, B., Hamirani, M., Chaudhry, N., Fatima, B., Husain, M., Naeem, F., & Chaudhry, I. B. (2014). Brief psychological intervention after self-harm: Randomised controlled trial from Pakistan. *The British Journal of Psychiatry, 204*(6), 462–470. https://doi.org/10.1192/bjp.bp.113.138370

Hwang, W.-C. (2006). The psychotherapy adaptation and modification framework: Application to Asian Americans. *American Psychologist, 61*(7), 702–715. https://doi.org/10.1037/0003-066X.61.7.702

Joel, D., Sathyaseelan, M., Jayakaran, R., Vijayakumar, C., Muthurathnam, S., & Jacob, K. S. (2003). Explanatory models of psychosis among community health workers in South India. *Acta Psychiatrica Scandinavica, 108*(1), 66–69. https://doi.org/10.1034/j.1600-0447.2003.01327.x

Kinderman, P. (2014). Get the message right: A psychosocial model of mental health and Wellbeing. In P. Kinderman (Ed.), *A prescription for psychiatry: Why we need a whole new approach to mental health and wellbeing* (pp. 30–47). Palgrave Macmillan UK. https://doi.org/10.1057/9781137408716_2

Laungani, P. (2004). *Asian perspectives in counselling and psychotherapy*. Psychology Press.

Leong, F. T., & Lee, S.-H. (2006). A cultural accommodation model for cross-cultural psychotherapy: Illustrated with the case of Asian Americans. *Psychotherapy: Theory, Research, Practice, Training, 43*(4), 410–423. https://doi.org/10.1037/0033-3204.43.4.410

Li, W., Zhang, L., Luo, X., Liu, B., Liu, Z., Lin, F., Liu, Z., Xie, Y., Hudson, M., Rathod, S., Kingdon, D., Husain, N., Liu, X., Ayub, M., & Naeem, F. (2017). A qualitative study to explore views of patients', carers' and mental health professionals' to inform cultural adaptation of CBT for psychosis (CBTp) in China. *BMC Psychiatry, 17*. https://doi.org/10.1186/s12888-017-1290-6

Lloyd, K. R., Jacob, K. S., Patel, V., St. Louis, L., Bhugra, D., & Mann, A. H. (1998). The development of the short explanatory model interview (SEMI) and its use among primary-care attenders with common mental disorders. *Psychological Medicine, 28*(05), 1231–1237.

Luhrmann, T. M., Padmavati, R., Tharoor, H., & Osei, A. (2015). Differences in voice-hearing experiences of people with psychosis in the U.S.A., India and Ghana: Interview-based study. *The British Journal of Psychiatry: the Journal of Mental Science, 206*(1), 41–44. https://doi.org/10.1192/bjp.bp.113.139048

McQueen, M., Blinkhorn, A., Broad, A., Jones, J., Naeem, F., & Ayub, M. (2018). Development of a cognitive behavioural therapy-based guided self-help intervention for adults with intellectual disability. *Journal of Applied Research in Intellectual Disabilities, 31*(5), 885–896. https://doi.org/10.1111/jar.12447

Menezes, A., & Moreira-Almeida, A. (2010). Religion, spirituality, and psychosis. *Current Psychiatry Reports, 12*(3), 174–179. https://doi.org/10.1007/s11920-010-0117-7

Mohr, S., & Huguelet, P. (2004). The relationship between schizophrenia and religion and its implications for care. *Swiss Medical Weekly, 134*(25–26), 369–376. 2004/25/smw-10322.

Naeem, F. (2012). *Adaptation of cognitive behaviour therapy for depression in Pakistan*. Lap Lambert Academic Publishing GmbH KG.

Naeem, F., Ayub, M., Gobbi, M., & Kingdon, D. (2009a, December 1). Development of Southampton adaptation framework for CBT (SAF-CBT): A framework for adaptation of CBT in non-western culture. *Journal of Pakistan Psychiatric Society*. http://www.pakmedinet.com/15940

Naeem, F., Gobbi, M., Ayub, M., & Kingdon, D. (2009b). University students' views about compatibility of cognitive behaviour therapy (CBT) with their personal, social and religious values (A study from Pakistan). *Mental Health, Religion & Culture, 12*(8), 847–855. https://doi.org/10.1080/13674670903115226

Naeem, F., Gobbi, M., Ayub, M., Kingdon, D., & Others. (2010). Psychologists experience of cognitive behaviour therapy in a developing country: A qualitative study from Pakistan. *International Journal of Mental Health Systems, 4*, 2.

Naeem, F., Ayub, M., Kingdon, D., & Gobbi, M. (2012). Views of depressed patients in Pakistan concerning their illness, its causes, and treatments. *Qualitative Health Research*. https://doi.org/10.1177/1049732312450212

Naeem, F., Habib, N., Gul, M., Khalid, M., Saeed, S., Farooq, S., Munshi, T., Gobbi, M., Husain, N., Ayub, M., & Kingdon, D. (2014). A qualitative study to explore patients', carers' and health professionals' views to culturally adapt CBT for psychosis (CBTp) in Pakistan. *Behavioural and Cognitive Psychotherapy*, 1–13. https://doi.org/10.1017/S1352465814000332

Naeem, F., Gul, M., Irfan, M., Munshi, T., Asif, A., Rashid, S., Khan, M. N. S., Ghani, S., Malik, A., Aslam, M., Farooq, S., Husain, N., & Ayub, M. (2015a). Brief culturally adapted CBT (CaCBT) for depression: A randomized controlled trial from Pakistan. *Journal of Affective Disorders, 177*, 101–107. https://doi.org/10.1016/j.jad.2015.02.012

Naeem, F., Phiri, P., Munshi, T., Rathod, S., Ayub, M., Gobbi, M., & Kingdon, D. (2015b). Using cognitive behaviour therapy with south Asian Muslims: Findings from the culturally sensitive CBT project. *International Review of Psychiatry (Abingdon, England), 27*(3), 233–246. https://doi.org/10.3109/09540261.2015.1067598

Naeem, F., Saeed, S., Irfan, M., Kiran, T., Mehmood, N., Gul, M., Munshi, T., Ahmad, S., Kazmi, A., Husain, N., Farooq, S., Ayub, M., & Kingdon, D. (2015c). Brief culturally adapted CBT for psychosis (CaCBTp): A randomized controlled trial from a low income country. *Schizophrenia Research, 164*(1–3), 143–148. https://doi.org/10.1016/j.schres.2015.02.015

Naeem, F., Phiri, P., Nasar, A., Munshi, T., Ayub, M., & Rathod, S. (2016). An evidence-based framework for cultural adaptation of Cognitive Behaviour Therapy: Process, methodology and foci of adaptation. *World Cultural Psychiatry Research Review, 11*, 67–70.

Naeem, F., Phiri, P., Rathod, S., & Ayub, M. (2019). Cultural adaptation of cognitive–behavioural therapy. *BJPsych Advances, 25*(6), 1–9. https://doi.org/10.1192/bja.2019.15

Naeem, F., Tuck, A., Mutta, B., Dhillon, P., Thandi, G., Kassam, A., Farah, N., Ashraf, A., Husain, M. I., Husain, M. O., Vasiliadis, H.-M., Sanches, M., Munshi, T., Abbott, M., Watters, N., Kidd, S. A., Ayub, M., & McKenzie, K. (2021). Protocol for a multi-phase, mixed methods study to develop and evaluate culturally adapted CBT to improve community mental health services for Canadians of south Asian origin. *Trials, 22*(1), 600. https://doi.org/10.1186/s13063-021-05547-4

NICE, N. I. of H. and C. E. (2014). *Psychosis and schizophrenia in adults: Prevention and management*. https://www.nice.org.uk/guidance/cg178/resources/psychosis-and-schizophrenia-in-adults-prevention-and-management-pdf-35109758952133

Podorefsky, D. L., Mcdonald-dowdell, M., & Beardslee, W. R. (2001). Adaptation of preventive interventions for a low-income, culturally diverse community. *Journal of the American Academy of Child & Adolescent Psychiatry, 40*(8), 879–886. https://doi.org/10.1097/00004583-200108000-00008

Rathod, S., & Kingdon, D. (2014). Case for cultural adaptation of psychological interventions for mental healthcare in low and middle income countries. *British Medical Journal, 349*, g7636. https://doi.org/10.1136/bmj.g7636

Rathod, S., Kingdon, D., Phiri, P., & Gobbi, M. (2010). Developing culturally sensitive cognitive behaviour therapy for psychosis for ethnic minority patients by exploration and incorporation of service users' and health professionals' views and opinions. *Behavioural and Cognitive Psychotherapy, 38*(05), 511–533. https://doi.org/10.1017/S1352465810000378

Rathod, S., Phiri, P., Harris, S., Underwood, C., Thagadur, M., Padmanabi, U., & Kingdon, D. (2013). Cognitive behaviour therapy for psychosis can be adapted for minority ethnic groups: A randomised controlled trial. *Schizophrenia Research, 143*(2), 319–326. https://doi.org/10.1016/j.schres.2012.11.007

Rathod, S., Gega, L., Degnan, A., Pikard, J., Khan, T., Husain, N., Munshi, T., & Naeem, F. (2018). The current status of culturally adapted mental health interventions: A practice-focused review of meta-analyses. *Neuropsychiatric Disease and Treatment, 14*, 165–178. https://doi.org/10.2147/NDT.S138430

Rhermoul, F.-Z. E., Naeem, F., Kingdon, D., Hansen, L., & Toufiq, J. (2017). A qualitative study to explore views of patients, carers and mental health professionals' views on depression in Moroccan women. *International Journal of Culture and Mental Health, 11*, 1–16. https://doi.org/10.1080/17542863.2017.1355397

Rojas-García, A., Ruíz-Pérez, I., Gonçalves, D. C., Rodríguez-Barranco, M., & Ricci-Cabello, I. (2014). Healthcare interventions for perinatal depression in socially disadvantaged women: A systematic review and meta-analysis. *Clinical Psychology: Science and Practice, 21*(4), 363–384. https://doi.org/10.1111/cpsp.12081

Rojas-García, A., Ruiz-Perez, I., Rodríguez-Barranco, M., Gonçalves Bradley, D. C., Pastor-Moreno, G., & Ricci-Cabello, I. (2015). Healthcare interventions for depression in low socio-economic status populations: A systematic review and meta-analysis. *Clinical Psychology Review, 38*, 65–78. https://doi.org/10.1016/j.cpr.2015.03.001

Sahin, N. H., & Sahin, N. (1992). How dysfunctional are the dysfunctional attitudes in another culture? *The British Journal of Medical Psychology, 65*(Pt 1), 17–26.

Shaikh, B. T., & Hatcher, J. (2005). Health seeking behaviour and health service utilization in Pakistan: Challenging the policy makers. *Journal of Public Health, 27*(1), 49–54. https://doi.org/10.1093/pubmed/fdh207

Spanhel, K., Balci, S., Feldhahn, F., Bengel, J., Baumeister, H., & Sander, L. B. (2021). Cultural adaptation of internet- and mobile-based interventions for mental disorders: A systematic review. *Npj Digital Medicine, 4*(1), 1–18. https://doi.org/10.1038/s41746-021-00498-1

Sutton, C. (2015). *Culturally adapted interventions for Latinos: A meta-analysis*. School of Graduate Psychology. http://commons.pacificu.edu/spp/1134

Sylvia, M., & Pfeifer, S. (2009). Delusions and hallucinations with religious content. In H. G. Koenig & P. Huguelet (Eds.), *Religion and spirituality in psychiatry* (pp. 81–96). Cambridge University Press. https://doi.org/10.1017/CBO9780511576843.007

Tam, P. W. C., Wong, D. F. K., Chow, K. K. W., Ng, F. S., Ng, R. M. K., Cheung, M. S. M., Choy, L. W., Dunn, E. L. W., & Mak, A. D. P. (2007). Qualitative analysis of dysfunctional attitudes in Chinese persons suffering from depression. *Hong Kong Journal of Psychiatry, 17*(4), 109.

Tateyama, M., Asai, M., Kamisada, M., Hashimoto, M., Bartels, M., & Heimann, H. (1993). Comparison of schizophrenic delusions between Japan and Germany. *Psychopathology, 26*(3–4), 151–158. https://doi.org/10.1159/000284815

van Loon, A., van Schaik, A., Dekker, J., & Beekman, A. (2013). Bridging the gap for ethnic minority adult outpatients with depression and anxiety disorders by culturally adapted treatments. *Journal of Affective Disorders, 147*(1–3), 9–16. https://doi.org/10.1016/j.jad.2012.12.014

Verghese, A. (2008). Spirituality and mental health. *Indian Journal of Psychiatry, 50*(4), 233–237. https://doi.org/10.4103/0019-5545.44742

Verghese, A., John, J. K., Rajkumar, S., Richard, J., Sethi, B. B., & Trivedi, J. K. (1989). Factors associated with the course and outcome of schizophrenia in India. Results of a two-year multi-centre follow-up study. *The British Journal of Psychiatry: the Journal of Mental Science, 154*, 499–503. https://doi.org/10.1192/bjp.154.4.499

Wallace, P. M., Pomery, E. A., Latimer, A. E., Martinez, J. L., & Salovey, P. (2010). A review of acculturation measures and their utility in studies promoting Latino health. *Hispanic Journal of Behavioral Sciences, 32*(1), 37–54.

Whitbeck, L. B. (2006). Some guiding assumptions and a theoretical model for developing culturally specific preventions with Native American people. *Journal of Community Psychology, 34*(2), 183–192. https://doi.org/10.1002/jcop.20094

Wykes, T., Steel, C., Everitt, B., & Tarrier, N. (2008). Cognitive behavior therapy for schizophrenia: Effect sizes, clinical models, and methodological rigor. *Schizophrenia Bulletin, 34*(3), 523–537. https://doi.org/10.1093/schbul/sbm114

Zafar, S., Syed, R., Tehseen, S., Gowani, S. A., Waqar, S., Zubair, A., Yousaf, W., Zubairi, A. J., & Naqvi, H. (2008). Perceptions about the cause of schizophrenia and the subsequent help seeking behavior in a Pakistani population – Results of a cross-sectional survey. *BMC Psychiatry, 8*(1), 56. https://doi.org/10.1186/1471-244X-8-6

Chapter 8
The Power Threat Meaning Framework and 'Psychosis'

Matt Ball, Gareth Morgan, and Maria Haarmans

8.1 Introduction

> **Box 8.1: Background Information About Matt**
> Matt was born in England. He grew up in the family home with his parents and three older siblings. His father was an engineer and mother a teacher. Matt was brought up as a Methodist and his parents were involved in the church and sports communities. He experienced his family and the local community as full of hypocrisy given that he saw a discrepancy between the stated rules and the actual actions of adults in the home, school, and wider society. Matt had a sense at an early age of being on the edge of the community. The area in which the family lived was strongly conservative and he experienced being 'different' as contentious. Matt lived in fear of violence within the family home following his parents' separation.
>
> Matt was sociable and sporty at his state school, excelling at football and badminton. Although he enjoyed sport, he also felt he had to achieve to be

(continued)

M. Ball
Humane Clinic, Adelaide, Australia
e-mail: matt@humaneclinic.com.au

G. Morgan (✉)
University of Leicester, Leicester, UK
e-mail: gsm23@le.ac.uk

M. Haarmans
University of Manchester, Manchester, UK
e-mail: maria.haarmans@manchester.ac.uk

J. A. Díaz-Garrido et al. (eds.), *Psychological Interventions for Psychosis*,
https://doi.org/10.1007/978-3-031-27003-1_8

Box 8.1 (continued)

accepted. He began to find school difficult following a number of events, including childhood sexual abuse within an institutional setting, a threat to his life, his parents' divorce, and ongoing violence and threats which had started at the age of around 8 that, included school and neighbourhood bullying.

Around the age of 13 or 14 years, Matt experienced what was later termed a 'psychotic' episode. He was taken out of class, frightened and distressed having experienced voices, and visions of people on fire and an entity that was trying to consume him and his classmates. The teacher took him to the school nurse but did not tell his family about the experience. Matt felt he had to conceal things from his friends and family. His schooling suffered and he began to use various drugs. These responses were framed by others as misbehaviour or laziness rather than a sign of distress.

Matt's teen years were chaotic. He left school with no qualifications. He took various short term jobs, continued his drug use, and often felt suicidal. Aged 20, he went to Australia and found himself homeless. He ended up living in a parkland in Perth, and again had 'psychotic' experiences. Here he was supported by some local Aboriginal people who invited him to stay with them. Although a White man who had never previously experienced racism, Matt was impacted by racial attacks he experienced as a consequence of being identified with the Aboriginal people with whom he had found community.

Matt spent a short period in an immigration detention centre, where he experienced additional voices, before being removed back to the UK. There he was admitted to a psychiatric hospital at the age of 21, experiencing voices and beliefs about being observed and followed via street cameras. These beliefs were regarded as 'paranoia' by mental health professionals. He was diagnosed with 'psychotic depression' and was given multiple psychiatric drugs (several at the same time) and ECT against his will. Matt experienced being placed in seclusion (when not detained) and was threatened with detention on a number of occasions when he tried to leave. Over the next 15 months, he had five admissions and received a number of additional diagnoses including 'schizophrenia' and 'drug-induced psychosis'. Matt's problems were mainly viewed through a diagnostic lens and mental health staff regarded him as someone who had little hope of recovery.

The language used by professionals to describe Matt, the first author's experiences in Box 8.1 are in keeping with the medical model of distress that is dominant in Western mental health services. From this perspective, experiences such as perceiving things others do not, or beliefs others regard as unusual or 'paranoid', are viewed as 'symptoms' of underlying 'mental illness' (Coles, 2013). This paradigm neglects the fact that such experiences are understood very differently in other parts of the world (Read et al., 2013c; Taitimu et al., 2018), and that the majority of people who have such experiences are not significantly distressed by them (Kråkvik et al., 2015; van Os et al., 2000). Further neglected is the evidence linking 'psychosis' with a whole range of adversities, inequalities, and trauma (Johnstone & Boyle, 2018a, Chp. 4). Although few Western professionals would claim 'psychosis' should be understood in purely biological terms,[1] the common application of the 'bio-psycho-social' model has been critiqued for relegating adversities to mere triggers of underlying 'pathology' (Boyle, 2020; Harper et al., 2021): For example, the adversities Matt survived were regarded as triggering a presumed 'biological vulnerability'. This in turn resulted in his so-called psychotic experiences being viewed by professionals as meaningless abnormalities to be cured.

We use this chapter to describe how the Power Threat Meaning Framework (PTMF; Johnstone & Boyle, 2018a, b) can support a very different approach; one that has potential to render 'psychotic' responses understandable through restoring the links between such experiences and various forms of adversity and oppression. We use quote marks around the term 'psychosis' to emphasise that it is a contested construct. We agree with the argument that research should focus on specific phenomena, rather than grouping a range of experiences together under problematic labels that risk being misread as synonyms of 'disorder' (Read & Bentall, 2013). Thus, throughout the chapter, we refer to experiences such as 'hearing voices' ('hallucinations' in medical model language) or 'beliefs that others regard as unusual/paranoid' ('delusions'). However, like the PTMF authors, we sometimes use 'psychosis' as a short-hand because of its frequent usage within research, and because it is widely recognised within Western cultures to describe '…experiences outside of generally shared reality…which others often find difficult to understand' (Johnstone & Boyle, 2018a, p. 15).

We begin the chapter by providing a brief overview of the development of the PTMF. We then describe the interrelated constructs of 'Power', 'Threat', 'Meaning' and 'Threat Responses', the latter being the category experiences such as hearing voices and unusual beliefs that tend to fall under within the PTMF. In each section, we consider factors relating to the onset of experiences that come to be regarded as 'psychosis' and then go on to consider how the responses of Western mental health services can present further threats that might replicate or reinforce adversities a person has survived. We describe how the PTMF might be used to develop narratives that take into account a person's strengths and conclude by considering some of the potential benefits of a PTMF approach. Throughout each section, we reference how content relates to Matt's experience in order to illustrate how the PTMF can support narrative development. A slightly different account of Matt's narrative, along with reflections, can be accessed via the PTMF website: https://www.bps.org.uk/power-threat-meaning-framework/resources-training.

The PTMF emphasises that cultural context is of central importance in making sense of all elements of power, threat, meaning, and threat responses (Johnstone & Boyle, 2018a). It is important to observe that all authors have been raised and educated within the Global North. Although we include some reference to the ways

[1] In the UK for example, Department of Health guidelines for 'psychosis and schizophrenia' recommend cognitive behavioural therapy for 'psychosis' and screening for trauma reactions (NICE, 2014).

different meanings will be assigned to experiences such as voice hearing in non-Western cultures, the content of this chapter is biased towards responses to 'psychosis' in the Western mental health services we have used, researched, or practised within. We also recognise that relevant threats associated with the criminal justice system are not well-considered in this chapter.

8.2 The Power Threat Meaning Framework

The PTMF (Johnstone & Boyle, 2018a) was developed by a team of around 40 people, a third of whom had used mental health services, including Dr. Jacqui Dillon and Dr. Eleanor Longden, both members of the core PTMF group and prominent activists for the hearing voices communities. The first iteration of the PTMF was the culmination of a 5 year project, funded by the Division of Clinical Psychology, and freely downloadable via the British Psychological Society (https://www.bps.org.uk/power-threat-meaning-framework). It was an attempt to develop an alternative framework to the dominant medical model paradigm for conceptualising distress; a paradigm which, in spite of billions of dollars worth of research, continues to lack empirical support or biomarkers for any functional psychiatric diagnoses (e.g. Johnstone & Boyle, 2018a, Chp. 1; Timimi, 2020). The authors of the PTMF instead took the evidence base linking adversity, inequality, and discrimination to various manifestations of distress as a starting position to explore whether it might be possible to distil different patterns from this empirical body of work. This evidence base clearly indicates that there are no simple 'cause and effect' relationships between adversity and manifestations of distress because most stressors are associated with a whole range of distress responses and are all shaped by their meaning to the person in distress (Cromby et al., 2013, Chp. 6; Johnstone & Boyle, 2018a, Chps. 4 & 6). Further, it is not possible to neatly separate out different causal influences because surviving one form of adversity (e.g. poverty) increases the likelihood of surviving further adversities (e.g. racism or abuse). Evidence also indicates a 'dose-response' effect whereby each additional adversity encountered exponentially increases the risk that a person will experience significant distress (*ibid.*).

The Framework was thus developed with the aim of restoring the link between distress and social injustice. In doing so, the Framework centres '*power*' in making sense of all human experience, not just presentations that come to the attention of the psy-disciplines. When '*power*' acts negatively on a person, it is regarded as presenting '*threats*' to a person's core needs. People are not seen as passive in this process, but are active in giving '*meaning*' to the threats they experience. Rather than seeing the different manifestations of distress as either 'symptoms' or mere effects of adversity, the Framework regards such experiences, including those that come to be classed as 'psychotic,' as '*threat responses*', things a person *does,* consciously or otherwise, in order to mitigate the threats posed by the negative operations of power.

The PTMF does not dismiss the centrality of biology in human experience. Indeed, there is a whole chapter concerned with this (Johnstone & Boyle, 2018a, Chp. 5). However, drawing upon decades of research that show that life experiences impact upon brain development, neurotransmitter activity (e.g. Read, 2013a), and even gene expression (e.g. Cromby et al., 2019), the Framework builds upon other models that challenge the false trichotomy between mind, body, and the environment (e.g. Read et al., 2014) to advance the evidence-based argument that our experiences are all embodied. Biology is regarded as mediating our experiences and influencing the meanings and responses we take to adversities, but is not regarded as causal in making sense of distress or troubling behaviour (notable exceptions include distress relating to physical pain).

Use of the framework is centred around the following six questions, although narrative construction rarely would proceed in a linear fashion, and it is not essential to use these exact words or phrases (see Sect. 8.3):

1. How is *power* operating in your life?/What has happened to you?
2. What kinds of *threats* does this pose?/How did this affect you?
3. What is the *meaning* of these situations and experiences for you?/What sense did you make of it?
4. What kind of *threat responses* are you using?/What did you have to do to survive?
5. What access to power resources do you have?/What are your *strengths*?
6. How does this all fit together?/What is your *story*?

As will become apparent, the elements of Power, Threat, Meaning, and Threat Responses are interrelated and not readily separated. However, the different factors are separated out in the PTMF for purposes of supporting narrative development.

8.2.1 Power – 'What Has Happened to You?' (How Is Power Operating in Your Life?)

Following the calls of survivor activists (e.g. Longden, 2013), the PTMF was developed with an aim of reorientating mental health professionals from asking '*what is wrong with you*?' to '*what has happened to you*' through drawing attention to various operations of power in a person's life. Drawing upon works of writers such as Foucault (1977), Bourdieu (2010), and Smail (2005), the PTMF authors present an understanding of power as something that acts *through* individuals, relationships, social structures, and institutions, rather than something that individuals possess (Boyle, 2020). Power supports security, enabling a person to influence their environment to meet their needs and interests (Johnstone & Boyle, 2018a, b, Chp. 6). This element of the PTMF is primarily concerned with the negative operations of power in a person's life, while the ways in which power has operated in enabling and protective ways are considered under strengths (see Sect. 2.5).

Table 8.1 shows one possible taxonomy of power with particular focus on operations of power commonly associated with experiences such as hearing voices and suspicious or unusual beliefs. Some of the forms of power will be more apparent to mental health professionals and people accessing services than others. For example, while most professionals would likely recognise the potential harms of Coercive and Interpersonal Power, Ideological Power tends to be neglected within formulations. However, this form of power is regarded as one of the most important within the PTMF because it relates to the control of meaning and thus enables other forms of power. Transmitted through all aspects of society, such as through media,

Table 8.1 A non-exhaustive taxonomy of power

Form of power	Examples of operations of power associated with increased prevalence of experiences such as voice hearing, suspicious beliefs, and unusual beliefs
Coercive Power: Power by force, using violence and aggression, or threats of aggression.	Bullying; victimisation; physical and sexual abuse/violence; threats of harm; war; forced displacement. Within mental health services: coercion to accept unwanted interventions (e.g. 'antipsychotic' medication), restraint & seclusion
Interpersonal Power: The power to support/not support others in a range of ways and to promote or deny relational security, support, love, and validation.	Discrimination; marginalisation; neglect; forced separation from attachment figures or dependents; bereavement; social isolation; reduced control over when and who one can have contact with; lack of trust and cooperation within a community
Legal Power: The use of the law to support or inhibit needs, protection, and justice.	Degree to which legal/safeguarding frameworks support a person to be safer from abuse or discrimination; degree to which attachment figures are supported with caregiving; racial profiling by law enforcers; stop and search powers; probation requirements; legal processes around children in care; compulsory hospitalisation/'interventions'; imprisonment; legal requirements to disclose 'mental health problems'
Economic and Material Power: The ability to acquire, control, or access economic and material resources. The inheritance or acquisition of additional material resources enables many other forms of power, including maintaining positions within social hierarchies.	Poverty; inequality; poor access to green spaces; people with devalued identities more likely to be housed in more deprived areas; homelessness
Social/Cultural Capital: Access to valued cultural resources such as education, knowledge, connections with high-standing individuals within a society.	Devalued within family/community; member of a devalued/oppressed group; living in poverty makes it harder to fit into socially valued roles; barriers to employment & education due to stigma and discrimination associated with diagnosis; less desirable as a romantic partner due to stigma associated with the diagnosis; people more likely to be fearful of the person due to stereotypes of violence

(continued)

Table 8.1 (continued)

Form of power	Examples of operations of power associated with increased prevalence of experiences such as voice hearing, suspicious beliefs, and unusual beliefs
Embodied Power: The embodied attributes which may or may not be valued within a given society, such as strength, physical health, fertility, appearance, and so on.	Adversity impacts upon brain development (c.f. traumagenic model of psychosis, Read et al., 2014); pain or physical illness; inability to manage day to day tasks without adequate support being provided; having a physical appearance or impairment that does not conform to socially constructed ideals for a given culture; having darker skin within racist societies that regard 'white' skin as 'the norm' (it is important to emphasise that Embodied Power should be understood as an interaction between bodies and social structures); impacts on cognitive functioning from drugs (prescribed or otherwise) or physical abuse; impairment due to ECT
Ideological Power: The control of meaning; this form of power is transmitted through all aspects of a given society.	Whiteness/institutionalised racism, white supremacy; patriarchy, ableism; heteronormativity; religious discourses; ideas about spirit possession; intersectional oppression discourses; discourses about 'madness' and 'mental illness'; neoliberal discourses that imply the poor deserve to be poor; imposition of disordered identities through diagnosis; difficulties attributed to genetics or 'disordered brains'; discourses about non-compliance with 'medication' being associated with increased risk; refusal to accept diagnosis regarded as sign the person 'lacks insight'; lived experience and adversity regarded as irrelevant by dominance of medical model understandings; voices and unusual beliefs regarded as 'symptoms' without meaning or function
Ecological Power (Morgan et al., 2022): The degree to which one's environment supports or inhibits key physical needs such as access to food and shelter, protection from extreme weather events. Also includes the degree to which a person can feel connected to nature and a person/community's ability to nurture local ecosystems.	Reduced access to green spaces; extreme weather events or displacement caused by climate breakdown

Adapted from Johnstone and Boyle (2018a, pp. 206–207)

education, advertising, interactions with peers, and so forth, Ideological Power can result in us coming to accept certain ways of being as 'normal', natural, or inevitable (Boyle, 2020; Johnstone & Boyle, 2018a).

Power and the Emergence of 'Psychosis' Research consistently shows that power inequalities are associated with distressing voices and unusual beliefs. There is strong evidence that negative operations of Coercive and Interpersonal Power, such as bullying, violence, sexual, emotional, and physical abuse, are associated with increased chances of voice hearing or suspicious/unusual beliefs (e.g. Bentall et al., 2014; Moskowitz et al., 2019; Varese et al., 2012). Abusers often intentionally target disempowered individuals, such as children or people with intellectual disability diagnoses because these people have reduced Social Capital and thus will be less likely to be believed if they speak out (e.g. Hollomotz, 2009; Warner, 2000). Adult abusers tend to be physically stronger than child victims (Embodied Power), who will be less able to stop abusive acts by physical resistance. Control of economic resources (Economic Power) or threats of harm to loved ones (Interpersonal Power) are also common within abusive relationships (Hamby, 2014; Postmous et al., 2012). Being placed into care as a child is another risk factor for 'psychosis' (e.g. Longden et al., 2016) that, like abuse, occurs within asymmetrical power relationships in which the child has little control over what is happening to them. Both being placed into care and being subjected to abuse increase the risk of exposure to further adversities (*ibid*). Further evidence for the relevance of asymmetrical power relationships comes from findings that people who are more distressed by voice or unusual belief content are significantly more likely to have been abused or have reduced Interpersonal and Social Capital Power compared to voice hearers with greater access to power resources (Bailey et al., 2018; Birchwood et al., 2004).

Being subjected to racism (e.g. Halvorsrud et al., 2019; Read et al., 2013b) or other forms of discrimination (e.g. Janssen et al., 2003) have also been linked to increased rates of 'psychosis'. That increased incidence of psychosis decreases for people from minoritised-ethnic groups when they live in areas with relatively high density of the same ethnic group suggests Social and Cultural Capital play a part in the elevated risk at the population level (e.g. das Munshi et al., 2012). Institutionalised discrimination results in intersectional barriers with, for example, people, from minoritised ethnic groups and people with intellectual disability diagnoses being less likely to have access to economic and community resources (Economic and Material Power) that would support escape from unsafe communities or relationships. Indeed, poverty has been described as 'perhaps the most powerful predictor of psychosis out of all the risk factors' (Read & Bentall, 2013, p. 266). As well as presenting threats to meeting basic physical needs, poverty is also associated with reduced Social Capital Power due to the devalued position of unemployed people and the working class within neoliberal societies that measure an individual's worth against status, possessions, and income (e.g. Timimi, 2020). The status quo is supported by Ideological Power, through discourses linked with legacies of colonialism, patriarchy, ableism, heteronormativity, humancentricism etc. that legitimise structural inequities; to make people think 'this is the natural way of the world' (c.f 'whiteness', e.g. Wood & Patel, 2017). Thus, whether a person is racially oppressed or benefits from institutional racism, neoliberal societies socialise people into regarding structural inequalities as inevitable, reflecting the natural order of things (c.f. internalised racism, ableism, etc.). The dominance of neoliberal ideals in supposedly meritocratic societies influences people to see poverty as a fault of the poor and wealth justified by merit: The structural inequalities and imbalances of other forms of power are obscured (Boyle, 2020).

Embodied Power is also relevant, as adversity, oppression, and abuse, particularly within the developmental period, impact upon brain development. For example, there is evidence indicating that adversity can result in changes to the brain that result in subsequent life events being more likely to be experienced as threatening or stressful (Read et al., 2014). The effects of power can be embodied in the impact of physical or sexual violence, as well as the processes involved in psychologically threatening operations of power that manifest in the way a person perceives and indeed experiences the embodied impact (van der Kolk, 2014).

Power and Western Mental Health Services Ideological Power operates to frame how experiences such as hearing voices or unusual beliefs are understood and responded to when people come into contact with services. 'Psychosis' and 'schizophrenia' are constructs that, since their creation, have been deployed by people in positions of power to classify and 'treat' the range of experiences such as voice hearing that have been coded 'abnormal' by Western psy-disciplines (Coles, 2013; Read & Bentall, 2013). While dominant discourses about 'mental (ill)health' and 'madness' may have already shaped how a person makes sense of experiences such as voice hearing before they access services, it is not until contact with mental health professionals that labels such as 'psychosis' or 'schizophrenia' are imposed. Diagnosis enables further use of Coercive and Legal Power, resulting in people being forced or persuaded to 'accept' medical interventions. While some people do report benefits from use of tranquilisers ('antipsychotics'), only around 20% of people report significant benefits (Division of Clinical Psychology (DCP), 2017). ECT has a similarly poor evidence base (Read et al., 2013a). These medical 'interventions' often result in reduced Embodied Power that in turn will impact how a person can respond to subsequent life stressors: ECT has been linked with memory and other cognitive problems (*ibid.*); while tranquiliser ('antipsychotic') use has been linked to tiredness, apathy, stiffness, problems in sexual functioning, muscle spasms, emotional flattening, sedation, cognitive impairment, and reduced brain matter (DCP, 2017; Moncrieff, 2013). Yet 'medication' remains the default response of mental health services in most Western nations, in part because of the operations of Ideological Power supporting the interests of psychiatry (e.g. O'Donoghue & Crossley, 2020) and the billion dollar pharmaceutical industry that continues to promote unsubstantiated claims that the drugs address 'chemical imbalances' and reduce risk (e.g. Davies, 2013; Moncrieff, 2013). We can see the intersection of Coercive, Legal and Ideological Power when people are chemically incarcerated or when professionals do not provide people with sufficient information about the effects and effectiveness of the drugs to enable informed consent. 'Consent' is further manufactured through the use of unsubstantiated claims about the legitimacy of 'mental illness' and the 'chemical imbalances' the drugs are marketed as addressing (*ibid.*).

Stigma and discrimination associated with imposed disordered identities result in decreased Social Capital, whereby a person's perspectives and wishes become more readily dismissed, compounding existing inequalities relating to, for example, poverty, racism, ableism, etc. While a diagnosis might support access to welfare benefits or legal safeguards, being identified with these labels results in barriers to employment, education, and opportunities to form relationships in which a person feels valued (e.g. Royal College of Psychiatrists, 2021). Consequently, a person's Interpersonal, Economic and Social Capital power resources are further depleted. Ideological Power again operates to justify these exclusionary practices and also supports the increased rates of incarceration due to dominant discourses that position such individuals as 'disordered', 'mad', or 'dangerous' (Morgan & Felton, 2013).

Given the subjectivity and unreliability of the 'schizophrenia' diagnostic criteria (Read, 2013b), power clearly plays a part in decisions about what beliefs constitute a 'delusion' or not: For example, widespread and dangerous denial of the threats of the climate crisis would not be regarded as delusional in spite of evidence to the contrary, simply because such beliefs are not regarded as unusual in Western society due to operations of Ideological Power that disconnect people from threats posed by climate breakdown (Morgan et al., 2022). Similarly, professionals who are not well-oriented to the social-realities of the people who have survived hate crimes will commonly label a person's concerns about victimisation as 'paranoid', while other beliefs labelled as 'delusional' will be rarely checked by services, in spite of there often being elements of truth in people's accounts (Harper, 2011). Similarly, people from non-Western cultures might be more likely to have their beliefs regarded as 'delusional' simply because they differ from the belief systems of the Western-educated professionals (Metzl, 2011). This decontextualised approach to assessment, in which a person's beliefs are not explored in relation to lived experience and culture, is aided by operations of Ideological Power that perpetuate the view that unusual beliefs are 'symptoms' of a biologically based disorder (Coles, 2013; Harper et al., 2021). The unquestioned assumptions that position White-Western belief systems as the norm (Wood & Patel, 2017) and racist discourses that perpetuate stereotypes about Black 'dangerousness' and 'madness' enable the perpetuation of institutionalised racism within mental health services (Metzl, 2011). In the UK, Black Caribbean and Black African people are five times more likely to receive a 'psychosis' related diagnosis, experience coercive pathways to care (e.g. police and criminal justice system; detention under the Mental Health Act), and receive biomedical as opposed to talking therapies (Bhui et al., 2018; Fernando, 2017; Halvorsrud et al., 2019; Read et al., 2013b). People with intellectual dis/abilities are also more likely to be prescribed drugs and restrictive interventions (Branford et al., 2019), while throughout history, labels of 'schizophrenia' and 'madness' have been deployed to incarcerate political dissenters (Fernando, 2017).

Power and Matt's Narrative Had professionals sought to connect with Matt and learn about some of the adversities he survived (Box 8.1 and Table 8.2), they may have recognised that the content of his voices and his beliefs about being monitored did not spontaneously emerge as 'symptoms', but could be linked to experiences of abuse, bullying, and significant threats to his life associated with his sense of being an outsider. Just as asymmetrical power relationships within the educational system resulted in Matt's communications of distress being framed as deficits in his character ('lazy', 'disruptive'), operations of power enacted through mental health professionals resulted in Matt internalising a 'disordered' identity through their medicalised framing of his threat responses. Ironically, Matt's concerns about being

Table 8.2 Operations of power Matt identified as relevant to his experience

Operations of power	Factors associated with the emergence of 'psychosis'	Responses by mental health services
Coercive/ power by force	Threats and violence in the home, school, and neighbourhood; sexual abuse	Coercion to take psychiatric drugs and ECT
Interpersonal	Bullying (school and neighbourhood); violence and threat inside and outside the family; criticism, invalidation of his views	Seclusion in hospital; reduced social network
Legal	Detention in immigration centre. Being removed to the UK	Detained against his will in a mental health ward; legal frameworks enabling coercion to take psychiatric drugs & ECT
Economic and material	Homelessness, lack of money, unemployment	Benefit recipient; barriers to employment due to diagnosis
Social/cultural capital	Despite a comfortable start in life, loss of status due to becoming homeless; Lack of opportunity due to interrupted schooling; discrimination towards the Aboriginal people he had found community with when homeless	Psychiatric patient and consequent lack of access to resources; invalidation of his views due to diagnosis
Biological/ embodied	Loss of sporting activities. Physical harm, e.g. physical neglect and poor nutrition while homeless	Psychiatric drugs including high doses and polypharmacy, ECT
Ideological power	As a child, impact of religion and conservatism, and sense of isolation due to non-conformity. Disagreeing with school rules and expectations. Ideological power enacted to silence Matt from speaking out about abuse	Imposition of identity of 'mental patient' and made to think of self as 'mentally ill'; in need of medical treatment

monitored were reinforced by the continual invasion of his privacy when an inpatient. At a time of acute crisis, Matt was subjected to forced detainment and coerced into taking drugs and ECT which reduced Embodied Power via sedation, disorientation, change in body shape, and appearance. The labels of 'schizophrenia' further impacted status and role in the community. Beginning to explore some of the ways that power operates negatively on an individual's life can support people to shift from making sense of problems in terms of a 'mental illness' identity to recognition of the multiple adversities a person has survived.

8.2.2 *Threat: 'How Did It Affect You?' (What Kind of Threats Does This Pose?)*

When power operates negatively, it poses threats to our abilities to meet core human needs, such as the need to feel loved and valued, to have proximity to attachment figures, to have our needs for food and shelter met, and our need to be safe from physical harm. Threat in the PTMF is thus inseparable from the operations of power.

Threats and the Emergence of 'Psychosis' As will be evident from the section above, many of the risk factors for experiences such as hearing voices or unusual beliefs relate to violence and abuse, which can present threats of physical danger, bodily invasion, powerlessness, loss of agency and control, and emotional overwhelm/dysregulation. The embodied experiences of sexual abuse may include ongoing physiological responses and altered bodily and sexual sensations (akin to what psychiatry calls 'somatic or olfactory hallucinations'), while dissociation during abuse can result in multiple situations triggering flashbacks that present threats in the present (van der Kolk, 2014). Being placed into care can be associated with threats of abandonment, powerlessness, rejection, and attachment loss, whilst experiences of discrimination and oppression can result in threats such as exclusion, marginalisation, 'othering', physical danger, loss or devaluing of social role, and material deprivation (see Johnstone & Boyle, 2018b, Chp. 4). This devaluing of a person's self-concept and identity can extend to the devaluing of a person's group identities, as was the case for Matt, who encountered threats due to the racism directed towards Aboriginal people he had become reliant upon during a time in his life he was particularly disempowered. Many people have linked experiences of unusual beliefs and voice hearing to threats associated with spiritual or existential crises (Clarke, 2013).

While voice hearing and unusual beliefs are primarily conceptualised as threat responses in the PTMF, it is recognised that such experiences can in themselves pose direct and indirect threats. For example, the content of voices will often replicate experiences of invalidation and blame of abusers in addition to reflecting social categories and structural inequalities in society (Haarmans et al., 2016). Talking out loud with voices or acting upon beliefs that others regard as bizarre can result in aggression or marginalisation from others.

Threats from Western Mental Health Services The negative operations of power associated with service responses often replicate the threats that led many users of services to seek support in the first place (Johnstone, 2000). Threats of epistemic injustice occur when a person's individual or cultural meaning-making is dismissed through the imposition of medicalised framings of their distress by relatively powerful professionals (Kinouani, 2019; Spivak, 1988). Such experiences not only mirror the threats of devaluing a person's self-worth and powerlessness associated with the silencing and dismissal of survivors of abuse or oppression (*ibid.*), but use of diagnostic language enables further dehumanisation and reduced clinician empathy (Lebowitz & Ahn, 2014; Pavon & Vaes, 2017). A person may experience further isolation, powerlessness, and lack of control if they are detained. Some may re-experience bodily threats if coerced into reliving trauma without sufficient attention given to developing threat responses that will support them in undertaking trauma-focussed work (Kezelman & Stavropoulos, 2012). Professionals who experience various domains of privilege risk perpetuating threats of marginalisation, stereotyping and othering in interactions with service-users, especially through not directly acknowledging systemic and institutional threats such as racism, sexism, ableism, and other forms of oppression and their impact on wellbeing (e.g. Haydon-Laurelet et al., 2013; Metzl, 2011; Pons, 2019; Warner, 2009).

Threats and Development of Matt's Narrative Table 8.3 shows threats Matt survived as a consequence of negative operations of power. As is often the case, the threats Matt survived prior to hospitalisation were replicated within the mental health system. For example, Matt had already been exposed to violence and was then subjected to ECT; Matt was already struggling to find his own identity rather than having others' views imposed on him, and subsequently had his identity defined by medical professionals and diagnostic language. Ironically, the replication of being watched and controlled in the mental health system could be seen as mirroring the sense of being watched and controlled in previous threat situations.

Table 8.3 Threats identified by Matt as relevant to his experiences

Type of threat (Johnstone & Boyle, 2018a)	Threats survived before entering services	Threats posed by mental health services
Relationships	Lack of emotional and physical safety, abandonment, rejection, shaming, isolation, invalidation	Lack of emotional and physical safety, shaming, isolation, not being heard by professionals
Emotional	Emotionally overwhelmed and despairing	Despairing, powerlessness
Social/ community	Isolation, rejection, bullying, invalidation, loss of social role and status, marginalisation	Invalidation, loss of social role and status, marginalisation, powerlessness
Economic/ material	Financial insecurity, lack of housing, unemployment, consequences of homelessness	Lack of housing choice, unemployable
Environmental	Living in unsafe areas	Confined to hospital, lack of choice in geographical location
Embodied/bodily	Unmet material needs, exposure to violence and sexual abuse	Impact of psychiatric drugs and ECT – weight gain, akathisia, sedation, cognitive impairment
Values, identity, and meaning-making	Discouraged from making own meanings, being heard, or finding own values and identity; dissent from social, community, and school norms; having meanings and identities imposed, including those associated with 'mental illness'.	Invalidation of personal ideas and perspectives of what was happening and the meanings of distress, including double bind like experiences, i.e. you have to take responsibility to get better, but you have a biological condition and you have to accept treatment. Discouraged from finding own values and identity; including spiritual, religious, sexuality related or other ideas to understand experiences. Having meanings and identities imposed, including those associated with 'mental illness'.

8.2.3 *Meaning: 'What Sense Did You Make of It?' (What Is the Meaning of These Situations and Experiences to You?)*

Meaning is regarded as the thread that holds the other aspects of the PTMF together as it mediates the relationship between threats and the specific threat responses a person enacts (Boyle & Johnstone, 2020). The term 'meaning' is understood differently to common usage in much Western psychology. For example, although it is recognised that individuals are active agents in making sense of their experiences, the PTMF authors draw upon the work of John Shotter to argue we are not free to interpret events as we please. Meaning is instead understood as being shaped and constrained by operations of power (predominantly Ideological Power) and the availability of shared language to describe experiences (Cromby, 2020; Johnstone & Boyle, 2018a, Chp. 3). Meaning is further constrained by memories of adversities we have survived (e.g. abuse perpetuated by people who are meant to care for us will impact on meaning-making of subsequent interactions with others claiming to care for us) as well as by function of the autonomic nervous system (high levels of arousal will impact upon meanings ascribed to particular threats in a given moment). Another difference is that the Framework does not regard meaning-making as occurring exclusively at the level of thought. Instead, it is recognised that meanings (e.g. shame) involve cognitive, affective, and bodily aspects that cannot readily be disentangled (*ibid.*). This conceptualisation is more congruent with the fact that some cultures do not differentiate between cognitions and emotions (Cromby, 2020). The broader understanding of meaning also supports recognition that young infants and adults with severe intellectual disabilities make meaning of their experiences even without verbal abilities (Skelly et al., 2017).

Meanings Associated with Emergence of 'Psychosis' The multiple threats associated with increased likelihood of 'psychosis' have been linked to various meanings in empirical research. Experiences of abuse, for example, in conjunction with various operations of ideological power deployed via abusers and society can result in meanings of shame, being unsafe, being powerless, of being contaminated/dirty/bad and so forth. Similarly, parental neglect has led to children developing a sense of being unworthy and undeserving, as well as a sense that others will not meet their needs (e.g. Johnstone & Boyle, 2018a; Warner, 2000). Experiences of discrimination, inequality, victimisation, and oppression can result in meanings of exclusion, shame, humiliation, entrapment, inferiority, worthlessness, powerlessness, anger, and injustice/unfairness (Johnstone & Boyle, 2018b). Highlighting the effects of internalised racism and patriarchy, Haarmans et al. (2016) found that racialised women reported racist voice content and almost all women, including White women, reported gendered insults.

Meanings Associated with 'Psychosis' Meaning-making of so-called psychotic experiences will be shaped by cultural and service level discourses. For many in the

Global North, meaning-making of voice hearing will be shaped by operations of Ideological Power that suggest experiences are signs of 'madness'. Such meanings are reinforced when relatively powerful professionals tell disempowered patients that their experiences are *caused* by a brain disorder. This form of epistemic injustice can have the effect of making an individual feel misguided if they had made sense of their experiences through a different lens. As was the case with Matt's experience, a person may internalise the disordered identity resulting in meanings of shame or defectiveness (Johnstone & Boyle, 2018b), supported by findings that so-called insight (conceptualised by researchers as indicating greater acceptance of one's 'schizophrenia' diagnosis) is associated with negative outcomes such as increased hopelessness (e.g. López-Moríñigo et al., 2012). Alternatively, a person may recognise the invalidation of their meaning-making by services, resulting in meanings of powerlessness, betrayal, anger, or fear.

Epistemic injustice might be more significant when imposition of medicalised understandings dismiss an entire community's sense-making of experiences. Indeed, the exportation of Western medical models to the Global South as part of Global Mental Health agendas has been critiqued as an extension of colonialist practices (Fernando, 2014; Summerfield, 2012). The view that voices or unusual beliefs are meaningless 'symptoms' is specific to the Western mental health service context and is understood differently in other parts of the world (Read et al., 2013c). It is not uncommon, for example, for experiences such as voice hearing or disconnection from reality to be regarded as signs of wisdom, as abilities to communicate with deceased ancestors or spirits (e.g. Taitimu et al., 2018). Consequently, people might experience meanings such as worthiness or gifted in relation to voice hearing, or they might have a sense of comfort and connection if they experience themselves conversing with a dead relative. Similar sense-making of visions or voices can occur for White people who identify with a Western-subculture (Clarke, 2013; DCP, 2017). The PTMF emphasises the importance of considering the way the cultural context will inform meaning-making and cautions against imposing different understandings upon people (Johnstone, 2019).

Supporting the PTMF position that meaning is embodied, recent research has indicated that specific instances of voice hearing often co-occur with perceiving things others cannot via other sensory modalities, bodily sensations (e.g. heaviness, tiredness), differing levels of arousal, and emotional sensations, to which participants attributed descriptive meanings such as 'fear', 'powerlessness', or 'boredom' (Melvin et al., 2021). Suspicious beliefs unsurprisingly can be associated with meanings of being unsafe and are commonly co-occurring with hyperarousal within bodies (Cromby & Harper, 2013). Other forms of unusual beliefs will have meaning for people and will make sense in the context of lived experience (e.g. Coles, 2013).

Meaning and Development of Matt's Narrative Meanings of shame and self-criticism were reinforced for Matt when professionals described him as 'mentally ill'. Matt internalised the disordered identity assigned to him and he came to experience himself as 'sick', 'abnormal', and 'unacceptable to society'. Matt consequently felt hopeless about future change and came to think that he was not capable of supporting himself. These meanings were not static, and at other times Matt resisted the imposition of a disordered identity. However, powerful professionals responded to Matt's resistance (threat responses) by labelling him as 'oppositional', 'non-compliant', and 'risky', resulting in Matt at times accepting their meaning that he 'lacked insight' into 'his illness', a meaning which not only implied defectiveness on Matt's part but simultaneously placed the professionals as the ones with the power to speak the truth about him. Had the professionals attended to the adversities Matt had survived and the meanings he had attributed to the experiences they regarded as 'symptoms', they might have been better able to recognise and respond to him as a whole person.

8.2.4 Threat Responses: 'What Did You Have to Do to Survive?' (What Kinds of Threat Response Are You Using?)

Thus far, we have considered Power, Threat, and Meaning in relation to the onset of voice hearing and unusual beliefs and the responses of Western mental health services. However, these types of experiences are primarily understood as *threat responses* within the PTMF; responses people have developed to survive or mitigate against the threats posed by the negative operations of power. Some threat responses may be protective in moments of acute threat. Others (e.g. isolating oneself) may be enacted as they limit exposure to potential threats, and yet others may be helpful as they enable access to power resources, for example, by supporting a person's position within social hierarchies, or facilitating inclusion within a community. Table 8.4 lists example threat responses grouped by some of the functions these responses might serve for different individuals. Many of the threat responses listed would be classed as 'symptoms' in medical-model understandings, including those often labelled 'psychotic'. However, responses such as compulsive overworking are rarely pathologised within overdeveloped Western nations. Use of a PTMF approach can thus support consideration of the more creative and unusual ways people can respond to a range of adversities (e.g. Matt's emigration to Australia, use of sport and itinerant lifestyle).

The threat responses a person enacts are influenced by the meanings ascribed to the threats, the culture the person lives within (different threat responses will be viewed differently across cultures), the intensity of the threats, and the power resources available to a person. Those with less power resources will have a more limited range of threat responses available to them. For example, a person living in poverty (i.e. lacking Economic Power) would be less able to go shopping for unneeded items (a response that is unfortunately widely celebrated within overdeveloped Western countries). Similarly, low Social Capital or Interpersonal Power would reduce opportunities for getting one's emotional and relational needs met by others, meaning we might adopt less socially sanctioned threat responses such as compulsive use of alcohol or substances, self-injury, 'anti-social behaviour', and so

Table 8.4 Example threat responses grouped by function

Function	Example threat responses (italicised text illustrates responses that often get labelled as 'psychosis' within the medical model)	Threat responses Matt utilised
Regulating overwhelming feelings	*Dissociation*, self-injury, *memory fragmentation*, bingeing and purging, differential memory encoding, *carrying out rituals*, intellectualisation, 'high' mood, low mood, *hearing voices*, use of alcohol and drugs, *compulsive activity of various kinds,* overeating, denial, *unusual beliefs,* projection, splitting, *derealisation*, somatic sensations, bodily numbing, shopping	Hearing voices, visual images, suicidal feelings, drugs and alcohol, leaving the country, finding communities to live among (a homeless community and a therapeutic community)
Protection from physical danger	Hypervigilance, insomnia, flashbacks, nightmares, fight/flight/ freeze, *suspicious thoughts*, *voice hearing,* isolation, aggression	Hypervigilance; suspicious beliefs about others' actions, voice hearing, itinerant lifestyle, non-adherence to medication
Maintaining a sense of control	Self-starvation, rituals, violence, dominance in relationships, *unusual beliefs*	Rebelling, rituals, saying what was expected and accepted, recognising threats through alternative means, i.e. unusual beliefs about being followed and watched, arguing with psychiatrist about medication, secrecy
Seeking attachments	Idealisation, appeasement, seeking care and emotional responses, use of sexuality, 'anti-social' behaviour, self-injury	Befriending the hospital priest and attending church despite no beliefs in the Christian ideology
Protection against attachment loss, hurt, and abandonment	Rejection of others, *distrust*, seeking care and emotional responses, submission, self-blame, interpersonal violence, hoarding, appeasement, self-silencing, self-punishment	Distrust, self-punishment, self-silencing, isolating self, at times not speaking, excelling at sport
Preserving identity, self-image, and self-esteem	*Grandiosity*, *unusual beliefs*, feeling entitled, perfectionism, striving, dominance, hostility, aggression, acquiring material goods, *voice-hearing*	Unusual beliefs; considering identity in 'obsessive' way, pretending to be 'okay', 'rebelling' in not accepting medical opinion
Preserving a place within the social group	Striving, competitiveness, appeasement, self-silencing, self-blame, acquiring material goods/wealth	Unusual expressions, expressing the words and behaviours that were considered acceptable. Excelling at sport, engaging in social groups, lying and concealing to find acceptance
Meeting emotional needs/ self-soothing	Rocking, self-harm, skin-picking, bingeing, alcohol use, overeating, compulsive sexuality	Drugs use, isolation, passivity (accepting others views) in health and other settings.
Communication about distress, elicit care	Self-injury, *unusual beliefs*, *voice-hearing*, self-starvation	Unusual beliefs, self-injury, voice hearing, seeing visions (as a child)
Finding meaning and purpose	*Unusual beliefs*, overwork, high moods	Unusual beliefs

Adapted from Johnstone and Boyle (2018a, p. 203)

forth. As well as being grouped by function, threat responses can be understood to be on a spectrum, from those that are more amenable to our control, even if difficult to stop (e.g. perfectionism, self-injury, use of alcohol) to those that are associated with the functioning of the autonomic nervous system and other bodily reactions that are not within our control (e.g. fight/flight/freeze responses; dissociation). We will be more likely to use the latter type of threat response when the intensity of the threats far outweighs the power resources we have available to protect us. The types of threat responses that get labelled as 'psychosis' fall towards this end of the spectrum, which is unsurprising given the severity of threats linked to these experiences, the asymmetrical power relationships these threats occur within, and the casual literature suggesting these threat responses are commonly associated with surviving multiple adversities (see Sects. 8.2.1 and 8.2.2).

Threat Responses That Are Labelled 'Psychosis' Perceiving things others cannot has been linked to dissociation, a threat response that occurs when a person protects against awareness of intolerable events by shutting off from what is happening to them, resulting in memories of experiences and events being encoded in fractured, unassimilated ways (Varese et al., 2012; Warner, 2000). These memories may come back in the form of voices of abusers or somatic sensations and may be experienced as emanating from elsewhere, or experienced as events happening to someone else and not oneself, in order to protect against overwhelming emotion or intolerable knowledge (Johnstone & Boyle, 2018a; Longden et al., 2012). Hearing or seeing things others cannot has likewise been linked to occasions when our abilities to 'source monitor' (i.e. to accurately make judgements about what is real or imaginary) are impaired (Bentall, 1990). High levels of arousal or states of altered consciousness brought about by various threats such as grief, abuse, violence, and the effects of sleep deprivation or drugs, all may make such judgements harder and we may then come to experience internal thoughts as voices, images, and so forth (DCP, 2017; Johnstone & Boyle, 2018a, p. 110). Source monitoring is regarded as more difficult when the content of the material is critical or highly distressing, as is often the case when surviving abuse or discrimination, because this content presents further threats and thus increases arousal. Experiencing the content as emanating from somewhere else, as opposed to one's own mind, may protect against threats of emotional overwhelm. Source monitoring will be further impaired when encountering situations associated with past adversity. Hearing voices in such circumstances may thus serve the function of protecting us from harm if their content warns us certain people or situations are dangerous, as was Matt's experience, and is common among people who have been groomed and thus are understandably wary of the intentions of others.

Of course, many people hear voices that say warm or supportive things. For some, these voices have been reported to serve functions of providing comfort, supporting emotional regulation, protecting against distress associated with the loss of a loved one, or to protecting against threats to identity (it is not uncommon for people to experience both critical and reassuring voices) (Parker et al., 2021). Perceiving things others cannot may also protect against threats associated with spiritual crises; however, we recognise that such experiences would unlikely be viewed as 'threat responses' in cultures that regard voice hearing as evidence of abilities to converse with spirits or deities.

Suspicious beliefs provide important protective effects for people who have been victims of psychological or sexual abuse, bullying, or discrimination as they can support reducing threats of being taken advantage of or harmed by others. Such beliefs risk being labelled 'paranoid' by professionals who might be overly suspicious of the rationality of a person's sense of threat, sometimes failing to recognise the threats of harm or invasions of privacy a person is enduring in their daily lives (Harper, 2011). Grandiosity or other unusual beliefs a person might have relating to abilities can serve to protect against threats associated with significantly compromised self-esteem and identity, whilst beliefs about persecution or being targeted could, for some, protect against threats of feeling unrecognised (it may be less painful to experience oneself as the centre of a conspiracy than as someone of seeming insignificance). Unusual beliefs may also serve functions of protecting against emotional overwhelm if the belief supports a person in remaining disconnected from other threats.

Threat Responses Associated with Surviving Mental Health Services Suspicious beliefs about the intentions of professionals claiming to want to help people accessing services are also understandable in the context of people's lived experiences. Such distrust can be understood as protective, especially when therapists use similar tactics as abusers to gain trust, such as warmth and praise (Warner, 2000), or when the power professionals have over people's lives replicates experiences of powerlessness or being controlled that a person has previously endured. Seemingly 'irrational' beliefs about professionals trying to poison a person when professionals tell patients the unsubstantiated claim that drugs correct 'chemical imbalances' in a person's brain also can be understood as protective, both in terms of protecting against lack of control and bodily invasion, and for protecting against unwanted side effects of the drugs. Intentional disengagement with services can thus be viewed as serving different functions for different people at different times. Resistance to accepting 'schizophrenic' or 'mental illness' labels can be understood as protecting against threats to further devaluate a person's identity and the subsequent consequences of a pejorative label (e.g. discrimination, exclusion, stigma) (Sayce, 1998).

Conversely, people may comply with what they believe professionals want them to do. In some cases, this might be because a person has learnt threat responses of appeasing to avoid harm by powerful others. Some survivors of psychiatric systems have described using acquiescence in order to be discharged from a service, sometimes affirming to professionals that they had been 'ill' but, thanks to the professional's input, they were now 'better' (e.g. Dillon, 2019; Johnstone, 2000). We might use compliance and acquiescence at times of crisis because deference to powerful others can serve to protect against feeling helpless or uncared for, whilest acceptance of disordered identities can offer hope for recovery and removal of threats associated with self-blame (Johnstone & Boyle, 2018b). Coming to accept the problem as being in one's biology or as part of one's identity can be less hurtful than connecting with ideas about attachment figures acting in harmful or neglectful ways, having to recall potentially overwhelming memories of past adversities, or feeling powerless in the face of oppression, inequality, and toxic societal structures (*ibid.*). However, as is evident in Matt and others' stories, seeing difficulties as a 'symptom' of a 'chronic mental illness' presents further threats associated with meanings of being 'abnormal' or 'disordered' (see Sects. 8.2.2 and 8.2.3; Delano, 2013, 2019; Longden, 2013).

Threat Responses and Development of Matt's Narrative Some of the threat responses Matt utilised to cope with the multiple adversities he survived are displayed in Table 8.4. Now that consideration has been given to the threats and meaning of these threats for Matt, what previously might have been regarded as meaningless 'symptoms' can be recognised as serving important functions. PTMF threat responses do not correspond to psychiatric 'symptoms', which is why we can include secrecy, trying to be accepted, and going to Australia as some of the creative ways Matt tried to survive. Matt's voices came to be understood by him as providing important messages about social and emotional conflicts, as well as warning him of danger and unsafe relational contexts. Beliefs about being monitored also served important functions of protecting against anticipated threats.

8.2.5 *Strengths: 'What Are Your Strengths?' (What Access to Power Resources Do You Have?)*

Recognising that a range of responses serve different survival functions for a person can support in the identification of *strengths*, the final interrelated element that feeds into narrative development (Johnstone & Boyle, 2018a, Chp. 6). Drawing attention to the ways in which even the most seemingly 'bizarre' responses are actually survival strategies can support recognition of a person's resourcefulness. The PTMF approach to attending to strengths also has parallels with trauma-informed practice (e.g. Warner, 2000) and the narrative approach of 'double-listening' (e.g. Guilfoyle, 2015), whereby seemingly insignificant or small responses in the face of extreme threats can be identified as acts of resistance. For example, developing a belief that one has superpowers, or experiencing periods of elated mood, can be recognised as a refusal to fully give into the many layers of invalidation and disempowerment a person may have endured. Recognition of threat responses such as rage or extreme low mood can indicate that there are values a person has that have been compromised by power imbalances; values that can be celebrated as strengths and utilised to identify other ways a person has enacted these values in their life (c.f. White, 2007, Chp. 2).

Strengths and Development of Matt's Narrative In spite of facing multiple adversities and considering suicide on a number of occasions, Matt is someone who has persevered and evidenced great courage – he is a survivor! Other strengths Matt has been able to identify include his intelligence, his sporting abilities, his sense of humour, rebelliousness, sociability, and ability to relate to others, including the Aboriginal community (a community that was culturally different to the one Matt had been raised within) and the many colleagues and people seeking support through the Humane Clinic he established.

8.3 Narrative Formation and Provisional Patterns

Through exploration of Power, Threat, Meaning, Threat Responses, and Strengths, a person may feel able to develop a narrative; a non-pathologising personal account of how they have resisted the operations of power in the ways they have (Boyle & Johnstone, 2020, Chp. 9). This integration of the interrelated elements into a single narrative is important because it enables a person to tell their story in the way they want to, which can be especially empowering for people labelled with 'psychosis' who often are denied the opportunity to author their own accounts within services (Geekie, 2013). Unlike diagnostic labels, narratives are fluid and we will tell different stories about ourselves to different people, whilst the narratives we develop will alter as we come to make new connections with regards to our experiences. For example, after developing his initial narrative with Lucy Johnstone (one of the PTMF lead authors), Matt experienced a unique reciprocity that he had not previously encountered. The experience of 'power *with*' rather than 'power *over*' facilitated Matt in developing connections that were meaningful for him, rather than accepting imposed perspectives of the professional. This led to a sense of trust and empowerment, which in turn supported Matt to find a voice to openly include childhood sexual abuse in a subsequent iteration of his narrative in a way that he had never previously felt able to do. For Matt, developing a narrative (Box 8.2) supported him in recognising the various different ways he had survived a range of threats, providing him with hope that a personally meaningful and useful story could be formed. These reflections on his own experiences have been valuable in enabling Matt to support others consulting with him at the Humane Clinic to make sense of their distress in terms of adversity, oppression, and abuse, whilst also drawing attention to their strengths and resistance. Matt's reflections on his own narrative development have further inspired subsequent work on the "Dissociachotic framework to supporting people with 'psychosis'" (Ball & Picot, 2021).

Box 8.2: Matt's Narrative

"I grew up in an environment that could be described as safe and comfortable. Despite the many privileges of this culture and environment, I felt estranged and different from those around me from an early age. This became more of a problem when I responded by keeping secrets and feeling disconnected from the social and cultural environment. I experienced a sense of hypocrisy from an early age and with the ongoing threats, was often confused by the contradictory narratives. I learned to 'fit in' enough through sport but also failed to complete education or find employment with any success and was often seen by others as not fulfilling my potential.

The sense of being trapped and then unintentionally making this worse for myself was constant. Not knowing whom I could connect with meant the secrets and reactions to the threats continued until I found I could not maintain the 'normal' any more. Suicide, and wondering whether this life was

(continued)

Box 8.2 (continued)

worth living, was a fairly constant internal dialogue, and I used drugs to manage the distress and fear.

In my teenage years the sense of isolation became increasingly difficult to manage. My response was to guess how I should behave in different situations to avoid further problems, but I also knew that I would be punished for certain actions. This felt a reasonable payoff as a way of protecting myself.

The labelling of diagnosis appeared to be a continuation of the convenient story of me being a problem – both socially and 'biologically'. Initially I accepted, or at least was powerless to challenge, the diagnostic narrative. I was aware that I was continuing the cycle of saying what I believed might be the most acceptable and least problematic (for me) set of 'truths' – this time to psychiatrists. But I became trapped in a narrative of 'illness' that led to vile medication reactions and subservience to the system, with apparently no way out.

Escaping the narrative of illness has created multiple opportunities in both my personal and professional life., I have found importance and meaning in personal relationships, being married with children especially important to me given the disruption to the relational safety in the context of adversities.

On a professional level the opportunity to take value from experiences that led up to the emergence of 'psychosis' and surviving the mental health system, has contributed to the development of a career as a Mental Health Nurse Practitioner and Psychotherapist. More recently I have developed an alternative conceptualisation of understanding 'psychosis', the Suicide Narratives approach, and I am setting up an alternative mental health service: The Humane Clinic (www.humaneclinic.com.au). Humane Clinic incorporates psychotherapy, training and the Just Listening Community – a community led alternative for people in emotional distress (www.justlistening.com.au)."

A person may want to consider their narrative in relation to the PTMF's provisional patterns. These are evidence-informed meta-narratives describing common patterns of meaning-mediated threat responses to particular operations of power (Johnstone & Boyle, 2018a, b). Unlike diagnostic labels, the patterns are not regarded as things a person can *'have'*, but describe the common ways people respond to similar negative operations of power. The patterns are not intended as a like-for-like replacement for psychiatric diagnoses. As such, there is no pattern for 'psychosis' or 'schizophrenia' because, as explained above, these experiences are understood as *threat responses* that serve different functions for people at different times. That said, because the patterns are derived from evidence that indicates certain forms of adversity are more likely to be linked with certain forms of threat responses, there are patterns that are more relevant for consideration by people who are troubled by unusual beliefs or voice hearing: We have relied heavily upon content within provisional patterns 1 (*Identities*), 2 (*Surviving rejection, entrapment, and invalidation*),

3 (*Surviving disrupted attachments and adversities as a child/young person*), and 6 (*Surviving social exclusion, shame, and coercive power*) to populate chapter content relating to the emergence of 'psychosis', while the sub-pattern *Being identified/identifying as 'mentally ill'* was central for our thinking about the impacts of mental health services (Johnstone & Boyle, 2018b). The PTMF authors acknowledge the Western context the patterns were developed within and posit that patterns will inevitably vary with culture and time given the role of Ideological Power in shaping meaning of both threats and threat responses (Johnstone, 2019; Johnstone & Boyle, 2018a). It is hoped that comparing one's narrative with the patterns will not only support a person in developing their own narratives, but will support normalisation of experience by supporting others to recognise that they are not alone in their experiences and responses. Patterns should always be shared tentatively and professionals should never enact epistemic injustices by asserting someone's experiences fit with a particular pattern (Boyle & Johnstone, 2020).

8.4 Conclusion and Implications

We have used this chapter to illustrate how, from a PTMF perspective, experiences labelled as 'psychosis' in the Global North can be more helpfully recognised as threat responses that are understandable in the context of a person's lived experience and positioning within complex networks of power. In centring power, the Framework has potential to support the development of personal narratives that are non-pathologising and that restore the links between threats and threat responses that are obscured through medical model practices (Boyle, 2020). Although we have focussed upon 'psychosis', it will hopefully be apparent that a PTMF approach would not centre on such experiences. To begin by focussing on 'psychosis' risks falling into the unhelpful trap of asking 'what is wrong with you?' and does not help in understanding and connecting with a person, nor appreciating their strengths. While it can be useful for people to explore the meaning of their voices and beliefs (Coles, 2013; Escher & Romme, 2010), professionals should avoid pathologising such experiences and recognise that such responses will be just some of many survival strategies and strengths a person will have utilised.

While we have described the PTMF elements separately, it is not advisable to work through the questions in a linear fashion. The process of developing narratives is nuanced and individualised and it is the sharing and discussion of the narrative between an individual and those supporting development that can facilitate shifts and connection. If professionals are developing narratives with individuals, this should be done in a collaborative dialogical way that gives careful consideration to the intersectional power dynamics between themselves and the person they are trying to support. Consideration should be given not only to 'what' is talked about, but also the 'how' these conversations will take place (c.f. Warner, 2009). Some people might find it easier to explore strengths early on, as this can be safer than discussing threats a person has survived with a relative stranger in a position of power. However, a focus on strengths may be too aversive for people if such a focus is too at odds with the negative meanings a person may have developed about themselves, or if such a process results in people feeling their difficulties are not being heard (Guilfoyle, 2015). The lead should be taken from the person seeking support, and narrative development should only ever be offered as an option for supporting making sense of experiences, never imposed (Johnstone & Boyle, 2018a).

Of course, professional input is not a requirement for narrative development and some people have reported finding benefit from working through the PTMF as an individual or within a peer support format (e.g. Griffiths, 2019; SHIFT Recovery Community, 2020). Indeed, the advantages of peer-support services have been long recognised by voice-hearing communities who have benefitted from making sense of experiences within more evenly balanced power relationships, away from pathologising services. Examples of lived experience led approaches that can be seen to have had a global impact include the Hearing Voices Movement (e.g. https://www.intervoiceonline.org/), the National Empowerment Centre (power2u.org) and Inner Compass, a psychiatric drug withdrawal community (theinnercompass.org). In Australia, the Humane Clinic has had early success with their 'Suicide Narratives' approach (Ball & Ritchie, 2020) and 'Just Listening' scheme (https://www.justlistening.com.au/), both of which are oriented towards supporting people who might be regarded as 'acutely psychotic' through providing non-pathologising spaces where volunteers actively listen. Conversely, professionals have reported benefits of using the PTMF to support more empathic understandings of individuals accessing services (c.f. 'team formulation', Johnstone, 2013). While there can be clear benefits for both staff teams and the people they support through development of non-pathologising understandings, use of the Framework in this way should be distinguished from narrative development, which should always be led by the person whom the narrative belongs to.

Finally, the PTMF has potential to orientate people experiencing distress and people providing services to consider ways a person might best be supported. Throughout the chapter, we have drawn attention to the evidence linking negative operations of power associated with a variety of adversities to the increased likelihood of distress from hearing voices or unusual beliefs, and how the responses of Western mental health services often replicate and present additional threats to people seeking support (Johnstone, 2000; Johnstone & Boyle, 2018b). It is thus not surprising that the evidence base indicates the greatest predictors of good outcomes for people labelled with 'psychosis' are those associated with increased power resources, such as connection with others, finding meaning in life and identities beyond those associated with being a 'patient', having control over key aspects of one's life, and having opportunities to education and employment (DCP, 2017). These findings likely relate to evidence that outcomes are generally better for people in the Global South, where it is more likely that social and community responses will be utilised over medical diagnosis and drugs (White et al., 2014). Consideration of the centrality of power on a person's experience can also motivate engagement in activism or survivor missions, which will not only be empowering for individuals but wider society; collective action has more potential to influence change to oppressive social structures than individual action (e.g. Holland, 2018; Smail, 2005).

References

Bailey, T., Alvarez-Jimenez, M., Garcia-Sanchez, A. M., Hulbert, C., Barlow, E., & Bendall, S. (2018). Childhood trauma is associated with severity of hallucinations and delusions in psychotic disorders: A systematic review and meta-analysis. *Schizophrenia Bulletin, 44*(5), 1111–1122.

Ball, M., & Picot, S. (2021). Dissociachotic: Seeing the nonpsychosis we share. *Journal of Humanistic Psychology, 63*, 0022167821993668.

Ball, M., & Ritchie, R. (2020). *Suicide narratives: Healing through knowing.* Retrieved from https://www.bps.org.uk/sites/www.bps.org.uk/files/Policy/Policy%20-%20Files/Humane%20Clinic%20-%20Suicide%20Narratives%202020.pdf

Bentall, R. P. (1990). The illusion of reality: A review and integration of psychological research on hallucinations. *Psychological Bulletin, 107*, 82–95.

Bentall, R., de Sousa, P., Varese, F., Wickham, S., Sitko, K., Haarmans, M., & Read, J. (2014). From adversity to psychosis: Pathways and mechanisms from specific adversities to specific symptoms. *Social Psychiatry and Psychiatric Epidemiology, 49*, 1011–1022. https://doi.org/10.1007/s00127-014-0914-0

Bhui, K., Halvorsrud, K., & Nazroo, J. (2018). Making a difference: Ethnic inequality and severe mental illness. *The British Journal of Psychiatry, 213*, 574–578. https://doi.org/10.1192/bjp.2018.148

Birchwood, M., Gilbert, P., Gilbert, J., Trower, P., Meaden, A., Hay, J., et al. (2004). Interpersonal and role-related schema influence the relationship with the dominant 'voice' in schizophrenia: A comparison of three models. *Psychological Medicine, 34*(8), 1571–1580. https://doi.org/10.1017/S0033291704002636

Bourdieu, P. (2010). The forms of capital. In I. Szeman & T. Kaposy (Eds.), *Cultural theory: An anthology*. Wiley-Blackwell.

Boyle, M. (2020). Power in the Power Threat Meaning Framework. *Journal of Constructivist Psychology*. https://doi.org/10.1080/10720537.2020.1773357

Boyle, M., & Johnstone, L. (2020). *A straight talking introduction to the Power Threat Meaning Framework*. PCCS.

Branford, D., Gerrard, D., Saleem, N., Shaw, C., & Webster, A. (2019). Stopping over-medication of people with intellectual disability, Autism or both (STOMP) in England part 1 – History and background of STOMP. *Advances in Mental Health and Intellectual Disabilities, 13*(1), 31–40. https://doi.org/10.1108/AMHID-02-2018-0004

Clarke, I. (2013). Spirituality: A new way into understanding psychosis. In E. M. J. Morris, L. C. Johns, & J. E. Oliver (Eds.), *Acceptance and commitment therapy and mindfulness for psychosis*. Wiley-Blackwell.

Coles, S. (2013). Meaning, madness and marginalisation. In S. Coles, S. Keenan, & B. Diamond (Eds.), *Madness contested. Power and practice*. PCCS Books.

Cromby, J. (2020). Meaning in the Power Threat Meaning Framework. *Journal of Constructivist Psychology*. https://doi.org/10.1080/10720537.2020.1773355

Cromby, J., & Harper, D. (2013). Paranoia: Contested and contextualised. In S. Coles, S. Keenan, & B. Diamond (Eds.), *Madness contested. Power and practice*. PCCS Books.

Cromby, J., Harper, D., & Reavey, P. (2013). *Psychology, mental health and distress*. Palgrave Macmillan.

Cromby, J., Chung, E., Papadopoulos, D., & Talbot, C. (2019). Reviewing the epigenetics of schizophrenia. *Journal of Mental Health, 28*(1), 71–79. https://doi.org/10.1080/09638237.2016.1207229

das-Munshi, J., Bécares, L., Boydell, J., Dewey, M., Morgan, C., Stansfeld, S., & Prince, M. (2012). Ethnic density as a buffer for psychotic experiences: Findings from a national survey (EMPIRIC). *British Journal of Psychiatry, 201*(4), 282–290. https://doi.org/10.1192/bjp.bp.111.102376

Davies, J. (2013). *Cracked: Why psychiatry is doing more harm than good*. Icon Books.

Delano, L. (2013). *The power of psychiatric diagnosis*. [Video]. https://www.youtube.com/watch?v=pHfzUAb57zo

Dillon, J. (2019). Names matter, language matters, truth matters. In J. Watson (Ed.), *Drop the disorder. Challenging the culture of psychiatric diagnosis*. PCSS.

Division of Clinical Psychology. (2017). *Understanding psychosis and schizophrenia*. British Psychological Society. Retrieved from https://www.bps.org.uk/what-psychology/understanding-psychosis-and-schizophrenia

Escher, S., & Romme, M. (2010). *Children hearing voices: What you need to know and what you can do*. PCCS Books.

Fernando, S. (2014). Globalization of psychiatry – A barrier to mental health development. *International Review of Psychiatry, 26*(5), 551–557.

Fernando, S. (2017). *Institutional racism in psychiatry and clinical psychology*. Palgrave Macmillan. https://doi.org/10.1007/978-3-319-62728-1

Foucault, M. (1977). *Discipline & punish. The birth of the prisons*. Penguin.

Geekie, J. (2013). Listening to the voices we hear. Clients' understandings of psychotic experiences. In J. Read & J. Dillon (Eds.), *Models of madness*. Routledge.

Griffiths, A. (2019). Reflections on using the Power Threat Meaning Framework in peer-led systems. *Clinical Psychology Forum, 313*, 9–14.

Guilfoyle, M. (2015). Listening in narrative therapy: Double listening and empathic positioning. *South Africa Journal of Psychology, 45*(1), 36–49. https://doi.org/10.1177/0081246314556711

Haarmans, M., Vass, V., & Bentall, R. P. (2016). Voices' use of gender, 'race', and other social categories to undermine female voice-hearers: Implications for incorporating intersectionality within CBT for psychosis. *Psychosis, Psychological, Social and Integrative Approaches, 8*(3), 203–213. https://doi.org/10.1080/17522439.2015.1131323

Halvorsrud, K., Nazroo, J., Otis, M., Brown Hajdukova, E., & Bhui, K. (2019). Ethnic inequalities in the incidence of diagnosis of severe mental illness in England: A systematic review and new meta-analyses for non-affective and affective psychoses. *Social Psychiatry and Psychiatric Epidemiology, 54*(11), 1311–1323. https://doi.org/10.1007/s00127-019-01758-y

Hamby, S. (2014). *Battered women's protective strategies: Stronger than you know*. Oxford University Press.

Harper, D. J. (2011). The social context of paranoia. In M. Rapley, J. Moncrieff, & J. Dillon (Eds.), *De-medicalizing misery*. Palgrave Macmillan. https://doi-org.ezproxy3.lib.le.ac.uk/10.1057/9780230342507_5

Harper, D. J., O'Donnell, E., & Platts, S. (2021). A "trigger", a cause or obscured? How trauma and adversity are constructed in psychiatric stress-vulnerability accounts of "psychosis". *Feminism & Psychology, 31*(1), 19–40. https://doi.org/10.1177/0959353520954313

Haydon-Laurelut, M., Nunkoosing, K., & Wilcox, E. (2013). Family therapy and dis/ableism: Constructions of disability in family therapy literature. *Human Systems: The Journal of Therapy, Consultation and Training, 24*(1), 146–158.

Holland, S. (2018). Psychotherapy, oppression and social action: Gender, race and class in Black women's depression. In R. J. Perelberg & A. C. Miller (Eds.), *Gender & power in families*. Karnac.

Hollomotz, A. (2009). Beyond 'vulnerability': An ecological model approach to conceptualizing risk of sexual violence against people with learning difficulties. *The British Journal of Social Work, 39*(1), 99–112. https://doi.org/10.1093/bjsw/bcm091

Janssen, I., Hanssen, M., Bak, M., Bijl, R., De Graaf, R., Vollebergh, W., et al. (2003). Discrimination and delusional ideation. *British Journal of Psychiatry, 182*(1), 71–76. https://doi.org/10.1192/bjp.182.1.71

Johnstone, L. (2000). *Users and abusers of psychiatry*. Routledge.

Johnstone, L. (2013). Using formulation in teams. In L. Johnstone & R. Dallos (Eds.), *Formulation in psychology and psychotherapy*. Routledge. https://doi.org/10.4324/9780203380574

Johnstone, L. (2019, February 24). *Crossing cultures with the Power Threat Meaning Framework – New Zealand.* [Blog Post]. Retrieved from https://www.madintheuk.com/2019/02/crossing-cultures-with-the-power-threat-meaning-framework/

Johnstone, L., & Boyle, M. with Cromby, J., Dillon, J., Harper, D., Kinderman, P., Longden, E., Pilgrim, D. & Read, J. (2018a). *The Power Threat Meaning Framework: Towards the identification of patterns in emotional distress, unusual experiences and troubled or troubling behaviour, as an alternative to functional psychiatric diagnosis*. British Psychological Society. Retrieved from https://www.bps.org.uk/sites/www.bps.org.uk/files/Policy/Policy%20-%20Files/PTM%20Framework%20%28January%202018%29_0.pdf

Johnstone, L., & Boyle, M. with Cromby, J., Dillon, J., Harper, D., Kinderman, P., Longden, E., Pilgrim, D., & Read, J. (2018b). *The Power Threat Meaning Framework: Overview*. British Psychological Society. Retrieved from https://www.bps.org.uk/sites/www.bps.org.uk/files/Policy/Policy%20-%20Files/PTM%20Overview.pdf

Kezelman, C., & Stavropoulos, P. (2012). *Practice guidelines for treatment of complex trauma and trauma informed care and service delivery*. Adults Surviving Childhood Abuse.

Kinouani, G. (2019). Violence under the guise of care: Whiteness, colonialism and psychiatric diagnoses. In J. Watson (Ed.), *Drop the disorder! Challenging the culture of psychiatric diagnosis*. PCCS Books.

Kråkvik, B., Larøi, F., Kalhovde, A. M., Hugdahl, K., Kompus, K., Salvesen, Ø., Stiles, T. C., & Vedul-Kjelsås, E. (2015). Prevalence of auditory verbal hallucinations in a general population: A group comparison study. *Scandinavian Journal of Psychology, 56*, 508–515.

Lebowitz, M. S., & Ahn, W. K. (2014). Effects of biological explanations for mental disorders on clinicians' empathy. *Proceedings of the National Academy of Sciences, 111*(50), 17786–17790.

Longden, E., Madill, A., & Waterman, M. G. (2012). Dissociation, trauma, and the role of lived experience: Toward a new conceptualization of voice hearing. *Psychological Bulletin, 138*(1), 28–76. https://doi.org/10.1037/a0025995

Longden, E. (2013). *The voices in my head.* [video]. TED. https://www.ted.com/talks/eleanor_longden_the_voices_in_my_head

Longden, E., Sampson, M., & Read, J. (2016). Childhood adversity and psychosis: Generalised or specific effects? *Epidemiology and Psychiatric Sciences, 25*(4), 349–359. https://doi.org/10.1017/S204579601500044X

López-Moríñigo, J. D., Ramos-Ríos, R., David, A. S., & Dutta, R. (2012). Insight in schizophrenia and risk of suicide: A systematic update. *Comprehensive Psychiatry, 53*(4), 313–332. https://doi.org/10.1016/j.comppsych.2011.05.015

Melvin, K., Crossley, J., & Cromby, J. (2021). The feeling, embodiment and emotion of hallucinations in first episode psychosis: A prospective phenomenological visual-ecological study using novel multimodal unusual sensory experience (MUSE) maps. *Clinical Medicine, 41*, 101–153. https://doi.org/10.1016/j.eclinm.2021.101153

Metzl, J. (2011). *The protest psychosis: How schizophrenia became a black disease*. Beacon Press.

Moncreiff, J. (2013). *The bitterest pills. The troubling story of antipsychotic drugs*. Palgrave Macmillan.

Morgan, A., & Felton, A. (2013). From constructive engagement to coerced recovery. In S. Coles, S. Keenan, & B. Diamond (Eds.), *Madness contested. Power and practice*. PCCS Books.

Morgan, G., Barnwell, G., Johnstone, L., Shukla, J., & Mitchell, A. (2022). The power threat meaning framework and the climate and ecological crises. *Psychology in Society, 63*, 3–109.

Moskowitz, A., Dorahy, M. J., & Schäfer, I. (Eds.). (2019). *Psychosis, trauma and dissociation: Evolving perspectives on severe psychopathology*. Wiley.

NICE. (2014). *Psychosis and schizophrenia in adults: Prevention and management, Clinical guideline [CG178].* Retrieved from https://www.nice.org.uk/guidance/cg178/chapter/1-Recommendations

O'Donoghue, T., & Crossley, J. (2020). A critical narrative analysis of psychiatrists' engagement with psychosis as a contentious area. *International Journal of Social Psychiatry, 66*(7), 724–730. https://doi.org/10.1177/0020764020934516

Parker, I., Schnackenberg, J., & Hopfenbeck, M. (Eds.). (2021). *The practical handbook of hearing voices: Therapeutic and creative approaches*. PCCS Books.

Pavon, G., & Vaes, J. (2017). Bio-genetic vs. psycho-environmental conceptions of schizophrenia and their role in perceiving patients in human terms. *Psychosis, 9*(3), 245–253.

Pons, J. (2019). How we can engage with race in a meaningful way for the people we work with, accessed 23/12/21 How we can engage with race in a meaningful way | MHT (mentalhealth-today.co.uk).

Poustmous, J. L., Plummer, S., McMahon, S., Murshid, N. S., & Sung Kim, M. (2012). Understanding economic abuse in the lives of survivors. *Journal of Interpersonal Violence, 7*(3), 411–430. https://doi.org/10.1177/0886260511421669

Read, J. (2013a). Biological psychiatry's lost cause: The 'schizophrenic' brain. In J. Read & J. Dillon (Eds.), *Models of madness*. Routledge.

Read, J. (2013b). Does 'schizophrenia' exist? Reliability and validity. In J. Read & J. Dillon (Eds.), *Models of madness*. Routledge.

Read, J., & Bentall, R. (2013). Madness. In J. Cromby, D. Harper, & P. Reavey (Eds.), *Psychology, mental health and distress*. Palgrave Macmillan.

Read, J., Bentall, R., Johnstone, L., Fosse, R., & Braken, P. (2013a). Electroconvulsive therapy. In J. Read & J. Dillon (Eds.), *Models of madness*. Routledge.

Read, J., Johnstone, L., & Taitimu, M. (2013b). Psychosis, poverty and ethnicity. In J. Read & J. Dillon (Eds.), *Models of madness*. Routledge.

Read, J., Magliano, L., & Beaven, V. (2013c). Public beliefs about the cause of 'schizophrenia'. In J. Read & J. Dillon (Eds.), *Models of madness*. Routledge.

Read, J., Fosse, R., Moskowitz, A., & Perry, B. (2014). The traumagenic neurodevelopmental model of psychosis revisited. *Neuropsychiatry, 4*(1), 65–79. https://doi.org/10.2217/npy.13.89

Royal College of Psychiatrists. (2021). *National clinical audit of psychosis – Employment spotlight audit 2021*. Healthcare Quality Improvement Partnership. Available from http://www.rcpsych.ac.uk/NCAP

Sayce, L. (1998). Stigma, discrimination and social exclusion: What's in a word? *Journal of Mental Health, 7*, 331–343.

SHIFT Recovery Community. (2020). Using the Power Threat Meaning Framework in a self-help group of people with experience of mental and emotional distress. *Journal of Constructivist Psychology*. https://doi.org/10.1080/10720537.2020.1773361

Skelly, A., [Anonymous], Fletcher, H., Flood, A., & Jones, L. (2017). *Incorporating attachment theory into practice: Clinical practice guideline for clinical psychologists working with people who have intellectual disabilities*. British Psychological Society. Retrieved from https://www.bps.org.uk/sites/www.bps.org.uk/files/Member%20Networks/Faculties/Intellectual%20Disabilities/Incorporating%20Attachment%20Theory%20Into%20Practice%20Clinical%20Practice%20Guideline%20for%20Clinical%20Psychologist%20working%20with%20People-%20who%20have%20ID%282017%29.pdf

Smail, D. (2005). Power, interest and psychology. *Elements of a social-materialist understanding of distress*. PCCS Books. ISBN 978 1 898059 71 4.

Spivak, G. C. (1988). Can the subaltern speak? In C. Nelson & L. Grossberg (Eds.), *Marxism and the interpretation of culture*. University of Illinois Press.

Summerfield, D. (2012). Afterword: Against 'global mental health'. *Transcultural Psychiatry, 49*, 1–12.

Taitimu, M., Read, J., McIntosh, T., & Ngā Whakāwhitinga. (2018). Standing at the crossroads: How Māori understand what Western psychiatry calls "schizophrenia". *Transcultural Psychiatry, 55*(2), 153–177. https://doi.org/10.1177/1363461518757800

Timimi, S. (2020). *Insane medicine*. Amazon. ISBN-13: 9798566925608.

van der Kolk, B. (2014). *The body keeps the score. Brain, mind and body in the healing of trauma*. Viking Press.

van Os, J., Hanssen, R., Bijl, V., & Ravelli, A. (2000). Strauss (1969) revisited: A psychosis continuum in the general population? *Schizophrenia Research, 45*(1–2), 11–20. https://doi.org/10.1016/S0920-9964(99)00224-8

Varese, F., Smeets, F., Drukker, M., Lieverse, R., Lataster, T., Viechtbauer, W., et al. (2012). Childhood adversities increase the risk of psychosis: A meta-analysis of patient-control, prospective-and cross-sectional cohort studies. *Schizophrenia Bulletin, 38*(4), 661–671.

Warner, S. (2000). *Understanding child sexual abuse: Making the tactics visible*. Handsell Publishing.

Warner, S. (2009). *Understanding the effects of child sexual abuse. Feminist revolutions in theory, research and practice*. Routledge.

White, M. (2007). *Maps of narrative practice*. Norton.

White, R., Jain, S., & Giurgi-Oncu, C. (2014). Counterflows for mental well-being: What high-income countries can learn from low and middle-income countries. *International Review of Psychiatry, 26*(5), 602–606. https://doi.org/10.3109/09540261.2014.939578

Wood, N., & Patel, N. (2017). On addressing 'Whiteness' during clinical psychology training. *South Africa Journal of Psychology, 47*(3), 280–291. https://doi.org/10.1177/0081246317722099

Chapter 9
Cognitive Behavioural Therapy for Psychosis

Rachel Manser and Louise Johns

9.1 Introduction

Cognitive behavioural therapy for psychosis (CBTp) is an adaptation of CBT for anxiety and depression, tailored for the needs of people with psychotic symptoms. While the therapy approach and format is generally the same, particular aspects of CBT are emphasised within CBTp, such as a greater focus on building trust and ensuring engagement (Brabban et al., 2016). There are some aspects of CBTp that are unique to this client group, such as 'working within' a client's belief system rather than requiring major belief change (Johns et al., 2014). The emphasis of therapy is on reducing distress and disruption from symptoms and working towards recovery goals. This chapter will outline fundamental aspects of CBTp, together with key therapeutic change strategies. While evaluating beliefs about anomalous or other experiences is an important part of CBTp, there are other factors that contribute to and maintain psychotic symptoms, and which clients would like help with in therapy (Freeman et al., 2019). We will illustrate the approach using examples from our clinical work.

9.2 Overview of CBTp Approaches

Cognitive behavioural therapy for psychosis (CBTp) is an evidence-based and recommended treatment in several national guidelines for schizophrenia and psychosis (Kreyenbuhl et al., 2010; National Institute for Health and Care Excellence, 2009, 2014; Royal Australian and New Zealand College of Psychiatrists, 2005). UK NICE

R. Manser · L. Johns (✉)
Oxford Health NHS Foundation Trust and University of Oxford, Oxford, UK
e-mail: rachel.manser@oxfordhealth.nhs.uk; louise.johns@psych.ox.ac.uk

J. A. Díaz-Garrido et al. (eds.), *Psychological Interventions for Psychosis*,
https://doi.org/10.1007/978-3-031-27003-1_9

guidance (National Institute for Health and Care Excellence, 2009) recommends that CBTp follows a treatment manual (based on a clinical trial) and includes at least one of the following: monitoring thoughts, feelings or behaviours in relation to symptoms; finding ways of coping; reducing distress; and improving functioning. Generic or 'first generation' CBTp includes a variety of therapeutic approaches to help with the problems that patients with psychosis wish to work on. Morrison (Morrison, 2017) describes their approach, outlining the format and change strategies used successfully in their treatment trials of CBTp in different patient groups, including those at high risk of developing psychosis, those with first episode psychosis, and those seen as having treatment-resistant schizophrenia (Morrison et al., 2011, 2014, 2018a, b). Developments in CBTp have involved evaluating discrete intervention components for specific psychotic symptoms, focusing on the processes involved in triggering and maintaining these symptoms (Freeman, 2011, 2016). CBT emphasises appraisal and behaviour as key to the development and persistence of the problem. Making changes in appraisals and behaviours, through new learning, is the main tool of change in all CBTp approaches.

9.2.1 *Appraisals of Experiences*

Cognitive behavioural models of psychotic symptoms state that it is not unusual experiences per se that cause distress, but the appraisal of these experiences as external, personally significant, and threatening (Bentall et al., 2007; Birchwood & Chadwick, 1997; Freeman et al., 2002; Garety et al., 2001, 2007; Morrison, 2001). Unhelpful coping and safety seeking behaviours maintain distress and poor functioning by preventing disconfirmation of negative appraisals (Gaynor et al., 2013; Heriot-Maitland et al., 2012). CBTp aims to break these maintenance cycles by helping people to make sense of their psychotic experiences in a way that promotes effective coping and functioning and counters negative appraisals of self and illness. Key alternative appraisals for patients are that they are safe and they have some control.

If acceptable to the patient, CBTp will target specific appraisals directly in therapy, which is the approach taken in Cognitive Therapy for Command Hallucinations (CTCH). This cognitive model of voices has clarified that appraisals of voice malevolence and omnipotence influence the voice hearer's affect and behaviour (Chadwick & Birchwood, 1994; Tsang et al., 2021). Compliance or appeasement behaviours in response to commanding voices occur when the hearer believes the voice has malevolent intent and the power to deliver the threat. CTCH aims to weaken beliefs about the power of voices to inflict harm on the voice hearer or others if commands are not obeyed, thereby reducing the hearer's motivation to comply. The therapy tests out the perceived power of the voice by examining evidence for the voice hearer's perceived lack of control over voice activity, the perceived omniscience of the voice (e.g. the apparent ability of the voice to predict the future), and the perceived capacity of the voice to carry out its threats for non-compliance (Byrne et al.,

2006; Meaden et al., 2013). In a randomised controlled trial (RCT) comparing CTCH with treatment as usual (TAU) over 9 months, the rate of voice compliance in the CTCH was significantly lower than in the TAU group at 18-months' follow-up (odds ratio 0·45) (Birchwood et al., 2014). This effect was matched by a change in the key target of the intervention, the appraisal of voices' power. A subsequent analysis confirmed that change in power beliefs at 9 months mediated the effect of therapy on compliance at 18 months (Birchwood et al., 2018a).

Understanding the appraisals of other types of voices is important for formulating the experience and identifying therapy targets. Using qualitative interview data, Sheaves (Sheaves et al., 2020) identified 21 reasons why patients with psychosis listen to and believe derogatory and threatening voices. These reasons grouped into six categories: to understand the voices; to be alert to the threat; normal instinct to rely on sensory information; the voices can be of people the voice hearer knows; the voices use strategies to capture attention; and patients feel so worn down that it is hard to resist the voice experience. Awareness of these reasons can help clinicians understand the patient experience and guide the CBT intervention.

9.2.2 Triggering and Maintaining Factors

Recent work has highlighted the different factors that trigger and maintain psychotic symptoms, and which offer additional therapeutic targets in CBTp. In a survey of 1809 patients with non-affective psychosis and severe paranoia and/or frequent voices, Freeman and colleagues (Freeman et al., 2019) found that patients had high levels of treatable problems such as agoraphobic avoidance, worry, reasoning difficulties, low self-esteem, and insomnia. Furthermore, patients wanted these difficulties to be treated. The authors' theoretical model of paranoia (Freeman, 2016) highlights these factors as causal mechanisms, and successful treatment of these difficulties can decrease paranoia. Freeman and colleagues have shown that reducing anxious avoidance (Freeman et al., 2016a), worry (Freeman et al., 2015a), low self-confidence (Freeman et al., 2014), insomnia (Freeman et al., 2015b), and reasoning bias (Garety et al., 2015) all lead to reductions in paranoia/persecutory delusions.

Alternative change strategies in CBTp are important as less than half of patients given first generation CBTp engage fully with the direct cognitive-behavioural techniques (Dunn et al., 2012), and many patients in the RCT of CTCH described fear of doing some of the therapy tasks to test the power of the voices (Birchwood et al., 2018b). Therapists may not need to work on appraisals in CBTp or may find this work easier when they come to it in therapy having worked on maintenance factors first. The Feeling Safe Programme for persecutory delusions (Freeman et al., 2016b) has combined the individual interventions targeting each maintenance factor into a full CBTp treatment. In the therapy, safety is relearned by entering feared situations after the influence of the maintenance factors has been reduced.

9.2.3 Evaluation of CBTp

A limitation of evaluating first generation (generic) CBTp is that therapy uses composite approaches in heterogeneous patient samples/clients with heterogeneous presentations of psychosis., and the therapeutic targets are not easily captured by a single primary outcome measure. Meta-analyses of these CBTp treatment trials have reported effect sizes in the small to moderate range (Bighelli et al., 2018; Turner et al., 2014).

Therapy approaches focused on specificity (targeting discrete factors causing or maintaining specific psychotic symptoms) have yielded higher effect sizes (Lincoln & Peters, 2018). Developments in CBTp have taken an 'interventionist-causal approach' (Freeman, 2011). In this approach, causation is ascertained by manipulation of the hypothesised causal mechanism and examination of the effect on the symptom of interest (Kendler & Campbell, 2009). In a systematic review of studies manipulating psychological processes potentially involved in psychotic experiences, Brown et al. (2019) identified the following mechanisms in patients with psychosis: worry and rumination, self-esteem, sleep, negative affect, reasoning biases, and beliefs about voices. Similarly, it has been argued that an interventionist-causal approach is necessary to untangle the relationship between trauma, PTSD, and psychosis (Brand et al., 2017).

In interventionist-treatment trials, there is a valuable combination of causal test and clinical test of specific treatment techniques (Brown et al., 2019). CTCH differed from generic CBTp as it was informed by a cognitive model of the psychological mechanisms involved in compliance with voices. This model proposed a single variable, which was the target of therapy and mediator of the outcome: the power differential between the voice and voice hearer. In addition, symptom-focused approaches are potentially more efficient than generic CBTp, and modular stand-alone interventions can be combined into a more comprehensive therapy (Freeman et al., 2016c). In the Feeling Safe Programme, patients chose treatment modules (e.g. worry, self-confidence, sleep) identified via assessment as being relevant to them. The Programme led to a significant end of treatment reduction in persistent persecutory delusions compared with befriending (Cohen's d –1·20) (Freeman et al., 2021).

9.3 Key Principles of the Therapeutic Approach

CBTp is formulation-driven, goal-directed, and uses cognitive behavioural interventions to disrupt key maintenance cycles. As with all CBT, the intervention occurs within the context of a warm, empathic, and collaborative therapeutic relationship, which is a prerequisite to effective therapy (Beck, 1979). However, there are differences from CBT for other conditions, not only in the theory-driven models that underlie formulations, but also in the emphasis of the work and therapeutic stance. When using CBT with people with psychosis, the therapist needs to have a greater focus on engagement, show open mindedness and genuine curiosity towards clients' beliefs, and empathy with their difficulties, together with a normalising and culturally aware approach to psychotic experiences and processes.

Therapy sessions follow the same structure as CBT for other conditions, with agenda-setting, followed by the main content of the session, including learning from between-session tasks, and ending with feedback and setting further between-session tasks. Phone calls, text messages, or emails can help to maintain hope and momentum between sessions. While number of sessions depends on progress towards therapy goals, sessions are usually weekly and between 16 and 26 in total (although may be fewer in early intervention for psychosis services). Further details of the CBTp approach and style are summarised elsewhere (Johns et al., 2014, 2020; Morrison, 2017). Here, we illustrate the key elements of CBTp using two examples* from our clinical work. We outline the progression of therapy with each client through the stages of CBTp:

(i) Engagement and development of a therapeutic relationship.
(ii) Assessment.
(iii) Establishing a shared problem and goal list.
(iv) Formulation.
(v) Interventions derived from the formulation.
(vi) Planning for the future/relapse management.

*These are hybrids of anonymised cases.

9.4 Bryan

Bryan, 23, is a Black male living with his parents in the outskirts of a city in which he grew up. His parents had a strong focus on achievement and working hard in order to provide for family. Growing up he was stopped and searched by the police on several occasions while his White friends tended to be left alone by the police. When he was working as an apprentice engineer aged 19, he was subject to verbal and racist bullying by a colleague and manager. He was finding it increasingly stressful and left the workplace before his placement had ended, which then made it difficult for him to find work. Many of his friends were working or studying at university. He became increasingly isolated, and for a period of time, he started hearing voices and sounds of what he assumed were people trying to break into his room. Following an altercation with his neighbours, during which Bryan threatened them with a knife, believing they informed the police about him being "a waste of space and probably dangerous", Bryan was admitted to his local psychiatric hospital. Since his discharge almost a year ago, he spends most of his time in his room, has lost touch with friends, and has started to believe more strongly that there is a police-run group who are trying to control his life and stop him from succeeding. On the rare occasions he goes out, he notices helicopters and people walking in pairs and assumes they are part of this conspiracy, and may, once they have enough information to know he will not succeed in life, take him away and kill him.

9.4.1 Engagement and Development of a Therapeutic Relationship (i)

Given that clients often present with issues of trust, often explicitly in the form of persecutory beliefs that others want to harm them, it is unsurprising that engagement is a key focus in CBTp. Sometimes clients may not wish to disclose aspects of their presentation, especially hallucinations, for fear of being re-hospitalised, particularly as hospitalisations are often experienced as traumatic (Berry et al., 2015).

To facilitate engagement, it is important that therapists are explicitly warm, non-judgemental, and collaborative in their approach. This includes, but is not limited to, using the client's terminology and beginning the therapy within their framework of meaning and beliefs. While the therapist usually conceptualises the problematic appraisal as a belief rather than reality, the client's reality is respected and the therapist matches the client's language. So, if Bryan describes an incident of perceived harassment, for example hearing scratching on his walls, this is discussed using the same language so *"when you heard your neighbours…"* rather than *"when you thought you heard your neighbours…"* An assertive outreach approach is more common, with therapists encouraging attendance at appointments, for example with text message reminders and offering home visits.

It is important to empathise frequently and to use explicit empathic comments, for example: *"'I'm sorry to hear that … that sounds really difficult for you … it sounds like you've been through an incredibly tough time"*, since clients with psychosis may misinterpret or fail to notice subtle non-verbal cues. To try to overcome issues of mistrust of services, it can be important for therapists to be clear about their intentions and capabilities as a therapist; notably, that CBTp is focused on the client's goals for their life and wellbeing rather than stopping voice hearing or changing beliefs per se. Therapists are usually part of these same health services and therefore may represent a mistrusted institution. For Bryan, who had negative experiences at the hands of predominantly White institutions, engagement is likely to take additional effort for a White therapist who is part of a similar service. An acknowledgement of this, as well as of the inherent power imbalance in therapy and services more widely, is often helpful. Therapist's self-disclosure tends to be used to a greater degree in CBTp to help engagement and reduce the power differential between therapist and client. Additionally, openness is important, notably about the limits of confidentiality and trust, for example what the therapy notes say, where they will be stored, and which aspects will be shared with other team members. The collaborative nature of CBT lends itself well to this open and direct approach.

It is an advantage if clients can understand and relate to the broad tenants of a CBT approach, for example that different thoughts can lead to correspondingly different emotions and behaviours. However, this is not necessary. Nor is it necessary for the client to have or gain 'insight' and see their experiences and beliefs as symptoms rather than reality. The CBTp approach meets the client where they are and uses their language and belief framework.

9.4.2 Assessment (ii)

Assessment begins with general questions to get an overview, followed by specific questions to build up a maintenance formulation *("What happened?... How did you make sense of that? ...How did you feel? ...How did you respond/what did you do to cope? ...What impact did that have?")*. A key part of CBTp assessment is clarifying experience-appraisal links. The 'intrusion' or experience may be an internal feeling or emotion, a hallucinatory experience, an external event (that may also have anomalous perceptual qualities), or a combination of these. The key is understanding the appraisal of the stimuli rather than distinguishing the type of experience. The assessment also clarifies the processes that maintain the appraisal and distress, particularly how the client responds in the moment, and the impact of this in both the short and long term. Clients should feel heard and understood, with you as their therapist viewing their concerns and reactions as understandable.

At CBT assessment, Bryan reports no longer hearing voices or other noises. This may be the case, but it is worth the therapist being aware that Bryan may not be reporting current voices due to fear of being readmitted to hospital. During the assessment, when trying to elucidate appraisals, the therapist asks gently about hallucinatory experiences:

Therapist: *So, from what you have told me, you know that this conspiracy against you is very active currently. I know from your notes that around the time you were in the ward you had been hearing noises of people trying to break in. I can only imagine how frightening that must have been. Is there anything like that happening at the moment which is giving you a clue about what these people are doing?*

Bryan: *No, I don't hear anything like that anymore.*

Therapist: *Fair enough, I just thought I would check. Let's look at what else is happening now.*

This is typical of the CBTp approach in that ideas are suggested tentatively and are withdrawn if the client is not receptive. Assessment is often a flexible and iterative process. At the time of assessment, Bryan said he did not hear any noises or voices, but later in therapy he said that when he was in his bedroom he heard almost constant tapping and scraping, which his parents had said they could not hear. This noise (auditory hallucination) was then incorporated into a re-formulation.

Questionnaire measures are used during the assessment process. These may be generic measures of distress and functioning for routine outcome monitoring (Fornells-Ambrojo et al., 2017), but can also be specific to the client's presenting issues and goals. Assessment of trauma and PTSD (Carr et al., 2018) is important because trauma is very common in this client group, pertinent to the formulation (Hardy, 2017; Morrison et al., 2003) and clients with psychosis are less likely to have been asked (Young et al., 2001).

9.4.3 Establish Shared Problem and Goal List (iii)

Collaboratively derived goals within CBTp will differ depending on the individual client and their presenting issues (Freeman et al., 2019). Goals may also differ depending on the timing of therapy. If a client is functioning well but has a fear of relapse, CBTp can focus on a relapse management plan to maintain their progress and help the client to plan how they might cope if difficulties were to re-occur (Gumley & Schwannauer, 2006).

The dialogue below shows the development of Bryan's goals and priorities in therapy:

Therapist: *So in terms of what we could look at together, you've said that you don't want things to carry on as they are at the moment, that you don't want these people who are following you to keep getting at you….*

Bryan: *Yeah, I mean if you could do that, but I don't think you'd have that level of influence over them.*

Therapist: *No, I know. It sounds like it's been a horrible time. If I could take that away from you or stop it happening, I would.*

Bryan: *It's been the worst time of my life. They won't stop harassing me.*

Therapist: *Absolutely, I can only imagine. So ultimately you want them to stop harassing you… Maybe we can think together about what we could do… If it were to stop, how would your life be different? What would you like to be doing that these events mean you're not able to do at the moment?*

Bryan: *I'd be back doing my apprenticeship, or maybe something better, but I'd be working for sure. But I can't even leave the house on my own. The level of surveillance is so intense.*

Therapist: *So would that be the first step towards that end goal of returning to your apprenticeship? Being able to leave the house?*

Bryan: *I mean it would be good if we could.*

Therapist: *We can see, can't we? There may not be but sometimes there are things we can do just to reduce stress, sometimes we are doing things that we don't realise are making us feel even more stressed than we need to be.*

Goals are then refined such that they are SMART and therefore progress (or lack thereof) can be measured and reviewed as therapy continues.

9.4.4 Formulation (iv)

Formulations can be complex with this client group and therefore formulation should be centred around the goals of the client rather than attempting an exhaustive understanding. Therapists may hold a separate formulation which encapsulates their broader understanding, but which they may not share with the client, for example because it differs from the client's perspective or includes aspects such as suspected trauma which the client is not yet ready to discuss.

The shared formulation would include appraisals of anomalous or other experiences and specific maintenance processes. It is important to develop idiosyncratic formulations with clients that are simple but also detailed enough to explain the maintenance mechanisms (which are the targets for therapy). Certain CBTp models highlight particular appraisals (Chadwick & Birchwood, 1994) or maintenance factors (Freeman, 2016) to pay attention to while assessing and formulating. Cognitive models and formulation of specific psychotic symptoms is a developing area, for example, the role of defeatist performance beliefs in negative symptoms (Rector et al., 2005) and the importance of the compensatory function in delusions of exceptionality (Isham et al., 2021).

The therapist develops and holds in mind the longitudinal part of Bryan's formulation shown in Fig. 9.1.

Formulations are presented in as much detail as is useful for the client at that stage of therapy and should not contain aspects that the client would disagree with. The longitudinal part of the formulation is not shared with Bryan at this stage as he firmly believes the persecutory belief not to have any relationship with his background experiences and core beliefs. Directly targeting Bryan's persecutory belief by discussing the evidence for and against his persecutory belief and evaluating alternative appraisals of his experiences could have a detrimental effect on Bryan. While he believes he is being targeted and while this belief causes him distress, the formulation suggests that his persecutory beliefs might also protect him from a

Background
High expectations from parents to behave well and earn well at work
Bullying at school
Black male, stopped by the police on several occasions as a young teenager

↓

Beliefs and assumptions
I need to work hard and be successful to gain approval
I stand out to (potentially dangerous) people
People in authority cannot be trusted

↓

Triggers
Bullying at apprenticeship, dropping out, seeing friends continuing to progress their careers
Subsequent isolation, disrupted sleep and voice hearing

↓

Presenting issues
Persecutory beliefs: 'I'm being followed and targeted, I could be taken away and killed'
Associated avoidance

Fig. 9.1 Longitudinal part of Bryan's formulation

more psychologically damaging explanation for his lack of career: that he is not good enough and his parents are not proud of him. Instead, working towards the goal of returning to work by reducing maintenance factors should allow Bryan to hold more positive beliefs about himself. His persecutory belief would then lose its function and may well diminish as a result.

Given Bryan's goal for therapy, and the evidence base for persecutory beliefs (Freeman et al., 2021), two key maintenance cycles that are contributing to his threat belief are mapped out with Bryan in session (see Fig. 9.2).

9.4.5 *Interventions Derived from the Formulation (v)*

Therapists draw upon a range of cognitive behavioural interventions to help the client reach their goal and disrupt the relevant maintenance cycle. While ultimately the aim of therapy is to change the appraisal to a less threatening and more empowered one (for example for Bryan this might be: *I am safe enough to return to work*), such a change in appraisal may not be addressed directly to begin with. Reviewing the maintenance formulation together in session, Bryan agreed to work on reducing worry, which felt a less daunting place to start making changes. Initial interventions are chosen by considering the client's preference and likelihood of achieving success quickly (which can enhance motivation, trust, and engagement in therapy).

Bryan introduced time-limited worry periods during the day and started lifting weights in his room as a way of directing his attention away from worry outside of these worry periods. This reduced his anxiety level and perception of serious threat and gave an early and easy win for therapy. Feeling calmer and having a sense of accomplishment through weight-lifting, Bryan felt ready to work on the next key maintenance process and consider reducing his avoidance of going out and safety seeking behaviours when out. Given that Bryan feared kidnapping and possible death, these behavioural experiments were negotiated and graded to make them feel

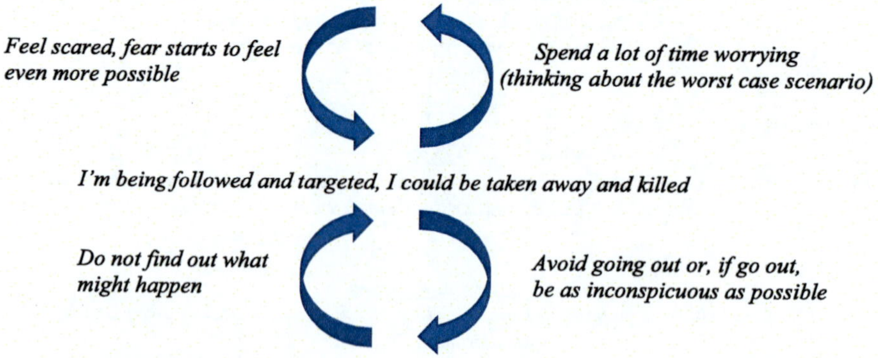

Fig. 9.2 Key maintenance cycles

as safe as possible. Once Bryan had completed a series of behavioural experiments to reduce anxious avoidance, both within and between sessions, an alternative safety belief was generated socratically as follows:

Therapist: *Bryan, we're reviewing our sessions and your progress today and I'm struck by how much more you are doing now. If we look at your maintenance diagram again, what do you notice?*

Bryan: *Because I've been going out I have seen what has happened. And it's been ok so far.*

Therapist: *Absolutely, you have done things that were feeling incredibly risky to do in terms of not just the likelihood of you being spotted but the likelihood that the harassment could worsen. Where would you say you are at with that now?*

Bryan: *I guess just that I can do a bit more than it seemed like I could do. They don't seem as focused on me, sometimes they are around but, even then, they usually leave me alone. They've had plenty of chances and they don't seem to be taking them.*

Therapist: *Absolutely. What do you take that to mean, both about them and about how safe you actually are, now that you have tested it out?*

Bryan: *That I am safer than I thought. They maybe aren't very effective or have other priorities. Maybe they are just keeping an eye on me but it seems like I can get out at least locally without too much harassment.*

Therapist: *That's brilliant, isn't it? So, you are safe to go out locally?*

Novice CBTp therapists might aim to change the client's delusional beliefs with good intention, but without considering whether such change is necessary for the client to reach their goals. Even when the formulation indicates that belief change would be helpful, minor changes may well be sufficient for the client to meet their goals (Johns et al., 2014) and be a more tractable therapy target. Offering an alternative belief too soon in therapy risks invalidating the client's past experiences and memories which the belief is based on (Janssen et al., 2003; Jun et al., 2018). It may also damage the therapeutic relationship and can result in the client defending their position more strongly.

9.4.6 Planning for the Future/Relapse Management (vi)

As with all CBT, final sessions focus on a therapeutic blueprint and plan for the future, which summarises progress in therapy and outlines CBT strategies to maintain, consolidate, or extend progress.

Positive CBT maintenance cycle formulations were drawn out for Bryan to record how he could continue to make helpful changes, as shown in Fig. 9.3.

We will consider how aspects of CBTp were tailored slightly differently with our second client example.

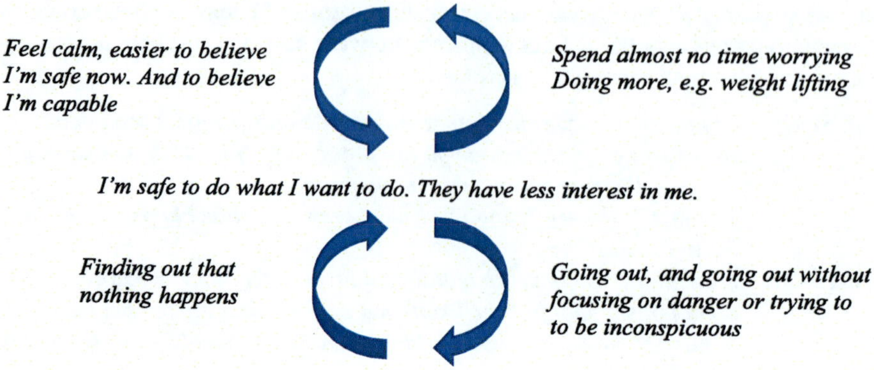

Fig. 9.3 Positive CBT maintenance cycles

9.5 Chrissy

Chrissy, 54, is a White female living in a small town with her longstanding partner. She was given a diagnosis of schizophrenia over 30 years ago and has had some ongoing contact with mental health services since that time. She has had a number of admissions to psychiatric units, but not for some years. Prior to her first contact with mental health services, she had ended her first romantic relationship, which had been one in which her partner was abusive. Having left this relationship, she experienced (undiagnosed) post-trauma reactions, hearing the voice of her ex-partner and starting to believe he still had control over her. Her mother took her to their family doctor and she was admitted to a psychiatric unit for 6 months and received a diagnosis of schizophrenia. She met her current partner around that time and they have been together since. Her partner has managed the household throughout their relationship and is protective of her. A referral for CBTp was prompted by her desire to become more active in her life, and also her partner becoming physically frailer and less able to provide care and support. Her fear of voices often prevented Chrissy from doing household chores and from leaving the house. She reported hearing one voice on a daily basis, usually threatening her ("If you go out, I'll kill you") or telling her not to do things ("Don't you dare make that cup of coffee").

9.5.1 Engagement and Development of a Therapeutic Relationship (i)

Voice hearing can make it more difficult for a client to concentrate on and remember session content, so reminders, prompts for the client to record the session on their phone to listen to it later, and more frequent in-session summaries can be helpful.

Due to current voices and often high levels of anxiety, therapists may need to ask more frequently how the client is tolerating the session. As Chrissy was open with the therapist that she was hearing a voice, this allowed the therapist to agree questions to ask her and her voice, for example *"Are you hearing anything now?... Can I ask what?...Would you like to wait a few minutes or ask him if it is ok for us to continue?"*

Chrissy had, over the years, formed an identity as a long-term patient, someone with 'chronic schizophrenia' and her expectation of achieving change in therapy was low. The therapist was explicit that she believed Chrissy had significant resilience, resources and skill, and held hope that therapy would result in positive change.

9.5.2 *Assessment (ii)*

While Chrissy had a trauma history, she did not meet criteria for current PTSD. Chrissy's therapy goal was to improve daily functioning, so assessment was tailored around her activity and hearing voices. Measures were given to understand Chrissy's experience of voices, relationship with her voice, and relevant beliefs about her voices and associated behaviours (Birchwood & Chadwick, 1997; Chadwick et al., 2000). An activity diary was completed between sessions to see Chrissy's current level of day-to-day activity and then generate a realistic goal to extend this.

9.5.3 *Establish Shared Problem and Goal List (iii)*

Chrissy had a clear aim to become more independent. The therapist asked questions to understand the current barriers to achieving this goal, illustrated in the dialogue below:

Therapist: *So you would like to be doing more, especially in the house. Can you tell me a bit more about what is stopping you at the moment?*
Chrissy: *This voice is, he just won't let me do more.*
Therapist: *Can you tell me more about him?*
Chrissy: *He sounds awful, really controlling and frightening.*
Therapist: *Gosh, that sounds awful for you. Do you know who he is?*
Chrissy: *To be honest, I've never really thought but he sounds like the first guy I was ever with, that was a grim relationship. He always said "Don't you dare!" and I knew that something would happen to me if he said that.*

Sometimes the client's goals are to stop their experiences happening, for example, to stop hearing voices or to stop (perceived) persecution. This was the case for Chrissy and was the only way she envisioned being able to do more. While as therapists we are ultimately aiming to change an appraisal about anomalous experiences, we are not aiming to stop the anomalous experience itself. This is similar to CBT in other areas, for example, for obsessive compulsive disorder or panic, we are not aiming to stop intrusive thoughts or physical sensations, respectively, but to change how they are appraised and responded to. These changes in appraisals and responses may lead to a reduction in the client noticing anomalous experiences (or intrusive thoughts or bodily sensations), but this is not the primary aim. The negotiated shared goal for Chrissy was as follows: *To be able to do daily chores (using dishwasher, cooking meals, washing clothes) and to meet my friend in the cafe once a week. To be 8/10 confident I can do this safely without my voice hurting me.*

9.5.4 Formulation (iv)

The shared maintenance formulation highlighted her appraisals about the power of the voice, leading to fear plus appeasement and compliance behaviours (see Fig. 9.4).

As Chrissy had disclosed and made a link between her voice and her experience of trauma, in a later session, the therapist added this information into the formulation and tentatively shared it with her (see Fig. 9.5).

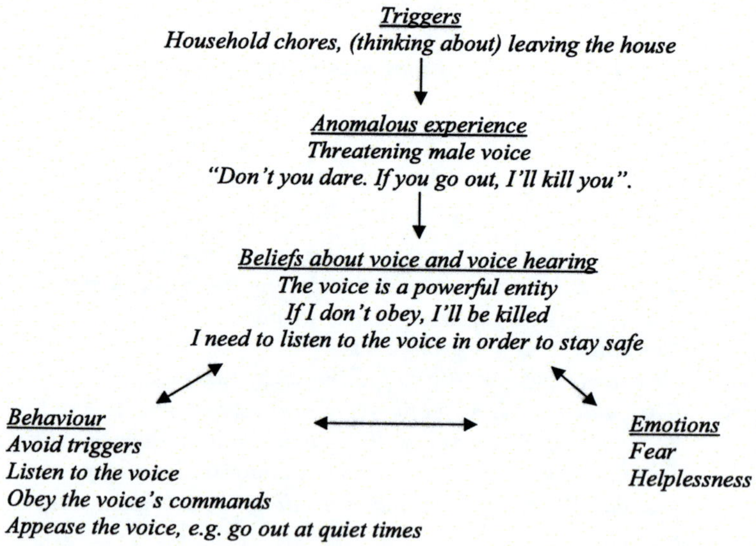

Fig. 9.4 Maintenance formulation. (Adapted from Morrison 2001)

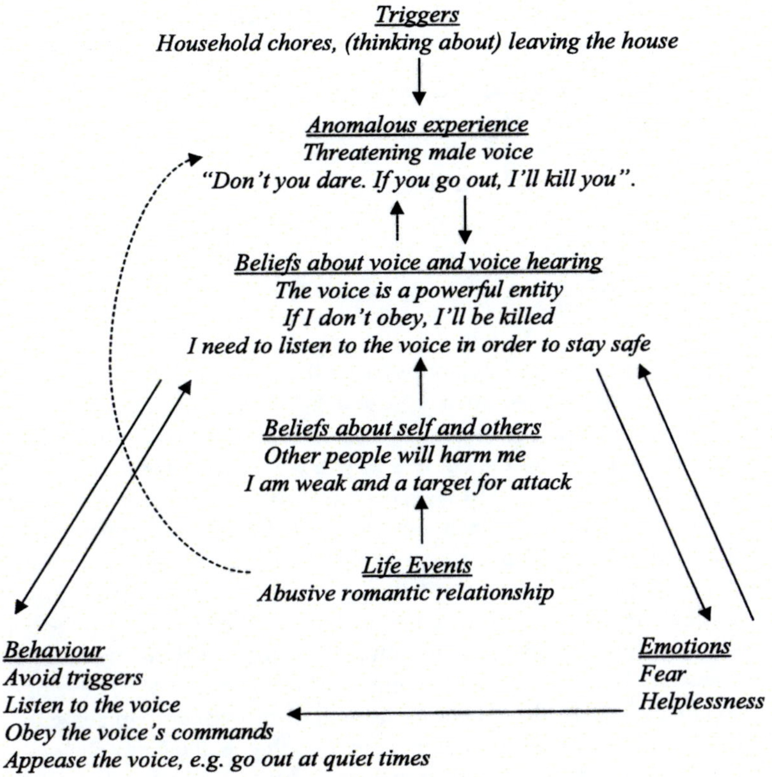

Fig. 9.5 Longitudinal formulation. (Adapted from Morrison 2017)

9.5.5 Interventions Derived from the Formulation (v)

Sessions started using the CTCH protocol (Meaden et al., 2013), enhancing coping strategies to build up Chrissy's sense of control and evaluating the power of the voice. The therapist and Chrissy spent some time discussing complex PTSD and some of the common sequalae of being a survivor of domestic abuse, leading to a new understanding that the voice was linked to her past trauma (Longden et al., 2012). This updated formulation offered an alternative (trauma-informed) appraisal of the voice. Chrissy accepted this possible alternative appraisal: *"Maybe my voice is related to my first relationship rather than being a powerful being"*. This shift in belief also meant she was more willing to test the power of the voice as therapy went on. Behavioural experiments allowed her to collect evidence that the voice gave empty threats, and nothing happened to her whether or not she obeyed. Her self-belief that she was weak and vulnerable also reduced, and she felt safe and empowered to do the things in life she wanted to.

9.5.6 Planning for the Future/Relapse Management (vi)

Given Chrissy's self-identity as a chronic and disabled patient, both within the home and the wider service, meetings were held jointly with her primary worker and her partner, in which Chrissy was empowered to outline her progress and how they could support her to continue with this.

9.6 Conclusion

CBTp is a client-centred and evidence-based therapy that aims to reduce distress and meet the goals of the client so they are able to live more fulfilling lives. Cognitive models identify a central role for appraisals of anomalous and other experiences, which therapy often focuses on, but in a way in which the current reality of the client is respected. Although not always specified in the cognitive models, formulation and intervention in CBTp will take into account the person's context and the function of delusional beliefs. This is reflected in the therapeutic approach, for example, considering the pros and cons of particular interventions and obtaining consent from the person to proceed, working within delusional beliefs to help the person to feel more in control, protecting the person's self-esteem, and linking change strategies to the person's goals. An interventionist-causal approach to the development of cognitive models of specific symptoms offers further promise to increase the precision and effect of therapy, with interventions targeting maintenance factors, including worry, negative affect, and cognitive biases. As with all therapies, CBTp must be done within the context of a good therapeutic relationship, in which the therapist is warm, open, and genuine. The therapist is curious, receives what the person communicates, validates the experience and distress, and works together with the client to make positive changes. It is a privilege to walk alongside our clients towards their recovery goals.

Disclaimer Clinical cases presented in this chapter do not include real names or personal information of real persons.

References

Beck, A. T. (1979). *Cognitive therapy and the emotional disorders*. Meridian Book.

Bentall, R. P., Fernyhough, C., Morrison, A. P., Lewis, S., & Corcoran, R. (2007). Prospects for a cognitive-developmental account of psychotic experiences. *The British Journal of Clinical Psychology/The British Psychological Society, 46*(Pt 2), 155–173. https://doi.org/10.1348/014466506X123011

Berry, K., Ford, S., Jellicoe-Jones, L., & Haddock, G. (2015). Trauma in relation to psychosis and hospital experiences: The role of past trauma and attachment. *Psychology and Psychotherapy, 88*(3), 227–239. https://doi.org/10.1111/PAPT.12035

Bighelli, I., Salanti, G., Huhn, M., Schneider-Thoma, J., Krause, M., Reitmeir, C., Wallis, S., Schwermann, F., Pitschel-Walz, G., Barbui, C., Furukawa, T. A., & Leucht, S. (2018). Psychological interventions to reduce positive symptoms in schizophrenia: Systematic review and network meta-analysis. *World Psychiatry, 17*(3), 316–329. https://doi.org/10.1002/WPS.20577

Birchwood, M., & Chadwick, P. (1997). The omnipotence of voices: Testing the validity of a cognitive model. *Psychological Medicine, 27*(6), 1345–1353. https://doi.org/10.1017/s0033291797005552

Birchwood, M., Michail, M., Meaden, A., Tarrier, N., Lewis, S., Wykes, T., Davies, L., Dunn, G., & Peters, E. (2014). Cognitive behaviour therapy to prevent harmful compliance with COMMAND hallucinations (COMMAND): A randomised controlled trial. *The Lancet Psychiatry, 1*(1), 23–33. https://doi.org/10.1016/S2215-0366(14)70247-0/ATTACHMENT/1B6515DE-0B69-4120-8252-1B68C1262280/MMC1.PDF

Birchwood, M., Dunn, G., Meaden, A., Tarrier, N., Lewis, S., Wykes, T., Davies, L., Michail, M., & Peters, E. (2018a). The COMMAND trial of cognitive therapy to prevent harmful compliance with command hallucinations: Predictors of outcome and mediators of change. *Psychological Medicine, 48*(12), 1966–1974. https://doi.org/10.1017/S0033291717003488

Birchwood, M., Mohan, L., Meaden, A., Tarrier, N., Lewis, S., Wykes, T., Davies, L. M., Dunn, G., Peters, E., & Michail, M. (2018b). The COMMAND trial of cognitive therapy for harmful compliance with command hallucinations (CTCH): A qualitative study of acceptability and tolerability in the UK. *BMJ Open, 8*(6), e021657. https://doi.org/10.1136/BMJOPEN-2018-021657

Brabban, A., Byrne, R., Longden, E., & Morrison, A. P. (2016). The importance of human relationships, ethics and recovery-orientated values in the delivery of CBT for people with psychosis. *Psychosis, 9*(2), 157–166. https://doi.org/10.1080/17522439.2016.1259648

Brand, R. M., Rossell, S. L., Bendall, S., & Thomas, N. (2017). Can we use an interventionist-causal paradigm to untangle the relationship between trauma, PTSD and psychosis? *Frontiers in Psychology, 8*(MAR), 306. https://doi.org/10.3389/FPSYG.2017.00306/BIBTEX

Brown, P., Waite, F., & Freeman, D. (2019). "Twisting the lion's tail": Manipulationist tests of causation for psychological mechanisms in the occurrence of delusions and hallucinations. *Clinical Psychology Review, 68*, 25–37. https://doi.org/10.1016/J.CPR.2018.12.003

Byrne, S., Birchwood, M., Trower, P., & Meaden, A. (2006). *A casebook of cognitive behaviour therapy for command hallucinations: A social rank theory approach*. Routledge.

Carr, S., Hardy, A., & Fornells-Ambrojo, M. (2018). The Trauma and Life Events (TALE) checklist: Development of a tool for improving routine screening in people with psychosis. *European Journal of Psychotraumatology, 9*(1), 1512265. https://doi.org/10.1080/20008198.2018.1512265

Chadwick, P., & Birchwood, M. (1994). The omnipotence of voices. A cognitive approach to auditory hallucinations. *The British Journal of Psychiatry, 164*(2), 190–201. http://www.ncbi.nlm.nih.gov/pubmed/8173822

Chadwick, P., Lees, S., & Birchwood, M. A. X. (2000). The revised Beliefs About Voices Questionnaire (BAVQ-R). *The British Journal of Psychiatry, 177*, 229–232.

Dunn, G., Fowler, D., Rollinson, R., Freeman, D., Kuipers, E., Smith, B., Steel, C., Onwumere, J., Jolley, S., Garety, P. A., & Bebbington, P. E. (2012). Effective elements of cognitive behaviour therapy for psychosis: Results of a novel type of subgroup analysis based on principal stratification. *Psychological Medicine, 42*(5), 1057–1068. https://doi.org/10.1017/S0033291711001954

Fornells-Ambrojo, M., Johns, L., Onwumere, J., Garety, P., Milosh, C., Iredale, C., Peters, E., Webster, A., & Jolley, S. (2017). Experiences of outcome monitoring in service users with psychosis: Findings from an Improving Access to Psychological Therapies for people with Severe Mental Illness (IAPT-SMI) demonstration site. *British Journal of Clinical Psychology, 56*(3), 253–272. https://doi.org/10.1111/bjc.12136

Freeman, D. (2011). Improving cognitive treatments for delusions. *Schizophrenia Research, 132*(2–3), 135–139. https://doi.org/10.1016/J.SCHRES.2011.08.012

Freeman, D. (2016). Persecutory delusions: A cognitive perspective on understanding and treatment. *The Lancet Psychiatry, 3*(7), 685–692. https://doi.org/10.1016/S2215-0366(16)00066-3

Freeman, D., Garety, P. A., Kuipers, E., Fowler, D., & Bebbington, P. E. (2002). A cognitive model of persecutory delusions. *The British Journal of Clinical Psychology/The British Psychological Society, 41*(Pt 4), 331–347. https://doi.org/10.1348/014466502760387461

Freeman, D., Pugh, K., Dunn, G., Evans, N., Sheaves, B., Waite, F., Černis, E., Lister, R., & Fowler, D. (2014). An early Phase II randomised controlled trial testing the effect on persecutory delusions of using CBT to reduce negative cognitions about the self: The potential benefits of enhancing self confidence. *Schizophrenia Research, 160*(1–3), 186–192. https://doi.org/10.1016/J.SCHRES.2014.10.038

Freeman, D., Dunn, G., Startup, H., Pugh, K., Cordwell, J., Mander, H., Černis, E., Wingham, G., Shirvell, K., & Kingdon, D. (2015a). Effects of cognitive behaviour therapy for worry on persecutory delusions in patients with psychosis (WIT): A parallel, single-blind, randomised controlled trial with a mediation analysis. *The Lancet Psychiatry, 2*(4), 305–313. https://doi.org/10.1016/S2215-0366(15)00039-5

Freeman, D., Waite, F., Startup, H., Myers, E., Lister, R., McInerney, J., Harvey, A. G., Geddes, J., Zaiwalla, Z., Luengo-Fernandez, R., Foster, R., Clifton, L., & Yu, L. M. (2015b). Efficacy of cognitive behavioural therapy for sleep improvement in patients with persistent delusions and hallucinations (BEST): A prospective, assessor-blind, randomised controlled pilot trial. *The Lancet. Psychiatry, 2*(11), 975–983. https://doi.org/10.1016/S2215-0366(15)00314-4

Freeman, D., Bradley, J., Antley, A., Bourke, E., DeWeever, N., Evans, N., Černis, E., Sheaves, B., Waite, F., Dunn, G., Slater, M., & Clark, D. M. (2016a). Virtual reality in the treatment of persecutory delusions: Randomised controlled experimental study testing how to reduce delusional conviction. *The British Journal of Psychiatry: the Journal of Mental Science, 209*(1), 62–67. https://doi.org/10.1192/BJP.BP.115.176438

Freeman, D., Bradley, J., Waite, F., Sheaves, B., DeWeever, N., Bourke, E., McInerney, J., Evans, N., Černis, E., Lister, R., Garety, P., & Dunn, G. (2016b). Targeting recovery in persistent persecutory delusions: A proof of principle study of a new translational psychological treatment (The feeling safe programme). *Behavioural and Cognitive Psychotherapy, 44*(5), 539–552. https://doi.org/10.1017/S1352465816000060

Freeman, D., Waite, F., Emsley, R., Kingdon, D., Davies, L., Fitzpatrick, R., & Dunn, G. (2016c). The efficacy of a new translational treatment for persecutory delusions: Study protocol for a randomised controlled trial (The Feeling Safe Study). *Trials, 17*(1). https://doi.org/10.1186/s13063-016-1245-0

Freeman, D., Taylor, K. M., Molodynski, A., & Waite, F. (2019). Treatable clinical intervention targets for patients with schizophrenia. *Schizophrenia Research, 211*, 44–50. https://doi.org/10.1016/J.SCHRES.2019.07.016

Freeman, D., Emsley, R., Diamond, R., Collett, N., Bold, E., Chadwick, E., Isham, L., Bird, J. C., Edwards, D., Kingdon, D., Fitzpatrick, R., Kabir, T., Waite, F., Carr, L., Causier, C., Černis, E., Kirkham, M., Lambe, S., Lister, R., et al. (2021). Comparison of a theoretically driven cognitive therapy (the Feeling Safe Programme) with befriending for the treatment of persistent persecutory delusions: A parallel, single-blind, randomised controlled trial. *The Lancet Psychiatry, 8*(8), 696–707. https://doi.org/10.1016/S2215-0366(21)00158-9

Garety, P. A., Kuipers, E., Fowler, D. G., Freeman, D., & Bebbington, P. (2001). A cognitive model of the positive symptoms of psychosis. *Psychological Medicine, 31*(2), 189–195. https://doi.org/10.1017/S0033291701003312

Garety, P. A., Bebbington, P. E., Fowler, D., Freeman, D., & Kuipers, E. (2007). Implications for neurobiological research of cognitive models of psychosis: A theoretical paper. *Psychological Medicine, 37*(10), 1377–1391. https://doi.org/10.1017/S003329170700013X

Garety, P., Waller, H., Emsley, R., Jolley, S., Kuipers, E., Bebbington, P., Dunn, G., Fowler, D., Hardy, A., & Freeman, D. (2015). Cognitive mechanisms of change in delusions: An experimental investigation targeting reasoning to effect change in paranoia. *Schizophrenia Bulletin, 41*(2), 400–410. https://doi.org/10.1093/SCHBUL/SBU103

Gaynor, K., Ward, T., Garety, P. A., & Peters, E. (2013). The role of safety-seeking behaviours in maintaining threat appraisals in psychosis. *Behaviour Research and Therapy, 51*(2), 75–81. https://doi.org/10.1016/j.brat.2012.10.008

Gumley, A., & Schwannauer, M. (2006). *Staying well after psychosis*. Wiley. https://doi.org/10.1002/9780470713303

Hardy, A. (2017). Pathways from trauma to psychotic experiences: A theoretically informed model of posttraumatic stress in psychosis. *Frontiers in Psychology, 8*(MAY), 697. https://doi.org/10.3389/FPSYG.2017.00697/BIBTEX

Heriot-Maitland, C., Knight, M., & Peters, E. (2012). A qualitative comparison of psychotic-like phenomena in clinical and non-clinical populations. *British Journal of Clinical Psychology, 51*(1), 37–53. https://doi.org/10.1111/j.2044-8260.2011.02011.x

Isham, L., Griffith, L., Boylan, A. M., Hicks, A., Wilson, N., Byrne, R., Sheaves, B., Bentall, R. P., & Freeman, D. (2021). Understanding, treating, and renaming grandiose delusions: A qualitative study. *Psychology and Psychotherapy, 94*(1), 119–140. https://doi.org/10.1111/PAPT.12260

Janssen, I., Hanssen, M., Bak, M., Bijl, R. V., de Graaf, R., Vollebergh, W., McKenzie, K., & van Os, J. (2003). Discrimination and delusional ideation. *The British Journal of Psychiatry, 182*(1), 71–76. https://doi.org/10.1192/BJP.182.1.71

Johns, L., Jolley, S., Keen, N., & Peters, E. (2014). CBT for people with psychosis. In *How to become a more effective CBT therapist: Mastering Metacompetence in clinical practice* (pp. 191–207). Wiley.

Johns, L., Isham, L., & Manser, R. (2020). Cognitive behavioural therapies for psychosis. In J. Badcock & G. Paulik (Eds.), *A clinical introduction to psychosis* (pp. 343–377). Elsevier. https://doi.org/10.1016/B978-0-12-815012-2.00015-8

Jun, H. J., Nam, B., Fedina, L., Smith, M. E., Schiffman, J., Link, B., & DeVylder, J. E. (2018). Paranoid beliefs and realistic expectations of victimization: Data from the survey of police-public encounters. *Schizophrenia Research, 199*, 326–332. https://doi.org/10.1016/J.SCHRES.2018.02.046

Kendler, K. S., & Campbell, J. (2009). Interventionist causal models in psychiatry: Repositioning the mind–body problem. *Psychological Medicine, 39*(6), 881–887. https://doi.org/10.1017/S0033291708004467

Kreyenbuhl, J., Buchanan, R. W., Dickerson, F. B., & Dixon, L. B. (2010). The schizophrenia Patient Outcomes Research Team (PORT): Updated treatment recommendations 2009. *Schizophrenia Bulletin, 36*, 94–103. https://doi.org/10.1093/schbul/sbp130

Lincoln, T. M., & Peters, E. (2018). A systematic review and discussion of symptom specific cognitive behavioural approaches to delusions and hallucinations. *Schizophrenia Research*. https://doi.org/10.1016/J.SCHRES.2017.12.014

Longden, E., Corstens, D., Escher, S., & Romme, M. (2012). Voice hearing in a biographical context: A model for formulating the relationship between voices and life history. *Psychosis, 4*(3), 224–234. https://doi.org/10.1080/17522439.2011.596566

Meaden, A., Keen, N., Aston, R., Barton, K., & Bucci, S. (2013). *Cognitive therapy for command hallucinations: An advanced practical companion*. Routledge.

Morrison, A. P. (2001). The interpretation of intrusions in psychosis: An integrative cognitive approach to hallucinations and delusions. *Behavioural and Cognitive Psychotherapy, 29*(3), 257–276. https://doi.org/10.1017/S1352465801003010

Morrison, A. P. (2017). A manualised treatment protocol to guide delivery of evidence-based cognitive therapy for people with distressing psychosis: Learning from clinical trials. *Psychosis, 9*(3), 271–281. https://doi.org/10.1080/17522439.2017.1295098

Morrison, A. P., Frame, L., & Larkin, W. (2003). Relationships between trauma and psychosis: A review and integration. *The British Journal of Clinical Psychology, 42*(Pt 4), 331–353. https://doi.org/10.1348/014466503322528892

Morrison, A. P., Stewart, S. L. K., French, P., Bentall, R. P., Birchwood, M., Byrne, R., Davies, L. M., Fowler, D., Gumley, A. I., Jones, P. B., Lewis, S. W., Murray, G. K., Patterson, P., &

Dunn, G. (2011). Early detection and intervention evaluation for people at high-risk of psychosis-2 (EDIE-2): Trial rationale, design and baseline characteristics. *Early Intervention in Psychiatry, 5*(1), 24–32. https://doi.org/10.1111/J.1751-7893.2010.00254.X

Morrison, A. P., Turkington, D., Pyle, M., Spencer, H., Brabban, A., Dunn, G., Christodoulides, T., Dudley, R., Chapman, N., Callcott, P., Grace, T., Lumley, V., Drage, L., Tully, S., Irving, K., Cummings, A., Byrne, R., Davies, L. M., & Hutton, P. (2014). Cognitive therapy for people with schizophrenia spectrum disorders not taking antipsychotic drugs: A single-blind randomised controlled trial. *The Lancet, 383*(9926), 1395–1403. https://doi.org/10.1016/S0140-6736(13)62246-1

Morrison, A. P., Law, H., Carter, L., Sellers, R., Emsley, R., Pyle, M., French, P., Shiers, D., Yung, A. R., Murphy, E. K., Holden, N., Steele, A., Bowe, S. E., Palmier-Claus, J., Brooks, V., Byrne, R., Davies, L., & Haddad, P. M. (2018a). Antipsychotic drugs versus cognitive behavioural therapy versus a combination of both in people with psychosis: A randomised controlled pilot and feasibility study. *The Lancet Psychiatry, 5*(5), 411–423. https://doi.org/10.1016/S2215-0366(18)30096-8

Morrison, A. P., Pyle, M., Gumley, A., Schwannauer, M., Turkington, D., MacLennan, G., Norrie, J., Hudson, J., Bowe, S. E., French, P., Byrne, R., Syrett, S., Dudley, R., McLeod, H. J., Griffiths, H., Barnes, T. R. E., Davies, L., Kingdon, D., & FOCUS trial group, S., … Tully, S. (2018b). Cognitive behavioural therapy in clozapine-resistant schizophrenia (FOCUS): An assessor-blinded, randomised controlled trial. *The Lancet Psychiatry, 5*(8), 633–643. https://doi.org/10.1016/S2215-0366(18)30184-6

National Institute for Health and Care Excellence. (2009). *Schizophrenia: Core interventions in the treatment and management of schizophrenia in primary and secondary care (update)*. Gaskell.

National Institute for Health and Care Excellence. (2014). *Psychosis and schizophrenia in adults: Treatment and management (CG178)*. National Institute for Health and Care Excellence.

Rector, N. A., Beck, A. T., & Stolar, N. (2005). The negative symptoms of schizophrenia: A cognitive perspective. *Canadian Journal of Psychiatry., 50*(5), 247–257. https://doi.org/10.1016/j.ahj.2005.01.046

Royal Australian and New Zealand College of Psychiatrists. (2005). Royal Australian and New Zealand College of Psychiatrists clinical practice guidelines for the treatment of schizophrenia and related disorders. *Australian and New Zealand Journal of Psychiatry, 39*(1–2), 1–30. https://doi.org/10.1111/j.1440-1614.2005.01516.x

Sheaves, B., Johns, L., Griffith, L., Isham, L., Kabir, T., & Freeman, D. (2020). Why do patients with psychosis listen to and believe derogatory and threatening voices? 21 reasons given by patients. *Behavioural and Cognitive Psychotherapy, 48*(6), 631–645. https://doi.org/10.1017/S1352465820000429

Tsang, A., Bucci, S., Branitsky, A., Kaptan, S., Rafiq, S., Wong, S., Berry, K., & Varese, F. (2021). The relationship between appraisals of voices (auditory verbal hallucinations) and distress in voice-hearers with schizophrenia-spectrum diagnoses: A meta-analytic review. *Schizophrenia Research, 230*, 38–47. https://doi.org/10.1016/J.SCHRES.2021.02.013

Turner, D. T., van der Gaag, M., Karyotaki, E., & Cuijpers, P. (2014). Psychological interventions for psychosis: A meta-analysis of comparative outcome studies. *American Journal of Psychiatry, 171*, 523–538. https://doi.org/10.1176/appi.ajp.2013.13081159

Young, M., Read, J., Barker-Collo, S., & Harrison, R. (2001). Evaluating and overcoming barriers to taking abuse histories. *Professional Psychology: Research and Practice, 32*(4), 407–414. https://doi.org/10.1037/0735-7028.32.4.407

Chapter 10
Person-Based Cognitive Therapy for Psychosis

Lyn Ellett

10.1 Introduction

Person-Based Cognitive Therapy for Psychosis (PBCT, Chadwick, 2006) is an integration of cognitive therapy and mindfulness, which emphasises understanding and reducing sources of distress, and promoting strengths and well-being. This chapter provides an integrated summary of the PBCT therapeutic approach. An overview of the four key therapeutic domains will be provided – symptomatic meaning, relationship to experience, schemata, and symbolic self, with accompanying case formulation models and key therapeutic techniques. Client and therapist work together in each of the four domains, with equal emphasis placed on working with strengths and distress. The domains are intentionally positioned alongside each other, promoting flexibility and movement between domains during therapy.

10.2 Symptomatic Meaning

This domain involves working directly with symptoms, such as paranoia and beliefs about voices (Chadwick et al., 1996). Working within this domain involves collaboratively exploring an individual's ability to decentre from their beliefs, which allows the individual not only to develop awareness of how their beliefs impact on behaviour and generate distress, but also to develop new meaning that enhances well-being.

L. Ellett (✉)
University of Southampton, Southampton, UK
e-mail: L.A.Ellett@soton.ac.uk

J. A. Díaz-Garrido et al. (eds.), *Psychological Interventions for Psychosis*,
https://doi.org/10.1007/978-3-031-27003-1_10

10.2.1 Formulation: ABC Framework

The main method for formulating symptomatic meaning and experience is the ABC framework. ABC formulation is a way of organising experience that clients find helpful and easy to understand. Use of the ABC formulation is flexible in PBCT – for example, it can be used as part of the assessment process, or to structure discussion of clients' experience. When using ABC formulations, it is important to isolate a specific situation where clients report that distress was high. Therapists are then able to draw out symptomatic meaning (e.g. images, thoughts, beliefs about voices & self, etc.), with associated emotion, behavioural urge/action, and body state. Consider the case of Simon, who experienced distressing voices and paranoid beliefs. Simon regularly heard voices telling him to harm his family. He believed the voices were powerful and controlling and felt scared when he heard them. He also experienced paranoid beliefs – for example, believing that his neighbours were deliberately tormenting him. This resulted in feelings of fear, anxiety, and powerlessness. Table 10.1 shows a summary of the ABC formulation, with examples that were developed with Simon during therapy.

10.2.2 Key Therapeutic Techniques

There are a number of CBT techniques that can be used when working therapeutically in the symptomatic meaning domain. These include: exploring goodness of fit of beliefs ('evidence'), including exploring doubt and generating alternatives, and planning and conducting behavioural experiments. They are briefly summarised here as they are discussed extensively elsewhere (see Chadwick et al., 1996).

10.2.2.1 Goodness of Fit ('Evidence') and Generating Alternative Symptomatic Meaning

Within PBCT, the starting point for assessing goodness of fit is always examining reasons that support individuals' beliefs – what is commonly referred to in the CBT literature as examining the evidence for the belief. Only when a full understanding

Table 10.1 Summary of ABC formulation with case example for paranoia and voices

Activating event or situation [A]	Beliefs [B]	Consequences [C]
At home on my own	My neighbours are deliberately tormenting me. They will try to harm me	Fear, anxiety, powerlessness Feels tense in body. Avoid leaving the house
Hears derogatory voice telling me to harm my family	Voices are powerful and control me If I do not do what the voices say, they will get worse	Try to resist what voices tell me to do Scared

of evidence for the belief has been gained, would the focus then turn to exploring elements of experience which are less consistent with beliefs, commonly referred to in the CBT literature as evidence against the belief. Part of exploring goodness of fit, or 'evidence', involves collaboratively exploring doubt with clients. This process begins by examining the client's capacity for doubt and includes client and therapist tentatively offering hypothetical contradictions (e.g. 'can you think of anything that would make you doubt this?'), which facilitates the development of alternative symptomatic meaning, or alternative explanations for experience. The symptomatic belief and alternative are assessed for consistency with the available evidence (i.e. goodness of fit) and usefulness (i.e. advantages and disadvantages of each). Within PBCT, we encourage clients to fully consider both alternatives.

10.2.2.2 Behavioural Experiments

Behavioural experiments are a method for testing hypotheses, and work best when they are formulated by clients and when there are clear predictions for both the symptomatic belief and the alternative. Their effectiveness is determined, at least in part, by the client's ability to be open to the possibility of disconfirmation, as well as confirmation. The effectiveness of any behavioural experiment is enhanced when the range of outcomes has been carefully considered beforehand. Ultimately, it is the client's choice to decide whether or not to carry out the experiment.

10.2.2.3 Accepting Fixity

Therapists are often faced with the situation of a client's belief being fixed. At these times, it is helpful for therapists to accept this - in PBCT, acceptance applies to the whole person, which includes their fixed beliefs. Although fixity can often be frustrating for therapists, it is actually informative – it reveals to the therapist that in this particular moment, change in the symptomatic meaning domain may not be posible. It may then be better to turn attention to working in one of the other domains. This facilitates flexibility and fluidity in the therapeutic process.

10.3 Relationship with Internal Experience

Within PBCT, mindfulness practice is used as the primary method for working within the relationship domain. By engaging in mindfulness practice, individuals learn to respond mindfully to psychotic sensations, rather than getting lost in reacting to them. Being more aware of psychotic sensations and their impact allows individuals to let go of their usual reactions which maintain distress, such as experiential avoidance and rumination. Decentred awareness and acceptance of present moment experience are the two main processes that support the reduction of distress and enhancement of well-being through mindfulness practice. This is facilitated by reflective learning (in which the role of the therapist is to draw out metacogntiive insights) and guided discovery both prior to, and following, mindfulness practice, as well as use of specific guidance during practice. Guidance during mindfulness practice and reflective learning both highlight key aspects of experience during meditation practice, for example that sensations come and go, and that nothing stays in awareness permanently. This facilitates the acquisition of metacognitive insights, as the therapist draws out what the client notices about the nature of sensations, and their reactions to them. This helps clients to gain awareness of how their relationship to (psychotic) sensations impacts directly on their current emotional state.

10.3.1 Formulation

When experiencing an unpleasant psychotic sensation (voice, paranoid thought, image, etc.), distress arises from indiviudals becoming lost in their (usual) reactions to it (Chadwick, 2006). Three main reactions have been identified that maintain distress– experiential avoidance, negative judgement, and rumination/confrontation (Chadwick et al., 2005). In contrast, responding mindfully to unpleasant psychotic sensations involves maintaining decentred awareness while being open to whatever is experienced, without reacting to it, or identifying with it. Consider the case of Julie, who heard distressing voices saying "you're bad, ugly and worthless" and "you can't do anything right, you'll never amount to anything". At the start of therapy, Julie tried to avoid/resist her voices and also avoided engaging in activities for fear of failure. She regularly confronted her voices by shouting and swearing back at them and also got lost in depressive rumination about them. She believed what the voices told her and consequently judged herself as bad. Through mindfulness practice, Julie learned to respond differently to her distressing voices by noting their presence (turning towards the difficult) and allowing them to be there (acceptance) and not getting caught up in her usual reactions to them (letting go). Figure 10.1 shows the mindfulness-based formulation that was developed with Julie during therapy.

10.3.2 Mindfulness Practice

Several adaptations to mindfulness practice have been suggested when working with people with distressing psychosis (Chadwick, 2006; Chadwick et al., 2005, 2009, 2011). First, practice time is limited to 10 min maximum, as most clients find this is the most that they can manage. Second, extended silences during practice are avoided – therapists give brief guidance or comments every 1–2 min. This is an important grounding method, and helps clients to decentre from voices, rumination, etc. and to reconnect with present experience with clearer awareness. Third, practice

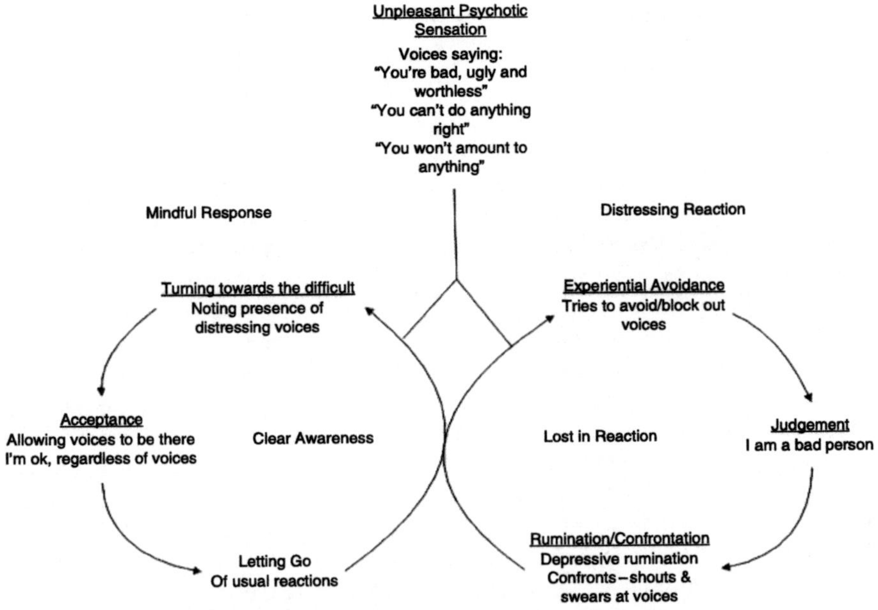

Fig. 10.1 Mindfulness formulation of distressing voices. (Reproduced from Morris et al., 2013)

outside sessions is not an essential requirement – audios of the 10-min guided mindfulness are provided, and practice is encouraged. In PBCT, the same 10-min guided mindfulness practice is used in every session.

10.4 Schemata

In PBCT, working within the schemata domain involves reducing distress directly linked to the individual's negative schema of self and others and enhancing overall well-being by developing positive self-schemata. In PBCT, there are four aims when working with negative schema. First, individuals increase awareness of the nature and characteristics of their negative schematic experience. Second, both client and therapist accept the negative self-schema. Third, to gain metacognitive insight about the nature of the negative self-schema, i.e. that it forms one aspect of the self, not *the entire* self. Fourth, reduce fear associated with negative schematic experience. Taken together, these four aims allow a new relationship with negative self-schema to be developed. When working with positive self-schema, the aim is to collaboratively draw out, maintain, and generalise positive schematic experience.

10.4.1 Formulation

Both positive and negative schemata are formulated in PBCT. Although schematic beliefs about self and others are incorporated into ABC formulations, it is also important to formulate them separately, as they are often extremely distressing and disabling. The emphasis when working in this domain is on acceptance of negative schematic experience as part of the self, rather than as defining the entire self. Equal importance is also placed on developing positive self-schema. In addition, the fact that positive and negative experiences of self are formulated using the same basic model facilitates the development of metacognitive insights that the symbolic self is made up of complex and conflicting experiences. Consider the case of Neil, who had a 10 year history of paranoid beliefs. Neil came to therapy believing that he was inadequate and a bad person, and that others were hostile and out to get him. He thought that others knew that he was unwell and therefore judged him negatively as a result. The future looked bleak and Neil believed that things would never change. Neil was afraid to leave his flat, as he believed that other people might harm him, and in particular might stab him. He would often spend time ruminating when he knew he would have to leave his flat (e.g. to buy food or attend appointments) and was hypervigilant of others when he did go out. During therapy, a number of rules for living were identified; Neil believed that if he let his guard down around others, and if they knew about his [mental health] history, they would judge him negatively and potentially harm him. This resulted in sustained periods of isolation and fear, in which he would avoid leaving his flat. Figures 10.2 and 10.3 are examples of Neil's NSS and PSS that were collaboratively developed during therapy.

10.4.2 Key Therapeutic Techniques

10.4.2.1 Two Chair Method

The two chair method is a key therapeutic technique for working in both the schemata and symbolic self-domains. It usually takes around 25–30 min, so can comfortably fit within a single therapy session. The rationale given to clients is that it provides an opportunity to explore both positive and negative experiences of self, and that it involves physically moving between two chairs. When the therapist has outlined the aims and process of two chair work, it is important to then check in with the client to see if they have any concerns about doing it. If concerns are raised, it is important that these are discussed fully and resolved prior to commencing two-chair work (Chadwick, 2003).

The first step in the process is for the client to briefly enact the negative self-schema. This is done briefly as negative experiences of self will be very familiar to clients and there is therefore no need to dwell on them for too long. Following the client's enactment, the therapist then provides an empathic summary of this

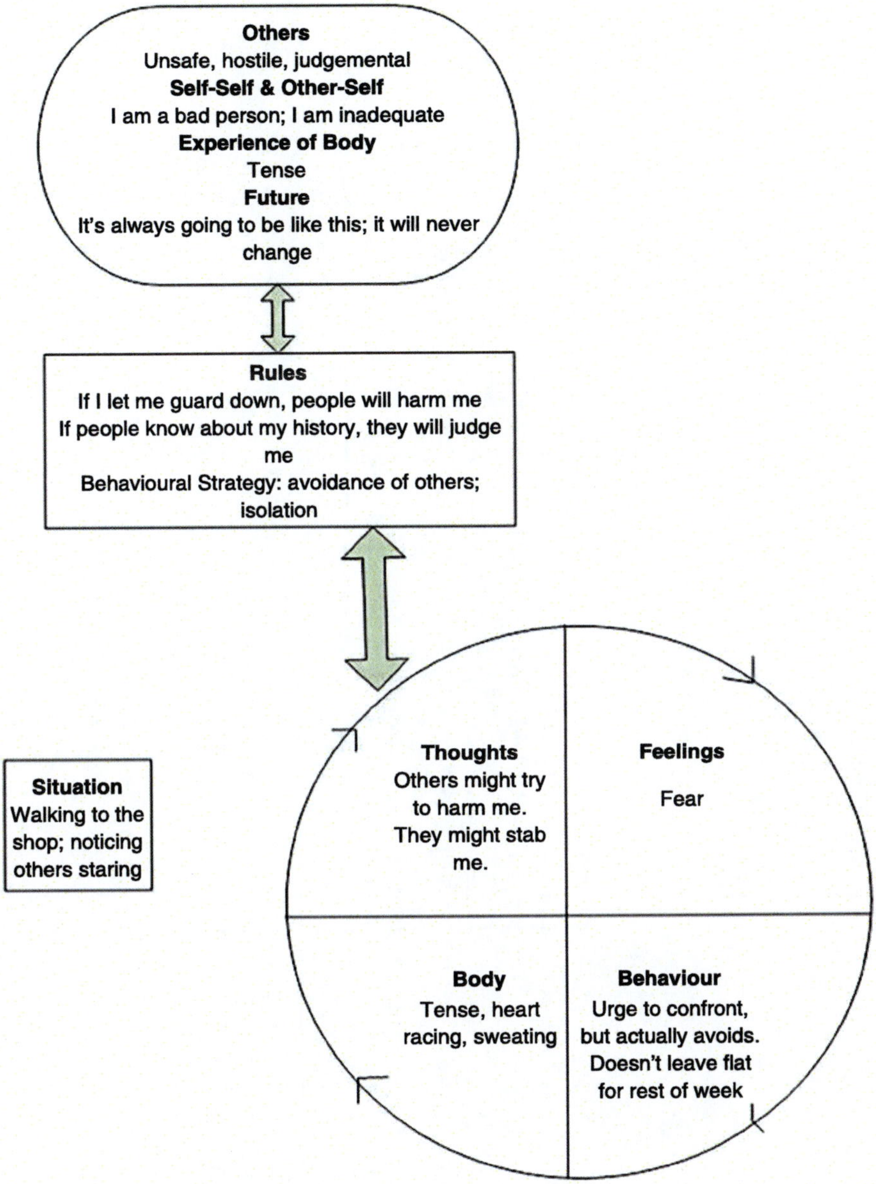

Fig. 10.2 Neil's Negative Self-Schema. (Reproduced from Morris et al., 2013)

negative experience of self. The client is then invited to move to the second chair; at this point, the therapist emphasises that the negative self-schema stays in the first chair. Following movement to the second chair, the client then articulates and 'lives' a positive self-schema. The therapist then facilitates acceptance of both schemata,

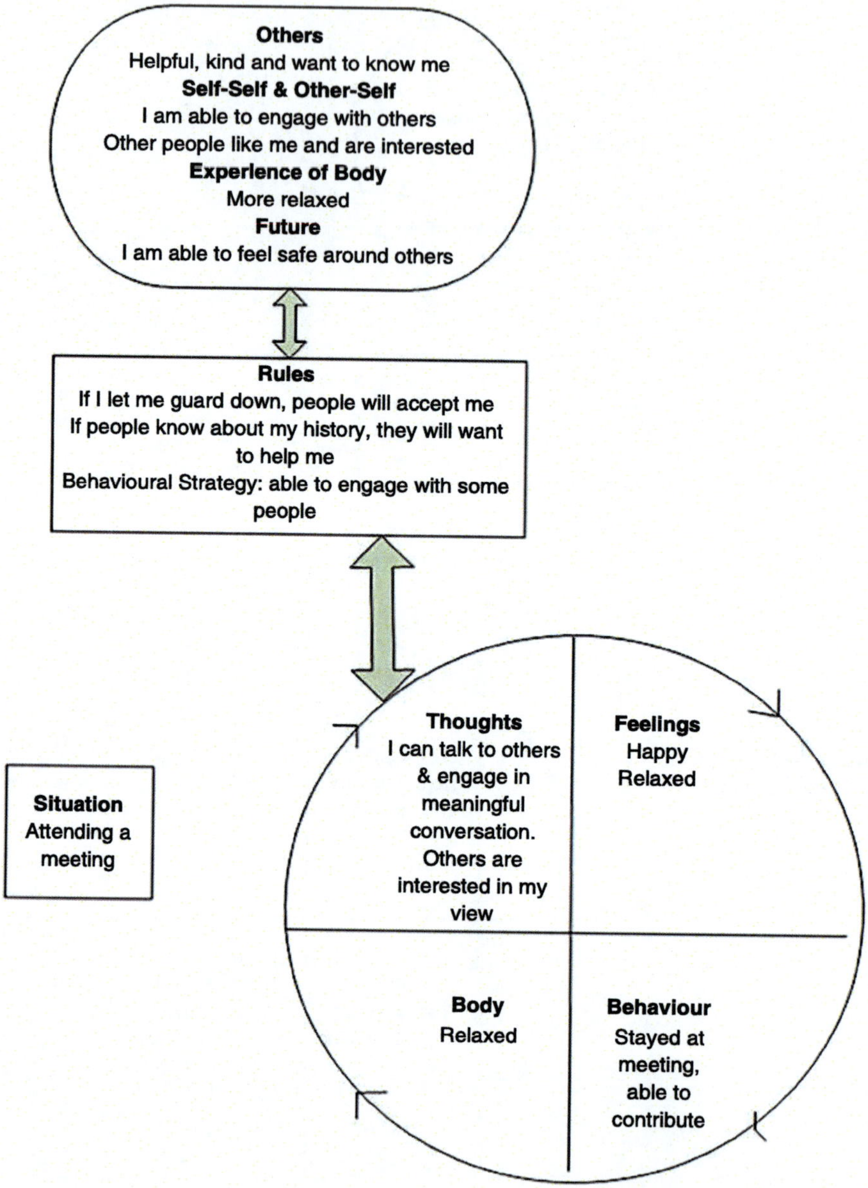

Fig. 10.3 Neil's Positive Self-Schema. (Reproduced from Morris et al., 2013)

and client and therapist together explore the complex and changing nature of the symbolic self. At the end of the two-chair process, it is important that the therapist checks in with the client, to ensure there are no continuing effects when the client returns to the chair in which the negative self-schema was enacted. To support metacognitive insight, maintenance, and generalisation, the 2-chair method needs to be seen as a flexible process, rather than a one-off task, which will often be used many times during therapy.

10.5 Symbolic Self

In PBCT, the symbolic self is a metacognitive model of self, which represents an integration of both positive and negative self-schematic experiences. The symbolic self brings awareness to, and facilitates acceptance of, the complex and changing nature of the experience of self. While most of us probably have moments of negative self-schematic experience, this does not tend to dominate or overwhelm our symbolic self. However, the more the person's experience of self is dominated by negative schematic experience, the more the focus of the symbolic self becomes restricted and overly negative – what Chadwick (2006) refers to as 'one dimensional'. It is common for the symbolic self of individuals with distressing psychosis to be one dimensional at the start of therapy; therapeutic work in this domain therefore involves bringing negative schematic experience into balance and elaborating and enhancing positive schematic experience, thereby 'opening out' the symbolic self and bringing awareness to, and acceptance of, the complex and changing nature of the self.

10.5.1 Therapeutic Techniques

Working with the dynamic nature of the symbolic self is achieved by: (1) bringing experientially into awareness the current focus of the symbolic self on the all consuming nature of the negative self chema; (2) enhancing and elaborating on positive self-schematic experience; (3) supporting acceptance of both the negative and position self-schemas as valid experiences of self; and (4) working directly to modify the symbolic self so that it is not solely defined by negative self-schematic experience, but also incorporates positive schemata of self and others. The purpose of working within the domain of the symbolic self is not to get rid of or change the negative self-schema in any way, but rather, the aim is to experience the negative self-schema as simply one aspect of self, not the entire self. By bringing the positive self-schema more into focus, therapists can facilitate reflection on, and experience of, the changing nature of the symbolic self. Therapists then emphasise that the client can either continue to be defined solely by their negative self-schema or commit to further development of the positive aspects of the symbolic self. This is mainly achieved using the two-chair method.

10.6 Conclusion

PBCT is a person-centred approach, with equal emphasis placed on working with distress and promoting strengths and well-being. In this chapter, an overview of PBCT for distressing psychosis has been provided. This has included consideration of the four key therapeutic domains – symptomatic meaning, relationship to experience, schemata, and symbolic self – including formulation models and key therapeutic techniques. PBCT has been shown to be beneficial for indiviudals with both voices and paranoia in RCTs (Chadwick et al., 2016; Ellett et al., 2020), in routine clinical practice (Dannahy et al., 2011; Jones et al., 2020), and more recently when delivered online in routine clinical practice (Ellett et al., under review).

Disclaimer Clinical cases presented in this chapter do not include real names or personal information of real persons.

References

Chadwick, P. D. J. (2003). Two chairs, self-schemata and a person-based approach to psychosis. *Behavioural and Cognitive Psychotherapy, 31*(4), 439–449.

Chadwick, P. D. J. (2006). *Person-based cognitive therapy for distressing psychosis*. Chichester.

Chadwick, P. D. J., Birchwood, M. J., & Trower, P. (1996). *Cognitive therapy for delusions, voices and paranoia*. Wiley.

Chadwick, P. D. J., Newman-Taylor, K., & Abba, N. (2005). Mindfulness groups for people with distressing psychosis. *Behavioural and Cognitive Psychotherapy, 33*, 351–359.

Chadwick, P. D. J., Hughes, S., Russell, I., Russell, D., & Dagnan, D. (2009). Mindfulness groups for distressing psychosis: A replication and feasibility study. *Behavioural and Cognitive Psychotherapy, 37*, 403–413.

Chadwick, P. D. J., Kaur, H., Swelam, M., Ross, S., & Ellett, L. (2011). Experience of mindfulness in people with bipolar disorder. *Psychotherapy Research, 21*(3), 277–285.

Chadwick, P., Strauss, C., Jones, A. M., Kingdon, D., Ellett, L., Dannahy, L., & Hayward, M. (2016). Group mindfulness-based intervention for distressing voices: A pragmatic randomised controlled trial. *Schizophrenia Research, 175*(1–3), 168–173.

Dannahy, L., Hayward, M., Strauss, C., Turton, W., Harding, E., & Chadwick, P. (2011). Group person-based cognitive therapy for distressing psychosis: Pilot data from nine groups. *Journal of Behaviour Therapy and Experimental Psychiatry, 42*(1), 111–116.

Ellett, L., Tarant, E., Kouimtsidis, C., Kingston, J., Vivarelli, L., et al. (2020). Group mindfulness based therapy for persecutory delusions: A pilot randomised controlled trial. *Schizophrenia Research, 222*, 534–536.

Ellett, L., Dannahy, L., & Chadwick, P. (under review). Engagement, clinical outcomes and therapeutic process in online mindfulness for psychosis groups delivered in routine care. *Psychology and Psychotherapy: Theory, Research and Practice*.

Jones, A. M., Strauss, C., & Hayward, M. (2020). A service evaluation of a group mindfulness-based intervention for distressing voices: How do findings from a randomized controlled trial compare with routine clinical practice? *Behavioural and Cognitive Psychotherapy, 49*(1), 76–90.

Morris, E. M., Johns, L. C., & Oliver, J. E. (Eds.). (2013). *Acceptance and commitment therapy and mindfulness for psychosis*. John Wiley & Sons.

Chapter 11
The Phenomenological Perspective and Metacognitive Psychotherapy in Addressing Psychosis

Gabriel Ródenas-Perea, Susana Al-Halabí, Félix Inchausti, and Eduardo Fonseca-Pedrero

11.1 Introduction

Psychotic experiences are part of human diversity and, because they are unique individual experiences, they cannot be understood in isolation from life circumstances or subjective experience (Cooke, 2017; Fonseca-Pedrero, 2019). Similarly, psychosis as a phenomenon of study is intrinsic to disciplines such as clinical psychology and psychiatry and is today one of the most widely studied phenomena in the field of mental health. From the beginning and even nowadays, psychosis—schizophrenia being the most representative—has been conceptualized as an illness that is biological in origin, the product of the expression of certain genes, dysregulation of neurotransmitters, or abnormal functional connectivity in brain regions. Despite the enormous amount of research over the last 50 years, there is yet to be found evidence of these supposed genetic or cerebral causes of psychosis and related disorders and some authors have indicated that we have still not managed to understand its causes or how it functions (Keshavan et al., 2011; Tandon et al., 2008). In this regard, it would perhaps be wiser to think about reasons not causes,

G. Ródenas-Perea
Servicio Andaluz de Salud, Seville, Spain
e-mail: gabriel.rodenas.sspa@juntadeandalucia.es

S. Al-Halabí
Department of Psychology, University of Oviedo, Oviedo, Spain
e-mail: alsusana@uniovi.es

F. Inchausti
Department of Mental Health, Servicio Riojano de Salud, Logroño, Spain
e-mail: finchausti@riojasalud.es

E. Fonseca-Pedrero (✉)
Department of Educational Sciences, University of La Rioja, Logroño, Spain
e-mail: eduardo.fonseca@unirioja.es

J. A. Díaz-Garrido et al. (eds.), *Psychological Interventions for Psychosis*,
https://doi.org/10.1007/978-3-031-27003-1_11

and at the same time understand psychosis as a response to the vicissitudes of life within the complex variety of human nature (Cooke, 2017; Fonseca-Pedrero, 2019). Psychosis, like any other psychological phenomenon, operates on a personal, phenomenistic, operant, linguistic, and contextual scale (Pérez-Álvarez & García-Montes, 2019).

Psychotherapy has been shown to be effective in addressing psychotic disorders (Leichsenring et al., 2022). Psychological treatments have been found to be beneficial to quality of life and personal development as well as to the reduction of "symptoms" and improved functioning. The treatments which are supported by the greatest amount of evidence and have been the most highly recommended are cognitive behavioural therapy (CBT) for psychosis and family interventions. It is worth mentioning that the NICE clinical guidelines (National Collaborating Centre for Mental Health, 2014) for managing psychosis recommend CBT as one of the main intervention options, even independently of medication. In recent years, new approaches to address psychotic "symptoms" have appeared, or old approaches have been recovered, including open dialogue, metacognitive therapy, and the phenomenological approach. These new and promising methods of intervention are still being analysed and evaluated, although they open the door to new ways of understanding psychosis and intervening in its "symptoms". This means there must be an approach focused on the person, on interpersonal relationships, on understanding experiences in the biographical context, on recovering the sense of *self*, and on giving a person back the scope of their life and thus escaping the trap of schizophrenia, without promising "a bed of roses" (Fonseca-Pedrero, 2019, 2021).

Within this context, this chapter explains the understanding of psychosis from a phenomenological perspective and the implications of that, outlining it in relation to the concept of metacognition. It presents the principles of phenomenologically oriented psychotherapy and introduces the characteristics of Metacognitive Reflection and Insight Therapy (MERIT), a psychotherapy that brings those aspects together. The chapter finishes with a summary and a description of a clinical case.

11.2 First-Person: Patient J.M

I am a 19-year-old male. I was born in a city in the north of Spain and grew up there in a middle-class family. Ever since I can remember, my childhood has been marked by my parents' work in the family restaurant. They expected me and my two siblings to help them in the kitchen and during service. If I had to describe my parents in two words, I would say that they were quiet and hard-working. I don't have any memories of them talking openly with me or my siblings about their feelings or thoughts, nor of me talking with them. I could also say that they are very strict, the kind of people it's better not to annoy. My two siblings are good students and have always been socially popular. They haven't had any physical or psychological problems as far as I know. In contrast, I suffered from ear infections and hearing problems from when I was little, and I had to spend a lot of time in hospital. Because of that, my school attendance was spotty and I never had close relationships with classmates. Socially, I've always felt unconnected. Despite my long absences from school, my grades were never affected. I can't remember ever being bullied or abused in school, but I was never part of any groups and I felt like a complete outsider. I spent breaks alone in the playground, usually reading. When other kids tried to get me to play with them, I was terrified of making a fool of myself or saying something embarrassing.

I made some friends in secondary school, but I generally preferred to be quiet and to keep apart. In the second year of upper secondary school [Bachillerato], I began to experience what I later learned to be psychotic "symptoms". I was convinced that my classmates and the people at school were talking about me and criticizing how I looked and what I wore. I heard them talking everywhere and even heard them whispering, although I was nowhere near them. I felt as if everyone was looking at me and judging me. Later, I began hearing voices in my head criticizing me all the time. At the time of the final exams, I had to be admitted to hospital by my parents, where they told me that I was suffering from paranoid schizophrenia and they gave me antipsychotic medication. I was discharged after 2 weeks and sent to my local mental health centre. After various visits to my psychiatrist, who adjusted my medication, I was sent to the clinical psychologist.

11.3 The Phenomenological Approach

Psychologists try to understand the experiences of the people who seek their help. This can be particularly difficult with people who are suffering psychotic symptoms, as this usually means dealing with unusual human reactions that are not shared by the majority. Karl Menninger used the metaphor of a fish on a hook to describe the behaviour of people with unusual difficulties, "When a trout rising to a fly gets hooked and finds himself unable to swim about freely, he begins a fight which results in struggles and splashes and sometimes an escape.... In the same way, the human stuggles ... with the hooks that catch him. Sometime he masters his difficulties; sometimes they are too much for him. The struggles are all that the world sees, and it usually misunderstands them. It is hard for a free fish to understand what is happening to a hooked one". Some professionals suggest that the way to break this deadlock might be to return, in the words of the founder of phenomenology, Edmund Husserl, "*to the things themselves*" (The Lancet Psychiatry, 2021). The phenomenological approach aims to be able to describe and understand experience, that is, understand the biographical context of the *self* and its circumstances. It is interesting for being able to describe the meaningful organization of people's experiences, expressions, and behaviours, proposing a narrative understanding of each individual. This narrative understanding relates the scenario of action with that of consciousness in order to make sense of people's experiences and behaviours (Stanghellini, 2010; Stanghellini & Lysaker, 2007). It is, therefore, a phenomenology that is interested in the interrelationship between experience, behaviour, and culture (Pérez-Álvarez et al., 2009). From this perspective, psychopathological syndromes are not mere associations of "symptoms", but rather express characteristic disorders of human existence and the *way-of-being-in-the-world* (Stanghellini & Mancini, 2017).

11.4 Psychosis as a Disorder of the Self or Ipseity

From a phenomenological perspective, and in line with the proposals from Parnas and Sass (2008; Sass & Parnas, 2003), psychosis and associated disorders can be understood as disorders of the experience of the self, or ipseity. Ipseity refers to the basic sense of *selfhood* as the core of one's own experience. This disorder affects the whole structure of the self, including the reflexive self, the narrative self, and the social aspects of the self. While the concept of schizophrenia as a problem of the brain involves a narrative of chronic illness that ends up being interiorized by sufferers and their families, schizophrenia as a problem of ipseity involves a narrative and a change of discourse towards oneself based on the recovery of the sense of self, where one contemplates leaving the condition behind (Davidson, 2003; Pérez-Álvarez et al., 2010; Hasson-Ohayon & Lysaker, 2021).

If we conceptualize the disorders on the psychosis spectrum as problems of ipseity, psychotherapeutic interventions should be aimed at restoring and strengthening the first-person experience and the sense of self, where intersubjective context and understanding are fundamental for a possible recovery. Phenomenology considers possible recovery to involve mutual recognition as people and the creation of shared meaning. The issue is re-establishing the weakened connection between feelings and interpersonal situations in the here and now and in the You and I relationship. This can be achieved through the therapeutic relationship (Stanghellini & Lysaker, 2007). If the therapeutic relationship creates the intersubjective context needed to re-establish ipseity, the hermeneutic relationship contributes to the creation of narratives that help reconstruct the sense of self (Pérez-Álvarez et al., 2010; Hasson-Ohayon & Lysaker, 2021).

With this approach, the patient has much to say and much to contribute. To begin with, the role of the clinician is not so much diagnosis but rather to be a participant who listens and tries to understand and make shared sense of particular experiences. It is not about trying to "indoctrinate" someone in the theory of ipseity, but instead it is about creating a holistic, intersubjective context in which it is possible to work together.

11.5 Ipseity and the Role of Metacognition

As indicated above, people who experience psychotic phenomena can find it difficult to construct an idea of what they have experienced psychologically and socially once those phenomena appear, and therefore may not be sure of how to respond or to manage them. They may also find that their place in the world and their relationships with others have changed or have become irreconcilable (Davidson, 2003; Firmin et al., 2021). One way of understanding these disorders in ipseity is to think of them as the result of problems in metacognition (Lysaker & Klion, 2017).

Metacognition is a complex set of processes that allow a person to have a sense of who they are in relation to others, what is happening now, what happened in the past, and what will happen in the future. The term means "thinking about thinking", but it also allows people to perceive the relationship between what they think, feel, and desire in order to then use that information to monitor and change their own behaviour adaptively (Dimaggio et al., 2020; Lysaker et al., 2020b; Moritz & Lysaker, 2018). In international samples, research has found that people with diagnoses of disorders on the psychotic spectrum experience a more fragmented sense of self and others compared to control groups and compared to others diagnosed with other mental disorders (Lysaker et al., 2020c). The highest levels of these kinds of metacognitive deficits have also been related to reduced awareness of the difficulties produced by the disorder (Lysaker et al., 2019), worse psychosocial functioning (Arnon-Ribenfeld et al., 2017), particularly in areas related to seeking intrinsically motivating activities, and difficulties in feeling and expressing emotions (Arnon-Ribenfeld et al., 2017; Dmitryeva et al., 2021; Lysaker et al., 2020c).

Metacognitive skills allow us to, for example, recognize the characteristics of others' behaviour and identify our own patterns of thinking or mental frameworks when it comes to understanding autobiographical interpersonal events (Vohs et al., 2015). When metacognitive processes work, they allow us to perform a variety of mental operations simultaneously, automatically, and adaptively. They also provide a flexible, multifaceted, multidimensional sense of oneself and the world in line with the changing needs of the context. This model of metacognition, in short, means a networked psychological process, with interdependent cognitive processes that cannot operate in isolation and which ultimately allow us to face life's psychological and social challenges (Inchausti et al., 2018).

When it comes to psychosis, this model suggests that metacognitive processes play a central role in recovery and that they occur and develop in a clearly intersubjective context. In other words, the beliefs of people with these types of experiences, no matter how elaborate, are formed in interpersonal situations over time, which means that they are representations that can be shared and recognized by others (Cortina & Liotti, 2010; Hasson-Ohayon, 2012; Tomasello et al., 2005).

In addition, metacognitive processes are organized hierarchically. People must be able to perform simple metacognitive tasks first (e.g. recognizing thoughts as their own) before performing more complex, holistic tasks (e.g. recognizing that thoughts and emotions are connected in day to day life). Therefore, if a process does not work properly, none of the higher processes will be able to function as they would need information from the lower level processes (Lysaker et al., 2005; Lysaker & Klion, 2017).

11.5.1 Metacognition in Patient J.M

Returning to the case of J.M, the negative "symptoms" and metacognition were evaluated before and after treatment using the Positive and Negative Syndrome Scale (PANSS) and the Metacognition Assessment Scale-Abbreviated (MAS-A) (see Table 11.1). J.M.'s scores in metacognition indicated that although he had few thoughts, he recognized that they were his and not from an external source, and he was able to differentiate between various cognitive processes such as desires, decisions, and memories. Nonetheless, he was not able to understand that his emotions and beliefs about himself and others could change over time. He also found it difficult to connect his thoughts and emotions both at the present and over time.

With regard to his ability to understand the minds of others, he recognized that other people had their own thoughts, but had difficulties differentiating different cognitive processes in others. He was unable to think about how others felt and seemed not to be able to form complex representations about other people's internal worlds.

In terms of his capacity for decentration, J.M.'s scores indicated that he was able to recognize that other people had lives which were independent of his, but he found it difficult to understand that there were different interpretations and points of view about a given situation. With regard to his mastery skills, J.M. recognized the existence of psychological problems. For example, he expressed his desire to take more initiative in his life. However, he was unable to suggest various alternatives to resolve his problems beyond calling his mother or sister to ask them what to do. This had also caused notable stress in the family, as J.M. was quite able to call his mother up to five times a day just to ask her advice.

11.6 Phenomenologically Oriented Psychotherapy

It is important to begin by recognizing something that may seem obvious, but is a sine qua non of the psychotherapeutic approach to psychosis: the therapeutic relationship. This is not solely the construction of a good therapeutic alliance or establishing a co-operative relationship, it is also about a thorough interpersonal meeting aimed at understanding the altered experience of *being-in-the-world* rather than repairing the supposed malfunction of a mechanistic system (Nelson et al., 2008). Much has been spoken about chemical imbalances, but the important thing in psychotherapy for psychosis is the "chemical aspects" of the therapeutic relationship. Validation, empathy, and curiosity in trying to understand a person's experience and accept it must be the basis underlying the process of working towards recovery (Davidson, 2003). In addition, the efforts of the therapist in constructing a sound therapeutic relationship must not be limited to just the beginning of the process; it should be reviewed and tended to throughout. Empirical evidence has shown the importance of monitoring and reviewing the different psychotherapeutic elements

Table 11.1 Structure of the Metacognition Assessment Scale-Abbreviated (MAS–A)

Level	Self-reflection	Understanding the mind of others	Decentration	Mastery
0	Complete lack of awareness of their own mental activity	Complete lack of awareness of others' mental activity	Thinking that one is the Centre of everything that happens	Lack of awareness of problems
1	Some awareness of their own mental activity	Some awareness of others' mental activity	Recognizing that other people have independent lives	Awareness of problems as insoluble
2	Awareness that thoughts are their own	Awareness that others have their own mental activity	Awareness that there are different ways of understanding a single event	Awareness of problems as something that can be solved but lacking responses
3	Differentiation of their own cognitive operations (thoughts, fantasies, memories, etc.)	Differentiation of others' cognitive operations (thoughts, fantasies, memories, etc.)	Awareness that facts are the result of multiple, complex factors	Passive responses
4	Differentiation of different emotional states	Differentiation of different emotional states in others	–	Help-seeking responses
5	Recognition that their own thoughts are fallible	Plausible supposition about the mental states of other people	–	Responses with specific actions
6	Recognition that desire is not reality	Complete descriptions of others' thinking over time	–	Responses with changes
7	Incorporation of their own thoughts and emotions into a narrative	Complete descriptions of others' thinking over their lives	–	Responses based on their own knowledge
8	Incorporation of various narratives recognizing patterns over time	–	–	Responses based on others' knowledge
9	Recognition of thoughts and emotions connected through their own life	–	–	Responses based on a broad understanding of life

Note. Adapted from Lysaker et al. (2005)

(including the therapeutic alliance), which can be key in achieving treatment objectives (Gimeno Peón, 2020).

Stanghellini and Lysaker identified four principles of phenomenologically oriented psychotherapy (Pérez-Álvarez et al., 2011):

1. *The importance of intersubjective disturbances*
   Intersubjective difficulties are the core of psychotic disorders rather than epiphenomena resulting from supposed neurobiological anomalies, psychodynamic conflicts, or idiosyncratic cognition (Nelson et al., 2008). As we explained above, understanding psychosis as a disorder of ipseity involves a disorder in the intersubjective arena, whether in a person's relationship with their symptoms or the experiences that they have getting on with others around them. In fact, better intersubjective participation in the world is understood to facilitate management of "symptoms" such as delusions and hallucinations. In this regard, the therapeutic relationship can provide a context in which a person's relationship with psychotic experiences can be changed, be it hallucinations (e.g. voices) (Pérez-Álvarez et al., 2008) or delusions (Ritunnano & Bortolotti, 2021), and those experiences can be given meaning and be incorporated into the person's own life story.
2. *Establish a shared interpersonal space*
   Shared interpersonal space refers to establishing mutual recognition as people, something which is necessary for restoring a first-person perspective and therefore the reappropriation of one's own experience. Phenomenologically oriented psychology does not have "internally" directed space, but instead is open in the "external" space between the therapist and the person. As Nelson et al. (2009) showed us, a therapeutic relationship ruled over by an attitude of concern about understanding the other and honest curiosity provides a space in which the patient can develop more robust pre-reflexive self-awareness while at the same time being a meeting in which they feel they are able to share their own emotional states and work to understand and be aware of others' mental and emotional states.
3. *Concentrate on the here and now, on the You and I relationship*
   The intent is to help the person to re-establish the connection with their current context. As Stanghellini and Lysaker put it, "psychotherapy can serve as a 'dialogical prosthesis' to help re-establish the lost connection between bodily feelings (emotions) and interpersonal situations". Although considering emotions as bodily sensations is not universally accepted, one might argue here the importance of corporality and intersubjectivity in phenomenology. The You and I relationship in psychotherapy is understood to mean the sensation of being there, a physical presence for the other which is mutual.
4. *Constructing shared meaning*
   This therapeutic method proposes the co-construction of stories which help to reconstruct a person's self, stories which need both internal and external consistency. While internal consistency is needed for the patient to develop meaningful understanding of their own psychological states, external consistency refers to

> the interpersonal aspects that make the narrative meaningful to others. The therapist acts as the arbiter, catalyst, and reference framework in meaningful narratives. It goes without saying that both the construction of dialogical prostheses and the construction of a shared vocabulary require a detailed, descriptive exploration of the structure of the person's experience. This ability gains meaning within the phenomenological framework and requires specific training to apply, as well as practice that is supervised by the therapist. Phenomenological psychotherapy is not simply listening to the patient and understanding them with sympathy and empathy, but rather, and above all, capturing essential experiences and offering personally meaningful interpretation. Stanghellini and Lysaker (2007) show that this intersubjective method can help those with schizophrenia to develop both a first-person perspective for themselves and a second-person perspective when they are with others, opening up a path to recovery.

Various psychotherapies have been developed for psychosis over recent years based on these principles (Hasson-Ohayon et al., 2021). Their therapeutic objectives have mainly focused on improving interpersonal functioning (Inchausti et al., 2018) and reducing psychotic "symptoms" (Salvatore et al., 2018; Vitzthum et al., 2014). Given the close relationship between phenomenology and metacognition in psychosis, in the following section we present Metacognitive Reflection and Insight Therapy, or MERIT, developed over the last 10 years by Paul H. Lysaker and colleagues (Lysaker et al., 2020a; Lysaker & Klion, 2017).

11.7 Starting Situation in Patient J.M

At the time of the first consultation, J.M. had been living independently in a shared flat for almost a year. With psychosocial support, he was able to successfully complete his Bachillerato exams and the university entrance tests and was able to start studying at university. At the weekends, he helped his parents in the family restaurant which allowed him to cover some of his living costs. His psychiatrist had stabilized his medication on low doses of Aripiprazol (10 mg/day). Nonetheless, the critical voices persisted, but with notably reduced impact, and his self-referential delusions disappeared completely. The same did not happen with the negative "symptoms", which progressively increased. Over time, there were increasingly noticeable signs and "symptoms" of alogia (sharp reduction in spontaneous language and content, frequent speaking blocks, and increased latency in responses), abulia (notable difficulties in making decisions, even simple day-to-day decisions, university attendance, and relating to others), and feelings of emptiness. Consequently, J.M. spent most of his time sitting in his room doing absolutely nothing. Despite wanting to interact with people, J.M. found himself almost completely isolated, except for the scant contact with his flat mates and his family. When he conversed with them, he had serious difficulties starting or maintaining conversations, he did not know what to say or ask and usually ended conversations quickly.

11.8 Metacognitive Reflection and Insight Therapy: MERIT

MERIT is an inclusive psychotherapy that combines the findings from the field of metacognition with the emerging psychotherapeutic models for recovery from psychosis. It's main objective is to help people with psychotic disorders to recover through stimulating metacognition. There are two core aspects of MERIT: (1) in order to encourage recovery it is essential to train those processes which allow people to develop a broad, flexible sense of self and of their world, in other words, metacognition; (2) people are able to improve their metacognition via a therapeutic relationship.

This therapy was created and developed in concert by clinicians from various countries with broad experience in long-term psychotherapy with people diagnosed with severe mental disorders. From that cooperation, MERIT has an inclusive concept of psychotherapy, which is why it sets out general principles to encourage change in people regardless of the preferred psychotherapeutic approach of the potential therapist. These principles aim to create an ideal relational context which encourages the development of metacognition rather than establishing a rigid set of psychotherapeutic techniques and activities. MERIT does not consider metacognition to be a discrete phenomenon which one can do or not, but rather an ordered continuum of psychological processes that a person can develop with time and practice.

As noted above, another central feature of MERIT is that people are able to improve their metacognitive skills in the context of a therapeutic relationship. Within the inclusive framework of metacognition, MERIT accepts that, as people can do more complex metacognitive tasks, they develop a better sense of themselves and the world, which encourages them to seek recovery.

MERIT sessions are governed by eight general principles which facilitate the promotion of metacognitive skills which have been damaged, weakened, or undeveloped. Each principle describes a quantifiable mental process that can occur regardless of the issue that the person brings to the session. All of the principles are conceptually and synergistically interrelated, but can be addressed and evaluated independently (Lysaker & Klion, 2017). The eight principles can be split into three subtypes (see Table 11.2).

11.8.1 Implications for Psychotherapy

Professionals working with patients with psychosis should follow at least five general principles which are summarized in Table 11.3 and outlined below:

1. *Process-oriented rather than content-oriented.* The clinician has to give up the attitude of being the "knowledge giver". In contrast it is the person, with their own experiences and difficulties, who will share their knowledge about what is happening to them. There should be a focus on how the person understands and

Table 11.2 Principles of Metacognitive Reflection and Insight Therapy (MERIT)

Subtype	Principle
Content	1. Talk about the person's present objectives, desires, and specific needs (or agenda). 2. Talk about the person's reactions to the therapist's thoughts, emotions, and behaviour as a consequence of the agenda (i.e. the transfer that produces counter-transfer). 3. Talk about the person's important life experiences via analysis of specific, minimally abstract autobiographical episodes during the session. 4. Talk about the psychological challenges arising from the three types of intersubjective content above.
Process	5. Reflect on and discuss the therapeutic relationship, as the context in which the person reflects about themself and others. 6. Reflect on and discuss the psychotherapeutic progress, both in terms of notable psychological results (e.g. improved self-esteem) and physical results (e.g. weight loss).
Super-ordinate	7. Think about themselves, others, and the world, in line with their current metacognitive abilities. 8. Examine skills of mastery (or problem solving) in line with their current metacognitive abilities.

Table 11.3 General principles for the clinical approach to psychosis

The clinician should be oriented towards...	The process (rather than the content). The objectives (rather than the problems). Recovery as an intersubjective phenomenon. Recovery as a changing phenomenon. Metacognition.

thinks about their psychopathological (their "symptoms") and psychosocial challenges (interpersonal, workplace, academic, occupational conflicts, etc.), which will involve access to complex, and occasionally painful biographical material.

2. *Objective-oriented rather than problem-oriented.* It is not just a person's difficulties that must be addressed, but also what they seek and what they want beyond the present "symptoms" and problems (the agenda of the person being treated). Ignoring an individual's objectives will make it harder to develop shared meaning of the recovery process. This does not mean unconditional support for the patient's agenda, but rather the construction of a dialogue that allows better understanding of the challenges underlying a potentially problematic treatment agenda.
3. *Oriented towards recovery as an intersubjective phenomenon.* The therapeutic relationship is the essential vehicle for encouraging and developing an ever richer, more flexible reflective dialogue.
4. *Orientation towards recovery as a changing phenomenon.* The treatment agenda can (and should) develop over the course of the recovery process. It should be accepted that treatment objectives can change unexpectedly.

5. *Orientation towards metacognition.* Any psychological intervention must adapt to the patient's capacity for reflection at any given moment and should systematically encourage the growth of metacognition, i.e. the skills of self-reflection, awareness of the minds of others (theory of mind), decentration (cognitive and emotional), and problem-solving.

11.9 Intervention with MERIT in Patient J.M

In this section we describe the psychotherapeutic intervention with J.M. and its results. The intervention was performed in a public mental health centre (CSM) by a clinical psychologist with extensive experience of psychotherapy with severe cases of psychosis and a resident psychologist intern (PIR) acting as co-therapist. The treatment followed the eight MERIT principles described in this chapter, as well as the general provisions of evidence-based practice and deliberate practice (Prado-Abril et al., 2017).

11.9.1 Principle 1. Talk About the Person's Objectives, Desires and Specific Needs (or Agenda) in the Present

When the clinical psychologist asked J.M. what he wanted to talk about in the first session, he responded with just "*I don't know*". It was as though he wanted to hand over all responsibility for what was to happen in the session to the therapist. In addition, he was clearly uncomfortable with long pauses in the conversation. The therapist asked him about his objectives in relation to the therapy. J.M. responded that he was only hoping that it would help him "*improve*" and be "*more normal, like everyone else*". He seemed to expect that it would also be the therapist who would tell him what he had to improve in order to be "more normal". With this attitude, J.M. put himself in a submissive role, dependent on the therapist, who he positioned in the role of the "expert". This made the therapist uncomfortable as they had to maintain the conversation and they had to decide what to talk about without asking questions that were too difficult at the same time as avoiding uncomfortable silences.

During the first few sessions, the therapist deliberately avoided being guided by this counter-transfer in order to try and make J.M. feel more at ease with the therapy and only dealt with superficial topics. Once J.M. felt more comfortable, the therapist chose to be explicit about their strategy in order to stimulate reflection, and in the next session asked:

T *What would you like to talk about today?*
JM *I don't know.*
T *You don't know what to talk about because you want me to decide.*

J.M. nodded silently and the therapist remained quiet. This seemed to make J.M. uncomfortable. The therapist continued reflecting on that:

T *Your mind is blank, you don't know what to talk about, but today I don't either, and you feel uncomfortable.*

JM (shyly) *Yes...(pause) I don't know what the proper things are to talk about. What do you think we could talk about?*

T *I don't know what the right topics are either, I don't know you very well... and I can't decide what's important to you. So I would really like it if you could decide yourself what you wanted to talk about today. I don't mind what we talk about, I'm sure any topic would be fine. I don't mind sitting in silence for a little bit while you think about what you'd like to talk about. Silence doesn't bother me in the slightest.*

This seemed to calm J.M. down, and after a few moments' silence, he was able to verbalize his fears of bringing up "stupid" topics and his fear that the therapist might criticize him. This led to a conversation about J.M.'s first objective or agenda: avoid being criticized by the therapist. Following this insight, the therapist decided to start all of the sessions the same way: "*What would you like to talk about today?*". This question continued to trigger J.M.'s fears of criticism in various sessions, but progressively he was able to reflect on his agenda: "*not doing anything wrong in the session and not being criticized by my therapist*". After 15 sessions, J.M. began to feel more relaxed and open, and by session 25, he was used to deciding the topics of conversation. From then on, when the therapist asked the question, J.M. would smile and say "*I knew you were going to ask me that!*", before beginning to verbalize what was on his mind that day, allowing himself and the therapist to be aware of his desires and intentions.

11.9.2 Principle 2. Talk About the Person's Reaction to the Therapist's Thoughts, Feelings, and Behaviour

The second principle of MERIT requires the therapist to share their thoughts about the person's behaviours and mental activities without invalidating their agenda. The objective is to help the patient develop better awareness of the mental states of the therapist. In the beginning in this case, the therapist avoided introducing their thoughts to make sure that there was enough space for the patient's mental state and agenda to appear. As noted above, J.M. began to share his internal state once he felt safe and free from possible criticism. This process allowed him to recognize what the therapist thought and it influenced how he spoke about himself. For example, in one session, he was able to verbalize how difficult he found it to occupy or entertain himself when he had no specific activity planned for the day.

JM *So, I feel like I have all this time in front of me and I don't know what to do... I don't know where to start... But I shouldn't moan, right? I should just get up and do something. Yes, that's what I should do...*

T *Do you think that's what I'm thinking now? That you shouldn't moan and you should get up and do something in this situation?*

JM *Yes, I complain too much but I don't do anything.*

T *In fact, I'm not thinking that at all. I'm thinking that it must be very hard for you to be in this situation, not knowing where to begin and feeling so lost.*

This triggered an interaction in which J.M. identified that he had, in fact, been using a phrase of his mother's ("*stop moaning and start doing something*") to second guess the therapists thinking. Again, this *insight* allowed him to question his hypothesis about the therapist's thoughts. After this *insight* was repeated various times over the sessions, J.M. finally became aware of his tendency to ascribe criticism and hostility not only to the therapist's thoughts, but also to the thoughts of others. From there, J.M. began to question his suppositions about the internal states of others rather than assuming them to be true unilaterally and was able to understand that a single situation can be read in many ways.

11.9.3 Principle 3. Talk About the Person's Important Life Experiences Through Analysis in the Session of Autobiographical Episodes

The third principle means that the therapist must work with detailed narrative episodes of the person's autobiographical events. The analysis of these events will ensure that the resulting narratives are connected to each other and not too abstract. This will help the patient to relate their thoughts and feelings over time.

Once J.M. identified his initial agenda, he was able to remember various episodes that were related to it. In one session, for example, he said that that week, he had felt like an outsider at a family party. The therapist and patient then reflected on the chain of events: how they began and unfolded, who knew, what they thought, and what they felt at the time. J.M. was able to explore how he had experienced that situation and was more aware of his thoughts and feelings at the party. With the therapist's help, he was also able to connect different events and situations over time and see how his thoughts and feelings were related in previous, similar social situations. In the final session, J.M. was able to integrate various previous narrative episodes in a detailed life history; this narrative included how his hearing problems in infancy had prevented him from attending school regularly and how this caused specific situations in which other children forgot about him or ignored him. These events led him to believe that he was boring and he began to reject social relationships. In high school, he continued being shy, withdrawn, and worried about not being accepted socially.

Similarly, he was able to talk about situations in which his siblings, who were very good at making friends, had made him feel socially inferior. This reinforced his belief that he was boring and that other people were not interested in him. These beliefs were evident when he began to hear critical voices in his head. This led him to withdraw even more and avoid social situations. He was convinced that he could not maintain friendships as he had never experienced that in his life. At the end of the therapy, he was able to understand that he had automatically accepted these beliefs without taking into account the important role of his hearing problems, school absence in childhood, the psychotic episode, and negative thoughts about himself when it came to making and keeping friends. In addition, he understood that his belief that other people did not want to be with him had led him to be isolated, which in turn made it more likely that others would not want to spend time with him. During the therapy, various strategies were discussed aimed at modifying this dysfunctional interpersonal pattern.

11.9.4 Principle 4. Talk About Psychological Challenges that Arise from the Three Previous Types of Content

Talking about challenges with J.M. happened naturally once he had clarified his agenda and had discussed various narrative episodes. At the beginning of the therapy, J.M. was already able to identify and express psychological problems, which made the therapist's job much easier.

In the fourth session, for example, after analysing an episode in which he had been alone in his room without doing anything, J.M. said, "*I wish I was able to entertain myself... I didn't know what to do...*". This led him to identify the psychological problem of feeling incapable of starting something, which he associated with thoughts of incompetence.

In general, patient and therapist must take enough time to identify the core psychological problems underlying the narrative episodes. In J.M.'s case, the idea that he was boring or his difficulties connecting with others were psychological problems that were repeated throughout the sessions. As he advanced with the therapy, J.M. was able to recognize these issues both in his agenda and in his narrative episodes, which allowed him to use this awareness to assess possible alternatives for dealing with his problems (Principle 8).

11.9.5 Principle 5. Reflection and Discussion About the Therapeutic Relationship

As mentioned above, working on the therapeutic relationship is fundamental, as it is the context in which the patient thinks about themselves and others in order to help improve their understanding of their maladaptive interpersonal patterns. As discussed in the first principle, J.M. usually put the therapist in the position of "expert" and himself in submission. The therapist had to deal with this pattern on various occasions over time, as well as manage their counter-transferal impulses to "rescue" him or solve his problems by telling him what to do or what to talk about. This pattern was addressed on various occasions by open, continued reflection about the therapeutic relationship. As a result of these reflections, J.M. became aware of his tendency to put himself in an inferior position, both with the therapist and with others, particularly his parents.

11.9.6 Principle 6. Reflection About the Psychotherapeutic Progress

So that the patient reflects on the progress of the session and the therapy, MERIT encourages the therapist to examine how the patient experienced the session. To that end, the therapist asked J.M. how they felt about the session at the end of each one. This was quite difficult for J.M. because of the intense fear he felt about being rejected by the therapist if he said anything critical. Consequently, when the therapist asked this question, J.M. would respond by saying that everything had been good and that he was satisfied, without truly reflecting on how the session had gone. The therapist had to address this fear directly and naturally, assuring him on various occasions that they would not be at all irritated or annoyed if J.M. said that anything had not been good. They also reiterated that the ultimate aim of this question was to improve the sessions, which is why it was important for J.M. to give honest answers rather than responding automatically. After 20 sessions, J.M. was able to cautiously begin expressing disagreement with some specific parts of the session. For example, on one occasion, the therapist made an incorrect consideration about J.M.'s thoughts. This caused an interruption in the conversation and made J.M. close off. When the therapist asked at the end of the session how it had been for J.M., he was able to reluctantly express the idea that he had felt he had not been understood and had felt disappointed with the therapist at that moment. The therapist reinforced J.M.'s honest *feedback* and apologized for what had happened. They also told J.M. that they tried as far as possible to understand J.M.'s perspective, but occasionally they were unable to do so and reiterated their intention to avoid any similar occurrence in the future. This reaction from the therapist was a very important corrective emotional experience that encouraged J.M. to more easily express his criticism and improved the clarity of the communication. This event also helped, in subsequent sessions, when dealing with difficulties of communication with other significant people.

11.9.7 Principle 7. Think About Oneself, Others, and The World

This principle means that the therapist stimulates skills of self-reflection and *insight* into the minds of others in line with, or slightly above, the current level of the person's metacognitive ability. The ultimate aim is for the patient to construct ever more developed, flexible thoughts about themselves and others. At the beginning of the therapy, J.M. was able to recognize his own thoughts but not his feelings. At times he reported feeling "uncomfortable" or that he "didn't feel right". The therapist had to encourage J.M. to dig into and label his emotions in the session and in his narrative episodes: "*You feel very sad. What do you feel exactly? Was it sadness or anger? Or both?*" or "*You seem to feel embarrassed because you don't have many thoughts today*". J.M. began to identify his emotions more often and was progressively deploying clearer, more detailed ideas about his feelings. The therapist also stimulated J.M. so that he understood that his thoughts changed over time and that his desires and intentions did not always become reality. At the end of the therapy, the therapist offered J.M. their thoughts about stimulating the connection between different thoughts and feelings in the present and over time. Over 40 sessions, J.M. made significant progress, which was not linear. This pattern of peaks and troughs (improvement, worsening, improvement) is common in metacognitive therapies with people with psychosis. Because of that, the therapist must be cautious about adapting their interventions to the patient's current level, as well as about identifying and managing their possible frustration in those troughs so that patients do not feel devalued or not understood. In J.M.'s case, when these setbacks were seen in the MAS-A, the therapist was able to identify and manage their counter-transferential responses to adjust their interventions to J.M.'s level.

In terms of awareness of the minds of others, at the beginning of the therapy, J.M. was able to identify that other people had independent thoughts, but was unable to distinguish between different cognitive operations. Owing to J.M.'s fear of being rejected by others, the therapist avoided reflecting on the minds of others in order to gain better awareness of J.M.'s internal states. It was only after various sessions that the therapist began to ask questions about what J.M. thought that they were thinking and even occasionally what others were thinking, expecting, or wanting in the narratives. As a result of these reflections, J.M. became more aware of his tendency to anticipate criticism of himself in the thoughts of others (principles 2 and 3). Nonetheless, at the end of the therapy, J.M. was still unable to produce clear pictures of other people's thoughts.

11.9.8 Principle 8. Reflection and Stimulation of Mastery Skills (Problem-Solving)

The final principle of MERIT aims for the therapist to stimulate the person's ability to use intersubjective information in the resolution of psychological problems. At the beginning of the therapy, J.M. was aware of the existence of problems, but the way he dealt with them was basically calling his mother or sister for advice. When J.M. understood that his thoughts could change over time and that there were multiple ways of interpreting the same situation, he made real advances in his abilities to solve his problems. The therapist tried to stimulate these skills with questions such as "*Is there another way of looking at this problem?*", "*What can you say to yourself in order to feel a little better?*", and "*How can you manage to maintain a positive view of this problem?*". For example, J.M. was able to realize that his view of himself as boring or uninteresting was interfering in his participation in social situations. This reflection helped him to think more flexibly about himself. On his own initiative, he made a list of topics of conversation that interested him and tried to update it every day. This helped him to initiate conversations and be more involved in social situations. However, the belief that he was boring kept reappearing, although he was able to begin questioning it and even occasionally adopt different points of view about himself. Similarly, he began to recognize how his belief that silence in a conversation meant the he was boring crippled him in conversations. To combat that, he convinced himself that he was not the only one responsible for conversations, and that occasionally silences happen naturally. This helped reduce the pressure he felt and helped him to relax and converse more naturally without freezing up.

11.9.9 Results

As we have been able to see, a central aspect of J.M.'s case was a sense of confusion and otherness about himself and others. This is closely related to the concept of ipseity that we examined at the beginning of the chapter. J.M.'s early experiences significantly affected how he constructed his perceptions of himself and others, and his ability to be involved in the world. During the treatment, these representations were clear, for example, the critical voices or the patterns and beliefs about himself as boring or uninteresting to others. Problems with metacognitive skills made it harder for J.M. to think about this way of understanding both his own experiences and mental processes and those related to the interpersonal arena, giving rise to complications in his everyday life. The work based on MERIT, with the importance placed on the therapeutic relationship, allowed J.M. to improve his metacognitive abilities, making him more aware of his thoughts and emotions, and thus allowing him to begin reconstructing his sense of *self*.

After finishing 40 sessions, two independent evaluators graded J.M. using the PANSS and MAS-A scales. This confirmed that his metacognition improved in the self-reflection, decentration, and mastery subscales. Similarly, his negative "symptoms" diminished generally, as indicated by the PANSS scores and the information from J.M. in the first person.

One important aspect of the therapy was that there was no increase in medication at any time, or hospitalization due to crises. In addition, J.M. did not need any additional treatment outside of the CSM (with psychiatrist, clinical psychologist, PIR, social worker, and specialist mental health nurse).

11.10 Current Scientific Evidence in MERIT

Although the data available so far are limited, it does point towards MERIT's viability, acceptability, and effectiveness for improving metacognition in people with severe mental disorders who are receiving treatment in natural clinical settings (Bargenquast & Schweitzer, 2014; de Jong et al., 2016; Vohs et al., 2018). A recent randomized clinical trial with 70 people diagnosed with schizophrenia replicated the positive results of MERIT for improving metacognition, and specifically self-reflection skills (de Jong et al., 2019). MERIT's impact on people themselves has also been examined. In a quantitative study, Lysaker et al. (2015) examined the effects on people receiving at least 1 year of therapy with MERIT or other support psychotherapy. The results indicate that MERIT, unlike support therapy, produced significant improvements in both a sense of agency and the capacity to tolerate and manage levels of distress that had previously been perceived as incapacitating.

In terms of effects at a personal level and the level of individual needs, MERIT has been found to be associated with a significant increase in the number of notable goals people set, both in early phases of severe mental disorders and subsequently (Arnon-Ribenfeld et al., 2018; Hamm & Firmin, 2016; Hasson-Ohayon et al., 2017; Hillis et al., 2015; Leonhardt et al., 2016, 2018; van Donkersgoed et al., 2016). Looking at people without awareness of the disorder, Vohs et al. (2018) randomly assigned adults with their first psychotic episode and poor insight to MERIT or to conventional treatment for 6 months. At the end of the trial, 80% of the participants who received MERIT completed their therapy and there were statistically significant improvements in objective measures of awareness of the disorder without that causing increased hopelessness or distress.

MERIT therapy is an example of operationalization and integration of phenomenological aspects and metacognitive work, which was illustrated by the clinical case of J.M.

11.11 Summary

This chapter sets out a view of human beings that cannot be broken down into a collection of organs and tissue, but is instead part of an external world which makes them a person. The approach proposed here does not confuse the organ with the organism and is a long way from the concept of psychosis as a merely physical phenomenon which fails to understand that a paranoid thought or a hallucination has meaning or sense. In contrast to the inertia that biomedical models bring to the understanding of the phenomenon of psychosis, the proposal here is of reflection and approaching its nature and necessary relocation. The traditionally predominant idea has been of psychosis as a "chronic mental disorder originating in the brain". However, in recent years there has been a gradual change in how psychosis is thought of and growing interest in the process of personal recovery. This process goes far beyond achieving the absence of clinical "symptoms" and is more focused on the person developing various skills that allow them to give meaning to what is happening to them and to find new meaning in their lives (Fonseca-Pedrero, 2019). To that end, there needs to be a change in the model; we need to move on from possible reductionist explanations and try to understand the process of psychosis within the individual's context and life story (Pérez-Álvarez et al., 2016).

Inevitably, this requires a change of mentality, and the attempt to understand people's experiences and ways of "being in the world" in order to decide what elements will make up part of the therapeutic work. Many authors suggest that this first-person emphasis is only possible if we re-engage with phenomenological perspectives. From phenomenology, understanding psychosis as a problem of the *self and* gives us the chance to understand it within the framework of people's relationship with their own mental and emotional states, and also in the external space of the interpersonal arena. In a complementary manner, metacognitive skills include all of the competencies needed to perform these processes and can be trained to help understand the nature of the lived experience and to give it meaning.

Considering psychotherapy from a phenomenological perspective for psychosis means understanding that all of the work aimed at restoring the *self* lies in the work "in" and "with" the therapeutic alliance. The shared space between therapist and patient is the ideal setting in which reflection can be encouraged about ourselves and others.

Ethical Statement This study was conducted in accordance with the Declaration of Helsinki. We obtained the patient's informed consent before publication. The patient grants his permission for his information to be published in this case report.

References

Arnon-Ribenfeld, N., Hasson-Ohayon, I., Lavidor, M., Atzil-Slonim, D., & Lysaker, P. H. (2017). The association between metacognitive abilities and outcome measures among people with schizophrenia: A meta-analysis. *European Psychiatry: The Journal of the Association of European Psychiatrists, 46*, 33–41. https://doi.org/10.1016/J.EURPSY.2017.08.002

Arnon-Ribenfeld, N., Bloom, R., Atzil-Slonim, D., Peri, T., de Jong, S., & Hasson-Ohayon, I. (2018). Metacognitive reflection and insight therapy (MERIT) among people with schizophrenia: Lessons from two case studies. *American Journal of Psychotherapy, 71*(4), 175–185. https://doi.org/10.1176/appi.psychotherapy.20180037

Bargenquast, R., & Schweitzer, R. D. (2014). Enhancing sense of recovery and self-reflectivity in people with schizophrenia: A pilot study of metacognitive narrative psychotherapy. *Psychology and Psychotherapy, 87*(3), 338–356. https://doi.org/10.1111/PAPT.12019

Cooke, A. (2017). *Understanding psychosis and schizophrenia*. The British Psychological Society.

Cortina, M., & Liotti, G. (2010). The intersubjective and cooperative origins of consciousness: An evolutionary-developmental approach. *Journal of the American Academy of Psychoanalysis and Dynamic Psychiatry, 38*(2), 291–314. https://doi.org/10.1521/JAAP.2010.38.2.291

Davidson, L. (2003). *Living outside mental illness: Qualitative studies of recovery in schizophrenia* (pp. 1–240). New York University Press. https://doi.org/10.1176/APPI.PS.55.9.1073-A

de Jong, S., van Donkersgoed, R., Pijnenborg, G. H. M., & Lysaker, P. H. (2016). Metacognitive reflection and insight therapy (MERIT) with a patient with severe symptoms of disorganization. *Journal of Clinical Psychology, 72*(2), 164–174. https://doi.org/10.1002/JCLP.22249

de Jong, S., van Donkersgoed, R. J. M., Timmerman, M. E., Aan Het Rot, M., Wunderink, L., Arends, J., van der Gaag, M., Aleman, A., Lysaker, P. H., & Pijnenborg, G. H. M. (2019). Metacognitive reflection and insight therapy (MERIT) for patients with schizophrenia. *Psychological Medicine, 49*(2), 303–313. https://doi.org/10.1017/S0033291718000855

Dimaggio, G., Ottavi, P., Popolo, R., & Salvatore, G. (2020). *Metacognitive interpersonal therapy: Body, imagery and change*. Routledge.

Dmitryeva, N., Chernov, N., Kostyuk, G., & Lysaker, P. H. (2021). Utilizing MERIT to promote recovery in schizotypal personality disorder: An illustrative case study. *Journal of Clinical Psychology, 77*(8), 1798–1806. https://doi.org/10.1002/jclp.23239

Firmin, R. L., Zalzala, A. B., Hamm, J. A., Luther, L., & Lysaker, P. H. (2021). How psychosis interrupts the lives of women and men differently: A qualitative comparison. *Psychology and Psychotherapy: Theory, Research and Practice, 94*(3), 704–720. https://doi.org/10.1111/PAPT.12317

Fonseca-Pedrero, E. (Ed.). (2019). *Tratamientos psicológicos para la psicosis*. Pirámide.

Fonseca-Pedrero, E. (Ed.). (2021). *Manual de tratamientos psicológicos. Adultos*. Pirámide.

Gimeno Peón, A. (2020). *Mejorando los resultados en psicoterapia: principios terapéuticos basados en la evidencia*. Pirámide.

Hamm, J. A., & Firmin, R. L. (2016). Disorganization and individual psychotherapy for schizophrenia: A case report of metacognitive reflection and insight therapy. *Journal of Contemporary Psychotherapy, 46*(4), 227–234. https://doi.org/10.1007/S10879-016-9326-7

Hasson-Ohayon, I. (2012). Integrating cognitive behavioural-based therapy with an intersubjective approach: Addressing metacognitive deficits among people with schizophrenia. *Journal of Psychotherapy Integration, 22*(4), 356–374. https://doi.org/10.1037/A0029576

Hasson-Ohayon, I., & Lysaker, P. H. (2021). *The recovery of the self in psychosis: Contributions from metacognitive and mentalization based oriented psychotherapy*. Routledge.

Hasson-Ohayon, I., Arnon-Ribenfeld, N., Hamm, J. A., & Lysaker, P. H. (2017). Agency before action: The application of behavioural activation in psychotherapy with persons with psychosis. *Psychotherapy, 54*(3), 245–251. https://doi.org/10.1037/PST0000114

Hasson-Ohayon, I., Cheli, S., & Lysaker, P. H. (2021). Emerging psychotherapeutic approaches to addressing self-experience in schizophrenia spectrum disorders. *Journal of Clinical Psychology, 77*(8), 1781–1785. https://doi.org/10.1002/jclp.23223

Hillis, J. D., Leonhardt, B. L., Vohs, J. L., Buck, K. D., Salvatore, G., Popolo, R., Dimaggio, G., & Lysaker, P. H. (2015). Metacognitive reflective and insight therapy for people in early phase of a schizophrenia spectrum disorder. *Journal of Clinical Psychology, 71*(2), 125–135. https://doi.org/10.1002/JCLP.22148

Inchausti, F., García-Poveda, N. V., Ballesteros-Prados, A., Ortuño-Sierra, J., Sánchez-Reales, S., Prado-Abril, J., Aldaz-Armendáriz, J. A., Mole, J., Dimaggio, G., Ottavi, P., & Fonseca-Pedrero, E. (2018). The effects of metacognition-oriented social skills training on psychosocial outcome in schizophrenia-Spectrum disorders: A randomized controlled trial. *Schizophrenia Bulletin, 44*(6), 1235–1244. https://doi.org/10.1093/SCHBUL/SBX168

Keshavan, M. S., Nasrallah, H. A., & Tandon, R. (2011). Schizophrenia, "just the facts" 6. Moving ahead with the schizophrenia concept: From the elephant to the mouse. *Schizophrenia Research, 127*(1–3), 3–13. https://doi.org/10.1016/J.SCHRES.2011.01.011

Leichsenring, F., Steinert, C., Rabung, S., & Ioannidis, J. (2022). The efficacy of psychotherapies and pharmacotherapies for mental disorders in adults: An umbrella review and meta-analytic evaluation of recent meta-analyses. *World Psychiatry, 21*(1), 133–145. https://doi.org/10.1002/wps.20941

Leonhardt, B. L., Benson, K., George, S., Buck, K. D., Shaieb, R., & Vohs, J. L. (2016). Targeting insight in first episode psychosis: A case study of metacognitive reflection insight therapy (MERIT). *Journal of Contemporary Psychotherapy, 46*(4), 207–216. https://doi.org/10.1007/S10879-016-9332-9

Leonhardt, B. L., Ratliff, K., & Vohs, J. L. (2018). Recovery in first-episode psychosis: A case study of metacognitive reflection and insight therapy (MERIT). *American Journal of Psychotherapy, 71*(4), 128–134. https://doi.org/10.1176/APPI.PSYCHOTHERAPY.20180032

Lysaker, P. H., & Klion, R. E. (2017). *Recovery, meaning-making, and severe mental illness: A comprehensive guide to metacognitive reflection and insight therapy*. Routledge. https://doi.org/10.4324/9781315447001

Lysaker, P. H., Carcione, A., Dimaggio, G., Johannesen, J. K., Nicolò, G., Procacci, M., & Semerari, A. (2005). Metacognition amidst narratives of self and illness in schizophrenia: Associations with neurocognition, symptoms, insight and quality of life. *Acta Psychiatrica Scandinavica, 112*(1), 64–71. https://doi.org/10.1111/J.1600-0447.2005.00514.X

Lysaker, P. H., Kukla, M., Belanger, E., White, D. A., Buck, K. D., Luther, L., Firmin, R. L., & Leonhardt, B. (2015). Individual psychotherapy and changes in self-experience in schizophrenia: A qualitative comparison of patients in metacognitively focused and supportive psychotherapy. *Psychiatry, 78*(4), 305–316. https://doi.org/10.1080/00332747.2015.1063916

Lysaker, P. H., Gagen, E., Wright, A., Vohs, J. L., Kukla, M., Yanos, P. T., & Hasson-Ohayon, I. (2019). Metacognitive deficits predict impaired insight in schizophrenia across symptom profiles: A latent class analysis. *Schizophrenia Bulletin, 45*(1), 48–56. https://doi.org/10.1093/SCHBUL/SBY142

Lysaker, P. H., Gagen, E., Klion, R., Zalzala, A., Vohs, J., Faith, L. A., Leonhardt, B., Hamm, J., & Hasson-Ohayon, I. (2020a). Metacognitive reflection and insight therapy: A recovery-oriented treatment approach for psychosis. *Psychology Research and Behavior Management, 13*, 331–341. https://doi.org/10.2147/PRBM.S198628

Lysaker, P. H., Kukla, M., Leonhardt, B. L., Hamm, J. A., Schnakenberg Martin, A., Zalzala, A. B., Gagen, E. C., & Hasson-Ohayon, I. (2020b). Meaning, integration, and the self in serious mental illness: Implications of research in metacognition for psychiatric rehabilitation. *Psychiatric Rehabilitation Journal, 43*(4), 275–283. https://doi.org/10.1037/PRJ0000436

Lysaker, P. H., Minor, K. S., Lysaker, J. T., Hasson-Ohayon, I., Bonfils, K., Hochheiser, J., & Vohs, J. L. (2020c). Metacognitive function and fragmentation in schizophrenia: Relationship to cognition, self-experience and developing treatments. *Undefined, 19*, 100142. https://doi.org/10.1016/J.SCOG.2019.100142

Moritz, S., & Lysaker, P. H. (2018). Metacognition – What did James H. Flavell really say and the implications for the conceptualization and design of metacognitive interventions. *Schizophrenia Research, 201*, 20–26. https://doi.org/10.1016/J.SCHRES.2018.06.001

National Collaborating Centre for Mental Health (UK). (2014). *Psychosis and Schizophrenia in Adults: Treatment and Management*. National Institute for Health and Care Excellence (UK).

Nelson, B., Yung, A. R., Bechdolf, A., & McGorry, P. D. (2008). The phenomenological critique and self-disturbance: Implications for ultra-high risk ("prodrome") research. *Schizophrenia Bulletin, 34*(2), 381–392. https://doi.org/10.1093/SCHBUL/SBM094

Nelson, B., Sass, L. A., Thompson, A., Yung, A. R., Francey, S. M., Amminger, G. P., & McGorry, P. D. (2009). Does disturbance of self-underlie social cognition deficits in schizophrenia and other psychotic disorders? *Early Intervention in Psychiatry, 3*(2), 83–93. https://doi.org/10.1111/J.1751-7893.2009.00112.X

Parnas, J., & Sass, L. A. (2008). Varieties of "phenomenology": On description, understanding, and explanation in psychiatry. In K. S. Kendler & J. Parnas (Eds.), *Philosophical Issues in Psychiatry: Explanation, Phenomenology, and Nosology* (p. 239). Johns Hopkins University Press.

Pérez-Álvarez, M., & García-Montes, J. M. (2019). La filosofía de la ciencia aplicada a la psicología clínica: pensando en psicosis. In E. Fonseca-Pedrero (Ed.), *Tratamientos psicológicos para la psicosis*. Pirámide.

Pérez-Álvarez, M., García-Montes, J. M., Perona-Garcelán, S., & Vallina-Fernández, O. (2008). Changing relationship with voices: New therapeutic perspectives for treating hallucinations. *Clinical Psychology & Psychotherapy, 15*(2), 75–85. https://doi.org/10.1002/CPP.563

Pérez-Álvarez, M., García-Montes, J. M., Cangas, A. J., & Sass, L. A. (2009). Defending a phenomenological-behavioral perspective: Culture, behavior, and experience. *Philosophy, Psychiatry, & Psychology, 15*(3), 281–285. https://doi.org/10.1353/PPP.0.0185

Pérez-Álvarez, M., García-Montes, J. M., & Sass, L. (2010). La Hora de la Fenomenología en la Esquizofrenia. *Clínica y Salud, 21*(3), 221–233.

Pérez-Álvarez, M., García-Montes, J. M., Vallina-Fernández, O., Perona-Garcelán, S., & Cuevas-Yust, C. (2011). New life for schizophrenia psychotherapy in the light of phenomenology. *Clinical Psychology and Psychotherapy, 18*(3), 187–201. https://doi.org/10.1002/cpp.716

Pérez-Álvarez, M., García-Montes, J. M., Vallina-Fernández, O., & Perona-Garcelán, S. (2016). Rethinking schizophrenia in the context of the person and their circumstances: Seven reasons. *Frontiers in Psychology, 7*. https://doi.org/10.3389/fpsyg.2016.01650

Prado-Abril, J., Sánchez-Reales, S., & Inchausti, F. (2017). En busca de nuestra mejor versión: pericia y excelencia en Psicología Clínica. *Ansiedad y Estrés, 23*(2), 110–117. https://doi.org/10.1016/J.ANYES.2017.06.001

Ritunnano, R., & Bortolotti, L. (2021). Do delusions have and give meaning? *Phenomenology and the Cognitive Sciences., 21*, 949. https://doi.org/10.1007/s11097-021-09764-9

Salvatore, G., Buonocore, L., Ottavi, P., Popolo, R., & Dimaggio, G. (2018). Metacognitive interpersonal therapy for treating persecutory delusions in schizophrenia. *American Journal of Psychotherapy, 71*(4), 164–174. https://doi.org/10.1176/APPI.PSYCHOTHERAPY.20180039

Sass, L. A., & Parnas, J. (2003). Schizophrenia, consciousness, and the self. *Schizophrenia Bulletin, 29*(3), 427–444. https://doi.org/10.1093/OXFORDJOURNALS.SCHBUL.A007017

Stanghellini, G. (2010). A hermeneutic framework for psychopathology. *Psychopathology, 43*(5), 319–326. https://doi.org/10.1159/000319401

Stanghellini, G., & Lysaker, P. H. (2007). The psychotherapy of schizophrenia through the lens of phenomenology: Intersubjectivity and the search for the recovery of first- and second-person awareness. *American Journal of Psychotherapy, 61*(2), 163–179. https://doi.org/10.1176/APPI.PSYCHOTHERAPY.2007.61.2.163

Stanghellini, G., & Mancini, M. (2017). *The therapeutic interview in mental health*. Cambridge University Press. https://doi.org/10.1017/9781316181973

Tandon, R., Keshavan, M. S., & Nasrallah, H. A. (2008). Schizophrenia, "just the facts" what we know in 2008. 2. Epidemiology and etiology. *Schizophrenia Research, 102*(1–3), 1–18. https://doi.org/10.1016/j.schres.2008.04.011

The Lancet Psychiatry. (2021). The things themselves. *The Lancet Psychiatry, 8*(3), 169. https://doi.org/10.1016/S2215-0366(21)00033-X

Tomasello, M., Carpenter, M., Call, J., Behne, T., & Moll, H. (2005). Understanding and sharing intentions: The origins of cultural cognition. *Behavioral and Brain Sciences, 28*(5), 675–691. https://doi.org/10.1017/S0140525X05000129

van Donkersgoed, R. J. M., de Jong, S., & Pijnenborg, G. H. M. (2016). Metacognitive reflection and insight therapy (MERIT) with a patient with persistent negative symptoms. *Journal of Contemporary Psychotherapy, 46*(4), 245–253. https://doi.org/10.1007/S10879-016-9333-8

Vitzthum, F. B., Veckenstedt, R., & Moritz, S. (2014). Individualized metacognitive therapy program for patients with psychosis (MCT+): Introduction of a novel approach for psychotic symptoms. *Behavioural and Cognitive Psychotherapy, 42*(1), 105–110. https://doi.org/10.1017/S1352465813000246

Vohs, J. L., Lysaker, P. H., Liffick, E., Francis, M. M., Leonhardt, B. L., James, A., Buck, K. D., Hamm, J. A., Minor, K. S., Mehdiyoun, N., & Breier, A. (2015). Metacognitive capacity as a predictor of insight in first-episode psychosis. *The Journal of Nervous and Mental Disease, 203*(5), 372–378. https://doi.org/10.1097/NMD.0000000000000291

Vohs, J. L., Leonhardt, B. L., James, A. V., Francis, M. M., Breier, A., Mehdiyoun, N., Visco, A. C., & Lysaker, P. H. (2018). Metacognitive reflection and insight therapy for early psychosis: A preliminary study of a novel integrative psychotherapy. *Schizophrenia Research, 195*, 428–433. https://doi.org/10.1016/J.SCHRES.2017.10.041

Chapter 12
Acceptance and Commitment Therapy (ACT): Contextual Therapy in the Approach to Psychosis

Bárbara Gil-Luciano, Francisco J. Ruiz, and Carmen Luciano

12.1 Acceptance and Commitment Therapy, or Contextual Therapy

Acceptance and Commitment Therapy (ACT; Hayes et al., 1999; Wilson & Luciano, 2002) is the main representative of the so-called contextual therapies due to its philosophical, theoretical, and empirical anchorage. This section will briefly review its philosophical roots and theoretical trunk, considering it as an application of Contextual Behavioral Science (Hayes et al., 2012, 2021).

12.1.1 Philosophical Anchorage of Contextual Behavioral Science: Functional Contextualism

Functional Contextualism (FC; Gifford & Hayes, 1999; Hayes, 1993) is the philosophical anchor on which Contextual Behavioral Science stands. FC is a form of pragmatism that tries to make more explicit the contextual pre-analytical assumptions of Skinner's Radical Behaviorism (Skinner, 1974). For this purpose, FC

B. Gil-Luciano (✉)
Universidad Nebrija, Madrid Institute of Contextual Psychology (MICPSY), Madrid, Spain
e-mail: barbaragil.luciano@micpsy.com

F. J. Ruiz
Fundación Universitaria Konrad-Lorenz, Bogotá, Colombia
e-mail: franciscoj.ruizj@konradlorenz.edu.co

C. Luciano
Universidad de Almería, Madrid Institute of Contextual Psychology (MICPSY), Madrid, Spain
e-mail: mluciano@ual.es

J. A. Díaz-Garrido et al. (eds.), *Psychological Interventions for Psychosis*,
https://doi.org/10.1007/978-3-031-27003-1_12

follows the classification of the world hypotheses of Stephen Pepper (1942). According to this, contextualism is a worldview that employs the root metaphor of action-in-context.

Contextualism considers that each event is inseparable from the historical and situational context in which it takes place and that, therefore, its complete understanding cannot be achieved by tearing apart its elements. This holistic view could lead contextualists to some immobility, as it is impossible to consider all the variables of the context in which psychological events occur. Being aware of this, contextualists allow selecting and analyzing parts of the context in which the psychological event takes place only as a means to achieve their pre-analytical goals, not to discover a preexisting reality. In other words, contextualism adopts a pragmatic truth criterion by which "truth" is defined in terms of its usefulness.

According to the pre-analytical goals pursued, there are multiple forms of contextualism (Hayes et al., 1993). Following the Skinnerian vision, FC proposes the pre-analytical objectives of prediction of and influence in psychological events. Adopting these objectives implies a radical departure from the predominant psychological models in which the explanation of a behavior (e.g., delusional behavior) through another behavior (e.g., experiencing auditory hallucinations) is accepted. Specifically, FC rejects the possibility that a psychological event is directly caused by another psychological event because this type of explanation would not allow progress in the pre-analytical objective of influence. As the psychologist cannot directly modify a psychological event, event-event causal explanations would not be "true" because they would not allow defining strategies to influence such events.

Conversely, FC holds that each psychological event must be explained in terms of contextual variables because these are the only ones that the psychologist can influence. Therefore, it is proposed that the relationships between events depend on contextual variables, even in those cases in which the event-event relationship is apparently causal.

12.1.2 Theoretical Anchorage of Contextual Behavioral Science: Laws of Learning and Relational Frame Theory

The trunk of Contextual Behavioral Science is constituted by the principles detected when performing an analysis that is consistent with the philosophical root represented by FC. Specifically, the trunk is mainly made up of the learning principles that explain the origin of the functions of psychological events, both directly and indirectly. In addition to the well-known learning principles (habituation/sensitization, respondent, and operant conditioning), the theoretical anchorage of Contextual Behavioral Science has been significantly expanded by the findings gathered under the label of the Relational Frame Theory (RFT; Hayes et al., 2001).

RFT is a very important leap in explaining human behavior because it has advanced considerably in providing a contextual-functional explanation of the generativity of language and cognition. For this explanation, RFT has not proposed a new learning principle. Instead, it has specified that derived relational responding is the basis of the generativity of human behavior and that relational responding is a set of purely functional operants, or generalized operants, learned through multiple exemplars with explicit contingencies provided by the verbal community.

During the last decades, a series of relational operants have been identified that involve relating stimuli through arbitrary cues such as coordination ("is," "is the same as," "is equivalent"), distinction ("is different from," "is distinct from"), comparison ("more than," "fewer than," "greater than," "less than"), hierarchy ("is part of," "contains"), perspective or deictic (I-you, here-there, now-then), causality ("if... then..."), etc. Establishing these relationships between stimuli (or framing stimuli) allows the derivation of new relationships and the transformation of their functions.

For example, ever since a child had a traumatic experience with a dog, he begins to experience intense fear and runs away from the situation when he sees a dog (or hears another person say "there is a dog"). If the child is shown a wolf and told that "wolves are *much more dangerous than* dogs," the aversive function associated with the word "dog," and the animal itself, will transform into the word "wolf" and the animal wolf. In this way, the child will react with even more fear and actions aimed at flight when hearing a person pronounce the word "wolf" or seeing a wolf. Note how, in this example, the reaction to the word "wolf" is explained in a functional-contextual way by mentioning how the current context (a person who says "wolf") actualizes functions related to the history of direct (aversive conditioning with a dog) and derived learning (establishment of an arbitrary relationship between "wolf" and "dog" through a comparison cue in a child who has learned to relate stimuli comparatively through multiple exemplars).

Given our interactions with the verbal community, human beings develop great fluency in framing stimuli through multiple types of relations, thus generating a myriad of derived stimulus relations and transformation of functions. This tremendously generative relational ability causes human beings to be in contact much more easily with appetitive and aversive functions than the rest of organisms. Following the above example, it is not necessary to see a dog to actualize explicitly learned aversive functions, but the mere sound of "dog," and even worse, of "wolf," can actualize them. Similarly, the same child can contact appetitive functions when he relates the beginning of December with the proximity of the Christmas holidays, or he can derive aversive functions when the feast of the Magi arrives because it implies going back to school soon.

As we discussed earlier, derived relational responding is the basis of the tremendous generativity displayed by human language and cognition. Thus, relational responding is involved in all complex human behavior such as problem-solving, self-regulation, analogical reasoning, perspective-taking and empathy, the creation of personal values, etc. Of course, understanding relational responding is vitally important to explain the generation of psychological problems, as well as therapeutic work. The following sections will be devoted to the latter issues.

12.1.3 Applications of Contextual Behavioral Science: Contextual Therapy, ACT

Metaphorically, the applications of Contextual Behavioral Science are ramifications supported on the trunk of knowledge of the laws of learning and derived relational responding, which, in turn, are anchored in the philosophical root represented by FC (Luciano, 2016). ACT represents the most recognized application in the clinical and health field due to its vast research volume (see https://contextualscience.org/state_of_the_act_evidence). Proof of this is the nearly 900 randomized clinical trials in multiple problems published as of January 2022. A review of the meta-analyses conducted on the efficacy of ACT can be seen in Gloster et al. (2020). This review concluded that ACT is effective in all the problems analyzed, including anxiety, depression, substance use, pain conditions, etc.

While the long-term aspiration of Contextual Behavioral Science is to define its applied models through principles derived from basic research (Hayes et al., 2021), the ACT model has traditionally been presented through the mid-level. These terms are halfway between technical terms and those coming from the common language. Specifically, mid-level terms are functional abstractions that serve as shortcuts to apply basic principles to complex applied fields (Vilardaga et al., 2009).

Next, we will briefly review the most popular form of presentation of ACT in mid-level terms and leave its explanation in basic terms for the next section. ACT is based on the model of psychopathology and behavioral ineffectiveness called psychological inflexibility – a behavioral pattern in which private experiences dominate action over contingencies related to personal values (Hayes & Strosahl, 2004). As shown in Table 12.1, psychological inflexibility consists of six interrelated processes: dominance of the conceptualized past or future, attachment to self-contents, fusion with the contents, avoidance of the contents, lack of values clarity, and inaction or impulsivity without a horizon of value. Likewise, the ACT model points out that psychological flexibility is a central process involved in mental health and behavioral effectiveness. This is defined as the ability to openly contact ongoing private experiences and respond with an action inserted in the direction of personal value (Hayes et al., 2006; Hayes & Strosahl, 2004). Psychological flexibility comprises six other mid-level processes: being in the present moment, acceptance, defusion, self-as-context, values, and committed action.

12.1.4 ACT in Basic Terms

In this section, we will review a conceptualization of psychological (in)flexibility that has been developing over the last decade in terms of basic processes (e.g., Luciano et al., 2012, 2021a, b; Törneke et al., 2016). For this purpose, we will begin by pointing out how joy and suffering are generated in verbal human beings.

Table 12.1 Mid-level processes involved in flexibility and psychological inflexibility according to the hexaflex model

Psychological flexibility	Psychological inflexibility
Acceptance: Actively and consciously contact the private experiences occasioned by own history without attempting to change their frequency or form, especially when doing so would generate psychological damage.	*Experiential avoidance*: A regulation pattern characterized by conscious attempts to avoid or escape unwanted private experiences.
Cognitive defusion: Deactivating unwanted functions of thoughts and private experiences to change how the person responds to them.	*Cognitive fusion*: Acting according to the immediate functions of private thoughts and experiences.
Contact with the present moment: Nonjudgmental contact with psychological and environmental events as they occur.	*Dominance of the conceptualized past or feared future*: Focusing on events that occurred in the past or may occur in the future.
Self-as-context: Sensation of the self as locus or perspective from which one can be aware of the flow of private experiences without being attached to them.	*Self-as-content*: Attachment to private thoughts and experiences related to the self.
Values: Chosen qualities of purposeful action that cannot be achieved as an object but can be contacted moment by moment.	*Lack of values clarity*: Dominance of pliant rule-following (source of reinforcement is social) or avoidant tracking (actions guided by obtaining relief from discomfort).
Committed action: Actions linked to chosen values.	*Inaction, impulsivity, avoidant persistence*: Actions disconnected from valued directions.

Based on Hayes et al. (2006)

As is known, we are born with a series of positive and negative primary reinforcers, fruit of our phylogenetic history as a species. Quickly, through the interaction between classic and operant conditioning, initially neutral stimuli begin to be conditioned to function as secondary and generalized reinforcers. The development of the relational operants discussed above will cause a much wider range of stimuli to acquire appetitive and aversive functions due to the transformation of functions through the various relational frames (e.g., coordination, opposition, comparison, etc.).

The complexity of the construction of verbal reinforcers increases as fluency develops in the hierarchical relational framework. Numerous reinforcers with an experiential base, both positive and negative, will begin to be inserted into increasingly abstract hierarchical networks (Luciano et al., 2021b). For example, a 6-year-old child for whom relating to other children through play has become reinforcing may begin to relate these activities to more abstract concepts such as "friendship," and this concept will have a series of characteristics such as playing together, telling secrets, trusting or defending each other from dangerous situations. From this moment on, the act of playing with a friend will not only involve the previous reinforcing interactions of play, but the child will also be able to contact hierarchical appetitive functions related to "having good friends," "building a friendship," or "being able to trust someone."

This construction of hierarchical positive reinforcers causes the source of joy and satisfaction to become increasingly symbolic and abstract. These hierarchical reinforcers organize other, more tangible, reinforcers and alter their functions. It also sets up objectives and goals that allow getting in touch with and "advance in the direction" established by the hierarchical reinforcer (e.g., make friends with the boy who plays soccer well, go to summer camp with my best friends, etc.). Similarly, the main sources of suffering become increasingly verbal and abstract until, typically, a hierarchical network of negative reinforcers is established that relates in opposition to the network of hierarchical positive reinforcers (Gil-Luciano et al., 2019; Luciano et al., 2021b). In this way, the child in our example may begin to suffer from events such as the impossibility of going to summer camp because it will imply "not becoming a better friend of his friends" or feeling that a friend prefers to play more with another boy than with him ("he is not such a good friend of mine," "he trusts the other boy more," "he only wants to be with me when the other boy is not there," etc.).

So far, we have reviewed the emergence of hierarchical or higher-order appetitive and aversive functions. However, contact with these functions in the form of private experiences is transitory. Thus, it is worth asking why some people develop a personally meaningful life and others a life tinged with suffering of a symbolic origin. The answer to this question lies in how we respond to our own behavior, including our private experiences. Specifically, Törneke et al. (2016) identified two main ways in which we respond to our own behavior.

The first kind involves responding according to, or in coordination with, the immediate discriminative functions of one's behavior. When it has aversive functions (e.g., thoughts or emotions related to hierarchical aversive functions such as "I can't trust him" or feeling rejected), the immediate discriminative functions are avoidance/escape. By responding in coordination with these discriminative functions, the person would engage in some form of experiential avoidance to diminish or eliminate such aversive functions. This type of response becomes problematic when, through multiple exemplars, a dominant relational functional class (or purely functional operant) is formed through which the person focuses on obtaining negative reinforcement and loses contact with actions and functions linked to hierarchical positive reinforcers. This relational functional class is what we call psychological inflexibility in middle-level terms.

In many learning histories, this inflexible relational functional class is dominated by a pattern of thinking that seeks to diminish the aversive functions of private experiences by achieving certainty about what may happen in the future (worry) and coherence or explanation about what happened in the past (rumination). The problem with this reflexive thinking pattern (usually referred to as repetitive negative thinking, RNT) is that it tends to prolong and intensify negative affect, which often actualizes discriminative escape functions that lead to multiple forms of experiential avoidance such as thought suppression, alcohol consumption, self-injurious behaviors, binge eating, or suicide attempts (Brailovskaia et al., 2021; Caselli, et al., 2013; Hughes et al., 2019; Nolen-Hoeksema et al., 2007; Wells, 2002). Additionally, involvement in RNT has tremendously counterproductive effects (Ruiz et al., 2020).

In the first place, it increases the complexity and extension of the relational networks involved in this process, thus facilitating the derivation of new thoughts that will function as discriminative or triggers to restart the process. Secondly, the derivation level of these networks is reduced, thus producing greater speed and automaticity in a future RNT episode. Finally, continued RNT reduces relational flexibility, leading to greater difficulties in disrupting the RNT process.

The second type of response to one's own behavior is to frame it hierarchically with the deictic "I"; in other words, to note one's own behavior as a transient event from a broad perspective of the self that contains any past, present, or future experience. This hierarchical framing allows the person to contact functions related to hierarchical positive reinforcers and behave in accordance with them. As can be seen, this way of responding is considerably more complex, but also more flexible than the previous one and leads to behavior mainly controlled by positive reinforcement. This type of response becomes an adaptive behavioral pattern when, through multiple exemplars, a dominant relational functional class is formed that allows the person to contact and guide their behavior according to functions linked to the hierarchical positive reinforcers built throughout their history (Luciano et al., 2021b). This relational functional class is called psychological flexibility in middle-level terms. According to this conceptualization, the goal of ACT is to shape the relational functional class of framing one's behavior hierarchically with the deictic "I" or psychological flexibility. Törneke et al. (2016) proposed three central strategies for its shaping (see also Luciano et al., 2021a, b) as a guide, without implying any particular order.

Strategy 1. Help the client contact the problematic consequences of the inflexible pattern. The objective of this strategy is for the client to contact experientially with the consequences of their inflexible pattern. For this purpose, through questions, the therapist guides the client to discriminate: (a) the main private experiences to which they respond inflexibly, (b) the types of inflexible responses they put into practice and how they develop over time, (c) their short-term consequences in terms of usefulness in reducing discomfort and advancing in personally valued directions, and (d) the long-term consequences in terms of chronic and extending discomfort and hindering progress toward valued directions.

Strategy 2. Help the client frame limiting private events hierarchically with the deictic "I" as an alternative functional class. This strategy consists of encouraging multiple interactions in which the patient frames the ongoing private events hierarchically with the deictic "I." The main relational processes involved in this strategy are (Luciano et al., 2011, 2021a; Ruiz et al., 2021): (a) framing private experiences (thoughts, sensations, etc.) through deictic cues (I-Here feeling my experience there as something to be observed); (b) framing experiences through hierarchical cues (I contain the experience, experience is a part of me, it is just something transitory that I am experiencing, etc.); (c) deriving rules that indicate valued courses of action (contained in the higher-order functions of positive reinforcement) and providing a regulatory function to the hierarchical framing of one's own behavior; and (d) hierarchically framing the choice made (I am the one who can choose, I have chosen to "be in charge," not my thoughts/emotions).

Strategy 3. Help the client clarify and amplify values as hierarchical positive reinforcers and select actions contained in that motivational context. The work in this strategy consists of helping the client to: (a) establish and/or come into contact with the hierarchy of positive reinforcers that have been established throughout their personal history in connection with actions chosen for their quality; (b) differentiate actions connected with hierarchical positive reinforcers from actions controlled primarily by reinforcement provided by others (e.g., continuously acting to please others even if the behaviors themselves do not have a personally valuable quality) and actions focused on immediate reinforcement, but whose long-term natural consequences do not allow progress toward valuable directions (e.g., pressing the work team to achieve a goal even at the cost of generating an environment that favors the subsequent break-up of the team); (c) identify concrete valued actions that allow progress in objectives symbolically contained in the hierarchy of positive reinforcers; and (d) identify difficulties in carrying out valued actions, promoting their integration from a hierarchical perspective of the self and flexible action when facing them.

These strategies can be seen as angles to shape psychological flexibility and not as rigid phases to be applied in order. In fact, to enhance the effect of the intervention, the three strategies should be addressed together as soon as possible. In this way, the client will learn to: (a) frame the ongoing private event hierarchically with the deictic I, (b) discriminate the inflexible behavioral tendency and its long-term consequences, (c) contact the functions linked to own values, and (d) engage in the action that, at each given moment, allows them to advance in valued directions.

12.1.5 ACT in Psychosis

Psychosis is usually described as the experience of a series of behaviors called positive symptoms (hallucinations and delusions) that are usually accompanied by other behaviors that are considered negative symptoms, such as social anhedonia, flat affect, emotional symptoms, etc. From a traditional perspective, it is usually understood that hallucinations and delusions are symptoms that must be reduced or eliminated to improve the quality of life of the person who experiences them. However, from a functional-contextual perspective, the presence of these behaviors does not necessarily constitute a clinical problem (Bach, 2004). As we discussed in the previous sections, these private experiences, although they may be frequent, are still transitory events to which people can (learn to) respond in different ways.

People with psychotic symptoms show a clinical problem not because they hear voices, but because they act according to the content of the hallucination, ruminate excessively on it, or try to control its emergence, engaging in counterproductive experiential avoidance strategies (suppression, substance use, etc.). Similarly, the person who presents delusional ideas does not have a problem due to *experiencing* these ideas but because of *behaving according to them.* The fact that hallucinations and delusional ideas tend to actualize discriminative functions to behave in a counterproductive way in the long run in people with psychosis does not mean that this necessarily has to be the case. Proof of this is that most people who experience hallucinations do not have psychological problems; they even tend to evaluate them as positive experiences. Similarly, the presence of ideas that do not correspond to reality is frequent in the general population (Oltmanns & Maher, 1988; Tien, 1991). As for negative symptoms, these are usually consequences of chronic experiential avoidance and the absence of behavior motivated by hierarchical positive reinforcers (values).

The goal of ACT in psychosis, as in any other problem, is to promote flexibility in how the person responds to hallucinations and delusions so that they can direct their behavior toward valued directions rather than in an unsuccessful struggle to reduce the aversive functions of these experiences. There are also pragmatic reasons to consider the increase in psychological flexibility as the objective of intervention in psychosis, given the high resistance to change shown by hallucinations and delusions and the tendency to reappear after periods of remission (Bach, 2004).

ACT work on psychosis does not deviate significantly from the typical implementation of this therapy. It is advisable, however, to bear in mind that it is probably necessary to implement strategies to facilitate the development of the intervention according to the intensity of symptoms, cognitive deficits, and communication skills (for more detail in this aspect, we refer the reader to O'Donoghue et al., 2018). We will discuss the path of clinical work in the next sections of this chapter.

12.1.6 Empirical Evidence of ACT in Psychosis

ACT has been evaluated as an intervention in psychosis for the past two decades. Specifically, the recent systematic review conducted by Jansen et al. (2020) found seven randomized controlled trials in which ACT-based interventions were tested in the United States, the United Kingdom, Canada, Sweden, and Australia. Although the results should be considered as preliminary, ACT has shown better results than treatment as usual in terms of rehospitalization (Bach & Hayes, 2002; Gaudiano & Herbert, 2006; Tyrberg et al., 2017), positive symptoms and discomfort related to hallucinations (Shawyer et al., 2017), and negative and emotional symptoms (Gumley et al., 2017; Spidel et al., 2018; White et al., 2011).

12.2 ACT Approach to Psychosis

12.2.1 Clinical Case: Ernest

Ernest, aged 47, comes to the consultation accompanied by his mother. He presents a report from the psychiatry unit with a diagnosis of Major Depressive Disorder of psychotic characteristics and recurrent episodes. But who Ernest is, what his suffering is, what he longs for, and what personal history surrounds him go far beyond this diagnosis.

Ernest spent his childhood tied to his mother's apron strings. This was his compass for what he did and why he did it. From his early years, he forged an intense dependence on his mother, as well as multiple widespread fears. His parents provided him with a constant context of protection from the world. His adolescence followed the same progression as his childhood, aggravated, among other things, by the characteristic complexity of interpersonal relationships at this stage. Also in this area of his life, his mother continued to direct his actions in his choices, for example, the how and when of his dealings with his peers and friends; as well as with girls. When his mother did not directly intercede in how her son could or should handle the things that happened to him, Ernest himself displayed the pattern of caution and cowardice developed in his childhood. On the other hand, his parents tried not to make excessive demands that he engage in his responsibilities – studies and household chores. They let him do whatever he felt like, trying to reduce any possible discomfort for him. In any case, he was not a bad student and finished his High School studies, without showing interest in any of the subjects or higher studies.

At the age of 18, he began his working life. He began working on his first and only job. His parents got him a post in a car factory located very close to home. In general, interacting with people other than his parents was difficult and uncomfortable for him, so he remained quite apart from any social life. At the age of 20, he had his first and only sexual relationship, which was traumatic for him because he was unsuccessful due to premature ejaculation and the girl's reaction. It happened in the bosom of an old group of classmates and friends, and the girl told them what had happened, mocking Ernest along with the others. From then on, he began to reduce attempts to socialize beyond what was strictly necessary, convincing himself of how complex and aversive human relationships were for him. Later, during most of his adulthood, he used to share very punctual moments with a group of coworkers with whom he shared some hobbies (running or role-playing championships). In his free time, he tended to immerse himself in the world of online video games, a world of fiction and fantasy that, as when he was a child and read, removed him from reality and transported him to a world of brave people.

Although comfortable and fluid in his work (operator on the assembly line), the monotony, solitude, and reduced intellectual demand of this job were gradually creating the conditions that led him to spend much of his time ruminating on his frustrations, worrying more and more about the future. His adult years passed without there being any more advancement or progression in his life except for time. From home, he went to work, and from work, back home. His mother did the household tasks and general chores (shopping, errands, paperwork, medical appointments, etc.) for him. At the age of 37, Ernest went to live alone in an apartment located very close to his parents' house through a real estate offer his father managed to achieve. His mother, however, continued to organize and do things for him. At the age of 42, Ernest began to request a series of sick leaves due to depression and decided to return to live with his parents, encouraged by his mother. In these circumstances, the company decided to terminate his contract and fire him. At that time, his mother was also diagnosed with a degenerative disease.

At this circumstantial point in his life, he began to have obsessions and ideas about catastrophes of all kinds and he also began to implement increasingly limiting behaviors. Suddenly, in his forties, Ernest came up against a feeling of helplessness, of facing an uncontrollable abyss, and a terrific fear of what might happen. These were feelings that, historically, all his life, he had managed to keep at bay through his way of functioning, but, now, they were triggered after losing his only job (of 27 years duration) and the detection of the degenerative disease of his mother, his only source of guidance, support, and protection so that nothing bad would happen to him. His greatest concern became very vivid: what did the future hold? who would take care of him? how was he going to survive?

Continuous thoughts and rumination surrounding the fear of being helpless began to take over his life, day and night. Thoughts about global and personal catastrophes became increasingly repetitive. He felt an intense fear due to the experience of these thoughts; he felt that some danger lurked at any moment. Through the Internet, he reached pages with examples about the causes of thoughts of this type, and the level of anguish and limitations they could produce, such as, for example, noticing "strange forces" that exerted mental power over people. He began to develop dissociative behaviors, complaints, laments, bodily states of very intense tension and, in the tensest moments, he began to appear on some nights in his parents' room with a kitchen knife (which he never seemed to remember the next morning). After episodes of great alteration, he would spend several days sleeping. He said that he noticed his thoughts aloud ("voices" of "cowards and brave people" who fight) and, after the increase in extreme behaviors and even idealizing suicide, the situation led to consulting a psychiatrist and the prescription of antipsychotics and cognitive-behavioral therapy, which he attended for a year and a half. The systematicity of the most problematic behaviors and the frequency of the "voices" were reduced. Following the psychological intervention, after his mother fell down at home, Ernest returned to the previous frequency of obsessions and severe behaviors. He refused to resume the previous intervention, and the mental health unit decided to refer his case.

The intervention that will be presented herein began at that point. At the time of the consultation, he was receiving an assigned financial benefit for mental disability, he continued living with his parents (who were very worried and worn out), and spent most of the day playing online video games, sleeping, and lying in bed ruminating, and talking aloud with his thoughts.

12.2.1.1 Functional Case Conceptualization

The pattern of psychological inflexibility, gathered from the information from the functional assessment, is described below.

Ernest had a very strong pattern of psychological inflexibility that was very limiting. Since his childhood, he had received a context of continuous caution about the dangers involved in the interaction with the world and with others, and constant support and help in the face of the slightest challenge, constantly deciding and doing things for him. He looked at the world and interacted with it through his maternal figure, directly or indirectly. He did it based on rules he had learned about the world, others, and himself. Of all of them, the one that seemed the most limiting was that "he was *incapable,*" thus, he needed *others* (until then, his mother) to show the way and set the favorable conditions to function and to avoid discomfort in the face of loneliness and uncertainty about what might happen. From this rule, other rules emerged, "The world is a dangerous and unsafe place, do not trust people's intentions," "The most important thing is to be calm and without upsets," "If something is difficult and involves a lot of effort, it might be bad for you, do not do it", "I am a person with a disabling disease, I have limitations," and so on. Frustration and fear of being helpless had been slowly and progressively emanating from the costs of the way he lived his life. The most problematic outburst occurred when his greatest fear became very present. The possible loss of his only source of support, security, and guidance (his mother), and losing the only support he had ever had, brought to the present the most aversive private events for him.

In the presence of such an intensity of suffering, Ernest resorted to his pattern of escape and avoidance, connecting his fears with thoughts of possible catastrophes. In this context, he began to consider his thoughts as *unbearable* "voices," external to him, in the face of which he resorted to increasingly limiting and greater escape and avoidance behaviors. His emotional lows in the face of these contents and his struggle to avoid discomfort produced a context of incapacity and anomaly directly associated with his history of overprotection and dependence, sustained by formal diagnoses of psychotic symptomatology and depression. This context chronified the coupling of his rules about the world and himself, multiplying them while increasing his discomfort, and he adjusted his responses to try to reduce it. Psychotropic drugs and psychological treatment to modify these thought networks reduced the "voices" and catastrophic thoughts and also the most dangerous responses of his limiting pattern. However, these changes took place apart from vital advances and progress that would have allowed him to build a pattern of interaction with himself that was effective in the long term, both in his facet of work and in the field of interpersonal relationships (friendships, possible partners, family, community …) and of personal care.

Ernest's pattern had come at a very high cost in interfering with his deep desires and interests, as will be seen later in the investigation of the pattern of inflexibility in the intervention process.

In the face of these rules, his pattern had been to keep clear from vital advances and progress, both in the area of his occupation (studies, work, various responsibilities) and in interpersonal relationships (friendships, possible partners, the possibility of starting a family, the social community in general). Overall, the pattern of psychological inflexibility in the functional X-ray shown in Table 12.1 of the following section can be seen in greater detail.

12.2.2 Approach to Contextual Therapy

The objective of ACT is always the same, no matter the profile of psychopathology, as, in all cases, the therapist's behavior will be adjusted to the patient's behavior with the same purpose: to build a repertoire of psychological flexibility. This is defined by interacting and responding to the thoughts and emotions that occur in each circumstance under the motivational function of value or personal meaning. As explained in the introductory section of the chapter, ACT has been presented in various ways over the last twenty years and, also, basic-applied research has shown part of the relational processes that are involved in the work carried out by the therapist and the patient (see the texts recently published in Luciano et al., 2021a, b). In this chapter, we will follow the trail of the processes or principal elements detected in the process of change. We will not delve into these processes here but instead, we will present the summary of the intervention following the three strategies that, as a whole, are oriented to build – or enhance – the pattern of psychological flexibility. (1) On the one hand, interactions aimed at helping the patient experience their pattern and limiting consequences will be presented, while opening a horizon of personal meaning. (2) On the other hand, interactions aimed at helping the patient to generate a space or observation point that allows them to experience their own behavior without becoming fused to their private events. (3) Furthermore, those strategies aimed at amplifying the central motivational function of personal life.

It is important to emphasize that the three clinical strategies of contextual therapy are not subject to any particular order, but instead, therapists can make use of them through multiple tools, adapting them elastically to their purpose. This is none other than to promote examples of flexibility so that a flexible pattern of responses is built, crowned with motivational functions of personal meaning. The clinician may choose to use multiple tools through physical exercises or imagination, metaphors, and variability in their interactions with the patient. The elasticity of the therapist's repertoire is aimed at producing flexibility in their patients. That is why a single or closed protocol will not be valid but instead, the action protocol of ACT is defined by its variability to adapt to the variability of behaviors that each patient will deploy in response to the therapist's behaviors.

Patients with a history of chronicity and inflexibility that impacts considerably their functionality usually require initial work on very basic skills to begin to "detach" from their own behavior. For example, in many of these cases, the degree of psychological inflexibility present in the session is so high that the therapist has to intervene to facilitate a minimum level of patients' detection of their own behavior. Thus, having produced some level of flexibility in session, the conditions would be established for other more complex clinical movements that allow the patient to detect their rules, their way of functioning, take charge of the effects of their pattern, and open and amplify horizons of personal meaning. In any case, both initially and later on, the intervention will revolve around generating flexibility in the face of private events (rules, emotions, etc.) that were triggering rigid and fused reactions. In the following sections, we will show the general lines of the process followed with Ernest.

12.2.2.1 First Steps to Produce Psychological Flexibility

Ernest's profile met the characteristics that we have indicated at the end of the previous section. For example, his behavior in session varied between examples of problematic behavior formally identified as manic episodes, dissociation when conversing with his symptoms, self-aggressions, emotional instability, etc., to which were added very reduced communication skills, and difficulty in maintaining attention. Whether due to the interference of the high degree of psychological inflexibility, or the effects of medication, these repertoires become the central point of the initial work. Inevitably, it becomes necessary to adapt each tool to build flexibility in the patient's behavior in such a way that, as in this case, very active short phrases and physical keys, and brief movements are used to catch the patient's attention. That is, interactions that, in other cases, could be redundant.

As mentioned at the beginning, the flexibility to be built in the face of thoughts-voices, delusions, hallucinations, and any private events of a very intense nature will alter the patient's relationship with them, how he responds, and what he pursues with it. From the beginning of the intervention, Ernest resorted in session to dissociating, ruminating at full speed "on a loudspeaker," crying uncontrollably, or self-harming (scratching wounds that he had made previously) when something evoked uncomfortable sensations and thoughts. At such times, it is very easy for the therapist to go into an orbit in which he can easily be influenced by the strong impact of some of the patient's behaviors, but he should take advantage of them to alter their function *in situ*. From the beginning, the therapist asked permission to work in a way that was most useful to the patient, warning him that he could interrupt at any time. In addition, the patient was ensured that the therapist would be with him, by his side, so that he could feel whatever he felt and think whatever he thought. In this context, the relationship between patient and therapist was marked by the integration and validation of all the thoughts and sensations that emerged, as a context of value that sustained the intervention.

When Ernest issued any of the behaviors indicated in the previous paragraph, movements were made aimed at making him respond flexibly. For example, (a) they sought to alter his inflexible behavior by directing the stimulating control towards the therapist, reminding him that (the therapist) was there with him, while he felt whatever he felt, and directly asking him to focus his gaze on the therapist, to focus on his voice, to feel his arm resting on the armchair, his feet on the ground, etc.; (b) maintaining his attention on the therapist, he was asked to say what he was feeling or thinking, the location of parts of his body right there, what he saw in the room, what those thoughts or emotions suggested; (c) through the patient's responses, he was trained to discriminate the context of who experienced those thoughts, who noticed them, along with the variability of private events, noticing that there were many sensations at that moment that he could feel, and that he was there to decide what he paid attention to and how he wanted to do it. If appropriate, (d) a flexible action was trained at that moment. Finally, the contingencies of having done so were noted.

These movements constitute one of the basic strategies of contextual therapy called, in mid-terms, defusion. As indicated in the introduction, they allow generating a space between oneself and one's private events to be able to turn one's attention towards actions that have a more relevant meaning. The literature of ACT and other contextual therapies offers numerous keys that can have the same function and which is none other than to generate, through different trials of this type (multiple trials), the foundations to build psychological flexibility in the face of painful or threatening content for the patient. Following the principles of discrimination, work can be initiated through neutral examples, that is, promoting neutral private events in deictic and hierarchical discrimination and, little by little, incorporating or provoking others that could provoke aversive or appetitive functions due to the patient's history.

Ernest was learning this repertoire. Multiple examples were made, either flexible or inflexible examples, as a way to build flexibility around private events. The frequency of flexibility began to increase, and this context cleared the way to work on other points, such as beginning to face the ways of coping he had used– and continued to use– on many occasions, and the interference that they had produced till now. This context opened the horizon to delve into how he could reorient his life, and on which personal meaning to base it.

12.2.2.2 Ernest, Caught in the Story About Himself

Gradually, the therapist began to help Ernest to contact his inflexible repertoire more broadly: what other ways did he have of dealing with his uncomfortable emotions and thoughts, what was their outcome, and what had been their outcome in his life, and whether they had interfered with something that was, or could be, relevant for him. This strategy is encompassed in the functional analysis and aims to help the patient become aware of the effects of their inflexible repertoire. Examining what his life was like now and what it had been like prior to these last years, Ernest stated that he missed his job and daily routine, and even his own space, like when he lived alone. Delving into what things he missed the most, he went on to point out that feeling useful and capable had been the things that he valued more than any other feeling. When asking him to compare in detail examples of situations in which he had come to feel something like this, Ernest broke down in a session, sobbing, and said that his biggest problems had always revolved around feeling weak and unable to live his life like everyone else seemed to. He spoke of his inability to identify and carry out valuable life goals, stating that "If at least I had something to hold on to now, maybe I would feel stronger about what is happening to my mother..." It was painful for him not to have been able to reach an intimate relationship with anyone except for his parents (including the possibility of having a partner), to have traveled, and to have developed in a more interesting job. They began to identify the private events that were old acquaintances when it came to setting up a barrier to opening up, like he said, "living outside the box." His history made him control those contexts and situations that would guarantee the comfort and security of not feeling threatened at all times. Underneath that was a central rule, about himself, as someone who was *unable to survive in conditions (feelings) of weakness and vulnerability*, therefore, *he had to escape and avoid contexts that generated them*. His family history would have been decisive to generate the armor of avoidance with which he walked through life. The conceptualization of the case presented in previous sections incorporates the information collected during this process.

Contextual therapy does not try to break the patient's coherence concerning the history they learned about what they *are* by discussing it and trying to modify it. Instead, it addresses the futile result of always behaving according to that history and the patient's own experience. Thus, the patient's most limiting ways to remain safe and sheltered from his feelings of incapacity and vulnerability were incorporated into the therapy. Figure 12.1 shows the functional schema of this pattern. Functional analysis movements are most effective if they are performed experientially, that is, taking advantage of clinical behavior *in situ* (when an example of the inflexible pattern is occurring in session) and leading the patient to contact the presence of their inflexible rules (private events), way of responding, and consequences. These movements will have to be repeated throughout the intervention because discriminating the pattern requires multiple, infinite examples in which it manifests to unify them as a problematic functional class. The objective is for the patient to manage to abstract the discrimination from his general tendency to behave under the mandate of the rigid rule prevailing according to his history. This, with care, allowed establishing the conditions to begin to move, with little big steps, in another direction.

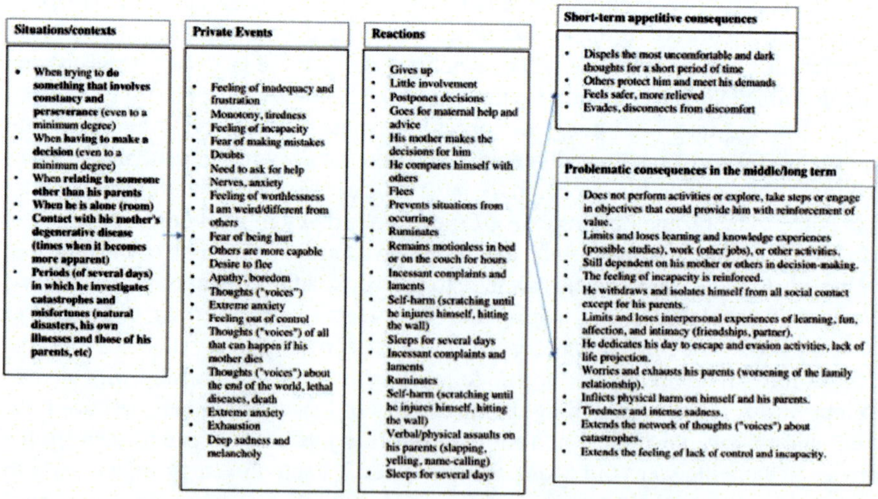

Fig. 12.1 Functional analysis of Ernest's pattern of psychological inflexibility

12.2.2.3 Investigating and Situating a Context of Meaning and Personal Value

Ernest had great difficulty not only making decisions, as he insisted, but also taking the initiative and exploring new paths. He did not find within himself what he wanted to do with his life but, instead, his answers were diluted by what his mother had insisted on throughout his life: avoid the evils that occur in many places and try to guarantee safety. Any possibility of exploring was stopped in its tracks by difficulty, effort, and fear that something would happen that would hurt him. This way of functioning had prevented contact with the natural contingencies of any interpersonal, academic, and labor process, or any other learning process. His need for his mother's support and guidance, or other sources of help, had been an inescapable link in his life. The process of contacting this mode of functioning began to make a dent in Ernest, to the point of beginning to consider "breaking the chains" with the avoidance armor he wore everywhere. He wanted to "live," but the private events in the face of what that could include were overwhelmingly present in session. It was necessary to delve into the motivation so that he could take charge of such fears.

Ernest felt that he was a person with a very low-profile life, a life that did not satisfy him and that produced a high level of frustration. Much of his frustration emanated from somewhere, and that place is usually made up of not cultivating something, of not living the life one would want—even if one had never tasted it. In one way or another, these are motivations of personal meaning; sometimes remote and sometimes derived, even from the omission with which one has lived. Motivations with true personal meaning are the directions of value and the drivers of behavior. Without exploring, amplifying, and continuously making this driver present, clinical change is unlikely and is not maintained over time. Patients with a history in which the context has been rigid in promoting rules and contingencies that match their adherence, accompanied by the corresponding derivations, are patients who learn inflexible behavior that becomes chronic over time. That is, it is not chronic patients, but chronic contexts that select one or another type of functioning. These are patients who have difficulty knowing what interests them, what they would like to do, what they would like to address, what trail they would like to follow to its end. Ernest's life story had not followed trajectories that were valuable to him, but were instead guided by the avoidance of fear; even less so since his entry into the "circuit of the diagnosis of psychotic mental illness." His fears, weakness, and incapacity, together with the suffering multiplied by the psychotic diagnosis, had acquired considerable strength and taken over the foreground to direct his life. Far, far back, diffuse, forgotten, or perhaps nonexistent, there was the possibility of doing something useful, of realizing some dream, and of functioning with some freedom.

A central premise derived from the basic-applied knowledge of RFT is also the premise in ACT that "something of immense value is at the epicenter of all suffering." The work on values in contextual therapy is not only based on exploring objectives or goals but fundamentally on the motivational context that gives meaning to the steps or actions. Therefore, the reinforcement of action lies in its meaning of value, especially when private events of considerable discomfort concur, such as those habitual ones in the case of Ernest. The process carried out to bring him into contact with such positive reinforcers of personal meaning also made Ernest come into contact with his inflexible pattern and its consequences: he said he felt trapped in his self-humiliation because of his dependence on his parents and his aggression toward them in moments of intense suffering when he felt useless, with nothing to do and no plan for anything, including establishing personal relationships. In contrast, the therapist's questions allowed Ernest to contact something deeper in himself and to indicate that, if he could, he would really want to be *useful, independent, loving, and brave.*

Multiple examples were practiced in session in which Ernest faced making small choices and carrying them out as if they were acts of courage and independence. It did not matter if they were significant actions but, instead, their significance lay in the fact that they were chosen, that he had to choose between two or three options, and he chose one without guaranteeing the result, he performed it, and exposed himself to the consequences. Soon it included exploring moments in his life to carry out actions guided by choice, courage, and independence, especially some actions that he performed under the custody and mediation of his mother. On the one hand, these steps were decisive, as he himself indicated later, in the learning process to build a new repertoire selected for contingencies of personal value. On the other hand, other steps began to be taken when teasing out the importance or meaning of Ernest's hobbies, past and present, no matter how insignificant they may seem to him. For example, concerning his preferences and their rationale, whether it was his favorite foods, video games, type of books, type of people, conversations, or what he was like that pleased him; the high school subjects that had captured his attention and why, and so on.

The exploration was not aimed at knowing formal details but, instead, trying to get Ernest to identify and experience what was of value at that time, even to imagine doing something in that direction and to feel whatever he felt. In other words, the exploration is carried out by investigating the quality of those interests that Ernest formulated and the actions that they implied. The quality highlighted the value reinforcers, while also allowing to know what dominance they might have in the face of problematic feelings and thoughts. The ACT literature is replete with questions and interactions that lead to these goals. For example: *"What do you like about what you are saying? Can you bring any of that here, what it made you feel? When you say that you have fun or that you enjoy reading that book, what is it that makes you enjoy it, what is in that story that grabs you so much? You say that you are caught by that character because he investigates and takes risks ..., what moves you when you are reading that he takes risks…?* Many of these questions are aimed at teasing out the feelings attached to the peaks of the reinforcers with personal meaning, to try to get the patient to contact, right there, the functions that come from actions performed, or possible future actions.

Gradually, a possible map was drawn with Ernest. The guide, or compass, were broad-spectrum motivations to which uncertainty and fears were inevitably linked.

Ernest wanted to be independent, helpful, loving, and brave. Later, he discovered other qualities, such as his interest in learning, or being diligent.

One move that proved useful was to create a metaphor with Ernest that could encompass all those qualities that he was discovering. To the question, *what might you look like if you saw yourself being brave, independent, diligent..?* he replied that it would be like being *"an eagle,"* mainly because of its freedom of movement and bravery. From there on, to aim every day to promote an *"Ernest-eagle"* was placed as the global horizon of work; a free, independent, useful, courageous Ernest, and so on. The metaphor started especially from his love of literature. He professed a true passion for adventure books. As a child, he had been passionate about reading and had continued this passion, also through video games. As a child, he recognized himself taking refuge for hours in books and adventure comics, which took him to parallel realities in which he enjoyed himself and admired how the characters challenged themselves until they managed to save themselves, or save others. In session, he was asked to tell some of these stories to explore possible reinforcers of value in reading, and evaluate possible extrapolations that could be found in some work or personal relationship. Through several movements like this and multiple exercises, a repertoire of discrimination of what possesses personal meaning was gradually sharpened, which Ernest recognized at the base of *his* identity.

This work involved the constant integration of the multiple thoughts and feelings that acted as barriers. Feelings of worthlessness, incapacity, shame, and failure *appeared* when exploring and amplifying actions with quality or value. However, the therapist did not engage in conversation with the patient's private events. Instead, he made him notice them, validating them, and placed Ernest in the perspective of his thoughts or emotions and actions. After this, the patient was asked for permission to *(up)hold* those feelings and continue to explore the value that could be located at the core of his pain or his fear.

The Ernest *"eagle"* dreamed of being able to have some job or occupation in which he taught children stories, either by reading them or teaching them some skill related to writing and imagination. On a personal level, he dreamed of being able to have a child and, beyond that, share that experience with a partner. He wanted to go back to living alone and contributing to his parents' support and security, rather than being a source of concern for them. He wanted to be more physically fit, to resume *running* (which also generated "eagle sensations": freedom, utility for the reward of effort...). This activity also used to be shared with colleagues from his previous work, and resuming the relationship with them was also something of great importance for Ernest, as it had been his only social source beyond the family.

Parallel to the systematic work of the experiential discrimination of the destructive function of his avoidant pattern, allowing contact with the consequences generated in the short and long term, several phases were organized in the intervention. We worked with Ernest on the "eagle" project at various times; always through personal choice, encouraging:

1. Contact with *value, independence, and affection* by reducing aid from his parents in basic domestic tasks: lunches, dinners, cleaning, and personal hygiene.

2. Contact with *courage, value, and independence* by helping and teaching children, collaborating with a children's volunteer association for children in need.
3. Contact with *affection, courage, and independence* when resuming the relationship with former coworkers, running, and other activities (with others or alone).

In the course of the process, Ernest drew future steps under the umbrella of that new Ernest: learn to drive, give support classes to disadvantaged children in reading and writing, become independent again in his own home, create a profile on dating websites, etc.

12.2.2.4 Clinging to a New Anchor in the Face of Emotional Relapse

During the process, emotional swings were an inevitable constant in the face of the strength of the sole and inflexible pattern of functioning. The therapist responded to the emergence of any of these emotions and thoughts with validation and invited the patient to relate to them inclusively, while making present whatever made personal sense. In the face of chronic patterns, it has been previously described that the whole process will be a constant dance between noticing inflexible examples and promoting flexible examples. What we present in this last section is the approach to an episode of relapse after several weeks, in which Ernest had begun to be present with his threatening thoughts, willing to feel his anguish *("in the form of a black fist, oppressor, in his chest,"* he verbalized), and breathe deeply while opening his eyes to focus on the small (but large) actions he had committed to doing.

The strong episode of relapse occurred in the wake of an interaction with his parents, in which his mother complained about Ernest's refusal to let her do things for him, as she had always done. For his part, his father reproached him for making his mother suffer despite her difficulties and warned him that he would always be a sick person who had to be cared for, that he would never be responsible because he had never shown courage. Ernest's worst thoughts were present.

Within seconds, Ernest entered a state of extreme anxiety to which he reacted by giving voice to his threatening thoughts, and to his old voices that *"he would do something bad if he didn't control his anxiety."* Ernest escaped to his room, shouting at his voices, and took an overdose of antidepressants. The episode ended with a mental health notice and transfer to the hospital. After a week, Ernest came to the session desolate, very depressed, and assuming that he could never lead another life, that he was condemned, and that he had thought about taking his own life again.

The possibility of a relapse is normal with long inflexible trajectories of patients like Ernest. On the one hand, in a contextual/functional view, relapses are *part of* building a new pattern. In fact, learning to live is not learning not to fall, but learning to *fall and get up*; that is our condition. On the other hand, contextual vision in therapy does not assume that building a pattern eliminates the previous one. Building a flexible pattern reduces the likelihood of inflexibly reacting to emotions and thoughts, but that requires a lot of training. Even in high doses, there may always be a time when the meaning of personal value could be clouded and, then, the patient may respond guided by the emotional obstacles present at that time. The need for practice in the flexible pattern, of multiple examples to build it, is something known at the level of basic research. Any pattern is an operant that is only constructed from multiple examples (see Luciano et al., 2021a, b). However, patients like Ernest, who carry a backpack of life defined by an inflexible pattern (that is, a functional operant that is not useful to them in the long run, even if it is useful to some degree because of its coherence), will need to take charge of the effects of relapse more than other patients and recover the rhythm of the flexible pattern at those moments.

Relapses like Ernest's produce stirrings of discomfort and thoughts of uselessness in the therapist. However, it is appropriate to apply the same medicine that the professional has to apply to his patient and react by showing his regret when noticing the patient's regret for what happened. In this case, what Ernest felt was validated, and an attempt was made to normalize his thoughts by remembering, once more, that living entailed this possibility: to feel even worse than at the beginning.

At first, Ernest said, *"I had no hope, I thought there was no solution... then I saw that there was a spark of light in the darkness... but, suddenly, everything has become much darker than before."* He argued that both the patient and the therapist were "wrong," and that ending his life would be the true act of bravery. The therapist sustained his own emotions upon hearing that and shared them with the patient. At the same time, he shared with the patient his joy at seeing him there, whole, showing his emotions and everything he thought. He invited Ernest to stop, to let the air flow between so many emotions, telling him to breathe deeply to feel whatever they had to feel right there, both of them. After a few minutes, he asked Ernest to look at him, Ernest burst into tears, and the therapist invited him to hold all that inside him, like weights that are put on us and are floating in us. And they remained that way for a few more minutes. In the end, both of them stated that they felt at a common point to *continue* working on building more flexibility.

The context of value of the interaction has been summarized by emphasizing that both therapist and patient are verbal human beings, who think and feel. The contextual therapist's way of being in session is to include their own private events, wrapping them in the value of what is important in their work – building the repertoire of flexibility in their patient. This session was one of the most important for Ernest in the direction of starting to be *another* Ernest.

12.3 Conclusions

Contextual therapy, or ACT, tries to break the patient's relationship with the problematic impact of their personal history, that is, with the thoughts or emotions that act as a barrier to a vital journey with meaning and personal value. In the chronic patient, as is often the case with a psychotic profile, the private experience of some private events called "psychotic" invites them to behave in very limiting ways. Progressively, the vital journey of these patients is directed by contents of the Self that revolve around disability, dependence, and weakness, forming a pattern of inflexibility that perpetuates and amplifies these private events. Contextual therapy affects the rupture of the pattern in the same way as in the face of any problem; adjusting the intervention process to the initial repertoire of psychological inflexibility of the patient in session. The refinement of contextual therapy based on the basic-applied research of the last decade allows focusing on three movements or strategies in the work towards the patient's psychological flexibility. Presented throughout this chapter, they involve an enormous elasticity that the therapist can use to adapt them according to the requirements of the context of each patient's repertoire. The purpose and the ultimate definition of building psychological flexibility is nothing more than to generate an alternative, flexible, and adaptive way of traveling down vital pathways that make sense and have personal meaning. Through the (necessary) emotional ups and downs of the intervention process, flexibility means that patient and therapist work in the same direction through multiple examples that make up a new repertoire. A new way of working, a course towards the lighthouse, explored and amplified, of personal meaning.

Disclaimer Clinical cases presented in this chapter do not include real names or personal information of real persons.

References

Bach, P. (2004). ACT with seriously mentally ill. In S. C. Hayes & K. D. Strosah (Eds.), *A practical guide to acceptance and commitment therapy* (pp. 185–208). Springer.

Bach, P., & Hayes, S. C. (2002). The use of acceptance and commitment therapy to prevent the rehospitalization of psychotic patients: A randomized controlled trial. *Journal of Consulting and Clinical Psychology, 70*, 1129–1139.

Brailovskaia, J., Margraf, J., & Teismann, T. (2021). Repetitive negative thinking mediates the relationship between addictive Facebook use and suicide-related outcomes: A longitudinal study. *Current Psychology*, 1–9.

Caselli, G., Gemelli, A., Querci, S., Lugli, A. M., Canfora, F., Annovi, C., et al. (2013). The effect of rumination on craving across the continuum of drinking behaviour. *Addictive Behaviors, 38*, 2879–2883.

Gaudiano, B. A., & Herbert, J. D. (2006). Acute treatment of inpatients with psychotic symptoms using acceptance and commitment therapy: Pilot results. *Behaviour Research and Therapy, 44*, 415–437.

Gifford, E. V., & Hayes, S. C. (1999). Functional contextualism: A pragmatic philosophy for behavioral science. In W. O'Donohue & R. Kitchener (Eds.), *Handbook of behaviorism* (pp. 285–327). Academic Press.

Gil-Luciano, B., Calderón-Hurtado, T., Tovar, D., Sebastián, B., & Ruiz, F. J. (2019). How are triggers for repetitive negative thinking organized? A relational frame analysis. *Psicothema, 31*, 53–59.

Gloster, A. T., Walder, N., Levin, M., Twohig, M., & Karekla, M. (2020). The empirical status of acceptance and commitment therapy: A review of meta-analyses. *Journal of Contextual Behavioral Science, 18*, 181–192.

Gumley, A., White, R., Briggs, A., Ford, I., Barry, S., Stewart, C., et al. (2017). A parallel group randomised open blinded evaluation of Acceptance and Commitment Therapy for depression after psychosis: Pilot trial outcomes (ADAPT). *Schizophrenia Research, 183*, 143–150.

Hayes, S. C. (1993). Analytic goals and the varieties of scientific contextualism. In S. C. Hayes, L. J. Hayes, H. W. Reese, & T. R. Sarbin (Eds.), *Varieties of scientific contextualism* (pp. 11–27). Context Press.

Hayes, S. C., & Strosahl, K. D. (Eds.). (2004). *A practical guide to acceptance and commitment therapy*. Springer Science & Business Media.

Hayes, S. C., Hayes, L. J., Reese, H. W., & Sarbin, T. R. (1993). *Varieties of scientific contextualism*. Context Press.

Hayes, S. C., Strosahl, K. D., & Wilson, K. G. (1999). *Acceptance and commitment therapy: An experiential approach to behavior change*. Guilford Press.

Hayes, S. C., Barnes-Holmes, D., & Roche, R. (2001). *Relational frame theory*. Kluwer Academic Publishers.

Hayes, S. C., Luoma, J. B., Bond, F. W., Masuda, A., & Lillis, J. (2006). Acceptance and commitment therapy: Model, processes and outcomes. *Behaviour Research and Therapy, 44*, 1–25.

Hayes, S. C., Barnes-Holmes, D., & Wilson, K. G. (2012). Contextual behavioral science: Creating a science more adequate to the challenge of the human condition. *Journal of Contextual Behavioral Science, 1*, 1–16.

Hayes, S. C., Merwin, R. M., McHugh, L., Sandoz, E. K., & A-Tjak, J. G., Ruiz, F. J., ... McCracken, L. M. (2021). Report of the ACBS task force on the strategies and tactics of contextual behavioral science research. *Journal of Contextual Behavioral Science, 20*, 172–183.

Hughes, C. D., King, A. M., Kranzler, A., Fehling, K., Miller, A., Lindqvist, J., & Selby, E. A. (2019). Anxious and overwhelming affects and repetitive negative thinking as ecological predictors of self-injurious thoughts and behaviors. *Cognitive Therapy and Research, 43*, 88–101.

Jansen, J. E., Gleeson, J., Bendall, S., Rice, S., & Alvarez-Jimenez, M. (2020). Acceptance-and mindfulness-based interventions for persons with psychosis: A systematic review and meta-analysis. *Schizophrenia Research, 215*, 25–37.

Luciano, C. (2016). Evolución de ACT [Evolution of ACT]. *Análisis y Modificación de Conducta, 42*, 3–14.

Luciano, C., Ruiz, F. J., Gil-Luciano, B., & Molina-Cobos, F. J. (2021a). Terapias contextuales [Contextual therapies]. In E. Fonseca-Pedrero (Ed.), *Manual de tratamientos psicológicos: Adultos* [Manual of psychological treatments: Adults] (pp. 167–199). Pirámide.

Luciano, C., Törneke, N., & Ruiz, F. J. (2021b, in press). Clinical behavior analysis and RFT: Conceptualizing psychopathology and its treatment. In M. P. Twohig, M. E. Levin, & J. M. Petersen (Eds.), *Oxford handbook of acceptance and commitment therapy*. Oxford University Press.

Luciano, C., Ruiz, F. J., Vizcaíno-Torres, R., Sánchez, V., Gutiérrez-Martínez, O., & López-López, J. C. (2011). A relational frame analysis of defusion interactions in acceptance and commitment therapy. A preliminary and quasi-experimental study with at-risk adolescents. *International Journal of Psychology and Psychological Therapy, 11*, 165–182.

Luciano, C., Valdivia-Salas, S., & Ruiz, F. J. (2012). The self as the context for rule-governed behavior. In L. McHugh & I. Stewart (Eds.), *The self and perspective taking: Research and applications* (pp. 143–160). Context Press.

Nolen-Hoeksema, S., Stice, E., Wade, E., & Bohon, C. (2007). Reciprocal relations between rumination and bulimic, substance abuse, and depressive symptoms in female adolescents. *Journal of Abnormal Psychology, 116*, 198–207.

O'Donoghue, E. K., Morris, E. M., Olier, J., & Johns, L. C. (2018) ACT for psychosis recovery: A practical manual for group-based interventions using acceptance and commitment therapy. .

Oltmanns, T. E., & Maher, B. A. (1988). *Delusional beliefs*. Wiley.

Pepper, S. C. (1942). *World hypotheses: A study in evidence*. University of California Press.

Ruiz, F. J., Luciano, C., Flórez, C. L., Suárez-Falcón, J. C., & Cardona-Betancourt, V. (2020). A multiple-baseline evaluation of acceptance and commitment therapy focused on repetitive negative thinking for comorbid generalized anxiety disorder and depression. *Frontiers in Psychology, 11*, 356.

Ruiz, F. J., Gil-Luciano, B., & Segura-Vargas, M. A. (2021, in press). Cognitive defusion. In M. P. Twohig, M. E. Levin, & J. M. Petersen (Eds.), *Oxford handbook of acceptance and commitment therapy*. Oxford University Press.

Shawyer, F., Farhall, J., Thomas, N., Hayes, S. C., Gallop, R., Copolov, D., & Castle, D. J. (2017). Acceptance and commitment therapy for psychosis: Randomised controlled trial. *British Journal of Psychiatry, 210*, 140–148.

Skinner, B. F. (1974). *About behaviorism*. Alfred A. Knopf.

Spidel, A., Lecomte, T., Kealy, D., & Daigneault, I. (2018). Acceptance and commitment therapy for psychosis and trauma: Improvement in psychiatric symptoms, emotion regulation, and treatment compliance following a brief group intervention. *Psychology and Psychotherapy: Theory, Research and Practice, 91*, 248–261.

Tien, A. Y. (1991). Distributions of hallucinations in the population. *Social Psychiatry and Psychiatric Epidemiology, 26*, 287–292.

Törneke, N., Luciano, C., Barnes-Holmes, Y., & Bond, F. W. (2016). RFT for clinical practice. In R. D. Zettle, S. C. Hayes, D. Barnes-Holmes, & A. Biglan (Eds.), *The Wiley handbook of contextual behavioral science* (pp. 254–272). Wiley.

Tyrberg, M. J., Carlbring, P., & Lundgren, T. (2017). Brief acceptance and commitment therapy for psychotic inpatients: A randomized controlled feasibility trial in Sweden. *Nordic Psychology, 69*, 110–125.

Vilardaga, R., Hayes, S. C., Levin, M. E., & Muto, T. (2009). Creating a strategy for progress: A contextual behavioral science approach. *The Behavior Analyst, 32*, 105–133.

Wells, A. (2002). *Emotional disorders and metacognition: Innovative cognitive therapy*. Wiley.

White, R., Gumley, A., McTaggart, J., Rattrie, L., McConville, D., Cleare, S., & Mitchell, G. (2011). A feasibility study of acceptance and commitment therapy for emotional dysfunction following psychosis. *Behaviour Research and Therapy, 49*, 901–907.

Wilson, K. G., & Luciano, C. (2002). *Terapia de aceptación y compromiso. Un tratamiento conductual orientado a los valores*. Pirámide.

Chapter 13
Acceptance and Commitment Therapy for Recovery from Psychosis

Daniel D. Simsion, Emma Caruana, and Eric M. J. Morris

13.1 Introduction

Finding purpose, meaning, and personal identity can be a long-term challenge for people who have experienced psychosis. Life can be impacted by unusual, distressing, and preoccupying experiences, along with challenges associated with negative symptoms such as amotivation and emotional flattening. The experience of attention, memory, and executive deficits may further increase difficulties in daily living. People with psychosis, their families and carers, as well as health practitioners, have identified psychological approaches as an important component of care and in supporting personal recovery. For some, it is a preferred alternative to the dominant medical paradigm where medication is the focus. Importantly, such psychologically-informed care and interventions should keep in focus the needs of the person and promote personal recovery (Leamy et al., 2011).

This chapter will outline how Acceptance and Commitment Therapy (ACT: Hayes et al., 1999, 2012) has been developed to support the personal recovery of people with psychosis. ACT is a contextual, third-wave cognitive-behavioural

D. D. Simsion (✉)
Victorian Institute of Forensic Mental Health (Forensicare), Melbourne, Australia

School of Psychology & Public Health, La Trobe University, Melbourne, Australia
e-mail: d.simsion@latrobe.edu.au

E. Caruana
School of Psychology & Public Health, La Trobe University, Melbourne, Australia
e-mail: e.caruana@latrobe.edu.au

E. M. J. Morris
School of Psychology & Public Health, La Trobe University, Melbourne, Australia

Northern Health, Melbourne, Australia
e-mail: Eric.Morris@latrobe.edu.au

J. A. Díaz-Garrido et al. (eds.), *Psychological Interventions for Psychosis*,
https://doi.org/10.1007/978-3-031-27003-1_13

therapy that presents a broad model for supporting the wellbeing, functioning, and quality of life for people across a diverse range of situations and experiences of problems. The ACT framework provides ways of understanding psychological distress, highlighting how people can respond to their life situations and inner experiences in ways that result in them becoming trapped and stuck in their suffering. It also suggests which psychological contexts may assist in helping people to find agency and purpose in responding to these circumstances, so that they break free of behavioural patterns that are unworkable. The ACT model suggests there are common processes across problems and disorders that can be attended to, to support people in making changes in their life. We will outline below how this general transdiagnostic model of psychological functioning can be extended to understanding the problems of psychosis and help inform pragmatic and effective ways of helping people pursue personal recovery.

In this chapter, we aim to provide the reader with an understanding of how ACT has been adapted for the needs of people with psychosis, including the key processes and goals of the intervention, modifications made to tailor techniques and language, and the formats that have been subject to empirical research thus far. We will outline the guiding principles of ACT for psychosis and provide several illustrations through case examples of how ACT can be used as a framework to support a person's recovery from psychosis. Finally, we will conclude with considering what are likely to be the next steps in the development of ACT as an intervention for people with psychosis.

13.2 Acceptance and Commitment Therapy

Acceptance and commitment therapy is a model of psychological therapy that seeks to change the relationship with unwanted experiences to promote increased valued action as a means of increasing quality of life and purpose. ACT has emerged from contemporary research and theory in behaviour analysis, developed as a cognitive-behavioural therapy informed by an operant learning account of language and cognition known as Relational Frame Therapy (Hayes et al., 2001). ACT emphasises skills in present moment awareness, active acceptance, mindfulness, and connection with chosen life direction (values) to help people to approach and engage with current challenges. ACT is based on the psychological flexibility model, a transdiagnostic framework that hypothesises that many challenges and problems are amplified through rigid and narrow behaviours that may serve purposes of controlling and avoiding unwanted emotions, sensations, and thoughts (experiential avoidance) or be guided unhelpfully by rules, expectations, and narratives (cognitive fusion), at the cost of responding effectively to what situations afford. The maintenance of problems through narrow and rigid behaviours performed repeatedly and seemingly less influenced by the long-term consequences is an important target of ACT, which aims to help people to make greater contact with the present moment, be open to the experiences they would usually seek to control and step back from the thoughts and stories that usually guide them, in order to connect with longer-term consequences for their behaviours (usually in the form of chosen life directions, or personal values). ACT therefore necessarily involves experiential learning, curiosity about experience, and awareness.

In ACT, the therapist encourages the client to bring a pragmatic perspective to bear in considering how their behaviour works in situations, having greater awareness of the costs of actions, both short-term and long-term, particularly in circumstances where the person's behaviour seems to serve purposes of experiential avoidance or is driven by cognitive fusion. The client is encouraged to consider whether their behaviours are resulting in them being able to act like the kind of person they would like to be, and if not, to consider what may be barriers to acting this way. Through problem-solving and reflection, the client is encouraged to consider whether active acceptance of unwanted experiences may allow for greater focus on doing things that are more aligned with their personal values. In these ways, the client is encouraged to notice their own lived experience of what works and what doesn't, judged by whether these ways of responding to situations let them act more consistently with the kind of person they would like to be.

The philosophy of science that underpins ACT, functional contextualism, provides a pragmatic perspective: what is considered true is what helps to advance a person's goals. Thus, actions, but also perspectives and narratives, can be evaluated within this framework, as to whether they help to serve the person's purposes in achieving their goals. It is not the presence of these experiences that matters. It is what the person does with them which is focused on. Rather than controlling or avoiding unwanted experiences, clients are encouraged to explore whether there is the possibility of acknowledging and reframing these as part of the experience of doing something that matters. Recasting unwanted experiences as something which is part of doing what matters is key – through making a moment be part of something, such as personal direction, there can be the possibility that different behaviours may occur, or that the client approaches the moment with curiosity, openness, and self-compassion.

ACT is an evidence-based psychological therapy. Meta-analytic reviews demonstrate that ACT is as effective as other CBTs (e.g. Ost, 2014; A-Tjak et al., 2015) and there is also a wealth of experimental, descriptive, and processes-based research providing support for the broad psychological flexibility model and the treatment components (Gloster et al., 2020). Moreover, the basic science account of language and cognition – relational frame theory – is showing empirical support and appears to be generative in terms of experimental evidence and applications (Dymond & Roche, 2013; Montoya-Rodriguez et al., 2017).

13.3 Acceptance and Commitment Therapy for People with Psychosis

ACT has been adapted to the needs of people with psychosis through both considerations of how the psychological flexibility model may account for the problems of distressing psychosis, as well as the broader influences upon development of cognitive-behavioural therapies for psychosis in understanding unusual experiences and how people respond and make sense of these. ACT for psychosis (ACTp) has been developed with an appreciation of the normalisation agenda and recovery-focused perspectives that have influenced CBTs over the last 30 years (e.g. Kingdon & Turkington, 1994; Chadwick, 2006; Garety et al., 2001). This includes acknowledging the limited utility of taking a disease/disorder perspective toward psychosis (e.g. Bentall, 1993) for the development of pragmatic psychological perspectives that can positively influence the care and support of people with psychosis.

Similar to other CBTs for psychosis, ACTp considers the person in context, seeking to understand how historical and situational factors have influenced a person's responses to their social environment, and what is important to the person in terms of their identity and goals. Unlike other CBTs which may take an information processing view of understanding a person's appraisals, emotions, and behaviour (e.g. Morrison, 2001; Garety et al., 2001), ACT is based upon a contextual perspective, where considering behaviour in context is key, from an operant learning perspective. This means that the ACTp therapist seeks to work with the client to understand what purposes their behaviours are serving and to help to find more effective ways of meeting their needs and making sense of themselves in light of their experiences.

This functional analytic perspective inherent to ACT means that the therapist is interested in understanding behaviour in context – the antecedents and the consequences, and the ways that the person is relating to their experiences. Importantly, within this framework, the experiences of psychosis themselves, along with other private experiences such as thoughts and emotions, are seen as behaviours. Thus, experiences of psychosis are therefore seen as complex behaviours that occur in contexts and have been shaped by consequences. By seeking to understand how the client makes sense of their experiences, and how this relating may also involve responses to the self that is having these experiences, there is the potential for collaborating to discover more flexible and effective ways of responding. This means that focusing on the person who is having unusual experiences and understanding what they desire, how their mind makes sense of what is happening to them, and their ways of coping with these experiences is the ideal way to be useful as an ACTp therapist.

The adaptations to the ways ACT is usually done are largely around considering the needs of people with psychosis and creating a context in interaction that may be therapeutic (experienced as psychologically safe and affirming). These considerations are related to being aware that many people with psychosis have experienced adversity and trauma and may have been subjected to controlling interventions from health-care providers. Approaching interactions in a trauma-informed way (Fallot & Harris, 2009; Mitchell et al., 2021) is essential – making it evident that the client has choice and influence over what happens in the sessions, that they will be respected, that the therapist is interested in learning about what works best for them. Some adaptations are also to consider the presence of cognitive difficulties and challenges with learning (such as if the client has memory difficulties or executive deficits). Similarly, some adaption is important to consider the impacts of being unable to pay attention in sustained ways, due to mental intrusions and preoccupying experiences, such as hallucinations.

13.4 ACT for Psychosis: Therapeutic Style

The style of how ACTp sessions are conducted therefore considers the above adaptations. We also think that there are a set of general principles that are important for the ACT therapist who is engaging people with serious mental health problems. These can be outlined in the following way: Appreciation – Connection – Addition – Construction:

1. *Appreciation*, of the person experiencing psychosis: the ACTp therapist responds to the client as a human being with a rich range of experiences and capacities, who is capable of values-based actions and compassion, and, like every person, is doing the best they can in the situations they find themselves in. The client is an equal partner in the collaboration being built in ACT sessions.
2. *Connection*, around the shared experience of being human: the ACTp therapist seeks to find ways to connect with the client around what it is like to be a human being – feeling, experiencing, caring, and being in the world trying to find meaning and purpose, just like the therapist. Where possible, the ACTp therapist highlights the common experiences of being human and is open about their own experiences and times of struggle (where this is useful to do for therapeutic ends).
3. *Addition*, of coping methods to what the person is already doing: The ACTp therapist seeks to understand how the client is actively coping with their experiences, including with unusual experiences and symptoms. The therapist seeks to understand how these ways of coping have been shaped by the person's history and opportunities, and what the person is trying to achieve when they cope in these ways. Exploration of further coping strategies is done alongside what the client is doing, as additions to the range of ways the client is coping. These coping methods are presented in the spirit of openness and curiosity, and a focus on successful living, based on personal values and goals, is kept as key throughout sessions.
4. *Construction*, of a life worth living today: The ACTp therapist seeks to acknowledge the challenges experienced and sacrifices the client may have made to do their best in coping with psychosis. Helping the client connect with their personal values may arise painful memories and feelings; there may also be challenges with connecting with past events and what the client has lost with their experience of psychosis. The ACTp therapist approaches values work with a sense of construction: conveying the perspective that the client can be supported to build things based on values in the here and now, and that this construction of the life worth living today is valuable in its own right. Values work is approached with a spirit of experimentation and curiosity, compassion, and openness. Whatever has happened before can be acknowledged while also promoting the stance that life can be lived in the here and now, and that there may be mileage in meaning being created each day, as it opens up possibilities and provides purpose.

13.5 Understanding the Challenges of Psychosis from a Psychological Flexibility Perspective

Central to understanding how to support people recovering from psychosis using ACT is considering how psychological inflexibility processes may be present when people are highly distressed, preoccupied, and/or impacted by unusual experiences and emotions. From the perspective engendered by the ACT model, it is not the presence of these experiences *per se* that is considered problematic, but rather the impact, which is amplified through psychologically inflexible ways of coping and responding. This perspective is informed by the knowledge that many people in the general community hold unusual ideas, hear voices, experience suspicion and paranoia, or have perceptions that are not shared with others, and do not require mental health treatment (Baumeister et al., 2017; Bebbington et al., 2013; Peters et al., 2016). While there may be qualitative differences between certain types of unusual experience for those who do not require care and those diagnosed with psychosis, it is also that there are differences in the ways people appraise and cope with these experiences that may be associated with distress and substantial impacts on functioning.

In ACTp, there are two ways of responding to these experiences which we are interested in. The first is cognitive fusion, that is taking the experiences and stories about them literally, using them as a guide for action. The other, potentially in an associated way to cognitive fusion, is whether these experiences are responded to with experiential avoidance. That is the person engages in strategies designed to eliminate or avoid experiencing these private events, such as when people may resist hallucinations, or become fearful and avoidant of places and people associated with persecutory beliefs. Experientially avoidant and/or cognitively fused relationships with experiences can be a focus of attention for clients, with associated worry, rumination, preoccupation, and 'tuning in' functioning as various ways to limit attention to the present moment. There can be a disconnection from personal values, if a person is preoccupied, avoiding or changing their behaviours based on unusual experiences; in a related way, there can be experiences of sense of self as different, confusing, or stigmatised that may contribute to the impact of unusual experiences.

An important consideration in the ACT approach to supporting recovery from psychosis is about the Self: how a person relates to themselves having experienced psychosis, how much capacity there is to respond with flexibility and compassion toward oneself, and fears about who one is, whether thoughts and feelings can be trusted, whether there is a sense of shame or humiliation about having been psychotic or experiencing mental health treatment for a serious mental health problem. People may internalise (be fused with) ideas of themselves as mad, unacceptable, untrustworthy, out of control, worthless, etc., due to their experience of psychosis and the treatment they have experienced. Chadwick (2006) described senses of self in the context of psychosis where a person can appraise being entrapped or engulfed by this identity: Thus, it is important in ACT for psychosis to attend to self-related processes that may be impacting the ability of the client to perspective-take about themselves and others, to find self-acceptance, or to imagine a future for themselves that involves a chosen identity (personal recovery).

A range of associated challenging emotions, moods, fears, and behaviours can make recovery from psychosis complicated. It is important for the ACTp therapist to consider the role that co-occurring depression, anxiety, trauma, substance use, and other mental health problems can play in being targets and consequences of psychological inflexibility. It is common for people with severe and enduring mental health problems to have histories of adversity and trauma that may have lasting impacts, along with associated experiences of social exclusion, discrimination, unemployment and financial problems, housing instability: These problems can be magnified for people who have a minority status(es) related to ethnicity, religion, sexuality, gender expression, and identity.

Finally, it is essential for the ACTp therapist to be sensitive to how the person with psychosis and their community makes sense of unusual experiences and behaviours, what explanations there are for these experiences, the ways people cope, and the cultural and social value of these. Frequently in Western, developed communities, the experiences associated with psychosis are stigmatised, with people who have these experiences subject to ostracism and discrimination. This stigma may mean that people are marginalised and their views subject to ridicule and invalidation. The first experiences of psychosis can occur during adolescence and young adulthood, times of developmental sensitivity, when self-identity, relationships, independence, and social roles are key tasks (Ben-David & Kealy, 2020). Periods of psychosis can disrupt developmental pathways, education and training, and social connections. Important tasks relating to personal agency and identity, valued social roles, and relationships can be disrupted by the experiences of psychosis and challenges in personal recovery.

We argue that the ACT model is consistent with frameworks for personal recovery. This is because ACT emphasises primary goals in supporting people to pursue personal meaning and purpose. The ACT model is consistent with the Connectedness, Hope, Identity, Meaning and Empowerment (CHIME) framework of personal recovery (Leamy et al., 2011), in multiple ways (Morris, 2018):

Connectedness: The pro-social approach of ACT orientates us towards connection with others, whether that be through our relationships, roles, striving to make a contribution, and/or recognising that as humans, we all struggle and suffer;

Hope: Hope is an active stance we can take towards our world: ACT promotes choices and actions focused on active engagement with life, rather than resignation or entanglement in unhelpful self-stories. The ACT approach is to acknowledge that feelings may come and go; our hopeful actions can be a way to change our world;

Identity (re-establishment of a positive identity): ACT encourages contact with self as awareness, noticing the process by which our minds create stories about ourselves. Instead of being entangled in the mind's judgements, we can observe whether these are useful for our chosen life directions. A 'flexible identity' in pursuit of values-based action is promoted, rather than self-consistency;

Meaning and purpose (finding meaning in life): Life's pain can be dignified as a part of doing the things important to us. Through acting on personal values, contact with meaning is increased;

Empowerment (encouraging self-management): In ACT we help people to be 'response-able', in other words to act on their values rather than their fear, through developing an open, compassionate stance towards their own experiences and themselves. People can be empowered by being encouraged to learn from their experiences.

ACT emphasises that wellbeing and thriving is promoted through engagement in actions that are personally meaningful. This means that these actions are personally defined, fulfilling purposes that the individual seeks in the moment. The ACT model promotes flexibility in ways of coping, in perspectives people take of themselves, in recognising that living involves contact with challenging circumstances, and finding ways to be flexible. At the heart of the ACT model is *psychological flexibility*, the capability that a person has to respond with openness to their experiences, recognise the opportunities of the current moment, and be in connection with their chosen life directions. The ACT model promotes learning from experience and does not have an implicit model of what a 'life lived well' involves, aside from promoting personal agency, connection with the social and physical environment one lives in, and how it may be advantageous to find and connect with personal sources of meaning and purpose. In these ways, the ACT model appears consistent with the notion of personal recovery.

13.6 Applying ACT: Open, Aware, and Active Skills

The ACT model can be described as a framework that helps the client and therapist to identify skills that can be strengthened, to enable greater psychological flexibility in daily life. There are various ways to talk about the organisation of these skills, from the six process Hexaflex model (see Hayes et al., 2006), to the ACT Matrix (Polk et al., 2016), to describing ACT as involving two processes – mindfulness and values-based behaviours (e.g. Flaxman et al., 2013). It can be useful to organise the skills that enable psychological flexibility in three groupings: Open, Aware, and Active.

Open

Open skills are about active acceptance and detached observation of thoughts and other experiences (cognitive defusion). With these skills the practitioner is seeking to help the client to find ways to observe their experiences from a stance of non-judgement and openness, exploring what it is like to simply be with feelings, sensations, thoughts, and other experiences. In ACTp, it is acknowledged that certain internal experiences are challenging to be open to (such as derogatory voices, paranoid thoughts, memories of trauma if they arise), and that the possibility of responding with active acceptance may be something to experiment with. The client is encouraged to notice whether a willingness to have experiences – not liking or wanting the experiences, but rather being open to them being there as part of doing things that matter, but not putting further focus or energy into them – opens up possibilities for responding and choosing actions that are more meaningful.

These skills are introduced through metaphors and experiential exercises: the client is encouraged to notice what happens with their ways of responding and coping with unwanted and preoccupying experiences when they engage in active acceptance – does this enable them to better approach doing the things that matter in life? Does this allow for new and different ways of acting and being that may be linked to the directions they want to go in their personal recovery? The Open skills can involve learning from the client how they understand their experiences and working collaboratively to find metaphors and conceptions that allow more personal agency in relation to the experiences (e.g. noticing the limits of what powerful voices can say and do to you; finding similarities between life experiences and how unusual perceptions and beliefs are responded to; trying on different perspectives and ways of acting toward experiences, such as learning to be assertive toward voices, or noticing a tendency toward jumping to conclusions and slowing down). Examples of methods of training Open skills are included in Table 13.1.

Aware

Aware skills are ways of developing present moment awareness and capacities to flexibly perspective-take, particularly around content and experiences related to the self. These skills are initially strengthened through 'noticing' exercises: brief and small practices around paying attention to the world around the client (such as with the senses) and anchoring attention by returning a focus back to an object, bodily experience, or the breath (whichever works for the client). The client is encouraged to share what they notice following these exercises, and the therapist encourages an observing and accepting perspective toward experiences. As these practices develop, the client is also encouraged to notice the changeable nature of the experiences they observe, as well as noticing a consistent observing perspective that is available through all these moments of 'noticing'. In ACT terms what may draw attention to is *self as process* and *self as observer*: This latter perspective, of I-HERE-NOW, may be cultivated as a useful anchor across changeable and sometimes intense and

Table 13.1 Examples of methods of training Open skills

Technique	Description
Leaves on a stream	Participants, through guided imagery, are encouraged to 'watch' their thoughts pass on leaves floating on a stream
Passenger on the bus	Participants are taught to see their private experiences as 'passengers' on the 'bus of life'
Think the opposite	Participants think a thought 'e.g. don't stand up' and then do the opposite action (e.g. standing up), highlighting that thoughts are just thoughts
Lemon, lemon, lemon	Participants repeat the word 'lemon' repeatedly over several minutes, examining how the indirect properties of the word become less prominent (e.g. its relationship to an actual lemon) and the direct properties become more prominent (e.g. the sound of the word)

confusing experiences – that throughout it all, noticed experientially, is a self that is consistent and unchanging because it can operate as the container of experience. This sense of self is that the observer may be illustrated with metaphors and analogies (such as the Sky and Weather metaphor; Harris, 2009) and is explored for whether this is pragmatic – does it help in terms of pursuing personal recovery, to be connected to a sense of self as an observer? Does this provide room experientially for a range of wanted and unwanted experiences, including aspects of personal history that may usually be struggled with, so that the person can have the flexibility to do the things that matter to them? Examples of methods of training Aware skills are included in Table 13.2.

Active

Active skills are about being able to construct and act upon chosen life directions (values) in ways that are flexible and allowing a person to learn from experience (committed action). The capacity to respond in different ways, doing what is most useful with what situations afford, and learning from experience is the hallmark of psychological flexibility. As can be seen in the descriptions of the Open and Aware skills above, the Active skills are woven through ACT for psychosis, with the reflection on progress toward valued directions being the pragmatic goalposts for conversations about ways of coping, skills to strengthen, and perspectives that may be useful. The ACTp therapist acknowledges the efforts the client puts into coping day-to-day and encourages them to consider their actions in the light of what matters to them over the longer-term, including the kind of person they would like to act like, based on what matters to them. This focus on personal recovery can mean that the Active skills may be about exploring different self-conceptions and narratives that help to make sense of life and allow for the opportunity of growth and meaning. Active skills here may be about learning to identify personal goals, to link them to wider valued directions, and to find pragmatic ways to pursue these goals. All of these opportunities may involve support and encouragement, particularly for clients who have not experienced much of a sense of personal agency through years of psychosis and treatment experiences that resulted in feeling entrapped, helpless, and/or lost. A common process in the Active work is about encouraging the client to notice their experiences and responses to them and to decide how they want to act

Table 13.2 Examples of methods of training Aware skills

Technique	Description
Mindfulness of orange	Take participants through guided mindfulness, focused on examining feel, smell and taste of an orange
Noticing the senses	Participants to notice five things they can see, four things they can feel, three things they can hear, two things they can smell, and one thing they can taste
Noticing in session	Participants are encouraged to notice their experiences, as they happen, during session
Mindfulness of the breath	Participants are taken through a guided mindfulness practice using the breath as an anchor

in the face of these, judging progress by whether these actions are progressing them in valued directions. Examples of methods of training Active skills are included in Table 13.3.

The Open – Aware – Active grouping allows for the practitioner and client to have a simple model to orient to as they are working together. As the ACT model applies to the practitioner as well, there are lots of opportunities for the therapist to model openness and awareness to the client, through responding in the moment during sessions, as well as sharing aspects of common humanity around suffering and efforts to act on chosen life directions (the use of self-disclosure in ACT for psychosis is discussed in a chapter in this volume by Nicholls, Newman, and Morris). We will now illustrate in the following case vignettes how ACT for psychosis can support recovery for people experiencing common challenges. These vignettes demonstrate how ACT can be applied to different presenting difficulties, as well as demonstrate how ACT can be applied flexibly based on the needs of those seeking support.

13.7 Case Example: David

David is a 42-year-old male who lives by himself and works part-time in the construction industry. David has been more distressed and preoccupied by his experience of hearing voices over the last 6 months. He describes hearing voices since he was a young person, and throughout his adult life, he has had periods where the voices have been less intrusive and manageable, and then times when the voices become nasty and controlling, louder, and more frequent.

David grew up youngest in his family; his father was a disciplinarian and held the children to high standards; there was a sense that the children should be doing well at school and getting a trade/profession as their parents had made sacrifices as immigrants. David's siblings performed well at school and enjoyed personal success, while David had a more troubled adolescence. David experienced bullying and exclusion at school due to stuttering and continues to lack confidence socially. He reports that he was given nicknames about the stuttering and found it hard to be

Table 13.3 Examples of methods of training Active skills

Technique	Description
Values card sort	Participants sort through a series of 'values cards' to identify which are most important to them
Committed actions	Through goal-setting, participants look at small steps they can take to act consistent with their values
SMART goal setting	Setting of goals that are specific, meaningful, adaptive, realistic, and time-bound
Heroes	Participants consider their heroes and the qualities they admire in those people. Discussion can then move to how participants can show these qualities

trustful of peers. David had a close relationship with his mother, who he felt was more loving and understanding about the troubles he experienced.

David enlisted in the armed forces after leaving school. His aspiration was to be in the navy; he passed through the assessment process on enlistment, however he found basic training too challenging, particularly socially – feeling he did not fit with other recruits, and found the discipline hard (including criticism, the amount of organisation required, the physical and mental demands). He left during training, believing he had let down himself and his family. After returning home David was unsure what he was going to do, and drifted for several months, spending time seeing old friends, smoking cannabis, and playing video games. He did not have a routine, playing games through the night and waking late in the day. David shared that he saw family members sporadically, as they did not share the same waking hours as he did.

David's first episode of psychosis was when he was 20 years old. He was living at home with his parents, unemployed, and spending his days playing video games and smoking cannabis. He started hearing voices and having thoughts that he was under surveillance by the government. He increasingly isolated himself to limit the surveillance; he became concerned that family members were part of what was going on. His mother shared her concerns for David with the family doctor – this led to a hospitalisation where he was diagnosed with schizophrenia and prescribed medication.

David has a few friends and contact with his siblings, a brother and sister. His parents are retired, quite elderly, and are cared for by the other siblings. David lives by himself, working intermittently as a manual labourer. On construction sites he is known as a quiet and good worker, but there can be times when he needs to take a break from being around other people. The foreman of the construction crew he works for is sensitive to this and can chat with David about when he needs to take a break.

David holds persisting persecutory beliefs of being targeted by government agencies for mind control experiments, designed to see what psychological punishment person can take before they lose control (by killing themselves). David believes that agents for the government are using high-tech devices to send signals to his mind (this is the source of the voices he hears) and that he is under regular surveillance. He believes he is an innocent person targeted as the government had records from his brief military service.

David has experienced several hospital admissions at times when more 'tortured' by the voices – believing that the voices are punishing him for shameful past actions. He can present feeling quite guilty, worried about punishment, disclosing that the voices remind him of regretful actions (nothing illegal or harmful to others). At these times, the voices give him commands to harm himself, which he resists by trying to appease them by denying himself pleasurable activities and seeking amends for his perceived misdeeds. Most of the time David is not so preoccupied by the voices. In these times, they occur with limited frequency, do not lead him to worry, and are not a source of persisting distress. He reports this is because the voices are different in quality to the distressing times, whispering rather than shouting, certain voices are not present (the torturers), and the content of the voices is less accusatory and condemning. David does not drink, but occasionally smokes cannabis recreationally – there is no other substance use.

13.7.1 Applying ACT to David

David participated in ACTp on the recommendation of his case manager. He reported a period of increasing worry and preoccupation, and the return of 'torturing voices', which had discouraged him from going to work and socialising. David reported that he had been taking medication as prescribed and had stopped his occasional use of cannabis. He expressed hope that he was not becoming unwell, but reported being fearful of what may happen next, including the possibility of ultimately ended up doing something he does not want to do (i.e., harm himself).

David had not previously been offered psychological therapy. In the first meeting the therapist met with him and the case manager, to discuss how the sessions would run, and what to expect. The therapist described being interested in understanding what mattered to David and how the voices and other experiences were acting as barriers to him living life the way he wanted to. David reported that he was unsure about what mattered, aside from not feeling so criticised and ashamed by what the voices were saying. He also reported that his focus right now was trying to ignore the voices when he can, and when he can't, trying to cope without getting too depressed.

The beginning sessions of ACTp were about the therapist getting to know how David coped with his voices, his fears and concerns, and the ways these experiences got in the way of him working and socialising. The therapist worked flexibly with David – there were sessions where David had trouble attending, due to how powerful the voices seemed or his suspicions about how others would act toward him as he travelled to the clinic. The therapist responded in an understanding manner and encouraged David to attend even if he found these experiences challenging.

Experiential Avoidance

David described coping with voices and worries by trying to block them by listening to music on his phone, although he found he could only listen to music without lyrics, as the torturing voices would include critical messages in the songs. David also coped when the voices were particularly critical by writing in a notebook, where he would write about pleasant memories and situations where he had felt that he had done things he was proud of. He stated that as he became more depressed, it was harder to feel positive about past events, or feel he was an acceptable person. David also reported that working helped him to cope by engaging in physical labour he had things to concentrate on and felt tired at the end of a day. This would help him to go to sleep earlier, and therefore having less time with hearing negative voices.

When David was having a 'bad day' he coped by staying in bed, trying to sleep through the day, with not much energy or enthusiasm to do things. When he did get up in the afternoon, David tended to then spend time listening to music, do some reading, or writing in his notebook.

Cognitive Fusion

David admitted living his life 'on hold', hoping that over the years the experiments and surveillance would stop, but this had never occurred. He did report periods of time when he had been less worried about this, times when he had been working more, having more of social life, but then something always happened to remind him that the experiment was still happening. This could be a random remark from a workmate or an acquaintance, or an occasion where David had felt that his tools or apartment had been disturbed, or just a sense that something was not right. David reflected that when his happened, he responded by withdrawing from others and worrying about what could happen next. He stated that he would also sleep less, spending more time checking around his apartment, and when he travelled outside, he would do things to ensure he was not being followed or having his belongings disturbed. David reported finding it hard to be present with doing things that matter, because part of his mind focused on scanning for threats. He shared how tiring it was with vigilance about harm from others.

Workability

The therapist engaged David in a review of how he was spending his time and sought to understand the various ways that he coped with the voices, the things he did to keep busy and feel better, and the times when he felt that he did not have the energy to do things for himself. The therapist asked David to reflect on the times when he really felt alive, when things were meaningful and important, when he felt that he was doing what matters. David appeared to struggle with this, stating that he did not have very much to be proud of, and that he was regretful about how the life's opportunities had passed him by. It was like he was living in limbo, hoping for the day when the surveillance and experiments would stop, so that he could live more freely to do what matters. There was a strong sense that living this way was unworkable, with David reflecting on the costs of vigilance to surveillance.

Function

The ACTp therapist formulated that, along with the patterns of *experiential avoidance* that David displays, there is a strong level of *coherence* to the beliefs of being the target of experimentation and surveillance, and with being a victim to powerful sources (such as the government agencies sending signals to his mind causing voices). The persecutory beliefs David holds and acts upon appear consistent with his experiences of unwanted attention and powerlessness he first experienced as a child (with bullying and family expectations) that have influenced how he tends to perceive himself in relation to others as an adult (as being weaker, a target of humiliation and shame: Iqbal et al., 2000; similarly finding voices to be omnipotent: Morris et al., 2014). David has *limited contact with personal sources of meaning and purpose*, due to the patterns of focusing his attention on avoiding and controlling threats, lack of closeness to others, and feeling that he needs to stay vigilant about losing control of his behaviour (an inaccurate rule he feels he needs to live by:

e.g. Torneke et al., 2008). It was planned to share this formulation with David and develop it further, to make sense of his experiences and guide how ACTp may help.

13.7.2 Intervention

Aware

The therapist carefully introduced David to present moment awareness skills, through first practicing this toward objects around him, then bodily sensations, and then finally to internal experiences including thoughts, memories, emotions, and the voices. Throughout these practices, David was encouraged to notice his experiences and the things that his mind was doing with these, and to do this as an observer of his experiences. This was challenging at times, and David would sometimes feel overwhelmed by the number and intensity of the experiences he was noticing. At these times, the therapist encouraged him to centre his attention on how he was sitting or standing, feeling the ground beneath his feet or the arms of the chair, so that David had a consistent 'place' to watch his experiences from. It was also important to offer these practices from a position of choice, the therapist emphasising to David that he could choose to disengage from a practice when he wanted to, and that the focus was just about 'noticing', rather than achieving any particular goal. David did stop practices several times in the early sessions: he was encouraged to share the experiences he was having, and the ways that he was responding to these. David was also encouraged to use these skills of noticing at other times, outside of the therapy sessions, to practice this way of relating to inner experiences. After practice over sessions David did report some occasions of 'more noticing' in day-to-day life: when going for a walk and noticing changes in a local park with the plants; when eating his favourite meal; when he was anticipating that the voices would comment on memories he was having (and noticing that what was said by the voices was not too upsetting).

The therapist worked with David to develop a shared formulation: it was important to validate David's feelings about what he believed was happening with the experimentation. The therapist indicated that these urges to be vigilant was understandable if you were concerned about the harm that could occur if you did not stay on guard. The therapist asked about what it was like in the short-term – seeking examples of times when David had needed to be vigilant – looking for any clues to confirm that active surveillance was occurring, such as hidden cameras and microphones in his flat. It was important for the therapist to understand the feelings, thoughts, and urges David experienced during these times. David also seemed concerned about whether the therapist believed him about these instances; there were occasions where the therapist and David 'agreed to disagree'. At these times, David reported disappointment that the therapist could not see things the way he did, although did say it was hard for people to understand if they had not been targets of surveillance too.

The therapist also invited David to reflect on what it has been like long-term to live with these suspicions. David stated that it was exhausting, that he felt angry about his life being disrupted, that it was unfair that he needed to stay alert to the experimentation. When asked, David indicated that he could not be sure whether surveillance was happening, especially when the voices were less punishing. He conceded there may have been occasions when he was mistaken, perhaps he had been too suspicious – however, acting as though things are OK felt too risky for David: he did not want to be fooled.

Active

The therapist also supported David to explore his chosen life directions (his values). This work focused on how David would like to act in different parts of his life: when he is spending time in his flat by himself, when he is working, when he is socialising with family members and friends, when he is out in his local community. In suggesting these areas of David's life, the therapist presented the idea that values are ways of finding meaning and purpose, even (or especially) when life has been challenging. This was contrasted with the meaning that life appeared to offer David otherwise – to just survive, to live as small as possible, to be vigilant but also limit commitment to others or the things that matter. The therapist asked David to consider whether this would be what he would choose life to be about, if he had a free choice: David said this definitely would not be the life he would choose and he did not feel he had much choice. He stated the pain of caring about things for them to be messed with or taken away seemed too much to bear.

The therapist engaged David in an exercise about remembering a moment in his life filled with meaning – the Sweet Spot exercise (Wilson, 2009) – providing several examples of these types of memories (doing something kind for another person; memories of being loved and cared for; a memory of appreciating something, a place, or a person, and being connected to your body). David shared a memory from his youth: spending time with his grandfather, collecting fruit in the orchard, and preparing a fruit salad for his family; what it had been like to just share time with his grandfather, listening to his stories. David described a particular memory – being on the veranda helping his grandfather to prepare the salad – what it was like to be preparing the food and the sunlight on the veranda. The therapist asked David to stay within this image and to connect with what was happening in his body, to connect again with what it was like to be there then. When asked what this moment meant David stated feeling close to his grandfather, that they had made something together for the family, that he enjoyed doing something useful. The therapist asked him what about the situation could be a purpose to guide his actions today. David said that while he was not close to others like he was with his grandfather, he did find something important in doing work that others relied upon. He stated that this is what made working important for him: many days he could see his labour made a difference, as he worked in a team of people constructing things. He reported that when he could not work due to mental health problems, this was something he missed. The therapist suggested that they note these reflections about what mattered and suggested to David there may be ways of heading in these directions, possibly even on days when it was hard to go to work.

Open

The painful work of connecting David more with what he cared about was done carefully through present moment awareness exercises and checking with him about experiences of doing this. Through engaging in exercises over sessions, and the therapist encouraging him to practice openness and curiosity to his emotions and mental experiences (through exercises like the Leaves on a Stream and metaphors like the Tug of War with the Monster), David appeared to be more actively accepting of a variety of feelings, including those arising when he felt suspicious or worried about the voices.

The therapist shared a perspective to develop the shared formulation – that due to David's unfortunate experiences as a young person with peers, he had learnt how being the focus of attention was hurtful, leading a person to feel rejected and ashamed. Could these powerful experiences when he was younger have become lessons learned about how life works, that he still lives by? David reflected on this, sharing with the therapist about the best ways to survive surveillance, voices and unknown others messing with you, through vigilance and avoidance. The therapist invited David to consider what the younger version of him would have wanted during these periods of being teased and rejected by peers – David stated that he would have wanted someone to be looking out for him, to protect him from the bullies, to have friends. Instead, he had to just cope by himself. The therapist validated that David had done the best that he could do in the situation.

Within the formulation, the therapist described the idea that thoughts and feelings can become familiar and frequent, so that new experiences are seen from this lens too. From this perspective, it is easier to continue to see the world as dangerous, to live with the rule 'it is better to be safe than sorry' through being vigilance, and that taking a chance to trust others becomes too risky to do. This idea of being a 'very familiar' story and one that keeps David 'playing it safe' was discussed over several sessions, with the therapist encouraging David to also notice it as a set of experiences that arise in his body and mind through his present moment skills.

A metaphor was offered – that David's concerns of surveillance and experimentation and the ways he had learned to live with these fears were like being caught in a spider's web, being entangled so that he felt he did not have much opportunity to move, and also that whatever he did would set off vibrations through the web, drawing attention to himself. It was like life needed to be lived with as little vibration as possible, for fear of something worse happening to him. Life's purpose had become to live as quietly as possible, to not stir up trouble, rather than it being about what he would *like* for his life to be about. It was sticky and strong, when he was caught up in a web of suspicion and worry. David stated that life was like being trapped, afraid of drawing more attention to himself, for fear of what would come... Interestingly, David said he had never seen who created the web (the spider?), with all these years of being worried of being stuck and worse things happening. The therapist reflected with David about whether this was the power of the web: making him fearful of things worse than being stuck (even if these things had not happened).

Steadily, David and the therapist worked on ways for him to find connection with his chosen life directions, even when he would experience upsetting voices and paranoid thoughts. David found that by being able to become more present he felt less panicky and anxious to seek safety, and more able to check things out, holding his suspicions a little more lightly. He also discovered that he was able to do more than 'play it safe' – by connecting more with his workmates and family members – particularly by doing things that linked to his values of contributing, making things, and acts of kindness. By practicing being present with these valued actions, David also reported that even if the experiment was happening, he was able to work to make the world a better place, which mattered most to him.

13.8 Case Example: Tom

Tom is a 23-year-old male. He was born into a high-achieving family, the eldest of three boys. His mother is a lawyer, and his father is a doctor. From an early age, there were high expectations that Tom would be as high achieving as his parents. When Tom met these high expectations, he was the centre of attention in his family and rewarded with praise, increased attention, and gifts. In contrast, when Tom did not meet these expectations, he was berated by his parents and compared unfavourably to his brothers. Tom's father did not show emotion or obvious signs of affection in front of the children, with most interactions focused on Tom's academic and sporting achievements. When Tom's father was angry, or intoxicated, he would often use violence against the children as a form of punishment. In contrast, Tom's mother's parenting style was varied, alternating between not engaging in any emotional expression and engaging in large amounts of emotional expression and praise.

Tom was generally a successful and popular child throughout his schooling, achieving high grades across most subjects. Tom was also successful in sports, becoming a skilled cricket player. However, despite these successes, Tom's parents continued to push him to achieve more. During high school, Tom began to experience high levels of anxiety, particularly around examinations, tests and sporting matches, with ongoing fears that he would perform poorly. Towards the end of his schooling, Tom commenced attending parties, increasingly consuming large amounts of alcohol at these events. Despite this, he achieved grades which were sufficiently high to enter a pre-medicine course at a prestigious university.

Tom's transition to university was characterized by a 'work hard, play hard' approach. This would involve significant periods of intense study (including 'all nighters'), broken up by period of intense 'partying', including recreational drug use, particularly marijuana, and binge drinking of alcohol. Following successful completion of the pre-medicine course, Tom then commenced studying medicine in a postgraduate course at age 22.

During his first year of studying medicine, Tom found the academic stress increasingly difficult to manage. This resulted in increased periods of intense, last-minute, studying, combined with increased alcohol and drug use during 'down times'. Increasingly, Tom's substance use would occur when alone, rather than with others. During this period, Tom started to develop a series of beliefs about being on a special mission to revolutionise the practice of medicine. At the same time, Tom began hearing a single male voice. This voice was initially very 'positive', encouraging Tom in his special mission. At this time, Tom managed these experiences by ignoring them when possible and by hiding them from those in his life.

As the first year of medicine progressed, Tom became increasingly stressed, relying more on periods of extreme studying, combined with alcohol and other drugs, to manage this. This resulted in him failing his second semester. Following this, Tom became increasingly pre-occupied with his mission to change the practice of medicine in the world and he begun devoting much of his time to this. He began speaking to his family about his special purpose and ceased his studies to focus exclusively on his mission. When his family expressed concern, he was largely dismissive of their worries. Initially, his family attempted to manage this without support, before eventually contacting the mental health crisis team who involuntarily admitted Tom to the local public mental health unit.

During this admission, Tom was prescribed Olanzapine. This helped in reducing the intensity of his pre-occupation with his voice and his beliefs; however, both remained. He also developed increasing depressive symptoms, including low mood and amotivation. The voice became increasingly 'negative', consistently pointing out how much of a failure Tom was. Once discharged from hospital, Tom became increasingly isolated, often ruminating about his behaviour while 'unwell' as well as his perceived failures. He managed this by attempting to ignore these experiences, by using drugs and alcohol and becoming increasing immersed in obscure theories of medicine. The voice started to initially make statements such as 'you're not worth having around' before graduating to commands to suicide. Several weeks after his discharge from hospital, Tom acted on these commands through taking a large number of paracetamol tablets with intent to suicide.

13.8.1 Applying ACT to Tom

Following his suicide attempt, Tom was referred to an ACTp therapist to provide increased support and for 'improved coping skills'. Initially, Tom was hesitant to engage in psychological intervention, making clear that 'there is nothing wrong with me', however agreed to 'give it a go'. With a focus on building collaboration, the ACTp therapist spent the initial part of the intervention working with Tom to gain a shared understanding of his current circumstances. From an ACT perspective, the therapist was particularly interested in exploring the role of two key contexts: experiential avoidance and cognitive fusion. There was also a focus on working with Tom to gain an understanding of the function of his behaviours and his experiences, and examining whether what he was doing was contributing him towards living a 'life worth living', as seen from Tom's own perspective. Given the role of suicidal behaviour in Tom's presentation, and the potential risk to life, the ACTp therapist was particularly attentive to understanding drivers of this behaviour in the early stages of treatment.

Experiential Avoidance

Tom's behaviours are indicative of the potential presence of multiple instances where experiential avoidance is contributing directly to his difficulties. During the initial phases of the ACTp intervention, Tom worked with the therapist to identify the range of experiences which he actively worked to avoid. This included his experiences of anxiety, thoughts of being a failure, his experiences of low mood, and the negative content of his voice.

Tom was also able to identify that he employs a range of strategies with the purpose of reducing the amount of contact he has with these unwanted private events. This includes the use of drugs and alcohol, which he noted had the effect of 'numbing out' his unwanted internal experiences. Tom also identified his attempts to 'ignore' his unwanted private events, particularly thoughts and voices, by focussing on other activities, such as intense studying, as having the goal of avoiding unwanted private events. Tom also noted using his encouraging voice as a tool to avoid unwanted experiences, ignoring the latter by focusing as much as possible on the former. Finally, as the intervention progressed further, Tom formulated his suicidal behaviour (discussed in more detail below) as also serving the function of helping him to escape his unwanted experiences.

The ACTp therapist was also be interested in the broader context for the development of Tom's experiential avoidance and helped Tom to explore this in the early stages of engagement. This included the history of this approach being reinforced during his early years, with Tom encouraged by his parents to present outwardly as successful and happy, regardless of his internal experience, with rewards (e.g. praise) associated with this. Tom also observed this behaviour growing up, both in terms of his father and, on occasions, his mother.

Cognitive Fusion

There is also a key role of cognitive fusion in Tom's presenting difficulties. Tom presented to the ACTp therapist with fusion with a series of cognitions and beliefs, including around beliefs of being a failure and beliefs around having a special purpose to change the practice of medicine. In the early stages of engagement, the ACTp therapist focused on supporting Tom to simply identify this process: Acknowledging that, at times, he sees these as the literal truth and acknowledges the associated behaviours, and this leads him to engage in (e.g. becoming pre-occupied with obscure theories of medicine and spending most of his time researching this).

Workability

When looking at the contexts of cognitive fusion and experiential avoidance, the ACTp therapist and Tom focused on the workability of these behaviours. This included an examination of whether these contexts are contributing to him moving towards the life he wants to live. For Tom, there is evidence that both experiential avoidance and cognitive fusion are contributing to significant relief from his unwanted private experience in the short-term, but are leading to significant difficulties in the long-term. Through these early discussions, the ACTp therapist was able to identify that there is evidence that these contexts are directly contributing to suffering and preventing Tom from living a rich and meaningful life, and thus were important to consider for formulation and intervention purposes.

Function

This vignette highlights the important role of understanding function when building an understanding of behaviours, including Tom's presenting 'symptoms'. Tom presents with some private experiences which he may experience as desirable and some which he may experience as aversive. Thus, they are likely maintained by different consequences. In both cases, it was important for the ACTp therapist to build an understanding of these behaviours through the lens of function and support Tom to also develop this understanding to assist him in making more overt choices about how he responds to different situations.

In terms of private events which he may experience as desirable, Tom presents with a preoccupation with beliefs associated with changing the world (these could sometimes be termed 'grandiose delusions') and a voice which sometimes delivers content consistent with these beliefs. The ACTp therapist, in their initial sessions, worked with Tom to build an understanding of these in terms of the function they served for Tom. With exploration, and examining his history of learning that failure is considered unacceptable, the therapist and Tom formulated these behaviours as being an escape mechanism from feelings of failure associated with the difficulties he was experiencing in his medical studies. That is to say, these experiences were maintained by helping Tom to avoid feeling like a 'failure', as well as by the associated positive feelings associated with having a 'special purpose'.

Tom also experiences private events associated with psychosis that he likely experiences as aversive (i.e., as unwanted). Notably, he at times experiences a voice which provides him with negative feedback and encourages him to withdraw from his friends and family. The ACTp therapist worked with Tom to explore this, understanding it within the context of the approach used by his parents to encourage him (i.e., berating him with a view to encouraging him to do better). Tom initially identified the voice as serving to motivate him. However, with exploration he was also able to identify a protective function of the voice, noting that it stopped him from taking risks which may lead him to engage in further failure. Tom was able to also see similar thoughts as serving similar functions as this voice.

In the early stages of engagement, the ACTp therapist also worked with Tom to build an understanding of his suicidal behaviour through the lens of function, building on the understanding as discussed under 'experiential avoidance'. The ACTp therapist and Tom were able to identify that he had been feeling unable to cope with the feelings associated with failure (named as 'shame' and 'embarrassment'). Thus, the suicidal behaviour had been driven by a last-ditch effort to escape these painful experiences. He was able to identify that this behaviour was also reinforced by an admission to the local mental health inpatient unit where he was able to 'take a break' from the challenges he was experiencing. Given the dangers associated with this behaviour, the ACTp therapist worked to build a more comprehensive understanding of the multiple drivers of this behaviour early on in the intervention to ensure Tom was empowered to identify and manage scenarios where he is at increased risk, while the therapist was also able to spot these and intervene as needed. Drivers of this behaviour included increases in 'negative' psychotic experiences (which were subject to their own functional analysis) as well a reduction in the positive experiences (e.g. the 'grandiose delusions'), associated with the use of medication. In Tom's case, there was also an important role of increased 'insight' in contributing to his recent suicidal behaviour (i.e., the medication led him to a reduction in 'protective' psychotic experiences, increasing his suicidality).

13.8.2 Intervention

Based on the above considerations of experiential avoidance, cognitive fusion, workability, and function, the ACTp therapist worked with Tom to build a comprehensive understanding of his behaviours in terms of the key ACT processes of open, aware, and active. This understanding was then used to jointly develop a plan for intervention. Initially, following gaining an understanding of Tom's behaviours, he was introduced to the Passengers on the Bus metaphor which was used to introduce key concepts and help with the development of a shared language between the Tom and therapist (e.g. private experiences came to be called 'passengers' during session). In short, this metaphor describes our private experiences as 'passengers' on our bus our life, which we are trying to drive towards where we want to go ('valued direction'). Different response styles to the passengers are shown to be unhelpful (e.g. arguing with them, listening to them) or helpful (e.g. acceptance). This also provided an introduction to Tom of each of open, aware, and active.

Active

Tom's history indicates a significant focus on pleasing others and achieving, because this is seen as something which 'must' be done. Upon exploration, there was little evidence that Tom was gaining internal satisfaction from his studies nor attending parties, but rather was doing these things because he felt they were 'what you have to do' to live a good life.

Given this, in combination with Tom's hesitancy to engage in intervention, the early work focused on building Tom's own sense of what his values were. In the initial stages of this intervention, Tom struggled to speak about his own values, linking them directly to his sense of failure and the associated pain. Thus, this work commenced by adding a layer of separation between Tom and values. This was done through exploration of Tom's heroes and what he admired about them. He identified a doctor, a family friend, who worked with Médecins Sans Frontières ('Doctors without Borders'), whom he had looked up to since adolescence. The ACTp therapist worked with Tom to identify exactly what he admired about this doctor through looking at specific behaviours he engaged in, with Tom identifying his compassion, persistence, and skill as being the key attributes he admired.

This then helped inform a discussion of how Tom could embody these behaviours in his own actions. While Tom initially identified larger goals (e.g. himself becoming a doctor and travelling to Africa to work), with support from the ACTp therapist, he was able to break this down into much smaller 'committed actions' which he could engage in to live these values. Tom's initial focus was on wanting to set goals which others saw and admired, rather than linking them to his values. Thus, the intervention also had a particular focus on building Tom's own sense of achievement and satisfaction from completing these goals. This included engaging in committed actions which were not witnessed by others in his life and then exploring these in detail during session (framed as an 'experiment' initially). Examples of early goals included making a small donation to a charity, reading an article on a new technology in medicine, and emailing his course co-ordinator to look at options for recommencing his studies with a reduced load.

Over time, and while working on the other ACT processes (open and aware, below), Tom was able to build on these initial committed actions, taking on more and more challenging goals, using his values as the compass to choose these. Unsurprisingly, while completing this work, Tom experienced a range of unwanted private experiences (including voices, emotions, and thoughts) which were addressed through focusing directly on the 'open' process of ACT.

Open

Tom presented with a range of strategies specifically focused on avoiding his unwanted private experiences (as discussed under 'experiential avoidance' and 'function', above). The initial parts of the intervention around 'open' with Tom involved exploring the benefits and costs of his efforts to avoid his unwanted private experiences (sometimes referred to as 'creative hopelessness' in ACT). This involved the ACTp therapist and Tom exploring three key questions: First, there was an examination he had already done to manage the unwanted private experiences (i.e. clearly identifying all the avoidance strategies being employed). Second, Tom and the ACTp therapist explored whether these strategies had actually worked, given how much effort was being committed to them. Tom identified that these strategies were highly effective in the short-term in that they provided temporary relief from his unwanted private experiences. However, he was also able to identify, from his own experience, that these strategies had been highly ineffective in the long-term, identifying that these behaviours ultimately served to make his difficulties worse. Finally, Tom was asked to consider the 'cost' of engaging in these strategies. Tom identified that these strategies had cost him 'almost everything'. Through the Passengers on the Bus metaphor, Tom was introduced to an alternative to his attempts to control, openness (termed 'willingness' in this intervention).

Open interventions targeted a range of Tom's experiences. Early on in the intervention, there was a focus on the voices and Tom's thoughts. Tom initially focused on identification of his unwanted private experiences, through simply naming them as 'passengers'. During sessions, the ACTp therapist would help Tom to identify his 'passengers in' the moment (e.g. 'I just noticed a shift in your facial expression. Has a passenger just shown up?'). Additionally, when reviewing each week during a session, Tom was asked to consider in given scenarios: who was driving the bus? That is, Tom explored times when he let his 'passengers' guide his behaviour and times he made a true choice, despite the presence of an unwanted 'passengers'. Over time, as patterns were identified in the 'passengers', Tom was able to name certain 'passengers' to more easily spot them. This included the 'suicide passenger' (i.e. auditory hallucination and thoughts telling Tom to die) and the 'fantasy passenger' (i.e. auditory hallucinations and thoughts which told Tom how amazing he was, about his special mission, etc.). Over time, Tom was able to more and more readily identify these passengers as a part of his whole experience, rather than as the absolute truth. This substantially lessened the impact of the experiences on Tom and allowed him to make more deliberate choices in the face of these experiences. Rather than choosing avoidance strategies, he was able to increasingly engage in active values-based actions, moving towards where he wished to go rather than away from things he was trying to escape. As Tom became more familiar with his frequent 'passengers', he was also able to also better understand them in terms of their function and see them within a context of his 'mind' working to attempt to help him. This increased his ability to respond openly to the experiences.

Tom also did similar work around his unwanted emotional experiences. This included considering them within the passengers on the bus metaphor, learning to name them in the moment (e.g. 'the shame passenger'), and learning to understand them in terms of function and purpose.

Finally, during this part of the intervention, the ACTp therapist worked with Tom to explore his strongly held beliefs (e.g. around having a 'special purpose' in the field of medicine). As with other cognitive-behavioural therapies, the ACTp intervention did not focus on the 'truth' of these beliefs, but rather on their workability. The ACTp therapist and Tom explored the benefits and costs of focusing on these beliefs. As the intervention progressed, Tom was also encouraged to see these beliefs within the broader range of his experience and in terms of their function (i.e. in this case, Tom identified that focusing on these beliefs helped avoid the emotion pain associated with not achieving as highly as he wished to). As the intervention progressed, and Tom began to build up values-based actions in other areas, his focus on these beliefs reduced significantly as they became a less central part of his experience and thus were given less and less attention.

Aware

Finally, the ACTp therapist worked with Tom to build his aware skills. As with all ACT interventions, there was overlap with the other processes in this section, and these skills were focused on in a non-linear fashion. That is to say, sessions jumped between focus on all three processes. One rationale for focusing on aware skills which was particularly important for Tom was improving his ability to track his own behaviour. That is, being more aware of the triggers for his behaviours (including his private experiences) and understanding their function, to allow him to make more active choices in any given moment.

For Tom, who remained passionate about engaging in physical activity, awareness was initially taught through focusing on paying attention to physical movement. During sessions, the ACTp therapist and Tom would engage in physical activities (stretching, jogging on the spot), but with specific instructions to pay attention to specific parts of the activity (e.g. focusing on the change in breath while jogging, focusing on the feet, noticing the feelings associated with a stretch). As Tom became more comfortable with these interventions, he decided to commence more formal 'meditation' practice using an 'app' on his phone between sessions, initially every other day before commencing daily practice.

Sessions also often involved 'check-ins' in any given moment, in which Tom would be encouraged to pay attention and notice what was happening in specific moments (including both private experiences and in the room). As the intervention progressed, Tom was able to increasingly engage in these 'check-ins' effectively, regardless of his emotional/mental state. This increased his ability to identify and allow private experiences (i.e. his open skills) and make choices to act on his values (i.e. his active skills).

Some aspects of Tom's presentation required some special consideration as they did not relate directly to psychosis specifically, but remained important part of the intervention.

Anxiety, Depression, and Substance Use

In addition to experiences directly linked to his psychosis, Tom presented with other difficulties including those associated with anxiety, depression, and alcohol and other drug use. These were important considerations when discussing an intervention plan with Tom and their relative importance determined by the impact they were having on Tom's ability to live a valued life. In this case, the substance use was seen as particularly important for Tom and thus a particular focus. However, as has been noted, while these behaviours were important to consider, they were considered within the same model (i.e., that of psychological flexibility and ACT) and were treated using the same 3 processes. Thus, while the intervention considered these important 'co-morbidities', the treatment itself did not need to be modified, except to incorporate these within the range of behaviours being examined.

Risk

Tom presented to the ACTp sessions following a recent suicide attempt. Given the risk to life of such behaviour, this was also an important part of the intervention, again considered within the framework of psychological flexibility and ACT. In the early stages of therapy with Tom, the ACTp therapist worked with Tom to build his ability to understand what had occurred and what had led to the attempt (i.e. using his aware skills) and built his ability to have the associated internal experiences without resorting to escape strategies such as suicide (i.e. using his open skills). This was then paired with a plan of what to do in the event of another crisis, built around his values, including seeking support and engaging in other activities he identified as helpful, such as exercise (i.e. using his active skills).

Medication
This vignette also highlighted the importance of the ACTp therapist understanding the function of behaviours, within the broader context of antipsychotic medication. Tom's suicide attempt occurred following the prescription of medication which had helped to ameliorate experiences that Tom had found desirable, and subsequently left him unable to cope with the resulting negative emotions. That is to say, the psychotic experiences had been serving a protective function for Tom in that they were helping him to avoid unwanted experiences that he was unable to otherwise cope with. Thus, the ACTp therapist worked closely with the medication prescriber to ensure that any changes/increases to medication were considered within this context.

13.9 Case Example: Maya

Maya is a 17-year-old non-binary young person (they/them pronouns), who lives with their mother Stacey and her new partner Chris, Maya's older brother Jaxon, and younger sister Zara. Maya recently dropped out of school, and they are currently single. Maya recently experienced a first-episode of psychosis.

Maya had experienced a gradual deterioration in mental state and functioning over the previous 18 months. Maya recently dropped out of year 11 at school, after having increasing difficulty with attendance and workload, and started to fail subjects. Prior to this, they enjoyed school, with particular strengths in creative arts and literature. Maya had worked hard to get good grades and took part in extra-curricular activities including drawing and writing classes.

Maya was a quiet, shy person, and had been bullied and excluded in primary school. As Maya entered high school, they discovered their interest in art and creativity, and through this connected with a small, though reliable, group of friends. Over the past 18 months Maya started to withdraw from these friends, in part as attendance at school and extra-curricular activities reduced. Maya also developed some worries that these friends didn't like them and believed they were excluding them from things and talking about them behind their back.

Maya had previously been in a 1-year relationship with Jorden, who Maya had met at art class, and were in the same friendship group. Maya reluctantly ended this relationship 6 months ago, after being sexually assaulted by Jorden. Maya was conflicted about the assault, and in part felt they 'asked for it'. Maya also felt the other people in the friendship group did not believe them, and lost these friends when the relationship ended.

Maya's parents separated when they were in primary school, due to physical and emotional abuse perpetrated by Maya's father, towards their mother Stacey. Maya's father was sexually abusive towards Maya and their younger sister Zara. Maya's mother found out about the sexual abuse towards Zara, and it was at this point that the separation occurred. Soon after separating, Stacey repartnered with Chris. Over the years, he has been staying more often at Maya's house, and Chris recently moved into the family home. Maya has become increasingly suspicious of Chris and worries he is trying to hurt them and Zara.

Maya was recently admitted to hospital after experiencing a first-episode of psychosis, and anorexia nervosa. As part of their experience of psychosis, Maya hears intense and distressing voices. There are three distinct voices – one providing neutral commentary and two with negative and demeaning content. The negative voices included themes of Maya being worthless and deserving punishment. They would also tell Maya that other people, particularly family and friends, disliked them and were trying to hurt them. Maya was experiencing episodes of dissociation, described as periods of feeling detached and disconnected from their body, at times in conjunction with flashbacks from past trauma. Maya's mother noted times when she would check on Maya, and Maya would not respond for several minutes. Often Maya would try and cope with distress and dissociation by withdrawing and self-harming, and this was increasing in the lead up to the hospital admission.

Several factors contributed to Maya's experience of dissociation: hearing distressing voices, gender dysphoria, and body image concerns. When Maya experienced loud and intense voices, commonly at times of heightened stress, dissociation would serve the function of 'switching off' the voices, blocking them out, as well as everything else in the external world. Maya experienced gender dysphoria, identifying as non-binary, and being distressed by primary and secondary sexual characteristics of their birth-assigned gender. Often Maya would become highly distressed when looking in the mirror as they did not identify with their reflection, and their body did not feel like their own. Additionally, as part of their experience of anorexia nervosa, Maya had body image concerns, believed they were overweight, and were preoccupied with losing weight. They also believed they did not deserve to eat and needed to be punished. Maya engaged in restricting food intake and purging behaviour to lose weight. Maya had lost a significant amount of weight due to their anorexia, and at the time of admission was medically compromised due to their low body mass index (BMI).

After a 3-week inpatient stay, Maya has been referred for ongoing outreach community support.

13.9.1 Applying ACT with Maya

Maya was reluctant to continue on medication commenced in hospital, due to suspiciousness about the medication, as well as significant distress associated with weight gain. Maya raised this with treating team, and together they developed a plan for Maya to stop medication, and for treatment to focus on engagement in ACT.

Maya and the therapist met to discuss what therapy may look like, and what Maya's goals for therapy were. Maya identified their main struggles were with ongoing voices, episodes of dissociation, and self-harming. They reported experiencing low mood, amotivation, poor sleep, and low self-esteem. Maya spent their days mostly in their bedroom watching movies and television, and sleeping. Maya also has two people they would connect with online, one who was also seeking professional mental health support, as well as a childhood friend. Maya was also continuing to restrict food intake and purge, and had ongoing body images concerns, which had been exacerbated by weight gain from antipsychotic medication. Maya was ambivalent about addressing disordered eating, though was open to discussing this further as they were aware they would need to return to hospital if their weight dropped and they became physically compromised and wanted to avoid this. Maya didn't feel their gender identity was accepted by their family, who continues to misgender them, and wanted to raise this with their family.

Maya and the ACTp therapist worked together to develop a shared understanding of Maya's struggles, using an ACT lens.

Experiential Avoidance

Maya described avoidance as one means of coping with distressing experiences. When Maya experienced negative voices or flashbacks from past trauma, they would work to shut them out; at its most extreme, this resulted in dissociation. Maya would be completely disconnected from their internal and external world, and Maya was unresponsive if others tried to communicate with them.

There were also forms of avoidance related to Maya's body image concerns and gender dysphoria, as well as disordered eating. Maya actively avoided looking at themself in the mirror or looking at photos of themself to avoid distress from gender dysphoria, and distress from their distorted perception of themself as 'fat' and 'ugly'. Maya aimed to control their weight by restricting their food intake – refusing food in efforts to avoid weight gain and fear of 'fatness'.

Maya also coped by withdrawing from life broadly – spending most days in their room watching movies and television, and sleeping. They had minimal interaction with their family and only an occasional conversation with friends online. They no longer engaged in creative endeavours.

Cognitive Fusion

Cognitive fusion was a common way that Maya engaged with their internal experiences. Maya was often fused with the voices, taking what they said as 'truth'. Maya would get 'sucked in' to what the voices were saying, believing them when they said Maya was 'worthless' and 'disgusting'. Similarly, Maya would get 'hooked' when eating disorder cognitions arose, such as 'you're fat' and 'you don't deserve to eat'. Maya also held conviction in their own beliefs about themself being worthless, and others being dangerous, and subsequently Maya 'hated' themself and was mistrustful and distanced from others.

Workability

When the ACTp therapist was exploring Maya's ways of coping with their experiences, the central questions that were considered were 'how is that approach going for you?' and 'is that helping you to live he life you want to be living?'. Maya reflected that on most occasions, cognitive fusion and experiential avoidance were not serving them well. When Maya got 'sucked in' to their voices and beliefs about themselves, it left them feeling flat and defeated, withdrawing from those things that

Maya identified as important – friendship and creative exploration. When Maya spent their energy avoiding and shutting out distressing experiences, they inevitably shut out the rest of the world too, for example via dissociation, or because all their energy was going into avoiding rather than doing things that mattered to Maya.

Function

A functional analysis of the voices was done collaboratively, and the voices started to be understood as symbolic of Maya's self-hate, internalised following past harm from others. The voices created a dynamic where Maya experienced others and the world around them as unsafe, consistent with their past life experiences. The voices were also acknowledged as somewhat 'protective', as they served to keep Maya withdrawn and distanced from others, which was helpful in protecting them from further hurt. However, this came at the cost of feeling disconnected from others.

There was exploration of the function of the eating disorder. Maya described it as a means for them to have some sense of control over their life, particularly when the voices and dissociation left them feeling out of control. Maya also identified when they felt thin, they felt less at risk of others hurting them, feeling 'almost invisible'. When they were at extremely low BMI, there were also physical and physiological changes which minimised sexual characteristics, thus reduced Maya's gender dysphoria.

Maya identified that their withdrawal to their room served the function of keeping themselves distanced from other people, which to Maya meant keeping themself 'safe'. This social separation also served to reduce Maya's struggle with self and identity – it minimised opportunity for misgendering and avoided social comparison around body image, as well as reducing exposure to stigma and alienation in the context of experiencing psychosis and anorexia nervosa – experiences Maya was ashamed of.

Open

One aspect of the therapeutic work was inviting Maya to explore whether responding to distressing experiences with a curious detached stance was helpful. Specifically, there was an experiential examination of whether Maya was better able to do things that mattered to them when they were able to defuse from distressing voices.

There was exploration of various ways Maya could respond to their voices. Commonly Maya would listen to the negative voices and believe what they were saying, which would leave Maya feeling alone, worthless, and mistrustful of others. It would contribute to Maya withdrawing to their room, and disconnecting from family, friends, and creative activities. When the voices were particularly loud and harsh, Maya's response was one of avoidance: Maya would dissociate, blocking out the voices, and the rest of the world along with them. The therapist engaged Maya in a creative hopelessness exercise (described in the 'Tom' vignette) and presented the idea that although Maya could not control the voices, Maya could choose their response to the voices. Alternative ways of responding were explored and practiced, including talking back to the voices, as well as Maya acknowledging the voices with a curious stance. Given the perceived omnipotence and of the voices, it was challenging to create some defusion. To assist this process, Maya and the therapist began to think of the voices like they were mean young children, after Maya shared that they reminded them of when their younger sister would have fights with their friends in primary school. Maya recalled the young children exchanging harsh words such as 'I don't want to be your friend anymore' and 'Eww, you're disgusting', or laughing at someone if they got an answer wrong in class. However, given the context of these words coming from young children, the words lost some of their sting, and Maya knew that young children did not yet know any better. This reframe of the voices made it possible for Maya to defuse and notice them with detached curiosity.

An experiment was done so Maya could experience which way(s) of responding to the voices felt most workable. This included trying listening to the voices and becoming fused with them, dissociating, talking back, or defusing. Through the experiment, Maya noted their distress associated with their voices was heightened by their fusion with the voices. The voices would hook Maya into their narrative of Maya being 'good for nothing' and others 'coming for you', and Maya's world would close in around them. Maya found the most workable response was to acknowledge them and notice what they were saying, while imagining them being a mean young child. The voices remained and content was unchanged; however, the voices lost some of their perceived power and control, and Maya was at times able to continue to engage in the world around them despite the voices.

Aware

At the commencement of the intervention with the ACTp therapist, Maya frequently was experiencing dissociation, feeling detached from themselves and the world around them. Dissociation is an almost complete temporary shutting off from the external world, including things that are meaningful, and people that matter. Thus, aware skills were identified as important skills to strengthen with Maya. The therapist and Maya normalised dissociation as a response that can develop following traumatic experiences. The therapist discussed with Maya the challenges that can arise when responses that may have been helpful THERE-THEN during past trauma may no longer be as helpful HERE-NOW, when the traumatic incident is no longer present, and instead the focus is on meaningful things such as creativity or connecting with others.

The therapist introduced grounding skills to help Maya manage during times of distress and dissociation. This included strategies using the five senses – such as splashing icy water on face, or chewing sour candy. Another skill was introduced to Maya to support them in developing present moment awareness, 'dropping anchor'. This involved in session practice when Maya started to become distressed and appearing to be 'zoning out'. The therapist would invite Maya to notice and acknowledge the thoughts and feelings coming up for them, re-connect with their body by stretching their arms and moving, noticing their body in the chair, and finally reconnecting with the room and people/activity around them. There was also teaching of simple prompts for Maya to continue practice out of session.

During therapy, the main focus was supporting Maya to be able to 'put on the brakes' and develop skills in being able to notice and flexibly respond to their internal experiences and the external world based on their values. There was not any deliberate focus on working directly with trauma content or flashbacks as this was contraindicated given Maya's mental state (i.e. this was expected to worsen the current situation).

Active

Since discharge from hospital, Maya had limited engagement with activities that meant something to them. The therapist invited Maya to engage in values exploration, and used this information to encourage behavioural activation, given the lack of structure to Maya's days, and lack of sense of ownership over their own life. This was done via both top-down and bottom-up approaches.

Using a top-down approach, perspective-taking was employed to invite Maya to think about what mattered to them prior to becoming unwell. Maya spoke about the importance of learning and creative expression and enjoyed activities such as art, writing, and reading. They also identified value in connecting with other people, including helping friends in need and being a role model for their younger sister. They had hoped to become a children's art teacher in future. From this, the therapist invited Maya to drill down to specific creative activities that would be possible to engage with now. This process was generative, and if desired, a large list of possible activities could be identified. As an example, Maya identified exploring their local parklands and finding a scene to paint as something they would find meaningful.

Using a bottom-up approach, the therapist asked Maya what they would do if they won a million dollars. Maya spoke about buying themself an art studio in an artist community, buying their sister a new bicycle that their sister has wanted for some time, and starting to save money for a possible overseas trip that they used to dream about with their childhood friend. From these specific tasks, the therapist invited Maya to describe what it was that mattered to them for each. From this exploration, key themes emerged of Maya valuing connection with others, creativity, and learning and discovery.

From this process, the therapist and Maya developed goals for Maya to start engaging in some values-based activities. Maya began to reflect that they noticed starting to have more energy and slightly lifted mood after engaging in activity. They also noted some sadness, as starting to re-engage in meaningful activity also served as a reminder of the lost time and experiences because of being unwell, as well as highlighting their reduced attention span compared to the past. This can be a common process when working with values in those whose life trajectory has been significantly impacted by an experience of psychosis. This may be especially so when this occurs during adolescence, a formative developmental stage.

Co-morbid Eating Disorder

The ACTp therapist introduced a central metaphor to frame the work – food as energy for the body necessary to engage in valued activity, just as a car needs fuel to make its journey. Psychoeducation was provided on the interplay between undernourishment, cognitive impact, and impact on experiences of psychosis. There was also discussion about the medical need for Maya to maintain stable weight to avoid further hospitalisation and medication.

Family sessions took place, to discuss how family could work together to support Maya at meal times. This included things such as encouraging family to sit and eat meals together, and Maya's mother seeking individual support to address her own body image and disordered eating issues. Maya had noticed their younger sister had started to express some body image concerns and engage in some disordered eating behaviour. This was explored in family sessions. In individual sessions, perspective taking was used to encourage Maya to consider their younger sister's experience of Maya's eating disorder and utilise Maya's care for their sister as motivation to address their eating disorder and work towards a healthier relationship with food and with their body.

Self and Identity

Given the various challenges Maya experienced with who they are, some targeted work occurred on the self. Firstly, the ACTp therapist introduced a self-compassion piece. This involved Maya writing a letter to themself; writing to themself from the perspective of a good friend, utilising Maya's strength as compassionate and caring for their friend who also experienced mental health struggles and inviting Maya to show that same care for themself.

The ACTp therapist also attempted to strengthen the process of 'self as context' – this is the concept that the self is an observer of experiences –serving as a container for internal experiences such as thoughts and feelings, but not being these internal experiences. For example, the ACTp therapist utilised perspective taking to support defusion from self-stories such as 'I am worthless' that Maya was fusing with. The ACTp therapist invited Maya to imagine themself as a small child, noticing that it was the same self looking out of through same eyes as Maya here and now in session. The therapist also invited Maya to notice that it is the same Maya during periods of wellness as unwellness, that they are a *container* for their psychotic and non-psychotic experiences, and they are not their experiences of psychosis. This helped to encourage flexible responding in response to Maya's feelings of shame, embarrassment, and internalised stigma about their mental health struggles.

Part of treatment also offered to Maya was connection to lived experience supports to help destigmatise experience of psychosis (e.g. hearing voices network, peer support worker), and Maya chose to engage with these supports.

Working with Young People

In the context of working with a young person, there is an emphasis on working with families and including families in treatment, given the developmental context. Family sessions occurred, to explore and work through the challenges Maya experienced relating to their gender identity. Maya used this space to discuss their distress when family misgendered them and create opportunity for family to learn more about gender and what being non-binary means (utilising a genderbread person as tool for discussion: Killermann, 2016), for the family to better understand Maya's experience. Family sessions also served to create space to explore family reactions to Maya's gender identity and encourage perspective taking among family members, as well as respectful open communication; also worked individually with Maya to consider where Maya could connect with others in a safe supportive space – explore youth services in LGBTQI+ community and referrals supported.

A separate family worker was involved to facilitate family sessions, to protect Maya's alliance with their individual therapist. In addition to above-described goals, family sessions were also a more general space for the broader family system to work through any questions, concerns, and challenges and support them in their understanding of Maya's struggles and facilitate a dialogue between Maya and their family on how family could best support Maya in their recovery.

13.10 Conclusion

ACTp can be a useful approach in supporting the personal recovery of people with psychosis. The underpinnings of ACT – inviting people to make space for experiences both positive and negative, in service of living the life they would like – align with the personal recovery framework. The therapeutic stance is collaborative, emphasising common humanity and the universal experience of suffering, which can be a useful approach for individuals with psychosis who have often had past experiences of being ostracised or pathologised and controlled by the medicalised health system and society broadly. The central processes of open, aware, and active lend themselves to addressing key challenges in psychosis – unusual and often distressing experiences, which tend to invite psychologically inflexible responses (e.g. avoidance, fusion) and commonly result in people withdrawing from meaningful engagement with the world and losing their personal identity in the process. ACT is transdiagnostic and inherently flexible, thus can be useful across a range of contexts and presentations of psychosis, as demonstrated by the case vignettes. With empirical evidence available, there is utility in psychological approaches such as ACTp to be routinely offered as a treatment option to individuals seeking support for psychosis.

Disclaimer Clinical cases presented in this chapter do not include real names or personal information of real persons.

References

A-Tjak, J. G., Davis, M. L., Morina, N., Powers, M. B., Smits, J. A., & Emmelkamp, P. M. (2015). A meta-analysis of the efficacy of acceptance and commitment therapy for clinically relevant mental and physical health problems. *Psychotherapy and Psychosomatics, 84*(1), 30–36.

Baumeister, D., Sedgwick, O., Howes, O., & Peters, E. (2017). Auditory verbal hallucinations and continuum models of psychosis: A systematic review of the healthy voice-hearer literature. *Clinical Psychology Review, 51*, 125–141.

Bebbington, P. E., McBride, O., Steel, C., Kuipers, E., Radovanovic, M., Brugha, T., Jenkins, R., Meltzer, H., & Freeman, D. (2013). The structure of paranoia in the general population. *The British Journal of Psychiatry, 202*(6), 419–427.

Ben-David, S., & Kealy, D. (2020). Identity in the context of early psychosis: A review of recent research. *Psychosis, 12*(1), 68–78.

Bentall, R. P. (1993). Deconstructing the concept of 'schizophrenia'. *Journal of Mental Health, 2*(3), 223–238.

Chadwick, P. (2006). *Person-based cognitive therapy for distressing psychosis*. Wiley.

Dymond, S., & Roche, B. (Eds.). (2013). *Advances in relational frame theory: Research & application*. New Harbinger.

Fallot, R. D., & Harris, M. (2009). *Creating cultures of trauma-informed care (CCTIC): A self-assessment and planning protocol*. Community Connections.

Flaxman, P. E., Bond, F. W., & Livheim, F. (2013). *The mindful and effective employee: An acceptance and commitment therapy training manual for improving well-being and performance*. New Harbinger Publications.

Garety, P. A., Kuipers, E., Fowler, D., Freeman, D., & Bebbington, P. E. (2001). A cognitive model of the positive symptoms of psychosis. *Psychological Medicine, 31*(2), 189–195.

Gloster, A. T., Walder, N., Levin, M. E., Twohig, M. P., & Karekla, M. (2020). The empirical status of acceptance and commitment therapy: A review of meta-analyses. *Journal of Contextual Behavioral Science, 18*, 181–192.

Harris, R. (2009). *ACT made simple*. New Harbinger.

Hayes, S. C., Strosahl, K., & Wilson, K. G. (1999). *Acceptance and Commitment Therapy: An experiential approach to behavior change*. Guilford Press.

Hayes, S. C., Barnes-Holmes, D., & Roche, B. (Eds.). (2001). *Relational frame theory: A post-Skinnerian account of human language and cognition*. Kluwer Academic/Plenum Publishers.

Hayes, S. C., Luoma, J. B., Bond, F. W., Masuda, A., & Lillis, J. (2006). Acceptance and commitment therapy: Model, processes and outcomes. *Behaviour Research and Therapy, 44*(1), 1–25.

Hayes, S. C., Strosahl, K. D., & Wilson, K. G. (2012). *Acceptance and commitment therapy: The process and practice of mindful change*. Guilford Press.

Iqbal, Z., Birchwood, M., Chadwick, P., & Trower, P. (2000). Cognitive approach to depression and suicidal thinking in psychosis: 2. Testing the validity of a social ranking model. *The British Journal of Psychiatry, 177*(6), 522–528.

Killermann, S. (2016). The Genderbread Person. *ESED 5234 – Master List*. 52. https://digitalcommons.georgiasouthern.edu/esed5234-master/52

Kingdon, D. G., & Turkington, D. (1994). *Cognitive-behavioral therapy of schizophrenia*. Guilford Press.

Leamy, M., Bird, V., Le Boutillier, C., Williams, J., & Slade, M. (2011). Conceptual framework for personal recovery in mental health: systematic review and narrative synthesis. *The British Journal of Psychiatry, 199*(6), 445–452.

Mitchell, S., Shannon, C., Mulholland, C., & Hanna, D. (2021). Reaching consensus on the principles of trauma-informed care in early intervention psychosis services: A Delphi study. *Early Intervention in Psychiatry, 15*(5), 1369–1375.

Montoya-Rodríguez, M. M., Molina, F. J., & McHugh, L. (2017). A review of relational frame theory research into deictic relational responding. *The Psychological Record, 67*(4), 569–579.

Morris, E. M., Garety, P., & Peters, E. (2014). Psychological flexibility and nonjudgemental acceptance in voice hearers: Relationships with omnipotence and distress. *Australian and New Zealand Journal of Psychiatry, 48*(12), 1150–1162.

Morris, E. M. (2018). Acceptance and commitment therapy. *In CBT for Psychosis* (pp. 79–97). Routledge.

Morrison, A. P. (2001). The interpretation of intrusions in psychosis: An integrative cognitive approach to hallucinations and delusions. *Behavioural and Cognitive Psychotherapy, 29*(3), 257–276.

Öst, L. G. (2014). The efficacy of acceptance and commitment therapy: An updated systematic review and meta-analysis. *Behaviour Research and Therapy, 61*, 105–121.

Peters, E., Ward, T., Jackson, M., Morgan, C., Charalambides, M., McGuire, P., Woodruff, P., Jacobsen, P., Chadwick, P., & Garety, P. A. (2016). Clinical, socio-demographic and psychological characteristics in individuals with persistent psychotic experiences with and without a "need for care". *World Psychiatry, 15*(1), 41–52.

Polk, K. L., Schoendorff, B., Webster, M., & Olaz, F. O. (2016). *The essential guide to the ACT Matrix: A step-by-step approach to using the ACT Matrix model in clinical practice*. New Harbinger Publications.

Törneke, N., Luciano, C., & Salas, S. V. (2008). Rule-governed behavior and psychological problems. *International Journal of Psychology and Psychological Therapy, 8*(2), 141–156.

Wilson, K. G. (2009). *Mindfulness for two: An acceptance and commitment therapy approach to mindfulness in psychotherapy*. New Harbinger Publications.

Chapter 14
Acceptance and Commitment Therapy for Psychosis in an Inpatient Context

Mårten J. Tyrberg and Brandon A. Gaudiano

14.1 Introduction

Our approach to acceptance and commitment therapy (ACT) for psychosis for inpatients is based on previous empirical work (Bach & Hayes, 2002; Gaudiano & Herbert, 2006; Tyrberg et al., 2017) combined with clinical experiences regarding the feasibility of various interventions. We find that the approach requires constant fine-tuning and that the key ingredient really is therapist flexibility based on an idiographic and functional case conceptualization of the individual patient being treated. This means that it is somewhat challenging to describe the approach in a standardized protocol manner or one-size-fits-all format. Rather, we would like to point to several central principles, each of which is subject to variation in terms of specific content, as all interventions need to be tailored to the context at hand.

While inpatient therapy is not necessarily different from outpatient therapy in essence, the setting requires some adjustments in terms of treatment delivery and its associated parameters. We have found that the work can be quite challenging, sometimes the feeling is one of having to use a shovel to get past layers of obstacles at the organizational, ward, and individual levels. Put another way, if traditional psychotherapy is white collar, inpatient therapy is blue collar. Geekie (2020) has poignantly described the work as trying to stay sane in insane places (referring here to the

M. J. Tyrberg (✉)
Region Västmanland, Centre for Clinical Research, Västmanland Hospital Västerås, Uppsala University, Västerås, Sweden
e-mail: marten.tyrberg@psyk.uu.se

B. A. Gaudiano
Butler Hospital and the Providence VA Medical Center, Brown University, Providence, RI, USA
e-mail: Brandon_Gaudiano@brown.edu

J. A. Díaz-Garrido et al. (eds.), *Psychological Interventions for Psychosis*,
https://doi.org/10.1007/978-3-031-27003-1_14

setting itself rather than the clinical issues). At the same time, therein lies much of the joy and satisfaction, as well as the potential to transform a crisis into an opportunity.

Flexibly adapting interventions to the context at hand is partly a question of understanding the patient, partly a question of understanding the particularities of the ward, and partly a question of understanding the organization in which they both reside. Folke et al. (2016) have summarized four overarching barriers to implementing psychological interventions in inpatient contexts. *Clinical* barriers refer to patients suffering from multiple and/or preliminary diagnoses, often presenting with problems of an acute nature. Meanwhile, most evidence-based protocols are diagnosis-specific and require cognitive capacities not always exhibited by inpatients. *Competence* barriers refer to the scarcity of psychotherapeutically trained staff on the typical ward and the difficulty of establishing training opportunities. *Culture* barriers refer to the fact that wards are often observational rather than interactional in nature, that interventions tend to be reactive rather than proactive, and that a medical rather than a psychological paradigm tends to direct the work. *Organizational* barriers refer to the risk of fragmented interventions, as admissions are often short and staffing unstable. It is our experience that these barriers summarize ward reality very well. At the same time, there is potential for them to be overcome, the key being flexibility on the part of the therapist, coupled with an understanding of and humility in relation to these very barriers.

A concrete example of how these barriers manifest themselves and how they might be handled follows. Paul, a middle-aged man with no previous psychiatry contacts, is admitted to a psychiatric ward after a serious suicide attempt. He is tentatively diagnosed with an unspecified depressive episode. The ward psychologist, who divides her time between several wards, first hears about the patient when she attends the ward round on Monday morning. She finds that the attending psychiatrist comes from a bank agency and is only there for a week. When starting rounds, the psychiatrist introduces himself and kindly says hello to the staff present (resident psychiatrist, intern physician, psychiatric nurse, assistant nurse, and ward psychologist). The round starts 15 min late. After spending around 10 min on introductions, small talk, and a short summary of ward routines, the round commences. The list of admitted patients and chart notes are displayed on a wall-mounted screen. The ward psychologist notices that most of the patients are the same as the previous week. She has ongoing interventions with a couple of them. She also notices a couple of new names, Paul being among them. The attending psychiatrist works through the names on the ward list quite fast, focusing on current medications, lab results, sleep, compulsory care restrictions, and whether any acute incidents have occurred during the weekend. The intern physician manages the computer, switching between lists of prescribed medicines, intake chart notes, and lists of lab results. When Paul's name comes up, the circumstances around his admission are briefly described by the nurse. The ward psychologist hears that this is a previously unknown patient and that during the weekend he has seemed eager to talk. She manages, before attention is switched to the list of medication, to ask if it would be suitable to offer Paul psychological interventions while on the ward. The attending psychiatrist stops and turns to look at the psychologist and asks, kindly: “I’m sorry, who are you again?”

This scene might certainly be frustrating for the psychologist. It is, however, a natural course of events on many wards, in the sense that psychological interventions are not seen as a natural part of the care package, and even as something of an anomaly. On many psychiatric wards, it is generally not expected nor planned for and hence not a topic that is covered in a typical round situation. Further, even after laying thorough groundwork over several months and informing the ward staff about the potential of inpatient psychological treatment, the arrival of a bank psychiatrist might efficiently put the psychologist right back at square one. We want to stress that none of this is due to ill intentions on anyone’s part. It is simply the lay of the land. For the stable staff on a ward, adapting to different attending psychiatrists on a sometimes weekly basis becomes tedious. Often, the resulting approach is to tend to the basics of the ward. Therefore, it is understandable that even though parts of the workforce are aware of the possibility of psychological interventions, their thoughts are elsewhere.

By definition, however, a barrier is not impossible to climb. If possible, knowing beforehand the staffing of the particular ward one enters is a great advantage and a way of leaping over some organizational barriers. It simply helps to know people’s names and who they are. Even with this information, patience is often required. It is tiresome to repeatedly introduce oneself and the nature of one’s services, but due to the organizational layout including unstable staffing, on many wards, this is required. Again, the overarching skill, we believe, is flexibility. It is required both in terms of one’s general professional stance and in terms of the treatment model one uses. If inpatients are to get access to psychological treatment, the psychologist ought to be ready to work in unconventional ways. This might include seeing a patient on very short notice, with little to no preparations (“It would be great if you could see this guy ASAP, he’ll probably be discharged this afternoon”). It might mean accepting to see a patient with a somewhat unclear purpose, rather than formulating the purpose as one goes along (“We really don’t understand this guy, could you help us out?”). Or it might mean seeing a patient with perhaps too clear a purpose (“Could you see this girl and give her some anxiety management skills?”). Given that one has the time, we have found that it is a good strategy to keep the threshold for taking on patients low. There is always something that can be done from a psychological standpoint, even if it is not always what is asked for. For this, a flexible model for psychological treatment is very helpful. We find that acceptance and commitment therapy (ACT; Hayes et al., 1999) is such a model.

14.2 Psychoses in the Inpatient Context

Typically, the psychosis patient admitted to an inpatient ward will be in an acute state. Often, this means exhibiting positive psychotic symptoms such as hallucinations, delusions, and disorganized thinking. In brief, hallucinations are defined as sensory perceptions in the absence of actual input; delusions are defined as false beliefs that are based on incorrect inferences about external reality; disorganized thinking is defined as disturbed thinking that affects language and communication (Bartek et al., 2020). Involuntary admissions are common for this patient group, adding to the challenge of delivering treatment, since the patient does not see it as necessary. The patient will sometimes exhibit both odd and aggressive behaviors on the ward, affecting both patients and staff. Staff on the ward need good verbal skills, so that volatile situations can be de-escalated. In some cases, seclusion or physically restraining the patient will be necessary, but this is considered a last hand option.

Often, the overall treatment plan when a patient with psychosis is hospitalized is to relieve the patient from the acute state, often using a combination of antipsychotic and antianxiety medication (Bartek et al., 2020). Besides pharmacological interventions, there is often need for stabilizing the patient's social circumstances. The so-called social determinants of health, including housing and food instability, un/underemployment, income inequality, adverse life experiences, discrimination/exclusion, and poor education access and quality, have historically been given short shrift in medical contexts and yet are major drivers of patient health and outcomes (Alegría et al., 2018). Luckily, many wards have access to social workers who can assist in housing matters, for example. In the early phases of treatment on the ward, the effects (including side effects) of the medication regimen are observed and treatment adjusted accordingly. It is advised that staff have a friendly and reassuring attitude and take into consideration possible cognitive deficits when interacting with the patient.

Several studies in both United States and European contexts (Bach & Hayes, 2002; Gaudiano & Herbert, 2006; Tyrberg et al., 2017) have shown that it is feasible to add psychotherapeutic interventions such as ACT for psychosis to the overall treatment of the ward as soon as the patient has improved somewhat from the acute state. In the aforementioned studies, patients were approached for inclusion as soon as they could understand the nature and purpose of the study. In other words, one can proceed quite quickly with offering psychotherapy on the ward. However, it is crucial that interventions are tailored to the needs, cognitive level, and pattern of symptoms of the individual patient.

14.3 The Open, Aware, Active Model

ACT is one of the so-called third-wave behavioral therapies (Hayes, 2004). While it shares many features with traditional cognitive behavioral therapy (CBT), it differs from it in terms of being more experiential than didactic and by focusing on second-order rather than first-order change. Many CBT protocols strive for changing the content of private experiences (e.g., the content of negative thoughts), while ACT strives for changing the person's *relationship* to private experiences.

ACT has demonstrated effectiveness in the treatment of many somatic and psychiatric conditions (A-Tjak et al., 2015; Hayes et al., 2006; Öst, 2008; Ruiz, 2010), with reported effect sizes that are generally in the medium range, which are consistent with those of other evidence-based psychological interventions for psychosis (Lincoln & Pedersen, 2019). With regard to psychosis, several randomized controlled trials (Bach & Hayes, 2002; Gaudiano & Herbert, 2006; Shawyer et al., 2012, 2017; Tyrberg et al., 2017; White et al., 2011) have investigated the effects of ACT. Results show both promising effects in terms of readmissions to inpatient care and symptom management, and challenges in terms of singling out the added effect of acceptance-based interventions over and above social support, medications, and other treatments that these patients typically receive. Generally, studies state that larger samples are needed. Recent reviews (Louise et al., 2018; Wakefield et al., 2018) likewise report that ACT for psychosis shows promise, but that further research applying a more stringent methodology is needed. At present, ACT for psychosis is deemed as having a modest level of research support by the American Psychological Association (n.d.) and the Australian Psychological Society (2018).

ACT is often described using the six processes of the so-called hexaflex (Hayes et al., 1999), namely acceptance, defusion, self as context, present moment focus, values, and committed action. Together, these processes work toward increased *psychological flexibility*, defined as "the ability to contact the present moment more fully as a conscious human being, and to change or persist in behavior when doing so serves valued ends" (Hayes et al., 2006, p. 7).

There has been some debate (e.g., Barnes-Holmes et al., 2016) as to the proper definitions and clinical utility of the six processes of the hexaflex, how they relate to and overlap each other, and to what extent they have been distinguished from each other using experimental research. In the clinical arena, usefulness is key. We have found that the open, aware, active model (Hayes et al., 2011; Oliver et al., 2013), which could be seen as a condensation of the six processes in the hexaflex, is a useful framework for the work we describe here. Open, aware, and active have been described as broad sets of response styles (Oliver et al., 2013) that can be fostered and trained. We find that this way of conceptualizing ACT is helpful as it brings its behavioral roots to the forefront by focusing on response classes. It thus describes three response classes (open, aware, active), which in turn combine to create the overarching response class of psychological flexibility, the fostering of which is the ultimate goal of ACT. As is the case with the six processes of the hexaflex, the three response classes of the open, aware, active model are interrelated and overlap each other. Distinguishing them from each other is a pragmatic matter.

The inherently unstable context of the inpatient ward calls for a flexible therapist, that can adjust their interventions to everchanging circumstances. Working in such an environment can be stressful and challenging, downright confusing at times. In other words, it is inevitable that during this kind of work, the therapist will experience a multitude of thoughts, feelings, and bodily sensations, while also carrying a psychological backpack of previous experiences, heritability, and rules that govern behavior. The therapist will feel worry, anxiety, anger, and frustration. They will experience thoughts such as "I'm no good at this," "I don't know what to say," and "This is too difficult." To put it plainly, the therapist is very much in the same situation as the patient. This might sound daunting. However, we find that it is ultimately a great advantage. It frees us up to use the open, aware, active model as a tool for ourselves as much as for our patients. If we as therapists can be mindful of our own status in terms of openness, awareness, and activity, we are capable to choose our interventions freely, rather than under the powerful spell of aversive control. Therefore, in the section that follows, as much weight will be given to open, aware, and active responses on the part of the therapist as the patient.

14.3.1 Open

Open refers to the extent to which we can allow experiences such as feelings, thoughts, voices, memories, perceptions, or bodily sensations to simply be there, without struggling with them by trying to change them, suppress them, or avoid them. Further, open deals with the extent to which we can observe our experiences at a distance, seeing them for what they are rather than what they claim to be (e.g., a thought as a string of words rather than objective truth). Acceptance, willingness, and stepping back are words that are often used to describe open responses.

It is tricky to approach the challenge of openness without trivializing or failing to acknowledge how difficult an open move can be for the patient. While the mental content of a psychosis patient is not necessarily different in kind from that of a reasonably healthy therapist (i.e., they are all experiences "under the skin" [Oliver et al., 2013]), it is certainly different in degree. Thus, before asking a patient to try openness by merely sitting with their imperative voices without acting on them, it is wise for the therapist to look back on their own experiences of sitting with difficult content. Likely, they will find that even content that is more lightweight (such as everyday worry) will rattle us and make us lose track of our path forward. Thus, we need to be humble and gentle when we ask patients to open up to experiences that are often perceived as life-threatening. Taking small steps is key. Meanwhile, there is dialectic tension here. It is extremely difficult to break patterns of avoidance in response to threatening content AND change needs to happen if the patient is to experience different outcomes than they have so far.

From the perspective of the therapist, being faced with the typical presenting complaints of a psychosis patient within the inherently complex context of the inpatient ward can prove challenging. Having had little time to prepare, being tired from a long working week, and perhaps juggling expectations from the ward team and the patient that are not aligned (e.g., "Help him develop insight" vs "Get me out of here"), the therapist will likely experience the pull of confusion and stress, among other experiences. Developing open responses is helpful here. Allowing uncertainty to be there, welcoming the thought that one is not properly prepared, willingly sitting with stories of frightening symptoms or heartbreaking life histories, and lightly holding the feeling of inadequacy are all such responses. Importantly, in each case one does not respond with openness because the experiences are wanted, but because they are there. If this is acknowledged, the chances improve that one will be able to choose an intervention freely, rather than prematurely leaping into problem-solving mode as an escape.

14.3.2 Aware

Being mindful, often defined as "paying attention in a particular way: on purpose, in the present moment, and non-judgmentally" (Kabat-Zinn, 1994, p. 4), is at the center of the aware response class. Put differently, it is about standing still here and now, and noticing what is there. Awareness is further about training a certain perspective (in ACT often referred to as self-as-context) from which all experiences are observed. In some sense, this perspective is about the distinction between having experiences and being them.

There is much in the mind of a typical patient with psychosis that pulls them from the present moment into the feared future or the failures of the past. Delusions, for example, have a way of painting the grimmest pictures of what might happen in the future. On a technical level, delusions often function as establishing operations in the form of rules (e.g., "I am under attack! I must protect myself at all costs, or else they will get me!"). This makes awareness a great challenge. A typical patient at an inpatient ward will also carry the burden of past failures (e.g., "I have tried everything, the medication doesn't work, and nothing helps. It has been like this my whole life and I'm a hopeless case. I might as well just end it"). This too makes awareness difficult, by constantly pulling the patient into the past and by reinforcing the perspective that mental content and self are one and the same. The challenge of awareness is a bit like when you first try to stand on a balance board. Inevitably, you will tip over in either direction (the future or the past). Awareness is like finding the balance. It is difficult, and it takes continuous training, but it can be accomplished.

The therapist must find the balance too. There is always the pull of the previous patient, the argument with one's teenage daughter during breakfast, the clumsy remark one made just seconds ago, the next patient one is late for, the presentation one has to prepare after lunch, the close relative that is struggling with breast cancer, or simply the sun shining outside, causing one's attention to wander. Adding to this, identifying with the feeling of being inadequate as a therapist rather than looking at such a thought as just more content, will rattle the board. When balanced, the therapist can pay deliberate attention to what is happening in the interaction with the patient and use what they experience to guide interventions. Awareness is not about never losing one's balance though, but rather about leaning back when it happens, as it inevitably will.

14.3.3 Active

The core of the active response class is the concept of values, which can be defined as freely chosen areas of life that are connected to patterns of action that give a sense of meaning, and that can coordinate behavior over time (Dahl et al., 2009). Activity refers to both being able to formulate one's values and acting in line with them. Ultimately, the active response class is what gives openness and awareness their raison d'être. Opening up to distressing content or staying present with pain is always in the service of values.

Many patients, and people in general, have become unaccustomed to talking or thinking about what is truly important to them. A lifelong struggle with difficult content will do that. There might be formulations that look like values, but on closer inspection, they will turn out to be about what is important NOT to have (e.g., "I just want a life without all this hassle and anxiety"). Active responses are about formulating freely chosen directions for life, that would be important irrespective of the presence of anxiety or other unwelcome content. Being curious, being a loving partner, being physically active, or being social are examples of such directions. In the midst of threatening experiences, however, such directions are like a compass needle that is stuck. Fostering active responses is like removing dirt from the compass so the needle can spin freely. Values are different from goals in that they, like a direction, cannot be accomplished. Working with activity is also about formulating concrete steps in a valued direction. In the inpatient context, this work is challenging in the sense that options for activity are quite limited. However, the pull of the overarching value can add some gold to an otherwise mundane behavior on the ward. Walking the length of a ward corridor can mean something, if it can be aligned with the overarching value of being physically active and taking care of one's body.

As therapists, we lose track of our values just as patients do. Unwelcome content such as frustration over the way the care system is organized, anger over the lack of funds for psychiatric care, or feelings of hopelessness triggered by a patient returning to the ward yet another time after a suicide attempt will cloud our vision. Stepping back from these experiences (openness) and taking a breath (awareness) might make it easier to take a look at our professional compass and remind ourselves of the heading – the answer to the question "How do I want to be in doing this job?" This, in turn, might pave the way for an active response such as leaving the desk, walking back out on the ward floor, and sitting down with a patient and listening attentively.

14.4 Central Principles

In the following, we would like to point to four principles that we have found useful in inpatient work with psychosis patients. We find that they form a framework for working that is concretely useful, and that provides ideas for specific interventions. The principles are all meant to be applied while standing on the foundation that is the open, aware, active model.

14.4.1 A Quick Way in Using Present Moment Awareness

There is an inherent paradox in inpatient work. On the one hand, psychosis is often a long-term condition, in some cases life-long. On the other hand, the inpatient context offers a very short time span for delivering interventions. The typical admission will range from 1 to 2 weeks (or even less in many cases in places like the United States). The challenge, thus, is quickly finding a way in – an opening for working with some small but significant part of a larger problem. This is also a matter of exploring the patient's motivation. Seeing as how the patient is admitted to a psychiatric ward, it is clear that something needs to change in their life. It is not uncommon though, that the patient's view on what this change entails differs quite significantly from that of the ward team. The challenge, for the therapist, is finding the change the patient is *willing* to make. We find that this is perhaps the most central challenge of all if inpatient psychotherapy is going to be successful.

Wilson (2008) has written about the importance of the therapist's noticing what happens in the here and now of the therapy room. Signs such as posture, tone of voice, quality of eye contact, pitch, way of sitting in a chair, and the movement of gaze might all be clues as to what is happening for the patient. It is our experience that focusing on such subtleties as much as the content of what the patient says is useful in the search for meaningful and feasible change. As the overarching goal of ACT is to foster psychological flexibility, staying on the lookout for subtle signs of rigidity often provides clues to where change needs to happen. In regard to people struggling with psychosis specifically, Serper et al. (2004) have mentioned specific signs that might be indicative of psychotic symptoms, such as looking in the corner of one's eye or to the side, abruptly interrupting one's speech, leaning one's head to the side in a listening pose, or unexpected laughter or smiling.

In our view, the importance of noticing and analyzing here-and-now signs is even greater in the kind of brief work that is done in the inpatient context. It is one of the ways of quickly finding a way in. To some degree, this thinking is akin to the basic premise of Functional Analytic Psychotherapy (Kohlenberg et al., 2009), a third-wave therapy related to ACT, which emphasizes being on the lookout for clinically relevant behaviors in the present moment within the context of the therapeutic relationship. Being quick also means allowing oneself to test out hypotheses as to what various behaviors might stand for. The challenge is to constantly connect however small and seemingly insignificant behaviors that one observes and formulate response classes. This is done using focused interviewing.

14.4.2 Focused Interviewing

Strosahl et al. (2012) have outlined a series of questions that are helpful in focusing in on a workable aspect of a larger problem. We have found them to be quite useful as a template for brief therapy work in a psychiatric inpatient context. We stress the word template here, arguing that the questions do not necessarily have to be asked verbatim or in a particular order. Rather, the goal is for these overarching questions to be answered during a conversation. The answers are useful building blocks for a functional analysis of the patient's struggle.

The first question, "What are you seeking?," aims to capture the presenting problem and what the patient would see as a successful outcome of treatment. With the second question, "What have you tried?," the therapist gathers information about past attempts at handling the problem. This includes the full range of previous experiences, including both prescribed solutions such as medication or past experiences of therapy and strategies that are typically considered as more problematic, such as overusing alcohol, self-harm, or suicide attempts. The third question, "How has it worked?," circles in on the functionality of previous problem-solving attempts, both short- and long-term. In some sense, when working in psychiatric inpatient care, we know beforehand that past attempts at problem-solving have not worked sufficiently, the patient being admitted is proof of this. However, it is important to maintain an open stance when doing this kind of interviewing. Curiosity, humility, and a generally nonjudgmental stance are suitable guiding stars. The fourth question, "What has it cost you?," is arguably the most important one, in terms of reaching the ultimate point of pain and opening up for alternative courses of action, much akin to the traditional ACT concept of creative hopelessness (Hayes et al., 1999). While it is painful to talk about what has gotten lost during a sometimes lifelong struggle of using various experiential avoidance strategies, it also opens up for alternatives. It is like reaching the bottom but being able to use it as a springboard for something new.

14.4.3 A Workable Metaphor

The use of metaphors is central to much ACT work (Hayes et al., 1999; Törneke, 2017). Its usefulness rests on the potential for relating well-known properties of a base to lesser-known properties of a target (Törneke, 2017). Thus, if used properly, metaphor can quickly elucidate a central struggle for a patient. In our experience, quickly establishing a workable metaphor is very helpful in inpatient work. It provides an easily accessible way into the central problem and allows for it to be talked about in a creative and playful way. It is further tightly connected to the function rather than the topography of behavior, and ideally sidetracks the common obstacle of rigid rule-following in favor of long-term values-based behavior.

In our experience, the firsthand choice ought to be using a metaphor that is derived from the patient's own words, and optimally created in the session. This increases the chances of being on target in terms of the central problem and maximizes the potential usefulness of the metaphor. Thus, the therapist ought to be on the lookout for descriptions that might be building blocks for a metaphor early in the very first session. One patient described the experience of using drugs to avoid his feelings in the past as being in a situation where you first believe you've seen the light at the end of the tunnel, only to realize all too late that it is a train bearing down on you shortly before the big crash. Other examples of metaphors we have encountered in patient work are how managing difficult thoughts and feelings is like handling a sticky ball, how finding one's direction in life is like lifting one's gaze from one's lap and looking straight ahead, how thoughts can be disturbing like when you lose focus while listening to an audiobook, and how keeping thoughts and feelings away is like keeping a monster in its cage. All of these suggest ways of speaking about the central challenge in effective ways ("So when you think back on that time when you tried to kill yourself, the ball is really big and super sticky"; "So in this situation we are talking about right now, what would lifting your gaze look like?"; "That really swept you away from the plot of the book"; "It sounds like the monster is really rattling the cage right now").

Not all patients easily provide such material, though. As a secondhand choice, therefore, the therapist can tentatively formulate a metaphor. Many times, the metaphor used will be created using a combination of the first- and secondhand choices. It is preferable, in our experience, that metaphors are relatively simple and short, using as much everyday language as possible. It is important to note that whether a metaphor is used at all is of course not interesting from the perspective of the patient. It is merely a way of speaking. This might be an obvious point for most readers, but we find that it is important to stress that the use of certain ways of speaking is completely a question of workability, as is all therapy work from a contextual standpoint. The power of the metaphor lies in its ability to cast light on something obscure and difficult to grasp, rendering it tangible. Whether the metaphor in question is elaborated and elegant or very simple is not important in and of itself. We prefer the latter, though. The workability of a metaphor can often be judged by staying present with the subtleties of the therapeutic moment. What happens in the patient's eyes when a metaphor is proposed? How does body posture shift? Are there traces of an incipient smile? However, for patients struggling with psychosis, it is important also to be aware of a tendency, on a group level, to show less overt emotional expressions compared to normal controls due to affective blunting, even though covertly emotions might be there (Myin-Germeys et al., 2000). This adds to the challenge of finding subtle confirmations that one is on the right track.

The original ACT manual (Hayes et al., 1999) contains many examples of useful metaphors, including the often-mentioned "passengers on the bus." In brief, it illustrates how handling one's thoughts, feelings, voices, or other troubling experiences (the target) is much like driving a bus with various threatening passengers on it, dictating where to drive in exchange for staying in the back of the bus rather than coming to the front (the base). This metaphor has been used successfully with people with psychosis, particularly in a group format (Butler et al., 2016). We have also found it to be useful as a tool in brief individual inpatient work (Tyrberg et al., 2017).

14.4.4 Physicalizing

People suffering from psychosis, especially schizophrenia, often exhibit cognitive impairments in the mild to moderate range (American Psychiatric Association, 2013; Heinrichs & Zakzanis, 1998; Vahia & Cohen, 2008). Deficits vary in nature and degree between individuals, but attention, working memory, learning, processing speed, and executive functioning are domains that are often affected. We have found that one useful way of addressing this vulnerability is using physicalizing exercises in a session. Using props, moving about in the therapy room, or using concrete properties of the therapy room has several benefits, one being that physicalization in itself facilitates focused attention and learning. Another benefit might be that it is simply something different than what the patient expects, with the novelty effect also promoting learning.

One physicalizing exercise we have found to be useful in this context is a simplified version of the lifeline (Dahl et al., 2009). If successful, it concretizes the findings from focused interviewing and results in a plan for behavior change in the vein of the active response style (i.e., connected to central life values). A central metaphor for the lifeline exercise is the compass, with the appeal of avoidance of different kinds being one of the magnetic poles, and values being the other. In a typical version of the exercise, the patient and therapist will stand up together in the middle of the therapy room. Using material from previous focused interviewing, they start to outline the two basic poles. Examples of avoidance behaviors (e.g., self-harm, overusing alcohol, rumination, suicidal ideation, isolation) are written down on sticky notes. Ideally, these are then placed on the floor in one of the corners of the room. Next, values are written down on additional sticky notes (e.g., being a loving parent, and being physically active). These are placed at the other end of the room, if possible near the door. The therapist and patient stand together between the two poles. When suitable, the pull of each pole is gently illustrated by nudging the patient in different directions. Next, obstacles such as voices, thoughts, or feelings are written down on more notes (e.g., a voice saying "You are worthless, you will never succeed"). By placing these in front of the patient while they are walking in their valued direction, it is illustrated how private experiences might be perceived as obstacles, making the patient turn in another direction. The physical narrowness of the corner where the avoidance pole is placed and the relative openness of the door where the values pole is placed can be creatively used for further concretization work.

We have found that using the compass as a central metaphor for this exercise fits well with the core tenet of the concept of values, namely that it is a constantly ongoing direction rather than an obtainable goal. It has also been useful to rely on the compass needle as a metaphor, pivoting in different directions depending on the pull from the poles. This pivoting is easily transferable to the patient and therapist turning in different directions in the room. While obtaining specific goals, which are often perceived as far away, might seem impossible to the patient, it is often quite feasible to merely turn and look in the direction of one's values. In future sessions, the opposite poles can also be referred to by simply pointing in different directions while talking about the patients' struggle ("So this really seems like a step in that direction, right?"). This being said, and in line with our previous reasoning, the exercise can be tailored in whichever way the therapist finds useful, using metaphors that fit the situation. The goal of the exercise is to formulate a realistic and concrete step in the valued direction, even if it means meeting difficult private content. We have found it useful to let the patient keep the sticky notes used in the exercise, extending it beyond the session. Inviting patients to carry the notes in their pocket while they go about their day can foster increased acceptance and openness. Next time, the patient can report on how it was experienced to carry difficult material while going about a typical day.

14.5 Connecting the Dots

The above principles are building blocks for a flexible inpatient psychotherapy model. Ideally, they will be used as needed, rather than in a structured protocol manner. We want to stress this idiographic stance because we believe it is central to adapting to the ebb and flow of the inpatient context. The principles may all be used during a single session, or over the course of several sessions. The overarching purpose is finding a change the patient is willing to make, that is in line with personally held values. The open, aware, active model with its focus on adaptive and useful response classes is seen as a foundation to stand on while applying the principles. In the following, the use of the principles will be illustrated with a patient case.

14.6 Case

14.6.1 Background

Mary was a 25-year-old woman diagnosed with a schizoaffective disorder. She was admitted to a psychosis ward following increasing concerns by her family and her outpatient contact person about her ability to handle ongoing auditory hallucinations. Mary had a long history of psychiatric care, with her first contact with child and adolescent psychiatric services in her teens, then struggling with self-harm. She had previously been treated with psychotherapy of various kinds, as well as different combinations of neuroleptics.

Currently, Mary was on sick leave from her job as an assistant nurse at a home for the elderly. She lived with her husband and child in a small house in the countryside. She liked being outdoors and spending time with her family and her two dogs. She had limited contact with friends, although she had a quite active social life when she was younger.

14.6.2 Formulation

In the assessment interview, Mary reported that she experienced a disturbing male voice giving her negative comments about her body, commenting on how she looked, and calling her "useless," among other things. She had a history of being bullied in her early teens, and to some extent recognized the content of what the male voice said from this period. Besides these auditory perceptions, Mary also had a clear inner image of the man giving her these comments – describing him as an older grey-haired man, with black eyes, tall and skinny. At times, the man almost felt like a ghost having invaded her, and having taken power over her thoughts. Not trusting the ghost-like man, Mary was afraid that her thoughts could hurt others. This caused a lot of shame, as she saw herself as a kind and peaceful person.

Mary had reluctantly agreed to be admitted to the ward, as she could see how difficult it had become for her to manage her everyday life. She missed her family while being on the ward, she felt isolated and hindered in terms of being able to go out. When asked what she hoped for with treatment ("What are you seeking?"), she stated that she wanted to find a way to be able to spend time with her family and being outdoors without being harassed by her voice. She wanted to come back to her job, at least to some extent. She also wanted to reconnect with some of her friends.

Exploring previous strategies ("What have you tried?"), Mary reported spending a lot of time and energy keeping her experiences in check, which she described as "keeping the lid on" (possibly a workable metaphor). This was done in various ways. She described how she was generally careful in all her movements and activities, as if she was afraid that any sudden changes would cause the lid to come off. At times, she had tried to let the experiences be and just relax, but this had increased her anxiety too much. Mary tried to appease the male voice in different ways. One of these was described as making herself small and unnoticeable. This meant speaking in a quite low and monotonous voice, hunching down when walking, lowering her gaze when meeting someone on the street, generally avoiding eye contact when speaking to someone, and huddling up when she sat down in a chair. All of these were described as ways of keeping the lid on. At times, as she also did during her period of self-harm, she cut herself as a way of placating the male voice.

Mary carefully monitored her thoughts, not wanting to risk thinking something bad about someone else. If such a thought entered her mind, she quickly tried to repress it and replace it with a kind thought. This was done regardless of what had happened to trigger a thought. This made her somewhat confused, as she had a hard time knowing right from wrong ways of behaving in relationships with others. She often opted for as passive a stance as possible, so as not to risk anything. This had caused many of her relationships to lose their meaning, and she had been seeing less and less people outside of her own family ("How has it worked?"; "What has it cost you?").

Further, Mary displayed some compulsive behaviors, such as arranging her chair in a very particular way before sitting down, being extremely careful when pouring a glass of water so as not to spill it, and keeping her room very tidy. On the ward, she was most often found either lying in bed in her room or standing still at one end of one of the long corridors.

Recently, Mary had spent quite a lot of time thinking about suicide. She felt the voices and her sense of being invaded by the ghost-like character was too much to bear. However, the love of her daughter and her relationship with her husband held her back. With regards to medication, Mary had at times experienced her medicines to work quite well, making voices and other experiences less impactful. At other times she had felt them to be of no use.

14.6.3 Flow of Treatment

In the first contact with Mary, a few things were noticeable in the nonverbal contact she gave. When walking down the corridor to the room where the session was held, she held her head down and kept her gaze fixed on the floor in front of her feet, seemingly trying to keep her body as still as possible while walking. When sitting down, she kept her head down and her gaze fixed in her lap, her shoulders hunched down, and her arms wrapped around her. She gave no eye contact. This pattern of overt behavior, together with the metaphor of keeping the lid on, was used as a quick way in. It was gently explored whether these behaviors were examples of keeping the lid on. Mary quickly confirmed this. A discussion followed with a focus on finding possible ways of carefully lifting the lid, while respecting Mary's earlier negative experiences of relaxing completely. It was clear that the balance between keeping the lid tightly shut and opening it slightly was delicate. From an early stage, however, she seemed open to discussing this as a possible avenue for change. In the section that follows, the therapist uses physicalizing.

Therapist: Would it be ok if we tried something different?
Mary: Um, sure.
T: Could we just stand up together, in the middle of the room? [Mary nods, and the therapist stands up and starts rearranging the furniture to make some space in the middle of the room.] We have talked for a while now about what your life has been like lately. It's clear you have really tried to handle the situation as best you can. At the same time, it's clear that it's difficult for you to really live your life as you would like to. It seems that you have lost more and more of your freedom to move.
M: Yeah, I really don't do much these days. It's bad.
T: It is, but it's not like you're doing this just to mess up your own life, right? It seems more like you struggle as hard as you can to keep it together.

One facet of the focused interviewing stance is to always assume that the patient has done their very best, given the circumstances and previous learning history. We find that this can remove some of the blame that makes it difficult for patients to stay aware in the present moment, as excessive self-criticism might risk balancing the board toward the past.

M: I do. But nothing seems to get better.
T: Right. It's even come to the point where you're sometimes thinking about ending it altogether.
M: Yeah. It's terrible. I hate to think about what that would do to my kid.
T: I can see that. At the same time, it kind of makes sense to end up there when you've tried everything. It's like being in an emotional dead-end.
M: I don't know what to do. What should I do?

For some of us therapists, such a direct question will cause a sort of tightening of the chest, a feeling of having to provide an answer. Perhaps to the extent that we do answer, by suggesting some course of action or training problem-solving, for example. Right here though, it might also be an option to pause for a bit, letting the tightness remain, responding with openness.

T: It's really difficult to know what to do. Let's look at that together. I wonder if we could make this all a bit more concrete, see if that helps. You've told me a lot about what you struggle with, how you've tried to handle all these difficult and frightening experiences that you have.
M: Nothing works.
T: So far it hasn't gotten better. Would it be ok if I jotted down some of those things on these sticky notes?
M: Yeah, sure.
T: Let's see, so you've told me how you really try to keep the lid on, in different ways. Making yourself small, being careful. Like not trying to upset in any way, keeping quiet, keeping your head down. You also told me how you're really careful when doing certain things, like keeping your room really tidy and keeping to a certain pattern when you sit down and eat. Almost like you can't make any mistakes. Would it be fair to say that's also a way of keeping the lid on?

Here, the therapist tries to connect various behaviors to common response classes (i.e., examples of keeping the lid on, and examples of handling the situation).

M: I guess, I mean, I think so.
T: And then you've described how you tend to retreat to your room here on the ward, like staying out of people's way.
M: Yeah. Feels better that way.
T: And then there's this difficult sense of not wanting to live any more, thinking about ending it. Would it be fair to say that's also a way of handling the situation?
M: Well, I suppose it is.
T: So if I go ahead and write "keeping the lid on", and then some examples of that, and then "staying out of people's way", and, if it's ok with you, "thinking about suicide". Ok if I write those things on a couple of notes?
M: It's ok.
[Therapist writes on notes. Holds them up in front of Mary.]
T: What's it like for you to see these things written down like this?

The therapist's aim here is to encourage present-moment awareness of difficult thoughts and feelings.

M: I don't know. It's bad, I guess.
T: It's bad.
M: Yeah. I don't know. I don't know what to do.
T: I think it's clear that you've done your best so far. But it's a struggle. I'm going to put these notes right over here in the corner for now. [Therapist places sticky notes on the floor in the corner of the room.] We've also talked about what you value in life, what's really important. You've told me how important your daughter is to you.

M: She is.

T: Spending time with your family. You've also talked about wanting to be more active, going for walks in the woods. Taking the dogs out for long walks. And also being active in your profession, coming back to work to some extent.

M: It's really hard, it feels like I can't do anything anymore.

T: Those things feel far away.

M: It's impossible.

T: From where you stand, it's really a long way to go. And then you've told me how you miss seeing some friends. Wanting to find your way back to some of those relations. I thought I would write some of those things down also.

The therapist aims for formulations that might work as directions (being active, nurturing relations), but also uses concrete attainable goals as concretizations of the overarching direction (going for walks, coming back to work). The risk when working with active responding is always the patient's sense that valued activities are too far away. This feeling must be validated, but at the same time, values ought to be used to convey that meaningful change is possible even from where the patient is standing right now.

M: Ok.

T: So if I write some of those things down as well on a couple of more notes. [Therapist writes "being a mother", "being physically active", "being a professional" and "nurturing relations" on notes and holds them up in front of the patient.] What is it like for you to see these things written down?

M: I don't know. It feels like I don't do any of those things. I can't.

T: It's been a while since life felt really meaningful. It's easy to lose track of what is really important. Tough thoughts and feelings will do that to you. I'm going to put these notes over here if it's ok with you. [Therapist places notes with values on the floor near the door of the room.] Would you come and stand with me here in the middle of the room? [Therapist and Mary stand in between the two sets of notes.]

Here, using their own awareness, it is essential that the therapist gets a sense of whether the patient is willing to experiment in this way. For some patients, standing next to the therapist will feel too uncomfortable. If the therapist is aware, this will be clear in the present moment of the session. To remain seated or to do the exercise in a different way altogether is completely fine. The aim is to provide the patient with a clear image of the present situation, and how it might be changed. In Mary's case, she seemed willing to go along, even though she preferred to still stand at a distance from the therapist. As the room where the session was held was quite spacious, it was possible to do it so that she was reasonably comfortable.

T: Let's see if we can make this a bit more concrete. It's like there's always a pull from different directions. So on the one hand, there are all these things that are important to you. [Points in the direction of values.] That's sort of a positive pull. But then, especially recently, stuff gets in the way when you try to move in that direction. Like those frightening voices that you've mentioned. They say really nasty things to you.

M: They do.

T: You've mentioned how they often call you worthless.

M: Yeah.

T: That's really tough to hear. Would it be ok with you if I wrote those words down on another note?

M: I guess. Sure.

T: [Writes "You're worthless" on a note. Holds it up in front of Mary.] What's it like for you to see those words written down?

M: I feel like it's true. I can't do anything.

T: It's really tough to feel like that. It seems to me that the situation is a bit like this. [Therapist places the note on the floor in front of Mary, in the direction of the values notes.] It's like when you try to even think about those things over there, this one gets in the way. What do you typically do when this happens?

M: I just want to get rid of it, make it stop. I have to make it stop.

T: Right. So standing here, facing this [points at the voice content note], what do you feel like doing?

M: [Turns away from it.] I want to run away I guess.

T: Right, and here are all of those things. [Subtly nods in the direction of the opposite set of notes.]. Would you be willing to just turn around and follow me a few steps over here? [Therapist and Mary turn towards the opposite notes and take a few steps.] You've told me how you spend a lot of energy trying to keep the lid on, making yourself small, not noticeable.

M: Yeah. I try to keep to myself, stay away.

T: That's understandable. But at the same time I wonder, when standing over here, what happens to those things over there? [Therapist points in the direction of the values notes.]

M: They're further away, I guess.

T: They're further away, and we have our backs turned against them. [Therapist and Mary walk back to the middle of the room.] I wonder if our work might first be about just acknowledging this tension, this pull from different directions. Sort of standing here in the middle and looking in different directions.

M: What do you mean?

T: I think just making room for the fact that life is like this might be a first step.

M: Ok.

T: Sometimes, stuff will show up that makes us turn away from what is important. Perhaps the challenge is not to never turn away, but to notice when we do it, and finding ways to turn back again. Would you be willing to explore that?

In the coming couple of sessions, the lifeline exercise was used as a starting point for discussing ways of experimenting with new behavior. For example, Mary's willingness to experiment with her posture was explored. Connecting back to the lifeline exercise, subtle adjustments of her posture were framed as possible steps in a valued direction. One example that was discussed was looking the therapist in the eyes instead of down in her lap. Mary felt this was too large a step. She was willing, however, to slightly change her huddled-up posture in the chair. Typically, she would sit with her shoulders hunched up, leaning forward a bit, with her hands in her lap, gaze directed at her hands. After a bit of discussion, it was agreed that she would try to lean back in the chair, placing her hands on the armrests. She did so and was encouraged to describe her experience. She reported that the male voice commented on her behavior, claiming that she was making a fool of herself. She also noted that it felt unusual to sit in this way. Despite the negative message from the male voice, Mary managed to remain in a leaned-back position. This was framed as still being directed toward values, an example of active responding. Mary noted that the voice remained but did not get stronger. She described the experience as still unusual and a bit uncomfortable, but also as interesting. She reflected that she had rarely moved outside of her comfort zone in this way before.

Next, the possibility of looking in some other direction than down in her lap was again discussed. Mary still found looking the therapist in the eyes too large a step but agreed to fix her gaze on a spot on the wall. When doing so, she noticed a similar feeling of unusualness as when leaning back. She also reported a strong urge to lower her gaze. However, she managed to keep it on the wall for a bit. Again, she reflected that it was interesting to step out of her comfort zone.

Step by step, and continuously connecting back to the opposite pulls demonstrated in the lifeline exercise, Mary was encouraged to try new behavior, to gently lift the lid, while continuing to be aware of whichever experiences this brought. When she was discharged from the ward, she was still struggling with difficult experiences. However, she reported having more options than before, and she was determined to keep trying to turn back to her values whenever she found herself lost.

14.7 Concluding Remarks

In this chapter, we described a flexible and practical model for delivering ACT for psychosis in an inpatient environment. We noted the many challenges encountered when doing this work, but also the numerous joys and rewards experienced along the way. On the one hand, it is true that conducting therapy with patients with psychosis on a ward entails providing care at a time when people are at their most distressed, impaired, and vulnerable. Admittedly, this can pose a great challenge. On the other hand, therein also lies the opportunity. We have shown how ACT can help patients with psychosis explore novel responses to potentially intractable problems that are fundamentally different from what they have been able or willing to try up to that point.

When done correctly, inpatient therapy comes with the potential for rapid change and growth that can be transformative for both the therapist and the patient. Further, the inpatient therapy process can provide both with a sense of freedom that is seldom glimpsed in routine outpatient work. Nevertheless, this work simultaneously demands more from therapists, who must closely attend to their own stance of openness and awareness to be successful in the endeavor. It is important to emphasize that in a behavioral therapy such as ACT, much of the learning in session comes through modeling from the therapist to the patient, along with the reciprocal feedback that is generated by the patient's responses as observed by a perceptive therapist. The challenging (and at times exhausting) nature of this work means that therapists delivering ACT for psychosis must also critically attend to their own self-care and foster self-compassion to remain healthy throughout the process.

One of the consistent findings from the research thus far is that inpatient ACT for psychosis produces reductions in subsequent rehospitalizations (Tonarelli et al., 2016). It would appear that, when effective, ACT is helping patients to respond differently to the same old problems when they encounter them again in the near future. Avoiding unnecessary rehospitalization can lead to a dramatically different life trajectory for individuals following their current hospital stay. Nevertheless, we also must humbly acknowledge that ACT for psychosis does not have all of the answers. There is much we still need to learn about how to most effectively and efficiently deliver ACT (and therapy in general) for this population. In the end, we wish to express our thanks and gratitude to the many patients whose willingness to share in this process has shaped and will continue to shape this effort as it evolves in the future.

Disclaimer Clinical cases presented in this chapter do not include real names or personal information of real persons.

References

Alegría, M., NeMoyer, A., Falgàs Bagué, I., Wang, Y., & Alvarez, K. (2018). Social determinants of mental health: Where we are and where we need to go. *Current Psychiatry Reports, 20*, 95. https://doi.org/10.1007/s11920-018-0969-9

American Psychiatric Association. (2013). *Diagnostic and statistical manual of mental disorders* (5th ed.). American Psychiatric Publishing.

American Psychological Association. (n.d.). *Acceptance and commitment therapy for psychosis*. Retrieved from: https://div12.org/treatment/acceptance-and-commitment-therapy-for-psychosis/

A-Tjak, J. G. L., Davis, M. L., Morina, N., Powers, M. B., Smits, J. A., & Emmelkamp, P. M. (2015). A meta-analysis of the efficacy of acceptance and commitment therapy for clinically relevant mental and physical health problems. *Psychotherapy and Psychosomatics, 84*(1), 30–36. https://doi.org/10.1159/000365764

Australian Psychological Society. (2018). *Evidence-based psychological interventions in the treatment of mental disorders: A review of the literature* (4th ed.). Retrieved from: https://psychology.org.au/getmedia/23c6a11b-2600-4e19-9a1d-6ff9c2f26fae/evidence-based-psych-interventions.pdf

Bach, P., & Hayes, S. C. (2002). The use of acceptance and commitment therapy to prevent the rehospitalization of psychotic patients: A randomized controlled trial. *Journal of Consulting and Clinical Psychology, 70*(5), 1129–1139. https://doi.org/10.1037/0022-006x.70.5.1129

Barnes-Holmes, Y., Hussey, I., McEnteggart, C., Barnes-Holmes, D., & Foody, M. (2016). Scientific ambition: The relationship between relational frame theory and middle-level terms in acceptance and commitment therapy. In R. D. Zettle, S. C. Hayes, D. Barnes-Holmes, & A. Biglan (Eds.), *The Wiley handbook of contextual behavioral science* (pp. 365–382). Wiley Blackwell.

Bartek, S., Kruger, T., & Casher, M. I. (2020). The inpatient with schizophrenia. In M. I. Casher & J. D. Bess (Eds.), *Manual of inpatient psychiatry* (pp. 1–27). Cambridge University Press.

Butler, L., Johns, L. C., Byrne, M., Joseph, C., O'Donoghue, E., Jolley, S., Morris, E. M. J., & Oliver, J. E. (2016). Running acceptance and commitment therapy groups for psychosis in community settings. *Journal of Contextual Behavioral Science, 5*(1), 33–38. https://doi.org/10.1016/j.jcbs.2015.12.001

Dahl, J. C., Plumb, J. C., Stewart, I., & Lundgren, T. (2009). *The art & science of valuing in psychotherapy*. New Harbinger Publications, Inc.

Folke, F., Kanter, J. W., & Ekselius, L. (2016). Integrating behavioural activation into acute inpatient services. *Journal of Psychiatric Intensive Care, 12*(2), 109–118. https://doi.org/10.20299/jpi.2016.xxx

Gaudiano, B. A., & Herbert, J. D. (2006). Acute treatment of inpatients with psychotic symptoms using Acceptance and Commitment Therapy: Pilot results. *Behavior Research and Therapy, 44*(3), 415–437. https://doi.org/10.1016/j.brat.2005.02.007

Geekie, J. (2020). On trying to stay sane in insane places. In M. Turel, M. Siglag, & A. Grinshpoon (Eds.), *Clinical psychology in the mental health inpatient setting* (pp. 138–147). Routledge.

Hayes, S. C. (2004). Acceptance and commitment therapy, relational frame theory, and the third wave of behavioral and cognitive therapies. *Behavior Therapy, 35*, 639–665.

Hayes, S. C., Strosahl, K. D., & Wilson, K. G. (1999). *Acceptance and commitment therapy. An experiential approach to behavior change*. The Guilford Press.

Hayes, S. C., Luoma, J. B., Bond, F. W., Masuda, A., & Lillis, J. (2006). Acceptance and commitment therapy: Model, processes and outcomes. *Behavior Research and Therapy, 44*(1), 1–25. https://doi.org/10.1016/j.brat.2005.06.006

Hayes, S. C., Villatte, M., Levin, M., & Hildebrandt, M. (2011). Open, aware, and active: Contextual approaches as an emerging trend in the behavioral and cognitive therapies. *Annual Review of Clinical Psychology, 7*, 141–168. https://doi.org/10.1146/annurev-clinpsy-032210-104449

Heinrichs, R. W., & Zakzanis, K. K. (1998). Neurocognitive deficit in schizophrenia: A quantitative review of the evidence. *Neuropsychology, 12*(3), 426–445.

Kabat-Zinn, J. (1994). *Wherever you go, there you are: Mindfulness meditation in everyday life*. Hyperion.

Kohlenberg, R. J., Tsai, M., & Kanter, J. W. (2009). What is functional analytic psychotherapy? In M. Tsai, R. J. Kohlenberg, J. W. Kanter, B. Kohlenberg, W. C. Follette, & G. M. Callaghan (Eds.), *A guide to functional analytic psychotherapy. Awareness, courage, love, and behaviorism* (pp. 1–20). Springer.

Lincoln, T. M., & Pedersen, A. (2019). An overview of the evidence for psychological interventions for psychosis: Results from meta-analyses. *Clinical Psychology in Europe, 1*, 1–23.

Louise, S., Fitzpatrick, M., Strauss, C., Rossell, S. L., & Thomas, N. (2018). Mindfulness- and acceptance-based interventions for psychosis: Our current understanding and a meta-analysis. *Schizophrenia Research, 192*, 57–63. https://doi.org/10.1016/j.schres.2017.05.023

Myin-Germeys, I., Delespaul, P. A., & deVries, M. W. (2000). Schizophrenia patients are more emotionally active than is assumed based on their behavior. *Schizophrenia Bulletin, 26*, 847–854. https://doi.org/10.1093/oxfordjournals.schbul.a033499

Oliver, J. E., Joseph, C., Byrne, M., Johns, L. C., & Morris, E. M. J. (2013). Introduction to mindfulness and acceptance-based therapies for psychosis. In E. M. J. Morris, L. C. Johns, & J. E. Oliver (Eds.), *Acceptance and commitment therapy and mindfulness for psychosis* (pp. 1–11). Wiley Blackwell.

Öst, L. G. (2008). Efficacy of the third wave of behavioral therapies: A systematic review and meta-analysis. *Behavior Research and Therapy, 46*(3), 296–321. https://doi.org/10.1016/j.brat.2007.12.005

Ruiz, F. J. (2010). A review of Acceptance and Commitment Therapy (ACT) empirical evidence: Correlational, experimental psychopathology, component and outcome studies. *International Journal of Psychology and Psychological Therapy, 10*(1), 125–162.

Serper, M. R., Goldberg, B. R., & Salzinger, K. (2004). Behavioral assessment of psychiatric patients in restrictive settings. In S. N. Haynes & E. M. Heiby (Eds.), *Comprehensive handbook of psychological assessment. Volume 3. Behavioral assessment* (pp. 320–345). Hoboken.

Shawyer, F., Farhall, J., Mackinnon, A., Trauer, T., Sims, E., Ratcliff, K., et al. (2012). A randomised controlled trial of acceptance-based cognitive behavioural therapy for command hallucinations in psychotic disorders. *Behavior Research and Therapy, 50*(2), 110–121. https://doi.org/10.1016/j.brat.2011.11.007

Shawyer, F., Farhall, J., Thomas, N., Hayes, S. C., Gallop, R., Copolov, D., & Castle, D. J. (2017). Acceptance and commitment therapy for psychosis: Randomised controlled trial. *British Journal of Psychiatry, 210*(2), 140–148. https://doi.org/10.1192/bjp.bp.116.182865

Strosahl, K., Robinson, P., & Gustavsson, T. (2012). *Brief interventions for radical change. Principles & practice of focused acceptance & commitment therapy*. New Harbinger Publications, Inc.

Tonarelli, S. B., Pasillas, R., Alvarado, L., Dwivedi, A., & Cancellare, A. (2016). Acceptance and commitment therapy compared to treatment as usual in psychosis: A systematic review and meta-analysis. *Journal of Psychiatry, 19*, 2–5.

Törneke, N. (2017). *Metaphor in practice. A professional's guide to using the science of language in psychotherapy*. New Harbinger Publications, Inc.

Tyrberg, M. J., Carlbring, P., & Lundgren, T. (2017). Brief acceptance and commitment therapy for psychotic inpatients: A randomized controlled feasibility trial in Sweden. *Nordic Psychology, 69*(2), 110–125. https://doi.org/10.1080/19012276.2016.1198271

Vahia, I. V., & Cohen, C. I. (2008). Psychopathology. In K. T. Mueser & D. V. Jeste (Eds.), *Clinical handbook of schizophrenia* (pp. 82–90). The Guilford Press.

Wakefield, S., Roebuck, S., & Boyden, P. (2018). The evidence base of Acceptance and Commitment Therapy (ACT) in psychosis: A systematic review. *Journal of Contextual Behavioral Science, 10*, 1–13. https://doi.org/10.1016/j.jcbs.2018.07.001

White, R., Gumley, A., McTaggart, J., Rattrie, L., McConville, D., Cleare, S., & Mitchell, G. (2011). A feasibility study of Acceptance and Commitment Therapy for emotional dysfunction following psychosis. *Behavior Research and Therapy, 49*(12), 901–907. https://doi.org/10.1016/j.brat.2011.09.003

Wilson. (2008). *Mindfulness for two. An acceptance and commitment therapy approach to mindfulness in psychotherapy*. New Harbinger Publications, Inc.

Chapter 15
Using Acceptance and Commitment Therapy Within a Functional Analysis Informed Therapy for Hearing Voices

Neil Thomas and Kim Morris

Auditory verbal hallucinations, commonly referred to as hearing voices, can occur as a persisting experience in a range of populations. Since the twentieth century, voice hearing has been most closely associated with schizophrenia (McCarthy-Jones, 2012), with particular forms of voice hearing being included among Schneider's influential first-rank symptoms proposed to define the syndrome. However, it has become increasingly apparent that persisting voice hearing experiences are encountered in a range of clinical populations, including being relatively common in the diagnostic groups of bipolar, major depression, borderline personality disorder, and PTSD, suggesting relevance as a transdiagnostic phenomenon (Larøi et al., 2012). Indeed, across these groups, the phenomenology of hearing voices is remarkably similar (Waters & Fernyhough, 2017). Experiences of voice hearing are also reported by a number of people with no mental health needs (Beavan et al., 2011; Johns et al., 2014), and may be considered a normative experience in some cultural groups (Larøi et al., 2014). This has given rise to contemporary conceptualisations of hearing voices as part of the spectrum of human experience, rather than as the manifestation of particular disease processes (Johns et al., 2014).

Nonetheless, hearing voices is an experience with which people often struggle. Whilst hallucinatory experiences vary from person to person, hallucination is, by definition, an experience that is as vividly real as a true perception, is experienced as uncontrollable and seems to have a life of its own (Slade & Bentall, 1988). People usually hear voices saying things related to themselves or what they are doing, typically in the form of voices talking to the hearer, or about them (McCarthy-Jones et al., 2014; Nayani & David, 1996). Whilst neutral content such as running commentary is characteristic for some people, negatively valanced content is most

N. Thomas (✉) · K. Morris
Swinburne University of Technology, Melbourne, Australia
e-mail: neilthomas@swin.edu.au

J. A. Díaz-Garrido et al. (eds.), *Psychological Interventions for Psychosis*,
https://doi.org/10.1007/978-3-031-27003-1_15

typical, with voices very often involving hearing criticism, threats to harm the person or others, or commands often to do harmful things (Larøi et al., 2019; Nayani & David, 1996; McCarthy-Jones et al., 2014).

15.1 Psychological Therapies for Hearing Voices

Understandably, hearing voices can be experienced as a highly distressing and distracting experience, and, as such, psychological therapies may have an important role in helping reduce the impact of hearing voices on distress and day-to-day functioning. The most established psychological treatment approach used for hearing voices is the broader intervention model of cognitive behavioural therapy for psychosis (CBTp). CBTp has been extensively studied in randomised controlled trials, typically with persisting positive symptoms including hallucinations, alongside delusions, as a target (van der Gaag et al., 2014). This trial evidence has led to it being widely recommended for people with psychotic disorders and experiences in clinical practice guidelines (e.g. National Institute of Clinical Excellence, 2010; Kreyenbuhl et al., 2010; Royal Australian and New Zealand College of Psychiatrists, 2015). Commonly used CBTp methods applied to hearing voices include enhancing coping strategies (Hayward et al., 2018), and cognitive restructuring of distress-related appraisals about the experience. These can include threat appraisals such as about losing control (Morrison, 1998, 2001), or reflect beliefs held about the person or entity from which the voices are arising (Chadwick & Birchwood, 1994). Chadwick and Birchwood (1994) highlighted that people typically regarded the voices being spoken by real others, holding extraordinary power over the individual, often with malevolent intentions, and proposed such beliefs drive voice-related distress. Hence beliefs about the extent of voice power, and control that the person has over the experience, are a particular target of cognitive restructuring in CBTp applied to voices.

As psychotherapeutic methods have progressed, there has been a range of further psychological interventions applied to help people who hear voices (Thomas et al., 2014). Whilst sometimes presented as alternative models, these are often intended as specialised components of broader therapy, and therefore compatible with a broader CBTp framework (e.g. competitive memory training, van de Gaag et al., 2012; exposure-based methods for associated trauma memories, Paulik et al., 2019; Brand et al., 2021). One notable trend has been a group of therapies that work with the experience that people have of the voices as agents or entities with whom they relate interpersonally (e.g. Craig et al., 2018; Hayward et al., 2014, 2017; Leff et al., 2013; Longden et al., 2021). A further major trend has been the third wave, or "acceptance and mindfulness-based," approaches, which we consider in more detail.

15.2 Acceptance and Mindfulness-Based Approaches

Third-wave approaches applied to hearing voices and/or psychotic experiences and include mindfulness programs (e.g. Böge et al., 2021; Chadwick et al., 2016; Louise et al., 2019; Strauss et al., 2015), acceptance and commitment therapy (ACT; e.g. Bach & Hayes, 2002; Gaudiano & Herbert, 2006; Shawyer et al., 2012, 2013; Thomas et al., 2013) and compassion-focused therapy (e.g. Braehler et al., 2013; Heriot-Maitland et al., 2019). These approaches share a common focus on changing clients' relationship, or patterns of interaction, with thoughts and their broader internal experience. This contrasts with modifying the content of thoughts and beliefs, as in cognitive therapy. Hence, applied to voices, rather than disputing what voices say, or modifying explanatory beliefs about voices, these approaches primarily aim to help the person to be less fused with, preoccupied with, and/or reactive to these experiences (Thomas, 2014, 2015).

ACT is one of the most widely studied of these approaches. A very simplified account of the theoretical basis of ACT is that, due to our evolved internalisation of language as verbal thought, much of our conscious experience occurs in relation to internal representations of events. Thus, imagining a feared catastrophe can elicit anxiety, thinking about a loss can elicit sadness, and dwelling upon past failures can generate shame. It is our interactions with these internal representations where human psychopathologies tend to arise (Hayes et al., 1999). In particular, we often engage in attempts to distract from or suppress these internal representations, which, due to their uncontrollability, can give rise to struggle which intensifies distress. We may also engage in broader forms of experiential avoidance that may narrow our range of experience and dominate our behaviour.

In relation to this, hearing voices is a notable experience in that it reflects a manifestation of internalised verbal representations, yet is experienced as a stimulus arising from, and often located in, external space. Thomas et al. (2013) conceptualised three layers of impact of the experience of voice hearing that may give rise to struggle. First, hearing voices is an intrusive, uncontrollable, inescapable sensory experience. This can intrude into and come to dominate awareness in ways akin to struggles with other sensory experiences such as chronic pain or tinnitus. Additionally, in the context of psychosis, the experience may be further associated with a subjective sense of being particularly salient or important which can make it particularly attention capturing.

Second, hearing voices is a verbal phenomenon, and the preponderance of negative emotional content, such as criticism, threats and harmful commands, involves the activation of broader internal representations that are personally highly salient. Third, hearing voices is typically experienced as interpersonally meaningful, experienced as if sentient others (Benjamin, 1989; Chin et al., 2009; Hayward et al., 2011). This can lead to hearers being drawn into internal dialogue with these experiences (Leudar et al., 1997), which may prolong engagement with them (Thomas, 2015). As voice content may be critical and threatening, patterns of reacting to voices with reciprocal hostility (e.g. internally shouting or swearing at voices) are particularly common (Hayward et al., 2020; Thomas et al., 2009), which may lead to increased arousal that may reinforce the experience.

Each of these layers of the experience – sensory, verbal and interpersonal – may be associated with struggle, distress and impacts on day-to-day life playing out. In the general ACT model, the antidote to struggle with aversive experience is *acceptance* – or willingness to experience things which are aversive – in combination with shifting from reactive responses to intentional behaviour in line with broader personal *values*. This is further supported by *defusion* exercises and skills, which highlight thoughts as internal representations distinct from environmental threats, and skills in engaging in *self as observer* of experiences, and awareness of the *present moment*, typically using mindfulness exercises. An array of experiential exercises and metaphors are used to support this work, such as those described in Hayes et al. (1999).

The emphasis on acceptance as an adaptive response to voices is notable as it has parallels with a principle of the Hearing Voices Movement (HVM, Corstens et al., 2014), a sociopolitical movement of people identifying as voice hearers and their supporters. The HVM was championed through early research of Romme and Escher (Romme & Escher, 1989; Romme et al., 1992) highlighting that non-clinical voice hearers typically reported accepting attitudes to the experience as being part of their life and were not distressed by the experience. This highlighted that acceptance of voices as part of one's experience may be an adaptive means of living with it, suggesting that this approach may have value to people with distressing voices as an alternative to the traditional paradigm of seeking to eliminate voices as a pathological symptom. Consequently, within the HVM, many people have accounts of learning to live with their voices adaptively by moving from attempts to get rid of voices to turning towards and exploring the experience (Corstens et al., 2014).

A challenge, however, is that the hostile negative voices that are most common in clinical populations are difficult for people to find ways to accept, and this is where the skills in acceptance and mindfulness-based therapies may be facilitative. Following the first applications to psychosis by Bach and Hayes (2002), our group in Melbourne has had an interest in developing and trialling (Shawyer et al., 2012, 2017) these approaches for helping people who hear voices, with an ACT protocol for voices summarised by Thomas et al. (2013).

15.3 An Integrative Therapeutic Framework for Hearing Voices

We have run a specialist voices clinic since 2006 offering psychological therapies to people who hear voices (Thomas et al., 2010; Paulik et al., 2020). In providing a specialist service we have a need to consider research evidence in combination with emerging innovations in practice, and, in particular, how to navigate an expanding array of therapeutic approaches. Whilst CBTp is best evidenced and has provided a useful overall model for practice with psychosis, specific elements for voices are less thoroughly operationalised, particularly if considering voices as a transdiagnostic phenomenon. Indeed, clinical experience in the Voices Clinic was that the best-operationalised cognitive targets for voices, such as perceived voice power, seemed to be the main source of distress for only some clients. In fact, many clients seen in the clinic were very insightful about their experiences, so much of the "psychosis"-focused cognitive work on developing alternative explanatory models has less well-aligned applicability. Many clients would say that they know the voices are being created by their minds, but they still find them intensely distressing. This suggests the potential for approaches with less emphasis on cognitive change. However, meta-analyses of other approaches (e.g. acceptance and mindfulness-based therapies, Louise et al., 2018; trauma-focused therapies, Brand et al., 2018) have not reported average effect sizes superior to those reported for CBTp. Indeed, experience in the clinic is that there is much individual variation in the applicability of most therapeutic approaches.

The development of therapeutic approaches that extend beyond the original CBTp model, but have a much less mature level of supportive evidence, suggests potential value in an integrative therapeutic framework that can flexibly accommodate innovations when working with hearing voices.

To do this, we have adopted a therapeutic model grounded in behaviour therapy – hence being consistent with both CBTp and third-wave therapies – which uses individual behavioural formulation to tailor therapy to the individual. This allows for the incorporation of broader therapeutic methods such as those from ACT. Heavily influenced by an early proto-CBTp approach developed by Tarrier (1992; Tarrier et al., 1990, 1993, 1998), the "Functional Analysis Informed Therapy for Hallucinations" (FAITH) model that we use in the Voices Clinic involves developing an individualised formulation of the patterns of antecedents and responses to episodes of hearing voices. The therapist seeks to understand variability in the experience, such as the onset and persistence of intermittently occurring hallucinations, and periods of increased (or decreased) intensity or distress associated with more continuous hallucinations. This draws on literature finding meaningful patterns of variation in hearing voices in response to identifiable antecedents such as noise levels, environmental stress, arousal, worry, rumination, and engagement in activity (Bell et al., 2022). It also draws on literature examining responses to hearing voices, including observations of meaningful but often inefficient engagement in coping strategies (Farhall et al., 2007), and tendencies to be drawn into hostile dialogue or relating to voices (Leudar et al., 1997; Thomas et al., 2009).

Because patterns of antecedents and response to this experience can vary substantially from person to person, therapy involves a collaborative process of developing individual formulation, or functional analysis, of experiences, used to consider potential ways to break out of unhelpful patterns that maintain distressing voice-hearing episodes. This is done on an ongoing basis as a focus of sessions to formulate recent episodes of hearing voices and identify potential exit points, similar to the chain analysis method used in dialectical behaviour therapy. This may be used both to problem-solve periods of especially challenging voices and to learn from episodes of voice hearing that had been dealt with well. Through this, the clients' adaptive behaviours are identified and applied more systematically, and new self-management behaviours are introduced as indicated. As well as incorporating preventative and coping strategies, this might include cognitive strategies ("what could you tell yourself?"), mindful responding, defusion, or practice of alternative ways of interacting with voices. In the session, exercises are used as much as possible. Over time the aim is to give the client a strong familiarity with the patterns occurring with their own voices, to know how to avert periods of escalating voice intensity and distress, and build up habitual ways of responding to voices that allow the person to live with hearing voices without it dominating their conscious experience and day-to-day lives.

15.4 Case Study – Chris

To illustrate the integration of ACT methods within a broader functional analysis model, we present a case description of therapy provided by the Voices Clinic to a client we refer to as Chris, who was seen over a course of 18 one-to-one sessions. Chris was a man in his early 20 s who had been experiencing persistent auditory verbal hallucinations for approximately 2 years prior to coming to the Voices Clinic. He primarily heard a single voice, which was male, older, of moderate loudness, and heard continually. The content was almost exclusively derogatory in nature, with occasional directive commanding content. Chris described the voice as "like a grandfather," stern, authoritative, and demanding high standards of achievement. He described the voice making bullying comments such as "you're not good enough…" or "you're not going to be able to do this well." The voice would also encourage suicide or behaviour with negative outcomes such as excessive alcohol consumption. Chris reported experiencing extreme distress associated with these experiences.

At the point of presentation, Chris had withdrawn from his apprenticeship and was not working, he had also parted from his long-term girlfriend and was finding it challenging to socialise. When at its worst, he described being very much "drawn into" the experience of the voice and withdrawing from the external environment. Prior to hearing voices for the first time, Chris had been playing sport at a high level which was no longer possible due to a significant injury. His participation in sport had involved daily training as well as competition, and he had described this as a significant part of his social life and identity. The loss of this resulted in a dramatic readjustment of how he spent his time.

Therapy commenced at the Voices Clinic using the FAITH framework. As Chris experienced hearing voices on a continuous basis, the functional analysis focused on the exploration of when voice content was noticeably more derogatory, loud, or escalated in any way, and/or when he was most distressed. During the first few sessions, multiple situations in which the voice was louder or more derogatory were identified. These included when socialising with friends, when undertaking a task that he wanted to achieve well and when trying to sleep. Further discussion revealed that these situations usually involved increased anxiety for Chris. This anxiety was fuelled by various factors such as feeling self-conscious or unsure of himself, feelings of guilt and failure associated with high standards of achievement, and rumination when trying to sleep. Anxiety in the social context became an issue for Chris partly due to a loss of social identity that had been enmeshed with his identity as a successful sportsperson. Chris also noted that his tendency to aspire to extremely high standards of achievement was, at least in part, fostered in the sporting environment. He had lost a significant source of validation and direction.

Chris also experienced voice content that would incite paranoid thoughts about being watched or talked about negatively by others. Antecedents for this type of voice content were situations such as walking in public or speaking to someone unfamiliar, for example, asking a question to a shop attendant. Similar to antecedents of escalating derogatory voice content, these circumstances also involved increased anxiety for Chris. These factors were drawn out in two overarching models of his difficulties with voices, illustrated in Fig. 15.1.

In addition to the responses included in these models, Chris would at times argue with or challenge the voice in an attempt to alleviate the distress from the experience. This approach tended to result in an escalation of the voice: Chris noted that the voice would get louder and angrier when challenged and if he tried to ignore the voice it would become very persistent and repetitive. If he asked questions such as "why are you saying this?," the voice would become annoyed that it was being questioned and either assert its authority or ignore Chris's questions.

Throughout the process of developing this shared formulation, Chris's personal conceptualisation of the voice content began to take shape. He noted that "sometimes he says he is helping me," and the voice "stems from my anxiety," observing that it reflected his worries but in a very exaggerated and severe way. Due to the central involvement of anxiety in Chris's voice-hearing experience, strategies for

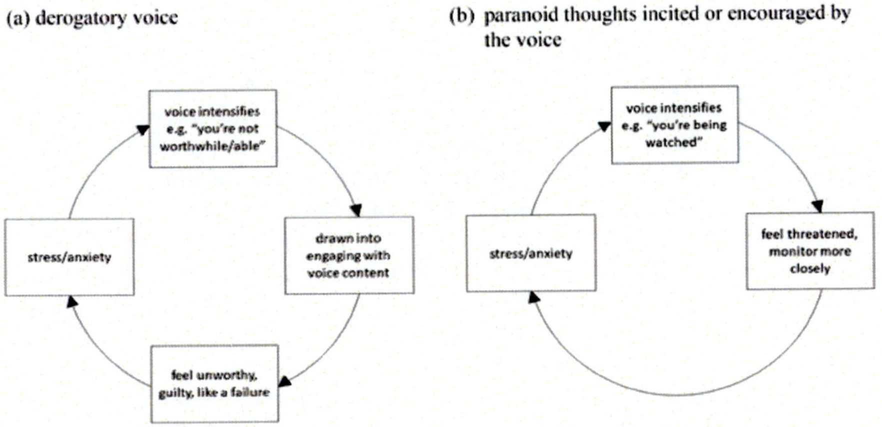

Fig. 15.1 Models of escalation of voice episodes informed by functional analysis. (**a**) Derogatory voice (**b**) Paranoid thoughts incited or encouraged by the voice

managing anxiety were a primary focus throughout sessions. This included psychoeducation about anxiety, identification of strategies for relaxation and reinforcement of regular practice of strategies. In addition to this, once chain analysis was completed for specific incidents of escalated voice hearing, time was spent collaboratively identifying "exits" from the spiral of anxiety and escalation. Some of the "exits" that Chris identified were changing what he was doing, engaging in a breathing exercise, having a shower, and exercising.

As Chris reported back about how he was going with putting into practice the strategies and "exits," an implementation challenge began to emerge. It became evident that strategies which could be viewed as achieved either successfully or not, would increase anxiety and the voice would escalate. For example, when Chris would attempt a breathing exercise with the goal of reducing anxiety, he would feel as though he had failed the exercise if he did not feel any relief from anxiety and the voice's derogatory commentary continued, which would, in turn, increase anxiety further. Imagery exercises were attempted; however, these also had the potential to backfire. When unable to conjure the suggested images, Chris would feel as though he were failing at the task and the voice would begin to interfere with comments about not doing it properly. For example, when attempting a "leaves on a stream" mindfulness exercise, Chris found that the leaves would not float down the stream but would stay still and stuck which would be commented on by the voice and thereby increase anxiety and feelings of failure.

In reviewing these patterns with Chris, we identified that focusing on trying to control the experience of hearing voices was becoming part of the cycles that were maintaining a struggle with hearing voices. We thought with Chris about considering finding an alternative way of responding to voices, paving the way for the integration of ACT methods. This concept was introduced to Chris using a "tug of war with a monster" metaphor (described in Thomas et al., 2013), where the option of "dropping the rope" was regularly reinforced as an alternative approach.

Values-focused work elicited values including maintaining strong positive relationships with friends and family, and hard work. Chris was already actively pursuing these values, however, with a significant level of distress. At this stage, Chris had started working with his father a few days a week, and he described "pushing through" despite often having significant anxiety and intense and derogatory commentary by the voice. This occurred both on the way to work and throughout the day. Chris also continued to spend time with friends on the weekends and work on his hobby of making furniture despite knowing that such activities would likely exacerbate his voice and anxiety. Identifying and discussing values allowed the goal to be redefined as moving towards what he wants in life despite the voice rather than trying to improve or reduce the experience of the voice. Although not explicitly stated this shift in goal was intended to assist with reducing the struggle with anxiety and the voice. It also created space for Chris to be proud of his achievements in areas he valued despite having to do so under distressing circumstances.

Defusion was introduced at this stage with the hope that, with practice, it would help reduce problematic engagement with the voice. Chris had reported a tendency to engage with the voice in his thoughts which had caused difficulty with concentration and could lead to escalation of the voice and anxiety. The concept of "bad news radio" was introduced as a way to refer to the voices, which fit with Chris's conceptualisation of the voice as an exaggerated and unhelpful reflection of his anxiety. This metaphor was utilised to encourage Chris to allow the voice to play on in the background while he continued with other valued endeavours.

Imagery methods for assisting with the understanding of defusion tended to be problematic due to the voice content interfering and undermining Chris's attempts to focus and grasp the concept. Therefore, helping to develop Chris's understanding of defusion was achieved over time via metaphors, diagrams, and discussion. The idea of observer-self and thinking-self was introduced and initially, Chris tended to liken the observer-self to observing work he was doing and struggled to differentiate between the observer-self and the thinking-self. Without the aid of mindfulness visualisation exercises, defusion proved difficult to grasp, however over time Chris's understanding began to develop. This was achieved by various methods such as visual aids including a cartoon diagram showing thoughts as separate from the self, Titchener's repetition (e.g. "lemon, lemon, lemon..."), and conceptualisation of thoughts as "just words" prior to meaning and emotion being attached to them. These concepts were described often in relation to "thoughts," but it was regularly reinforced that they could extend to voice content, and thoughts and voice content were at times discussed interchangeably.

Metaphors were often integrated with the functional analytic formulation that was developed during earlier sessions. For example, Chris had a hobby of furniture building and had previously enjoyed seeing his work take shape. Unfortunately, his ability to enjoy his work was increasingly sabotaged by the voice which would criticise and make comments about him and his work not being good enough. Chris had developed an understanding that in circumstances involving an element of achievement, internalised high standards would exacerbate the voice's derogatory content. This awareness allowed him to improve on his ability to take a "step back" from these comments and reconceptualise as "bad news radio."

Once it became clear that Chris's understanding of defusion had developed well, the concept of "choice points" and becoming "hooked" by thoughts, feelings or the voice was introduced. This became a common way for the discussion to be framed, particularly when discussing events that occurred between sessions and were often helped with the visual aid of a choice point diagram. Chris developed skills in identifying his choice points and both utilising strategies identified during functional analysis and recruiting his observer-self to help get himself "unhooked." It was noted that becoming hooked by anxiety or the voice would usually involve becoming stuck in a spiralling situation as described by the functional analysis models in Fig. 15.1. At this point, Chris had reported that he wished to reconcile with his ex-girlfriend but was very anxious about how this might go. Increased anxiety in association with new experiences and changing circumstances was regularly normalised during sessions. Work then focussed on "making room" for anxiety and practicing becoming "unhooked" from anxiety. Again, without the aid of visualisation such as the ACT "expansion" exercise, this was achieved by other methods. The concept of "leaning into" the anxiety and allowing it to be there while he continues with what is important to him, was frequently promoted. Chris was also encouraged to take inventory of the physical sensations of anxiety like a "curious scientist". The goal of this activity was to reduce fear of the feeling of anxiety and assist with creating distance or "unhooking" from it. There was also frequent discussion about how the feeling could exist at the same time as Chris could continue to do something he valued. There were some hiccups with the practice of "leaning into" anxiety, and it was identified that during this practice, Chris was hoping the anxiety would reduce. It was important to regularly reinforce that the goal was simply to be curious and approach with an exploratory attitude.

Chris was a very driven individual and working from a values-oriented perspective seemed to suit him well. He had strongly held values in relation to positive relationships with friends and family and achievement in work and leisure. During the early stages of his treatment at the Voices Clinic, Chris had already started to re-engage with some of these areas of life including spending time with friends and starting work, which he persisted with, despite often tolerating high to extreme levels of anxiety and distress associated with voice hearing. Chris was fortunate to live with his family whom he described as very supportive and encouraging which assisted him to stay engaged with his values and associated goals. The therapeutic goal of sessions with the Voices Clinic was primarily distress reduction and gently assisting him to shift focus from fixing the problem (making the voice stop) to pursuing a meaningful and fulfilling life despite the voice. Sessions included regular discussion of the previous week's events and associated challenges, which were informed by the functional analytic formulation, with the focus driven by his values.

Towards the end of sessions with the Voices Clinic, Chris described having arrived at a point of knowing the voice would be there but having decided to "move on" and "take action" anyway. His ability to disengage from the previous problematic spirals of anxiety and escalating voice causing increasing anxiety was becoming easier and more habitual. Whilst the voice remained present, he referred to it as not being "too bad". At this point, he had begun a full-time apprenticeship with his father's business, he had reconciled with his ex-girlfriend, was exercising regularly, and frequently spending time with friends. Reengaging with these valued areas of life, presumably increased Chris's sense of achievement and self-esteem, which likely also assisted with reducing anxiety. By the final session with the Voices Clinic, Chris reported that he felt equipped and enthusiastic about continuing his recovery on his own and getting on with life.

15.5 Discussion

This case study illustrates the potential for ACT methods to be integrated within an individualised formulation-based therapy for hearing voices. ACT methods were particularly indicated in this case because of the behavioural repertoire of attempting to control the experience of hearing voices operated as part of the maintaining cycle, which made a simple self-management or coping enhancement approach difficult to effect change. Whilst behaviours that Chris could engage in that would help to reduce voice-related distress were identified, the intention behind their application required a different framing in order to be effective, which was supported by the experiential exercises on acceptance, defusion and values. This enabled him to use the strategies that had been discussed earlier in therapy and do so without being drawn into a cycle of unsuccessfully trying to forcibly suppress either the voices or related anxiety, which appeared to exacerbate the overall problem. In this way, ACT methods were supportive of the overall therapeutic approach, and enabled progress that appeared otherwise difficult to achieve.

A question arising is whether a pure ACT approach from the outset would have been equally successful. Whilst we do not know how therapy would have progressed in this case, the work on shared formulation provided the opportunity for socialisation into a shared understanding of how patterns of voices were being maintained, providing a rationale for exploring alternative ways of responding to them. This may be supportive of establishing a stronger therapeutic alliance, and stronger buy-in to the application of methods that are a significant shift from existing ways of coping. Qualitative data from a randomised controlled trial of a focused one-to-one ACT intervention for persisting positive symptoms (Shawyer et al., 2017) was that clients sometimes felt a disconnect between ACT exercises and their own experiences (Bacon et al., 2012). Anecdotal therapist experience from that trial was also that ACT could be confronting for many participants by threatening an established equilibrium of just getting by. We speculate that additional time on building a shared formulation may be important groundwork that enables a rationale for adopting a different approach to be developed, allowing ACT methods to be used more effectively.

Finally, the use of ACT within a functional analytic framework enables integration with a broader behavioural therapeutic model. This offers a coherent approach to clients for presentation of different therapeutic methods that allow for individualisation of therapeutic approach, beyond less voice-specific CBTp models, whilst also grounding the overall intervention in an empirically-supported framework that offers a balance between evidence-based practice and individualisation of therapy.

Disclaimer Clinical cases presented in this chapter do not include real names or personal information of real persons.

References

Bach, P., & Hayes, S. C. (2002). The use of acceptance and commitment therapy to prevent the rehospitalization of psychotic patients: A randomized controlled trial. *Journal of Consulting and Clinical Psychology, 70*, 1129–1139.

Beavan, V., Read, J., & Cartwright, C. (2011). The prevalence of voice-hearers in the general population: A literature review. *Journal of Mental Health, 20*, 281–292.

Bell, I. H., Cartner, S., & Thomas, N. (2022). *Examining predictors of fluctuations in hallucinations using ecological momentary assessment: Systematic review*. Manuscript submitted for publication.

Benjamin, L. S. (1989). Is chronicity a function of the relationship between the person and the auditory hallucination? *Schizophrenia Bulletin, 15*, 291–310.

Böge, K., Hahne, I., Bergmann, N., Wingenfeld, K., Zierhut, M., Thomas, N., et al. (2021). Mindfulness-based group therapy for in-patients with schizophrenia spectrum disorders: Feasibility, acceptability, and preliminary outcomes of a rater-blinded randomized controlled trial. *Schizophrenia Research, 228*, 134–144. https://doi.org/10.1016/j.schres.2020.12.008

Braehler, C., Gumley, A., Harper, J., Wallace, S., Norrie, J., & Gilbert, P. (2013). Exploring change processes in compassion focused therapy in psychosis: Results of a feasibility randomized controlled trial. *British Journal of Clinical Psychology, 52*, 199–214. https://doi.org/10.1111/bjc.12009

Brand, R., McEnery, C., Bendall, S., Rossell, S. L., & Thomas, N. (2018). Do trauma-focused psychological interventions have an effect on psychotic symptoms? A systematic review and meta-analysis. *Schizophrenia Research, 195*, 13–22. https://doi.org/10.1016/j.schres.2017.08.037

Brand, R., Bendall, S., Hardy, A., Rossell, S. L., & Thomas, N. (2021). Trauma-focused imaginal exposure for auditory hallucinations: A case series. *Psychology and Psychotherapy: Theory, Research and Practice, 94*, 408–425. https://doi.org/10.1111/papt.12284

Chadwick, P., & Birchwood, M. (1994). The omnipotence of voices: A cognitive approach to auditory hallucinations. *British Journal of Psychiatry, 164*, 190–201.

Chadwick, P., Strauss, C., Jones, A. M., Kingdon, D., Ellett, L., Dannahy, L., & Hayward, M. (2016). Group mindfulness-based intervention for distressing voices: A pragmatic randomised controlled trial. *Schizophrenia Research, 175*, 168–173. https://doi.org/10.1016/j.schres.2016.04.001

Chin, J. T., Hayward, M., & Drinnan, A. (2009). "Relating" to voices: Exploring the relevance of this concept to people who hear voices. *Psychology and Psychotherapy, 82*, 1–17.

Corstens, D., Longden, E., McCarthy-Jones, S., Waddingham, R., & Thomas, N. (2014). Emerging perspectives from the hearing voices movement: Implications for therapeutic and research practice. *Schizophrenia Bulletin, 40*(Suppl. 4), s285–s294. https://doi.org/10.1093/schbul/sbu007

Craig, T. K., Rus-Calafell, M., Ward, T., Leff, J. P., Huckvale, M., Howarth, E., et al. (2018). AVATAR therapy for auditory verbal hallucinations in people with psychosis: A single-blind, randomised controlled trial. *Lancet Psychiatry, 5*, 31–40.

Farhall, J., Greenwood, K. M., & Jackson, H. J. (2007). Coping with hallucinated voices in schizophrenia: A review of self-initiated strategies and therapeutic interventions. *Clinical Psychology Review, 27*, 476–493. https://doi.org/10.1016/j.cpr.2006.12.002

Gaudiano, B. A., & Herbert, J. D. (2006). Acute treatment of inpatients with psychotic symptoms using acceptance and commitment therapy: Pilot results. *Behaviour Research and Therapy, 44*, 415–437.

Hayes, S. C., Strosahl, K. D., & Wilson, K. G. (1999). *Acceptance and commitment therapy: An experiential approach to behavior change*. Guilford Press.

Hayward, M., Berry, K., & Ashton, A. (2011). Applying interpersonal theories to the understating of and therapy for auditory hallucinations: A review of the literature and directions for further research. *Clinical Psychology Review, 31*, 1313–1323.

Hayward, M., Berry, K., McCarthy-Jones, S., Strauss, C., & Thomas, N. (2014). Beyond the omnipotence of voices: Further developing a relational approach to hearing voices. *Psychosis, 6*, 242–252. https://doi.org/10.1080/17522439.2013.839735

Hayward, M., Jones, A. M., Bogen-Johnston, L., Thomas, N., & Strauss, C. (2017). Relating therapy for distressing voices: A pilot randomized controlled trial. *Schizophrenia Research, 183*, 137–142. https://doi.org/10.1016/j.schres.2016.11.019

Hayward, M., Jones, A. M., Berry, C., & Strauss, C. (2018). Brief coping strategy enhancement for distressing voices: An evaluation in routine clinical practice. *Behavioural and Cognitive Psychotherapy, 46*, 226–237.

Hayward, M., Schlier, B., Strauss, C., Rammou, A., & Lincoln, T. (2020). Construction and validation of the approve questionnairs: Measures of relating to voices and other people. *Schizophrenia Research, 220*, 254–260. https://doi.org/10.1016/j.schres.2020.03.003

Heriot-Maitland, C., McCarthy-Jones, S., Longden, E., & Gilbert, P. (2019). Compassion focused approaches to working with distressing voices. *Frontiers in Psychology, 10*, Article 152. https://doi.org/10.3389/fpsyg.2019.00152

Johns, L. C., Kompus, K., Connell, M., Humpston, C., Lincoln, T. M., Longden, E., et al. (2014). Auditory verbal hallucinations in persons with and without a need for care. *Schizophrenia Bulletin, 40*(Suppl 4), S255–S264.

Kreyenbuhl, J., Buchanan, R. W., Dickerson, F. B., Dixon, L. B., & Schizophrenia Patient Outcomes Research Team (PORT). (2010). The Schizophrenia Patient Outcomes Research Team (PORT): Updated treatment recommendations 2009. *Schizophrenia Bulletin, 36*, 94–103. https://doi.org/10.1093/schbul/sbp130

Larøi, F., Sommer, I. E., Blom, J. D., Fernyhough, C., Hugdahl, K., Johns, L. C., et al. (2012). The characteristic features of auditory verbal hallucinations in clinical and nonclinical groups: State-of-the-art overview and future directions. *Schizophrenia Bulletin, 38*, 724–733.

Larøi, F., Luhrmann, T. M., Bell, V., Christian, W. A., Deshpande, S., Fernyhough, C., et al. (2014). Culture and hallucinations: Overview and future directions. *Schizophrenia Bulletin, 40*(Suppl. 4), S213–S220. https://doi.org/10.1093/schbul/sbu012

Larøi, F., Thomas, N., Aleman, A., Fernyhough, C., Deamer, F., & McCarthy-Jones, S. (2019). The ice in voices: Understanding negative content in auditory verbal hallucinations. *Clinical Psychology Review, 67*, 1–10. https://doi.org/10.1016/j.cpr.2018.11.001

Leff, J., Williams, G., Huckvale, M., Arbuthnot, M., & Leff, A. (2013). Computer-assisted therapy for medication-resistant auditory hallucinations: Proof-of-concept study. *British Journal of Psychiatry, 202*, 428–433.

Leuder, I., Thomas, P., McNally, D., & Glinski, A. (1997). What voices can do with words: Pragmatics of hallucinations. *Psychological Medicine, 27*, 885–898. https://doi.org/10.1017/s0033291797005138

Longden, E., Corstens, D., Morrison, A. P., Larkin, A., Murphy, E., Holden, N., et al. (2021). A treatment protocol to guide the delivery of dialogical engagement with auditory hallucinations: Experience from the talking with voices pilot trial. *Psychology and Psychotherapy, 94*, 558–572. https://doi.org/10.1111/papt.12331

Louise, S., Fitzpatrick, M., Strauss, C., Rossell, S. L., & Thomas, N. (2018). Mindfulness- and acceptance-based interventions for psychosis: Our current understanding and a meta-analysis. *Schizophrenia Research, 192*, 57–63. https://doi.org/10.1016/j.schres.2017.05.023

Louise, S., Rossell, S. L., & Thomas, N. (2019). The acceptability, feasibility and preliminary outcomes of an individual mindfulness intervention for hearing voices. *Behavioural and Cognitive Psychotherapy, 47*, 200–216. https://doi.org/10.1017/S1352465818000425

McCarthy-Jones, S. (2012). *Hearing voices: The histories, causes and meanings of auditory verbal hallucinations*. Cambridge University Press.

McCarthy-Jones, S., Trauer, T., Mackinnon, A., Sims, E., Thomas, N., & Copolov, D. (2014). A new phenomenological survey of auditory verbal hallucinations: Evidence for subtypes and implications for theory and practice. *Schizophrenia Bulletin, 40*, 231–235. https://doi.org/10.1093/schbul/sbs156

Morrison, A. P. (1998). A cognitive analysis of the maintenance of auditory hallucinations: Are voices to schizophrenia what bodily sensations are to panic? *Behavioural and Cognitive Psychotherapy, 26*, 289–302.

Morrison, A. P. (2001). The interpretation of intrusions in psychosis: An integrative cognitive approach to hallucinations and delusions. *Behavioural and Cognitive Psychotherapy, 29*, 257–276.

National Institute for Health and Clinical Excellence. (2010). *Core interventions in the treatment and management of schizophrenia in adults in primary and secondary care* (Updated ed.). British Psychological Society and Royal College of Psychiatrists.

Nayani, T., & David, A. (1996). The auditory hallucination: A phenomenological survey. *Psychological Medicine, 26*, 177–189.

Paulik, G., Steel, C., & Arntz, A. (2019). Imagery rescripting for the treatment of trauma in voice hearers: A case series. *Behavioural and Cognitive Psychotherapy, 47*, 709–725. https://doi.org/10.1017/S1352465819000237

Paulik, G., Thomas, N., Glasshouse, E., & Hayward, M. (2020). Being a scientist-practitioner in the field of psychosis: Experiences from voices clinics. In J. Badcock & G. Paulik (Eds.), *A clinical introduction to psychosis: Foundations for clinical psychologists and neuropsychologists* (pp. 615–636). Academic. https://doi.org/10.1016/B978-0-12-815012-2.00026-2

Romme, M. A. J., & Escher, S. D. (1989). Hearing voices. *Schizophrenia Bulletin, 15*, 209–216.

Romme, M. A. J., Honig, A., Noorthoorn, E. O., & Escher, S. D. (1992). Coping with hearing voices: An emancipatory approach. *British Journal of Psychiatry, 161*, 99–103.

Shawyer, F., Farhall, J., Mackinnon, A., Ratcliffe, K., Sims, E., Johnson, L., et al. (2012). A randomised controlled trial of acceptance-based cognitive behavioural therapy for command hallucinations in psychotic disorders. *Behaviour Research and Therapy, 50*, 110–121. https://doi.org/10.1016/j.brat.2011.11.007

Shawyer, F., Thomas, N., Morris, E. M. J., & Farhall, J. (2013). Theory on voices. In E. M. J. Morris, L. C. Johns, & J. E. Oliver (Eds.), *Acceptance and commitment therapy and mindfulness for psychosis* (pp. 12–32). Wiley. https://doi.org/10.1002/9781118499184.ch2

Shawyer, F., Farhall, J., Thomas, N., Hayes, S. C., Gallop, B., Copolov, D., & Castle, D. (2017). Acceptance and commitment therapy for psychosis: Randomised controlled trial. *British Journal of Psychiatry, 210*, 140–148. https://doi.org/10.1192/bjp.bp.116.182865

Slade, P., & Bentall, R. (1988). *Sensory deception: A scientific analysis of hallucination*. Johns Hopkins University Press.

Strauss, C., Thomas, N., & Hayward, M. (2015). Can we respond mindfully to distressing voices? A systematic review of the evidence for engagement, acceptability, effectiveness and mechanisms of change for mindfulness-based interventions for people distressed by hearing voices. *Frontiers in Psychology, 6*, Article 1154. https://doi.org/10.3389/fpsyg.2015.01154

Tarrier, N. (1992). Management and modification of residual positive psychotic symptoms. In M. Birchwood & N. Tarrier (Eds.), *Innovations in the psychological management of schizophrenia: Assessment, treatment and services* (pp. 147–169). Wiley.

Tarrier, N., Harwood, S., Yusopoff, L., Beckett, R., & Baker, A. (1990). Coping strategy enhancement (CSE): A method of treating residual schizophrenic symptoms. *Behavioural Psychotherapy, 18*, 283–293.

Tarrier, N., Beckett, R., Harwood, S., Baker, A., Yusupoff, L., & Ugarteburu, I. (1993). A trial of two cognitive-behavioural methods of treating drug-resistant residual psychotic symptoms in schizophrenic patients: I. Outcome. *British Journal of Psychiatry, 162*, 524–532.

Tarrier, N., Yusupoff, L., Kinney, C., McCarthy, E., Gledhill, A., Haddock, G., & Morris, J. (1998). Randomised controlled trial of intensive cognitive behaviour therapy for patients with chronic schizophrenia. *British Medical Journal, 317*(7154), 303–307.

Thomas, N. (2015). A model for the development of acceptance and mindfulness–based therapies: Preoccupation with psychotic experiences as a treatment target. In B. Gaudiano (Ed.), *Incorporating acceptance and mindfulness into the treatment of psychosis: Current trends and future directions*. Oxford University Press.

Thomas, N., McLeod, H. J. & Brewin, C. R. (2009). Interpersonal complementarity in responses to auditory hallucinations in psychosis. *British Journal of Clinical Psychology, 48*, 411–424. https://doi.org/10.1348/014466509X411937

Thomas, N., Rossell, S., Farhall, J., Shawyer, F., & Castle, D. (2010). Cognitive behavioural therapy for auditory hallucinations: Effectiveness and predictors of outcome in a specialist clinic. *Behavioural and Cognitive Psychotherapy, 39*, 129–138.

Thomas, N., Morris, E. M. J., Shawyer, F., & Farhall, J. (2013). Acceptance and commitment therapy for voices. In E. M. J. Morris, L. C. Johns, & J. E. Oliver (Eds.), *Acceptance and commitment therapy and mindfulness for psychosis* (pp. 95–111). Wiley. https://doi.org/10.1002/9781118499184.ch7

Thomas, N., Hayward, M., Peters, E., van der Gaag, M., Bentall, R. P., Jenner, J. M., et al. (2014). Psychological therapies for auditory hallucinations (voices): Current status and key research directions. *Schizophrenia Bulletin, 40*(Suppl. 4), s202–s212. https://doi.org/10.1093/schbul/sbu037

van der Gaag, M., van Oosterhout, B., Daalman, K., Sommer, I. E., & Korrelboom, K. (2012). Initial evaluation of the effects of competitive memory training (COMET) on depression in schizophrenia-spectrum patients with persistent auditory verbal hallucinations: A randomized controlled trial. *British Journal of Clinical Psychology, 51*, 158–171. https://doi.org/10.1111/j.2044-8260.2011.02025.x

van der Gaag, M., Valmaggia, L. R., & Smit, F. (2014). The effects of individually tailored formulation-based cognitive behavioural therapy in auditory hallucinations and delusions: A meta-analysis. *Schizophrenia Research, 156*, 30–37. https://doi.org/10.1016/j.schres.2014.03.016

Waters, F., & Fernyhough, C. (2017). Hallucinations: A systematic review of points of similarity and difference across diagnostic classes. *Schizophrenia Bulletin, 43*, 32–43.

Chapter 16
The Use of Therapist Self-Disclosure in Acceptance and Commitment Therapy for Psychosis

Julia Nicholls, Ellie Newman, and Eric Morris

In this chapter, we will describe how therapist self-disclosure can be an important feature of the acceptance and commitment therapy (ACT) approach to supporting the recovery of people with psychosis. We will guide the reader through a brief introduction to acceptance and commitment therapy as adapted for psychosis, present an overview of therapist self-disclosure as a commonly used tool in psychotherapy, including what is known from the research literature and then discuss the purposes of therapist self-disclosure in ACT. We will illustrate these using examples, with scripts of interactions from both individual and group ACT for psychosis. Finally, we will discuss considerations in using therapist self-disclosure in ACT for psychosis.

16.1 Acceptance and Commitment Therapy

Acceptance and commitment therapy is a model of contextual intervention, identified as part of the third wave of cognitive and behavioural therapies (CBT). ACT is based on an operant learning approach to language and cognition (Relational Frame

J. Nicholls (✉)
Alfred Health, Melbourne, Australia
e-mail: julia.nicholls@alfred.org.au

E. Newman
Peninsula Health, Melbourne, Australia
e-mail: ellienewman@phcn.vic.gov.au

E. Morris
School of Psychology & Public Health, La Trobe University, Melbourne, Australia

NorthWestern Mental Health, Melbourne, Australia
e-mail: Eric.Morris@latrobe.edu.au

J. A. Díaz-Garrido et al. (eds.), *Psychological Interventions for Psychosis*,
https://doi.org/10.1007/978-3-031-27003-1_16

Theory) and is grounded in functional contextualism as a philosophical stance. This philosophy has a pragmatic approach to supporting the pursuit of meaning through actions in the service of personal goals. People engaging in ACT are encouraged to orient to personally-defined qualities of actions in the service of greater life meaning.

ACT therapists seek to strengthen skills in psychological flexibility, which is the capacity to be aware of the present moment and open to the experiences that arise, while changing or persisting in actions guided by personal values (Hayes et al., 2012). Psychological flexibility is considered a fundamental capability to support health, meaning and effectiveness: A body of evidence demonstrates that psychological flexibility is associated with greater well-being and skilled behaviour across multiple contexts in the population (Kashdan & Rottenberg, 2010) and can be considered a public health target (Gloster et al., 2017).

ACT has been researched as a trans-diagnostic and process-based model (Hofmann & Hayes, 2019), with evidence across a range of populations, problems and situations for its effectiveness and theorised processes of change (for reviews see Hayes et al., 2006; A-tjak et al., 2015; Gloster et al., 2020). People engaging in ACT are supported to develop greater psychological flexibility through practising skills in active acceptance, mindfulness, observation of thoughts and feelings, connection with personal values and commitment to meaningful behaviours across situations. The psychological flexibility skills are considered in a functional way: The form of these skills is less important, rather it is about the behavioural processes they promote, focused on transformation of functions (purposes) as an aim. Thus, ACT usually involves the client learning to approach avoided situations, experiences and people, through a transformed relationship to feelings and thoughts that previously have been barriers to action. It is typical in ACT for people to be supported to change their relationship to unwanted feelings and thoughts, through practising acceptance and openness to these experiences, in the service of doing things that matter (guided by personal values).

The ACT model emphasises experiential learning and engagement in actions that are based on chosen life directions (values). People are encouraged to consider whether their ways of coping to both their outer worlds (situations, relationships with others) and inner worlds (feelings, sensations, urges, memories, etc.) are workable, that is, are enabling contact with meaning and purpose in ways that are personally chosen. If through reflection a person finds that their ways of coping are not workable, they are encouraged to explore whether there are other ways of acting and consider what may be barriers to this. These barriers can be due to circumstances and opportunity; an important set of barriers can be when ways of responding are focused on over-control and avoidance of inner experiences (experiential avoidance) and/or rigidly guided by rules, beliefs and stories that limit responding in different ways (cognitive fusion). These psychological contexts – experiential avoidance and cognitive fusion – are considered important when engaging people in ACT, as they seem implicated in the maintenance of unhelpful and distressing ways of responding to experiences over the long term (while also being understandable and socially supported, through the language processes identified in Relational Frame Theory: Hayes et al., 2001).

Experiential learning in ACT is about encouraging the person to attend to the ways that language (rules, thoughts, narratives, how things are related together) may lead people to act in ineffective ways, to not learn from experience, or to pursue goals that make sense but do not work in practice. The ACT therapist supports the person to notice what their direct experience is showing them about how things work and to contrast this with what their mind says should happen (the mind is treated as a separate part of their experience, which can be observed). Experiential learning is enhanced in ACT through the cultivation of skills in being flexible with attention, particularly broadening attention through acceptance and openness and deliberately noticing the effects of chosen behaviours in everyday life. The person is encouraged to try a pragmatic approach to living where it is useful – noticing times when it is more useful to hold thoughts and ideas lightly, to embrace uncertainty and learn from direct experience (especially when overthinking or following rules has been found to be problematic).

The ACT model suggests that it is understandable that human beings suffer through processes that are usually hidden in language, the very capability that has allowed our species to overcome challenges, cooperate and have impact on our environment to an unprecedented degree (compared to other species). Due to our capacity to be influenced by language humans are unfortunately able to suffer in ways beyond the challenges of the current moment, being able to re-experience painful past events and to imagine feared futures. The ACT model suggests that while humans cannot free themselves of language's processes, they can become more aware of its effects and have greater capacity to choose to be less influenced by language processes where this is useful. Typically in ACT this is done through cultivating the ability to be more in the present moment, to draw attention to when language is less workable as a tool and to support learning through direct experience and openness to uncertainty. As the ACT therapist is not outside of the effects of language in their own lives, a common humanity perspective is offered, where both the therapist and the client can observe and share what it is like to both notice judgement and be aware of this as a process. In this way, it is typical for the ACT therapist to share their own experiences of what they notice during the process of therapy, as a means of modelling openness to experience, fostering connection with the client and promoting awareness of the processes of language 'in flight' during sessions.

16.1.1 ACT for Psychosis

ACT has been adapted for people with psychosis, in both individual and group forms. ACT for psychosis can address a number of needs, including relapse prevention and rehospitalisation (Bach & Hayes, 2002; Gaudiano & Herbert, 2006), depressive episodes (White et al., 2011; Gumley et al., 2017), to enhance coping with distressing positive symptoms and command hallucinations (Shawyer et al., 2012, 2017) and to foster personal recovery and quality of life (Johns et al., 2016; Jolley et al., 2020). ACT for psychosis aims to help people to respond to unusual and preoccupying psychotic experiences with flexibility, especially when this enables them to engage in actions guided by personal values. ACT is a mindfulness-based intervention (MBI), promoting an open, accepting and curious stance toward personal experiences, through the practice of present-moment awareness in various forms. Mindfulness-based interventions for psychosis have shown good signs of being efficacious: Recent meta-analyses suggest that MBIs show benefits, particularly for overall symptomatology, rehospitalisation and depressive symptoms, with indications that group interventions may be advantageous (Louise et al., 2018; Jansen et al., 2020).

The ACT model has been conceptualised for the needs of people with psychosis, while remaining fundamentally the same – there is a focus on promoting psychological flexibility and understanding where and how inflexibility impacts a person's life. The ACT therapist is oriented toward helping the person with psychosis to explore whether approaching situations with flexibility (an open, aware and active stance) helps them to engage in actions that are personally meaningful and support personal recovery. The ACT for psychosis framework promotes personal recovery in ways consistent with the CHIME model (Leamy et al., 2011): Through psychological flexibility skills, there is the promotion of connectedness, hope, identity, meaning and empowerment (Morris, 2018). This approach of engaging in guided discovery about the pragmatism of the ACT stance is key in working with people with psychosis: For reasons we discuss below, it is important for the ACT therapist to be sensitive to the ways that people with psychosis can experience alienation, stigma and invalidation.

The adaptations of the ACT approach for people with psychosis are around pace, use of language, greater sensitivity and understanding around the challenges of living with a severe mental health problem and flexibility on the therapist's part to fluctuations in client presentation. Although there is heterogeneity in the presentations and capacities of people with psychosis, there are several adaptations made to the usual way ACT is done, in order to be more engaging for people living with persisting challenges associated with serious mental health problems. Typically, this means that the ACT therapist may use simpler language, more repetition of metaphors and ideas, to engage with the client at a pace to suits them, being more flexible about the length and format of sessions and to lead experiential exercises with a more talkative style to better ensure that the client does not lose track or become overly confused (which may happen in mindfulness exercises that involve long pauses: for details, see Butler et al., 2016).

ACT therapists also need to be sensitive to the experiences of alienation, stigma and invalidation that people with psychosis can experience, particularly for those that have persisting positive symptoms, recurring episodes and/or long-term involvement with mental health services. Some people with psychosis can experience social exclusion and have limited social support, have experienced discrimination and can find it challenging to trust others due to symptoms such as paranoia, but also due to histories of trauma, abuse and neglect. Being seen as a person with psychosis may be associated with ostracism and stigma: There may be a sense of anger and/or shame about this treatment from others. Finally, people with psychosis may have experienced invalidation in various ways, including being considered 'mad' and so treated as untrustworthy in terms of their reports of experiences and beliefs. This means that ACT therapists may need to spend more time building rapport, seeking to understand the perspectives of the client and demonstrating that they are a trustworthy and reliable person, before there is the opportunity for other therapeutic activities.

The ACT therapist seeks to find ways to foster common humanity in the therapeutic relationship, promote trust through openness about what they are thinking and feeling, and model the ACT stance toward noticing, active acceptance of experiences and embracing uncertainty. With the client's lived experience at the core of the work, it becomes essential then to explore what is learned experientially, through both the exercises, metaphors and moments of the therapeutic sessions, and also what is discovered by engaging in values-based actions out in the world. For these reasons, it is very important that ACT therapist has an openness about their own experiences and intentions, which can be demonstrated through the use of self-disclosure in sessions.

16.2 Introduction to Therapist Self-Disclosure

Therapist self-disclosure (TSD) is a commonly used tool in the therapeutic relationship, with over 90% of therapists reporting the use of TSD in some way (Henretty & Levitt, 2010). Despite this, TSD is seldom addressed in clinical training and has been minimally researched over the years, though interest in this area is growing. Therapist self-disclosure is generally defined as verbal 'statements that reveal something personal about the therapist' (Hill & Knox, 2001, p. 413). In this chapter, we will refer to two types of TSD, as they are both used distinctly in the ACT model. The first form of TSD is termed *extra-therapy disclosure*. This form of disclosure encompasses verbal information that is shared about the therapist's life outside of therapy (Hill et al., 2018, p. 446). For example, when teaching a client about values and goals, a therapist might make an extra-therapy disclosure and share 'my goal is to go to the gym twice each week, which is in line with my value of maintaining health and well-being'. The second form of TSD is termed *present-moment disclosure*. Present-moment disclosure is defined as any therapist-initiated expression of 'thoughts and feelings related to therapists' in-session (i.e. present-moment) experiences' (Levitt et al., 2016, p. 3). For example, when using present-moment disclosure, the therapist might want to strengthen noticing skills and may say to their client, 'I just noticed I am worrying if I am talking too much, what was happening for you when I was talking?'. In this chapter, we will not be addressing non-verbal disclosures, such as the wearing of a wedding ring, or disclosures initiated by the client. Rather, we will focus on deliberate process-driven TSD used as part of ACT for psychosis.

The use of TSD differs by therapeutic orientation and has evolved over time. Historically, Freudian and traditional analytic definitions of TSD dictated that the analyst should not share any personal information about themselves (Freud,

1912/1958). In contrast, approximately 50 years later, humanistic therapists advocated for use of TSD as it was viewed as a way to humanise the therapist, encourage the client to share in therapy and to foster a genuine therapeutic relationship (Henretty et al., 2014). Farber (2006) reviewed the use of TSD across a range of psychotherapies and found that most therapists sit somewhere between the traditional analytic approach and complete self-disclosure. In terms of deciding what to self-disclose, research suggests the decision is typically influenced by therapist comfort level, previous experiences of TSD either as therapist or client, the norms of colleagues (Farber, 2006) and the therapist's theoretical orientation (Carew, 2009). In ACT, TSD forms a part of the intervention 'if and when it's likely to be beneficial to the client in the service of normalisation, validation, promoting self-acceptance, or enhancing the therapeutic relationship' (Harris, 2009, p. 235) or when it is likely to 'move the client forward in some way' (Westrup, 2014, p. 51). The multiple functions of TSD in ACT for psychosis will be discussed later in this chapter.

There have been several methodological challenges in researching the impact of TSD on clients to date. Firstly, there are many different ways to define TSD, with some studies looking exclusively at extra-therapy disclosures and others at present-moment disclosures, whereas other studies have not distinguished between disclosure types. Further, many studies have investigated the effects of TSD in analogue studies (i.e. asking non-clinical samples to imagine a therapy situation), rather than in real therapy relationships, which makes it difficult to know how well the findings from these studies map onto real-life therapy situations (Henretty & Levitt, 2010). To date, one meta-analysis has been conducted which looked at the impact of extra-therapy and present-moment disclosures within therapeutic relationships (see Hill et al., 2018). Overall, it was found that the use of extra-therapy and present-moment disclosures enhanced the therapeutic relationship, improved client mental health, resulted in gains in insight and overall perceived helpfulness. Present-moment disclosures specifically resulted in the client opening up and sharing their present-moment experiences within the therapeutic relationship. Despite the aforementioned limitations within the clinical literature, other studies have overwhelmingly found benefits when contrasting disclosing therapists to non-disclosing therapists in terms of client likelihood to disclose information and a favourable perception of the therapist (Henretty et al., 2014; Ziv-Beiman et al., 2016). Whilst research in the area of TSD among people with psychosis is scant, there are early promising signs, with those participating in a group therapy for psychosis reporting TSD reduced the 'them and us divide' between therapists and clients and made 'exercises appear more relevant' (Brownell et al., 2015).

16.2.1 The Use of Therapist Self-Disclosure in ACT for Psychosis

Surprisingly, despite TSD being a feature of the ACT model, TSD has yet to be formally researched in ACT and research is underway to address this gap in the literature. Therapist self-disclosure is used across all key ACT therapy components, including mindfulness, experiential exercises and values-based action. Whilst there are many ways to use extra-therapy and present-moment disclosures across these different therapy components, in ACT for psychosis, there are common ways these forms of TSD are utilised. Firstly, extra-therapy disclosures are typically used in order to share the therapists' psychological experiences, such as examples of psychological inflexibility, for example, sharing with our client that we too experience anxiety and get caught up in worrying thoughts. Secondly, we also use extra-therapy disclosures to share our personal values and how we act upon these in our own lives, for example, 'when I connect with my value of creativity by painting, I feel really present and engaged'. With regard to present-moment disclosures, we use this form of TSD primarily when we are practising exercises and sharing our reactions, for example, when practising a mindfulness exercise, the therapist might share 'I noticed my mind was quite busy during that exercise, what did you notice?'.

In the group setting, it is commonplace to make more frequent extra-therapy and present-moment disclosures than in the individual setting. This is due to the fact group facilitators actively participate in the experiential exercises each session (see Example 16.1) and share their personal experiences through sharing their homework, such as movement towards valued actions.

Example 16.1: Present-Moment Disclosure in Group Therapy for Psychosis

Group Therapist: *What did everyone notice during that mindfulness of breath exercise?*

Participant 1: *I felt relaxed*

Group Therapist: *Thank you for sharing, it's great to hear that today you noticed feeling relaxed during the exercise. Did anyone notice anything else?*

Participant 2: *I couldn't do the exercise, I got distracted*

Group Therapist: *It sounds like you had a busy mind today during the exercise, is that right?*

Participant 2: *Yeah, I was thinking a lot and couldn't focus on what you were saying at all*

Group Therapist: *Thank you for sharing your experience. Some days you might find it easier for your mind to stay on track but other days you might notice that your mind is really busy and it's more difficult. Mindfulness is like that, so when we practice it is simply about noticing what our experience is in that moment. Today for me, I noticed thoughts that I wasn't speaking at the right pace but then I came back to noticing you all here in this room with me and I was able to continue to lead the exercise.*

Example 16.2: Extra-Therapy and Present-Moment Disclosures in Individual Therapy for Psychosis

Client: *I feel really far away from my values right now, the more we talk about them the more I realise I'm not living by them.*

Therapist: *I'm noticing sadness showing up (present-moment disclosure) when I hear you be hard on yourself because I know how hard you are working on your value of personal development, which I can clearly see when you engage in these sessions with me.*

Client: *But it's true – I'm not living by my most important values. I'm unfit, barely socialise and have no job.*

Therapist: *Sometimes it can be really hard when we talk about our values, because it can lead to the realisation that we aren't living fully by our. I want to reassure you that these thoughts are completely normal and I can really relate with what you are saying. I want to share with you that when I first learned about ACT and started applying it in my own life, I had similar thoughts to you right now (extra-therapy disclosure).*

Client: *Really?*

Therapist: *Yes really. I noticed self-critical thoughts that I wasn't being the daughter I wanted to be, or as healthy as I wanted to be. I suppose it's because when we look at our values it highlights areas of our life that are really important to us but know that it isn't possible to be acting perfectly in line with all of your values at a given moment in time. While I know looking at values is hard, I think focusing in on what's truly important to you will help you to take steps towards a greater sense of purpose and vitality in your life, we just need to take it one step at a time. I know this is the approach that helped me. How does that sound?*

Client: *That sounds good, thanks for sharing!*

Hence, there is a distinction between the individual and group setting, given in the individual setting you would be less likely to have this formal sharing structure in place.

In individual therapy, the therapist will still make present-moment and extra-therapy disclosures (see Example 16.2) with the purpose of progressing the client forward in some way.

16.3 Understanding Therapist Self-Disclosure in ACT Through the Learning Principles of Relational Frame Theory

As described earlier, ACT is an application of Relational Frame Theory (Hayes, 2004), an operant learning account for how language and cognition influence human behaviour.

Below we will describe the various purposes that TSD is used to promote psychological flexibility in ACT for psychosis. Before we do this, it is useful to share some ideas about how the therapeutic processes of change underpinning ACT can be understood in terms of basic learning principles. While a presentation of how Relational Frame Theory can inform the approach therapists take is beyond the scope of this chapter (see Villatte et al., 2015 for a book-length treatment of this), we do think there are a couple of principles to illustrate. We hope this will enable the reader to better understand why TSD can be an important component in the psychotherapeutic approach ACT offers.

In contextual behavioural therapies, a key process is *transformation of stimulus functions*, where the functions of one stimulus alter the functions of another, according to the derived relation between the two, without additional training (Dymond & Rehfeldt, 2000). This process allows for the ways that clients and therapists use language to transform what may be avoided or experienced as overwhelming to that which can be approached and accepted; for people to be able to relate psychological experiences to metaphors and analogies that may allow for new discoveries and ways of responding that were previously inaccessible. This process is a hallmark of ACT: Examples are when metaphors are introduced that map (relate) to the client's direct experience of a problem (such as the Tug of War or the Passengers on the Bus metaphors: Hayes et al., 2012), or when the connection to long-term sources of meaning, such as personal values as chosen life directions, enable the client to access sources of motivation and purpose, where unwanted experiences (such as hearing derogatory voices) may be part of a larger life direction (an altered relationship to voices, e.g. Thomas et al., 2013).

Therapist-self-disclosure is when the therapist shares their own experiences and narratives to promote psychological flexibility for the client/ participant. While there are many ways of relating stimuli that can be used (see Foody et al., 2014), such as in opposition (the opposite of), distinction (different from), spatially (over, under, here, there), temporally (now, then), hierarchically (this is part of that), a common type of relating that occurs with TSD is *coordination*. This is where the therapist shares an experience that may be 'similar to' the issue being discussed, or to the client's direct experience. This coordination can hopefully illustrate similarities that increase the rewarding nature of what is being illustrated (if this is needed), or alter how the original issue is being related to (if alternate ways of responding may be useful).

Using TSD may serve to make the therapeutic context more rewarding (reinforcing) for the client – again, through the client having greater access to the therapist's inner experiences in these present-moment disclosures, or through the relatability of what the therapist demonstrated in extra-therapy disclosures, it may be more salient to the client that the therapeutic relationship (or group context) is one that is psychologically safe (friendly, trustworthy, respectful and allowing choice). This increased coordination between the therapist and the client may usefully alter how a group or individual therapy is experienced, and open further possibilities for experiential learning.

In present-moment disclosures, we can see how this coordination can occur where the therapist may model ways of responding to their own emotions, thoughts, sensations and other inner experiences, that are otherwise less visible to the client.

This modelling may encourage the client to also act toward their own experiences in a similar way (a coordination) and discover experientially what this is like. Further, present moment and extra therapy disclosures may assist the client to perspective-take about how another person experiences their own mind: Hopefully, this coordination may help people who have felt alienated from others to find a connection with the therapist and other group members, transforming what could be avoided (such as coming to sessions) to something that is approached and engaged with.

16.4 Therapist Self-Disclosure in Working with People with Psychosis

The ACT therapist in working with people with psychosis has an openness about their own experiences and intentions, and considers the individuals' case conceptualisation for how TSD might be beneficial to the client and their presenting difficulties. While we acknowledge the functional underpinning of TSD may vary, generally speaking, the use of TSD is particularly important in working with people with psychosis and serves a number of purposes and functions central to the ACT model:

- To strengthen the therapeutic relationship
- To build common humanity, to promote trust through openness
- To bring acceptance and nonjudgmental awareness to distressing experiences, that is, model the ACT stance towards noticing and openness to experiences
- To strengthen perspective-taking, and to promote committed action through values-driven behaviour

In this section, we review each of these components in turn, focusing on how we use extra-therapy disclosure and present-moment disclosure in sessions.

16.4.1 Strengthening the Therapeutic Relationship

Meaningful therapeutic connection, regardless of theoretical orientation, is a crucial part of any psychological intervention for psychosis; and research has found the quality of therapeutic relationship to be a causal factor in determining whether or not people benefit from therapy (Wright et al., 2009). Thus, the ACT therapist places great importance on spending time to build rapport and promote trust through openness, with TSD used as a deliberate move towards connection and authenticity in the therapeutic relationship.

The ACT therapist aims to relate to the person with psychosis in a kind, curious, open and supportive manner demonstrating genuine interest and appreciation of the person, and their life, while capitalising on opportunities for modelling non-judgemental awareness and being present with the 'whole person' and their experiences. Therapist self-disclosure here acts as a scaffold for relating, and the beginning of strengthening the therapeutic relationship.

Extra-therapy disclosure of personal and therapy-relevant values in both individual and group ACT for psychosis is one way of strengthening rapport and creating a foundation for collaboration and a safe therapeutic environment; together we are identifying and defining values that are important to 'us' and how we can show this in our behaviour, in the therapeutic space and in our work together (Example 16.3).

Example 16.3: Extra-Therapy Disclosures to Promote Valuing and Strengthening the Therapeutic Relationship in Group Therapy for Psychosis

Group therapist: *we will invite you to share your experiences in the group. It will be great if you are willing to talk about what you noticed in the group, but it is OK to pass on this. We value choice, and want you to know that everything in the group is an invitation, which you might 'try out'.*

We want to spend the next few moments, setting up some ground rules for our group, what do you think will be important in our work together?

Participant: *Respect for others?*

Group therapist: *Great! And how might we show respect to others in the group?*

Participant: *not talking over others, and taking turns. I've been in groups before like that, and sometimes you just can't get a word in.*

Group therapist: *great so if we let everyone have a say, take it in turns, and try to not talk over others? What else?*

Participant: *don't judge others. I already do it to myself.*

Group therapist: *Thank you for sharing! I know what it feels like when I get caught up in my own judgmental thoughts, like you aren't doing this bit right! Just now, so I can certainly relate to this one. But reminding myself I am here with you all now, because I value connection, even if I notice the thought I'm stuffing this up.*

So how can we show, 'don't judge others' in our behaviour?

Participant: *I guess we could just listen and be kind?*

Group leader: *great, so listening to others, being present and showing kindness towards others experiences, without putting words to them. How does that sound?*

One last ground rule we haven't covered, which is important to us, is confidentiality. We want this group to feel as safe as it can for you, and it is important that we keep what's said in the group, within the group. What do you think?

Here we are using TSD to promote the early construction of valuing and purpose in therapy; while strengthening rapport by reinforcing a shared experience and fostering trust and connection (Example 16.3).

16.4.2 To Promote Trust Through Openness

Therapist-self-disclosure that demonstrates authenticity and transparency in the relationship is particularly important for people with psychosis and aids in promoting trust through openness. Authentic and transparent use of TSD aims to display flexibility and openness, while sharing experiences of vulnerability (thoughts, feelings, choosing, valuing) and willingness to tolerate ambiguity, with the function of promoting acceptance from the beginning of the therapeutic engagement. When people with psychosis come into therapy, they may be in a vulnerable position and doubt the authenticity of the therapist, the benefits of or reason for engaging in therapy and fear the consequences of opening up due to previous experiences (such as negative reactions to their expression of psychotic symptoms in helping settings) – this makes way for the foundations of an unequal relationship.

The ACT therapist employs TSD as a tool to increase transparency and provide opportunities to see how another person's mind works, by deliberately and openly sharing values and vulnerabilities, to promote levelling and equalising within the therapeutic relationship and reduce the power differential between the 'them-and-us'. Use of extra-therapy disclosures from the therapist's own life and present-moment disclosures of thoughts and feelings related to the therapist's experiences in the session aims to increase connection to the common human experience, reduce a sense of alienation (feeling less isolated in an experience) and tackle stigmatisation. By using TSD, the ACT therapist is sharing their humanity, and modelling acceptance of the human experience. By sharing our humanity, we can normalise a person's experience and validate them, while also showing compassionate behaviour towards them (Howe, 2011).

16.4.3 To Build Common Humanity

ACT therapists need to be sensitive to the experiences of stigmatisation, alienation and invalidation that people with psychosis can experience. For some people with psychosis enduring stigmatisation and alienation can lead to feelings of shame, and engagement in behaviours (experiential avoidance) that may increase the impact of their difficulties on their lives, including isolation, a reluctance to open up to others, seek help or engage in treatment. Use of TSD to build the common humanity perspective when working with people with psychosis is important. We do not think the struggles of people with psychosis are fundamentally different to the struggles of any other human being. While the struggles of people with psychosis may manifest in ways that are profoundly disabling and likely garner social disapproval, from an ACT perspective, these experiences are seen as a variant on the theme of what it means to be a human being. The ACT therapist practices from the perspective of Martin Buber (1923) called 'I and thou' and uses TSD to build the common humanity perspective in session.

The ACT stance, centres on the premises of a close therapeutic relationship, however, we know that for some people with psychosis opening up and connecting with others, can understandably be feared. It is important to recognise that many people with psychosis have had their fair share of challenging experiences that can contribute to psychological inflexibility; with high levels of childhood maltreatment, it is understandable that as an adult they may struggle with connection and intimacy, due to enduring mistrust and fears of vulnerability. Traditional psychoanalytic schools of thought encouraged therapists to be a 'blank slate' and the person knows nothing of the therapist's internal world. However, the ACT stance embodies that closeness requires an openness of both parties, and this is particularly important when working with people with psychosis. If the person with psychosis knows nothing of the therapist's internal world – nothing about what they care about or what gives their life meaning, and nothing about how they truly think and feel – then they do not have a close relationship, and the reluctance to open up continues. Use of TSD aims to normalise the commonality of the shared human experience, that we too get caught up in our minds and at times can struggle with life. Through sharing parts of ourselves, we aim to model socially appropriate dyadic social reciprocation, trust, openness and vulnerability, in the hope to foster and strengthen the therapeutic relationship – truly embodying that ACT stance. 'A fellow human being who, like us, gets caught up in their mind and ends up struggling with life' (Harris, 2009).

16.4.4 To Bring Acceptance and Non-judgemental Awareness to Distressing Experiences

The ACT therapist uses TSD when working with people with psychosis as a function to validate and normalise the person's experience by enhancing their awareness of and connection to the common humanity – not being alone in their experience. Essentially, we want to communicate and convey that their responses are understandable given their experiences or situation at the time, and you as the therapist are not dissimilar. It is important to be mindful that your attempts to normalise through self-disclosure do not enhance the person's fusion with the experience, but rather provide opportunities for perspective-taking and modelling more flexible and compassionate responses to ourselves as therapists, and to the person, we are working with. Regardless of the target function, it is always important for therapists to observe the effects of TSD. Equally, it is important to highlight that the approach of common humanity is not to trivialise or minimise the client's experiences (Morris,

2018), but rather to share in their experiences of being human (feeling, thinking, choosing and valuing).

16.4.5 Open: Modelling the ACT Stance Towards Experiences, Choices and Actions

Extra-therapy disclosures and present-moment disclosures are used to model the ACT stance towards experience, choices and actions, and highlight the impact of unwillingness and psychological inflexibility. People with psychosis may experience symptoms that increase the likelihood of responding to them with more suppression or avoidance, and less acceptance. The use of TSD becomes particularly important here. The ACT therapist through extra-therapy disclosure and present-moment disclosure shares things that keep them in a struggle, such as thoughts, or feelings regarding themselves, or their past, and how getting caught up in or fused with thoughts and feelings has acted as barriers to living out their values (Example 16.4). Here, the common humanity piece is important.

From here, the ACT therapist may use extra-therapy disclosure to highlight the different ways of responding to private experiences (listening to, fighting and struggling with, suppressing/avoiding); while highlighting the cost of unwillingness. The particular dimensions which require acceptance, and choice, become clear; and the therapist in a compassionate and empathetic way, highlights the alternative way of being with their experience; 'what am I willing to make space for, to have a long for

Example 16.4: Present-Moment Disclosure and Extra-Therapy Disclosure Modelling the ACT Stance Towards Experiences, Choices, and Actions (Open, Aware, Active)

Client: *I nearly didn't come today!*

Therapist: *can you tell me a little about what can up for you today, that tried to get in the way of you coming?*

Client: *well, I thought I couldn't do it, you know, all those people on the tram looking at me, following me, not getting off my case.*

Therapist: *yeah, okay, that sounds really tough, really scary stuff. Tell me, what feelings came up for you.*

Client: *I just felt scared, and then sad.*

Therapist: *I can see there were difficult feelings that came up for you. and some really sticky thoughts, trying to hook you and pull you in. But you got here today, despite all that. How did you do that?*

Client: *yeah, I guess I remembered what we kind a tried with that clip board, you know, like I noticed that I was getting hooked by all these thoughts, and*

listening to them you know. But I, I remembered what you told me about that time you, you wanted to go to that thing with your friends, and you had thoughts too, and that you were scared.

Therapist: *Great noticing, it sounds like you were really able to notice what your mind was saying, and notice feelings coming up for you and there was something similar about our experience, we can both worry about what other people think, and feel scared. You also mentioned feeling sad, and I noticed my mind wondering about that as it sounds different.*

Client: *well yeah, it is I guess. I noticed I felt sad and I noticed a heavy feeling in my stomach because for a moment there I didn't come, and I was on the same old road again, you know. Not doing things that are important to me. Like coming here, because, I want to have friends.*

Therapist: *whoa, yeah, I think this sadness is really important, I noticed a heavy feeling in my stomach too. When you thought about not coming today, sadness showed up for you, and it sounds like you made a little bit of room for that. You did a great job of noticing, and sounds like you made a fair bit of room for it to still get here today.*

Client: *well, I figured, this guy isn't going anywhere, like your guys haven't have they? So maybe I can come, even though this guy is here all the time. Because making friends is important to me, I haven't had any since school and if I keep listening to this guy all the time, well he will just keep me on round-about going in circles, with a broken indicator.*

Therapist: *yeah, nice, well done. And, I can so relate, it's not nice having these guys along for the ride. Each time I have a gathering to go to my passengers come to the front of the bus and tell me all sorts of things like 'don't do it', 'you have nothing good to say', 'no one is interested in you', 'you will be a sweaty anxious mess'. But like you today, I just notice that 'thanks mind', 'good job mind', have a little fun with it 'ah haaaa the drama lama' and accept that they are going to come up, that's what passengers do. But I remind myself, that being a good friend is important to me, like you today; I value friendships and want them in my life. Which for both of us means showing up to our passengers, leaning into them, making a little room for them on the bus, maybe installing a few extra seats or converting it into a stretch bus and going and connecting anyway!*

Client: *yeah, I just noticed my mind screaming ' yeah but its not easy!', like really, really loud. And I just want to tell it such up. Or chuck the clip board away – out the window.*

Therapist: *ah ha, yes. I'm noticing that my mind is coming up with all sorts of stories about that now too, and I notice felling a strong urge to want to fight with them, maybe even listen and just quit. But I wonder if we can both just notice this now, together, coming back to our body and breath… And I wonder if we can be willing to climb to the peak of the mountain, knowing that there may be another swamp ahead that could also be hard to cross?*

the ride, and accept what shows up without engaging with it, or making attempts to change it, while choosing to base my actions on what is personally important to me'. In Example 16.4, the ACT therapist uses extra-therapy disclosures and present-moment disclosures to model, stepping back from experiences in session (defusion), willingness and strengthening the acceptance perspective. The 'clipboard exercise', 'swamp metaphor' and 'passengers on a bus' metaphor can be helpful in demonstrating giving up the struggle (i.e. experiential avoidance and control) and represent the idea of stepping back from the literal context of language, and the active and aware embracement of acceptance/willingness (opening up) and choice as an alternative response. Even when distressing internal experiences (passenger's, i.e. thoughts, feelings, memories, urges, sensations) are bothering us. Through the use of therapeutic dialogue and TSD, the ACT therapist provides an opportunity to see how another person's mind works, by deliberately and openly sharing values, and vulnerabilities ' I don't need to eliminate or get rid of these experiences in order to live a rich and meaningful life'. While TSD is used to model the ACT stance towards experiences, choice and action, the ACT therapist presents acceptance and willingness not as a solution, but rather as 'an addition to the tool kit.

16.4.6 Aware: Strengthen Perspective-Taking

The self as context or the 'observing self' is the perspective from which all internal experiences are observed and held. Self as context (the constant you) provides the basis for adopting acceptance/willingness as a way of approaching experiences. For people with psychosis strengthening perspective-taking and present-moment focus is important, with psychosis often considered as a lack of present-moment focus – a break with reality (the present) via hallucinations/and or delusions (Oliver et al., 2013).

Everyone's reality is self-defined, and not so concrete, therefore, we are all in our own reality. Present-moment disclosure is utilised by the ACT therapist, by modelling noticing experiences and not passing judgement on thoughts, feelings, memories, sensations or urges. From an ACT perspective, behaviour based on attachment to thoughts or avoidance of feelings can lead to narrow experiences and a detachment from one's external surroundings or values. Hallucinations and delusions are common in people with psychosis, and constant, can make being present with relationships, and interventions extremely difficult. Being present is a central process to dropping the struggle, accepting one's own experience, and taking a step back from thoughts. In Example 16.4 the ACT therapist uses present-moment disclosures in session to strengthen the perspective-taking of the person with psychosis, and highlights learning to be here now, and being present is a skill that takes practice.

16.4.7 *Active: Promote Committed Action Through Values-Driven Behaviour*

Implementing consistent actions can be challenging for people with psychosis because of the emotional reactions that the process can evoke and the realisation of remoteness from connecting with values. With the latter in mind, ACT therapists acknowledge the distress associated with connecting with values and normalise the confronting nature of struggling with identifying values and what they want their life to be about. As such, in working with people with psychosis we promote focusing on the process of 'valuing' in one's actions instead of achieving a particular narrow outcome in itself, and encouraging noticing thoughts, feelings, memories, urges or sensations that show up and how they were responded to (Oliver et al., 2013).

Many values can be difficult to connect with, and take persistence and patience, thus, use of extra-therapy disclosure can help highlight the ongoing process of working towards personal goals in the service of greater life meaning, and promote value as a process of meaning, regardless of a specific outcome.

16.5 When Should I Use TSD in ACT for Psychosis?

On the whole, the literature indicates that extra-therapy and present-moment disclosures are helpful clinical tools with clear benefits to clients. Despite this, ACT therapists need to be mindful of when we decide to use these disclosures, as TSD is most helpful when it is in the best interest of the client. In addition to seeking supervision, there are a number of important considerations that can help decide when it is appropriate to disclose.

Using TSD in the early stages of therapy with clients with psychosis can be beneficial to build trust (Ruddle & Dilks, 2015). One reason for this is that clients with psychosis may experience paranoia and be concerned regarding the therapist's intentions, such as whether they are monitoring their sessions or asking questions for particular reasons. Hence therapists sharing information about themselves and what is happening at a given moment in their mind can build trust and help clients feel connected. One way to introduce TSD to clients is through the use of metaphors, such as the 'Two Mountains' metaphor (Hayes et al., 1999). In this metaphor the therapist explains:

> *Imagine that you and I are climbing our own mountains of life. These two mountains sit across from one another in a valley. From my mountain I can see different paths you might be able to take to get you to where you want to go, but it's not as though I've reached the top of my mountain and am looking down on you. I am on my own journey.*

Use of this metaphor, as early as the first session, provides a rationale to the client for the use of TSD, thus gaining informed consent for its use. This helps ensure that it comes as no surprise when the therapist shares their own struggles or experiences as part of the therapeutic process.

As part of considering when to disclose in therapy, it is important to consider the ACT processes you are trying to strengthen. For example, are you trying to teach your client experiencing psychosis about defusion from their paranoid thoughts? In this case, it may be helpful to emphasise this point by sharing an example of when you became cognitively fused and how you became defused. The therapist might say, 'I notice that when I do public speaking my mind becomes caught up in worry about what others think about me, so I label those thoughts the 'judgement story' and then I return my focus to what is happening around me using my senses. This strategy helps me to do public speaking, which is important to me as part of connecting with other people. What might you be able to label your worrying thoughts when they show up when you are trying to socialise?'.

When you have shared any type of TSD with a client it is important to directly observe whether this disclosure helps or hinders them. For example, do they ask you more questions about your experience (thus shifting the focus to you), or are they able to use the example to apply the skill to themselves and make some form of progress in therapy? This may give you an indication as to whether for this particular client TSD is supporting their development, or whether it is causing the client to focus too much on you. It is also of utmost importance to check your intentions for using extra-therapy or present-moment disclosures. To check in on your intention, you can ask yourself whether you are noticing your own urges to share something about yourself, or if is it to better the client's situation (Westrup, 2014).

Lastly, it is important to note that there are times when the use of extra-therapy and present-moment disclosures are more prescribed in ACT for psychosis, so the therapist does not need to make as many decisions about when they will make such disclosures. For example, in ACT for psychosis groups, the facilitator role includes present-moment disclosures through reflection on exercises during the group (e.g. mindfulness exercises) and extra-therapy disclosures through actively participating in and sharing their out-of-session practice. Despite this, there is still room for therapist discretion in reducing or increasing the frequency of TSD as appropriate. In our experience, TSD is more beneficial in the early stages of group therapy as clients are building trust and rapport with each other and facilitators. TSD in the early stages of the group helps to model sharing of experiences and participation whereas as the group progresses, TSD can be decreased as the participants become more active in sharing their own experiences and engaging with one another.

16.6 Challenges with TSD and Common Pitfalls

The use of extra-therapy and present-moment disclosures, while beneficial, do not come without their challenges as clinical tools. One of the reasons for this is that there is no one size fits all approach. There are many considerations, as noted earlier in this chapter, that the ACT therapist needs to reflect on prior to making disclosures and despite best intentions, the disclosure may not have the desired effect. In one such situation, an extra-therapy disclosure could inadvertently invalidate a client who perceives their struggle to be distinct from the therapist who is sharing with the intention of normalising the client's experience. For example, a client who has experienced psychosis may feel the therapist doesn't understand their experience when they share that they have experienced intrusive thoughts, as this falls short of having a shared experience of psychosis, 'It's kind of like my therapist has a broken finger and my whole arm is broken, and she says, "But you know, we're the same"' (Audet & Everall, 2010, p. 336).

TSD is also a greyer area compared to other clinical tools. This can increase anxiety in using TSD and thus limit its use, especially considering the little attention given to TSD in training and supervision (Westrup, 2014). For example, in contrast to directing a client through a mindfulness exercise which is a standard part of ACT intervention, deciding whether to share how much you struggle with applying mindfulness in your own life requires careful deliberation as to whether this information is likely to be of benefit to the client and progress them forward in some way.

While it has been found in research that most experiences of extra-therapy and present-moment disclosures are positive there have also been reports of negative effects. Hill et al. (2018) reported negative effects in up to 30% of cases included in their meta-analysis. It is clear that for some clients, hearing about the therapist's life outside of therapy or their present-moment reactions in the therapeutic space is not as beneficial. As yet, we do not know who these people are. Thus, these interventions can often be helpful but sometimes can have unwanted effects. This reinforces the need to use disclosures both judiciously and in a process-driven manner.

Lastly, it is important to acknowledge that TSD may make the client feel compelled to act in line with what the therapist discloses in therapy. Through fear of persecution, being wrong, or being different to the other, a client may feel it is safer to keep differences between you and themselves smaller. This may be the case in situations where therapists are working with culturally and linguistically diverse populations. Hence it is pivotal that therapists are aware of their own cultural lens and the impact of this on what they share using extra-therapy and present-moment disclosures. In terms of the literature, Hill (2014) noted that in non-Western cultures present-moment disclosures can be experienced as disrespectful and invasive, whereas extra-therapy disclosures can be particularly important for clients from culturally diverse backgrounds who are seeking reassurance that the therapist is someone who can be trusted. In a recent study conducted among people with psychosis from black and ethnic minorities, TSD was found to be particularly important in terms of aiding trust and the overall relationship with the therapist (Phiri et al., 2019). One of the limitations of current research is that it has predominantly been published in English and conducted in the United States, making what we currently know about the effect of TSD on clients with diverse backgrounds very limited (Hill et al., 2018). To address this current gap in knowledge, it can be useful to take a stance of humble curiosity when it comes to your client's cultural perspective and utilising TSD. One such approach is to check in with your client about their perception of TSD when used to assess the impact as part of the therapy process.

At this point in time, we do not know who exactly extra-therapy and present-moment disclosures are not helpful and not helpful for. Whilst there are no risk-free disclosures it is also a risk to say nothing and not disclose given the range of potential benefits to connect with our clients with psychosis and foster progression in therapy. Research continues and will shed more light on the who, what, when and where to disclose over time.

16.7 Conclusion

In acceptance and commitment therapy we seek to connect with people through the shared experience of being human: that each of us feels, thinks and acts in our world, that our capacity to remember and imagine brings with it joys and sorrows, that finding personal meaning and purpose in life is a common challenge. To support the personal recovery of people with psychosis, the ACT model provides a framework for the skilful use of therapist self-disclosure. Present-moment and extra-therapy disclosures can strengthen the therapeutic relationship, model the skills to promote psychological flexibility, bring changes in perspective and make visible a useful common humanity that can otherwise be hidden when people are entrapped or entangled by the experiences of psychosis. Together we may be able live life more fully.

Disclaimer Clinical cases presented in this chapter do not include real names or personal information of real persons.

References

A-tjak, J. G., Davis, M. L., Morina, N., Powers, M. B., Smits, J. A., & Emmelkamp, P. M. (2015). A meta-analysis of the efficacy of acceptance and commitment therapy for clinically relevant mental and physical health problems. *Psychotherapy and Psychosomatics, 84*(1), 30–36.

Audet, C., & Everall, R. (2010). Therapist self-disclosure and the therapeutic relationship: A phenomenological study from the client perspective. *British Journal of Guidance and Counselling, 38*(3), 327–342. https://doi.org/10.1080/03069885.2010.482450

Bach, P., & Hayes, S. C. (2002). The use of acceptance and commitment therapy to prevent the rehospitalization of psychotic patients: A randomized controlled trial. *Journal of Consulting and Clinical Psychology, 70*(5), 1129.

Brownell, T., Schrank, B., Jakaite, Z., Larkin, C., & Slade, M. (2015). Mental health service user experience of positive psychotherapy. *Journal of Clinical Psychology, 71*(1), 85–92. https://doi.org/10.1002/jclp.22118

Buber, M. (1923). *Ich und Du* [I and Thou]. Insel Verlag.

Butler, L., Johns, L. C., Byrne, M., Joseph, C., O'Donoghue, E., Jolley, S., Morris, E. M. J., & Oliver, J. E. (2016). Running acceptance and commitment therapy groups for psychosis sin community settings. *Journal of Contextual Behavioral Science, 5*(1), 33–38. https://doi.org/10.1016/j.jcbs.2015.12.001

Carew, L. (2009). Does theoretical background influence therapists' attitudes to therapist self-disclosure? A qualitative study. *Counselling and Psychotherapy Research, 9*(4), 266–272. https://doi.org/10.1080/14733140902978724

Dymond, S., & Rehfeldt, R. A. (2000). Understanding complex behavior: The transformation of stimulus functions. *The Behavior Analyst, 23*(2), 239–254.

Farber, A. B. (2006). *Self-disclosure in psychotherapy*. The Guilford Press.

Foody, M., Barnes-Holmes, Y., Barnes-Holmes, D., Törneke, N., Luciano, C., Stewart, I., & McEnteggart, C. (2014). RFT for clinical use: The example of metaphor. *Journal of Contextual Behavioral Science, 3*(4), 305–313.

Freud, S. (1958). The dynamics of transference. In J. Strachey (Ed.), *The standard edition of the complete psychological works of Sigmund Freud* (12th ed., pp. 97–108). Hogarth Press (Original work published 1912).

Gaudiano, B. A., & Herbert, J. D. (2006). Acute treatment of inpatients with psychotic symptoms using acceptance and commitment therapy: Pilot results. *Behaviour Research and Therapy, 44*(3), 415–437.

Gloster, A. T., Meyer, A. H., & Lieb, R. (2017). Psychological flexibility as a malleable public health target: Evidence from a representative sample. *Journal of Contextual Behavioral Science, 6*(2), 166–171.

Gloster, A. T., Walder, N., Levin, M. E., Twohig, M. P., & Karekla, M. (2020). The empirical status of acceptance and commitment therapy: A review of meta-analyses. *Journal of Contextual Behavioral Science, 18*, 181–192.

Gumley, A., White, R., Briggs, A., Ford, I., Barry, S., Stewart, C., Beedie, S., McTaggart, J., Clarke, C., MacLeod, R., & Lidstone, E. (2017). A parallel group randomised open blinded evaluation of acceptance and commitment therapy for depression after psychosis: Pilot trial outcomes (ADAPT). *Schizophrenia Research, 183*, 143–150.

Harris, R. (2009). *ACT made simple*. .

Hayes, S. C. (2004). Acceptance and commitment therapy, relational frame theory, and the behavior therapy. *Behavior Therapy, 35*(4), 639–665. https://doi.org/10.1016/S0005-7894(04)80013-3

Hayes, S. C., Strosahl, K., & Wilson, K. G. (1999). *Acceptance and commitment therapy: An experiential approach to behavior change*. Guilford Press.

Hayes, S. C., Barnes-Holmes, D., & Roche, B. (Eds.). (2001). *Relational frame theory: A post-Skinnerian account of human language and cognition*. Kluwer Academic/Plenum Publishers.

Hayes, S. C., Luoma, J. B., Bond, F. W., Masuda, A., & Lillis, J. (2006). Acceptance and commitment therapy: Model, processes and outcomes. *Behaviour Research and Therapy, 44*(1), 1–25.

Hayes, S. C., Strosahl, K. D., & Wilson, K. G. (2012). *Acceptance and commitment therapy: The process and practice of mindful change*. Guilford Press [Traducción española Desclée de Brower, 2018].

Henretty, J. R., & Levitt, H. M. (2010). The role of therapist self-disclosure in psychotherapy: A qualitative review. *Clinical Psychology Review, 30*(1), 63–77. https://doi.org/10.1016/j.cpr.2009.09.004

Henretty, J. R., Berman, J. R., Currier, J., & Levitt, H. M. (2014). The impact of counselor self-disclosure on clients: A meta-analytic review of experimental and quasi-experimental research. *Journal of Counseling Psychology, 61*(2), 191–207. https://doi.org/10.1037/a0036189

Hill, C. E. (2014). *Helping skills: Facilitating exploration, insight, and action* (4th ed.). American Psychological Association.

Hill, C. E., & Knox, S. (2001). Self-disclosure. *Psychotherapy: Theory, Research, Practice, Training, 38*(4), 413–417. https://doi.org/10.1037/0033-3204.38.4.413

Hill, C. E., Knox, S., & Pinto-Coelho, K. G. (2018). Therapist self-disclosure and present-moment disclosures: A qualitative meta-analysis. *Psychotherapy, 55*(4), 445–460. https://doi.org/10.1037/pst0000182

Hofmann, S. G., & Hayes, S. C. (2019). The future of intervention science: Process-based therapy. *Clinical Psychological Science, 7(1)*, 37–50.

Howe, E. (2011). Should psychiatrists self-disclose? *Innovations in Clinical Neuroscience, 8*(12), 14–17.
Jansen, J. E., Gleeson, J., Bendall, S., Rice, S., & Alvarez-Jimenez, M. (2020). Acceptance-and mindfulness-based interventions for persons with psychosis: A systematic review and meta-analysis. *Schizophrenia Research, 215*, 25–37.
Johns, L. C., Oliver, J. E., Khondoker, M., Byrne, M., Jolley, S., Wykes, T., Joseph, C., Butler, L., Craig, T., & Morris, E. M. (2016). The feasibility and acceptability of a brief Acceptance and Commitment Therapy (ACT) group intervention for people with psychosis: The 'ACT for life' study. *Journal of Behavior Therapy and Experimental Psychiatry, 50*, 257–263.
Jolley, S., Johns, L. C., O'Donoghue, E., Oliver, J., Khondoker, M., Byrne, M., Butler, L., De Rosa, C., Leal, D., McGovern, J., Rasiukeviciute, B., & Morris, E. M. J. (2020). Group acceptance and commitment therapy for patients and caregivers in psychosis services: Feasibility of training and a preliminary randomized controlled evaluation. *British Journal of Clinical Psychology, 59*(4), 524–551.
Kashdan, T. B., & Rottenberg, J. (2010). Psychological flexibility as a fundamental aspect of health. *Clinical Psychology Review, 30*(7), 865–878.
Leamy, M., Bird, V., Le Boutillier, C., Williams, J., & Slade, M. (2011). Conceptual framework for personal recovery in mental health: systematic review and narrative synthesis. *The British Journal of Psychiatry, 199*(6), 445–452.
Levitt, H. M., Minami, T., Greenspan, S. B., Puckett, J. A., Henretty, J. R., Reich, C. M., & Berman, J. S. (2016). How therapist self-disclosure relates to alliance and outcomes: A naturalistic study. *Counselling Psychology Quarterly, 29*(1), 7–28. https://doi.org/10.1080/09515070.2015.1090396
Louise, S., Fitzpatrick, M., Strauss, C., Rossell, S. L., & Thomas, N. (2018). Mindfulness-and acceptance-based interventions for psychosis: Our current understanding and a meta-analysis. *Schizophrenia Research, 192*, 57–63.
Morris, E. M. J. (2018). Acceptance and commitment therapy. In C. Cupitt (Ed.), *CBT for psychosis: Process-orientated therapies and the third wave*. Routledge.
Oliver, J. E., Joseph, C., Byrne, M., Johns, L. C., & Morris, E. M. J. (2013). Introduction to mindfulness and acceptance-based therapies for psychosis. In E. M. J. Morris, L. C. Johns, & J. E. Oliver (Eds.), *Acceptance and commitment therapy and mindfulness for psychosis*. https://doi.org/10.1002/9781118499184.ch1
Phiri, P., Rathod, S., Gobbi, M., Carr, H., & Kingdon, D. (2019). Culture and therapist self-disclosure. *The Cognitive Behaviour Therapist, 12*(25), 1–20. https://doi.org/10.1017/S1754470X19000102
Ruddle, A., & Dilks, S. (2015). Opening up to disclosure. *The Psychologist, 28*(6), 458–461. https://thepsychologist.bps.org.uk/volume-28/june-2015/opening-disclosure
Shawyer, F., Farhall, J., Mackinnon, A., Trauer, T., Sims, E., Ratcliff, K., Larner, C., Thomas, N., Castle, D., Mullen, P., & Copolov, D. (2012). A randomised controlled trial of acceptance-based cognitive behavioural therapy for command hallucinations in psychotic disorders. *Behaviour Research and Therapy, 50*(2), 110–121.
Shawyer, F., Farhall, J., Thomas, N., Hayes, S. C., Gallop, R., Copolov, D., & Castle, D. J. (2017). Acceptance and commitment therapy for psychosis: Randomised controlled trial. *The British Journal of Psychiatry, 210*(2), 140–148.
Thomas, N., Morris, E. M., Shawyer, F., & Farhall, J. (2013). Acceptance and commitment therapy for voices. In E. M. J. Morris, L. C. Johns, & J. Oliver (Eds.), *Acceptance and commitment therapy and mindfulness for psychosis*. Wiley.
Villatte, M., Villatte, J. L., & Hayes, S. C. (2015). *Mastering the clinical conversation: Language as intervention*. Guilford Publications.
Westrup, D. (2014). *Advanced acceptance and commitment therapy: An experienced practitioners guide to optimizing delivery*. .

White, R., Gumley, A., McTaggart, J., Rattrie, L., McConville, D., Cleare, S., & Mitchell, G. (2011). A feasibility study of acceptance and commitment therapy for emotional dysfunction following psychosis. *Behaviour Research and Therapy, 49*(12), 901–907.

Wright, J. H., Turkington, D., Kingdom, D. G., & Basaco, M. R. (2009). *Cognitive-behavior therapy for severe mental illness: An illustrated guide*. American Psychiatric Publishing | American Psychiatric Association Publishing.

Ziv-Beiman, S., Keinan, G., Livneh, E., Malone, P. S., & Shahar, G. (2016). Immediate therapist self-disclosure bolsters the effect of brief integrative psychotherapy on psychiatric symptoms and the perceptions of therapists: A randomized clinical trial. *Psychotherapy Research, 27*(5), 558–570. https://doi.org/10.1080/10503307.2016.1138334

Chapter 17
Acceptance and Recovery Therapy by Levels for Psychosis (ART): A Context-Centred Model

Horus Laffite, Juan Antonio Díaz-Garrido, Raquel Zúñiga, María Francisca Martínez-Huidobro, and José Luis Hernández-Fleta

17.1 Introduction

Acceptance and recovery therapy by levels of impairment for psychosis (ART) proposes a multidisciplinary, recovery-oriented model of intervention. ART attempts to overcome the limitations encountered by other psychotherapeutic approaches to Psychotic Spectrum Disorders (PTSD) by adapting the therapy to the psychosis and the person, rather than the psychosis to the therapy and its postulates.

ART is based on the principles of functional contextualism, as well as on acceptance and commitment therapy (ACT), and therefore has a wide range of psychotherapeutic tools and resources at its disposal. Moreover, the flexibility that the contextual perspective permits allows for the redefinition and adaptation of strategies and techniques from other psychological currents. However, the novelty that ART brings is the adaptation of psychotherapeutic processes, strategies and tools to the level of cognitive and functional impairment that a person with PTSD may present. Adaptation to impairment is aimed at complementing and enhancing interventions to the individual needs of the person with psychosis throughout the different moments and difficulties they may experience, facilitating the continuity of care from an interdisciplinary perspective.

H. Laffite (✉) · J. A. Díaz-Garrido · M. F. Martínez-Huidobro · J. L. Hernández-Fleta
Hospital Universitario de Gran Canaria Doctor Negrín, Las Palmas de Gran Canaria, Spain

R. Zúñiga
Hospital Universitario de Canarias, San Cristóbal de La Laguna, Spain

J. A. Díaz-Garrido et al. (eds.), *Psychological Interventions for Psychosis*,
https://doi.org/10.1007/978-3-031-27003-1_17

17.2 The Need for a Paradigm Shift in Psychosis

The history of PTSD largely corresponds to the history of schizophrenia, which begins with Emil Kraepelin and his *dementia praecox* (Hoff, 2012). Kraepelin proposed a dual taxonomic model, which still enjoys considerable influence today, that differentiated between manic-depressive psychosis and dementia praecox. The evolution of both followed what was called the "Kraepelin rule," that is, manic-depressive psychosis had a good prognosis, while dementia praecox stood out for its poor prognosis, with severe cognitive and behavioural impairment (Jablensky, 2010).

According to Eugen Bleuler (1911), the term *dementia praecox* was inadequate, as impairment often did not appear early or even did not occur at all (Jablensky, 2010), so he proposed using the term schizophrenia or the group of schizophrenias. Bleuler distinguished between fundamental and accessory symptoms. Fundamental symptoms are those that are present continuously (Bleuler, 1993), and therefore characterise the schizophrenias, while accessory symptoms may or may not appear in the schizophrenias. The fundamental Bleulerian symptoms correspond to a large extent to what we nowadays consider as negative symptomatology, whereas the accessory symptoms correspond to positive symptomatology.

Kurt Schneider's (1946) psychopathological contributions were a turning point for the conceptualisation of schizophrenia when his work was belatedly rediscovered by English-speaking psychiatry, where due to misunderstandings or ignorance of the author's context, the definitions of first-rank symptoms were reworked (Hoenig, 1982) and dogmatised in a self-interested way to emphasise the primacy of first-rank symptoms (positive symptomatology) and the action of antipsychotic drugs as a panacea for psychosis.

However, Kurt Schneider did not contemplate that first-rank symptoms were of greater importance for the course and prognosis than second-rank symptoms (negative symptomatology), but only referred to their specificity to pragmatically distinguishing and diagnosing schizophrenia (Hoenig, 1982).

This biased and partial Schneiderian interpretation pathognomises the first-rank symptoms and makes them the most characteristic and important manifestation of psychosis, being incorporated by the main diagnostic criteria manuals, until their most recent versions (ICD-11 and DSM-5), extending to the research and academic field, relegating the understanding and treatment of PTSD to delusions, hallucinations and associated dopaminergic theories.

In this way, the medical-biological and pharmaco-centric models, with the focus restricted to positive symptoms, have marginalised other aspects that are fundamental in PTSD, such as negative symptomatology and impairment (cognitive and functional), which precisely do not respond to or worsen with pharmacological treatment.

Proposing a change in the approach to people with PTSD from a perspective focused on "mental illness" to one focused on functional recovery represents a new conception of health, where the symptom loses importance in favour of functionality, adaptation, and inclusion of the person in the community.

From an empirical position, cognitive impairment is considered a central feature (Anda et al., 2019; Sheffield et al., 2018), with some authors proposing its potential as an *endophenotype* of psychosis (Burdick et al., 2006) and even as a predictive factor of its emergency (Sheffield et al., 2018). Moreover, cognitive impairments present predictive capacity when it comes to psychosis' expression and recovery, as well as level of functionality (Islam et al., 2018).

Cognitive impairments have been widely observed from early stages of PTSD and all cognitive functions studied have been shown to be in deficit, finding, among others: significantly lower general cognitive performance (Engen et al., 2019; Stramecki et al., 2019), marked variation in processing speed from prodromal stages, deficits in executive functions, as well as in sustained and alternating attention (Engen et al., 2019), reduced attentional span (Stramecki et al., 2019), memory alteration, both verbal and visual memory, as well as in prospective memory (Liu et al., 2017).

Another essential aspect to consider is the deficits in social cognition, which have been shown to be relatively stable and present in all phases of schizophrenia (Fan et al., 2019), with no studies in relation to other PTSD. As a result, there may be difficulties in interpreting complex social situations, as well as in understanding emotions, resulting in difficulties in establishing and maintaining interpersonal relationships. Difficulties in metacognition have also been described, at all stages, regardless of the presence of positive or negative symptomatology (Shakeel et al., 2020; Trauelsen et al., 2016), including deterioration in the ability to monitor one's own behaviour (Koren et al., 2006), make aware (Langdon et al., 2001) and form complex ideas for understanding one's own life in a longitudinal development (Berna et al., 2011).

The cognitive functions described are of enormous importance because of their mediator role in social and adaptive functioning (Davies et al., 2017), as well as in the use of psychotherapeutic interventions, so that the adaptation of psychotherapy to cognitive/functional impairment is an essential axis of the treatment in psychosis that has not been taken into sufficient consideration.

17.3 Basis of Acceptance and Recovery Therapy by Levels for Psychosis (ART)

ART is theoretically positioned from a *functional and transdiagnostic contextual framework,* based on *Acceptance and Commitment Therapy (ACT)*. Based on these assumptions, psychotherapeutic strategies are adapted and incorporated according to the level of cognitive and functional impairment of the person.

Approaching the difficulties that appear in PTSD as behaviours with an adaptive function in the person's environment (functional contextualism), and in global terms as a *disorder of the self or ipseity* (transdiagnosis), (Sass & Parnas, 2003), makes it easier to move away from stigmatising and reductionist labels that imply understanding psychosis simply as a chronic and deteriorating brain disease.

ART presents an *interdisciplinary* vocation, which seeks to involve in practice all professionals and the person's environment in its own process of recovery and search for values. In general, interventions in psychosis are based on the harmful differentiation and division between hospital treatment and rehabilitation (Shepherd, 1998), which hinders the integrity of the treatment, the coverage of the initial phases and life transitions (Vallina, 2003), and this distinction unfortunately also extends to clinical and functional aspects, with priority being given to the former. The flexible and adaptable nature of ART to the clinical and functional evolution of the person facilitates its application by all staff, in different contexts (hospital, outpatient, community and residential) and according to the needs of the person at different times, areas and vital dimensions, guaranteeing the continuity of care.

17.3.1 The Use of Metaphor in Psychosis

Metaphor is one of the fundamental therapeutic strategies of ACT, which has also been shown to be useful in PTSD. However, it is not possible to refer to the use of metaphor in psychotherapy without making a brief reference to the Theory of Relational Frames (TRF), developed as a theory of human cognition and language by Hayes et al. (2001).

TRF posits that people develop early the ability to establish patterns of relationships (frames) between different stimuli which, through the reinforcement of numerous and repeated experiences in different contexts (personal history), acquire the capacity to generate new learning through the derivation of functions (operant conditioning). This human characteristic greatly facilitates adaptation to the environment, as it allows one stimulus to acquire or alter the functions of another, even when no direct experience with that stimulus has been maintained (Valdivia & Luciano, 2006). Moreover, this learning capacity also applies to emotional experiences (Dougher et al., 1994), as will be discussed in the section on dealing with delusional activity.

Despite the great adaptive advantage of learning by function derivation, it can also be counter-productive when *verbal rules* are created which, if rigidly followed, can become the main source of behavioural regulation for the person and end up generating inflexibility and insensitivity to contingencies (cognitive fusion).

Metaphor, understood from TRF, consists of a derivation of functions between different events or relational networks based on a coordination relationship, either by similarity or equivalence. The importance of the use of metaphors in psychotherapy lies on their ability to promote self-observation and perspective on the relationship between the I-content and behaviour, in order to subsequently intervene on behaviour (Foody et al., 2014).

However, difficulties may arise in the approach to PTSD when using metaphors. These difficulties may be related to difficulty in understanding symbolic content (literalism), or that interpretations of metaphors contain a special or unusual personal significance, leading to an alternative function derivation that reinforces the content of the delusion or hallucination. In addition, the presence of possible impairment of cognitive functions and metacognition, as well as the psychotic symptomatology itself (including affective symptomatology), must be taken into consideration as circumstances that may also limit the understanding of metaphors. Therefore, it is necessary to make some considerations prior to the application of metaphors in psychosis.

McCurry and Hayes (1992) identified three components that seem to influence the functioning of metaphors:

- *Memorability*. Associated with several factors, such as: the number of interpretations that can be derived from; their ability to be associated with different sensory experiences, as well as the availability of subsequent discriminative signals.
- *Comprehensibility*. Metaphors are more understandable, generalisable and better remembered when they are drawn from everyday objects and common situations present in the person's life.
- *Aptitude*. Aptitude has to do with therapeutic quality and appropriateness.

The inclusion of common physical properties improves the aptitude of the analogy and facilitates derivation (Ruiz & Luciano, 2015) and this effect is also found when personal values are included. Furthermore, metaphors that specify relations between a particular (discriminative) behaviour and obtaining positive reinforcement, allowing the establishment of a rule with augmentative function, would be more effective than those that do not specify these augmentative functions (Sierra et al., 2016).

From our point of view, the metaphorical aptitude described by McCurry and Hayes (1992) can be differentiated into three subcomponents:

- *Temporal aptitude*. Related to the temporal moment that takes into account the therapeutic relationship, as well as the clinical situation of the person.
- *Functional aptitude*. Metaphors are effective if they contact the functional and topographical class of the person's avoidance.
- *Phenomenological aptitude*. The best metaphors are those that start from the person him/herself and possess non-arbitrary properties.

The components of memorability, comprehensibility and aptitude of the metaphor are, moreover, complementary to the person's *aptitude* as an active constructor/receiver of the metaphor. McCurry and Hayes (1992) already pointed out as a requirement of the metaphor that it should be "consistent with the developmental level of the client," a concept whose vagueness can be resolved when we consider its relationship with measurable and operable neurocognitive functions.

We must keep in mind that the therapeutic relationship means an emotionally relevant framing that can amplify the effects of metaphors, both in a positive and negative sense. Therefore, the use of metaphor can also be dysfunctional. In this regard Foody et al. (2014) referred to several errors in the application of metaphors that can be detrimental, such as (a) presenting a metaphor too early or not fully formed, (b) presenting a metaphor that does not have precise control over the person's derivations, and therefore makes alternative referrals possible, (c) the person does not feel understood or validated in their suffering.

In summary, when working with people with PTSD it is essential to adapt metaphors, with particular care being taken with abstract metaphors. The adapted and functional metaphor in psychosis has to be practical in relation to the context, concerns, interests and values of the person, as well as oriented towards changes in behaviour and functionality. The use of metaphors that fit the vital context will not only facilitate understanding and recall but also its generalisation.

17.3.1.1 A Metaphor as a Guide to the Recovery Process in Psychosis

The establishment of a central or guiding metaphor is particularly useful when initiating a prolonged therapeutic process with an individual or group, as it will serve as a framework to contextualise the difficulties (of the treatment and of the clinical process itself) within a valuable direction, as well as to help the therapist to focus quickly and easily on the therapeutic goals. Morris (2019) proposes the use of the central metaphor as a scaffold for the activities, exercises and the rest of the secondary metaphors that will be added in therapy subsequently.

Characteristics of the core metaphor include: (a) it should be easily remembered, (b) capture the essence of the person's problems and (c) be repeated throughout the sessions. A commonly used core metaphor is that of "Passengers on the Bus" (O'Donogue et al. 2018). Our team uses the metaphor of "the storm" (Díaz-Garrido et al., 2021) as an analogy for the process experienced by a person suffering from a psychotic episode, with its various phases and manifestations.

17.3.2 Attachment and the Therapeutic Relationship

The therapeutic alliance is the starting point of the recovery process. However, achieving and maintaining attachment with people with PTSD can be complex (Shattock et al., 2018). These difficulties may arise from the symptomatology itself but also from the person's attachment history. Insecure attachment (Lavin et al., 2020) and trauma (Bloomfield et al., 2021; Wells et al., 2020; Croft et al., 2019) have been consistently described as risk factors for developing PTSD. However, the potential for therapeutic alliance establishment and symptomatic and functional recovery remains (Berry et al., 2018). Therefore, addressing insecure attachment through the establishment of a warm and compassionate therapeutic relationship, as well as through interventions aimed at regulating alterations of the I-content in favour of the I-context, must become a primary goal of the psychotherapeutic intervention.

The difficulty for the establishment of the therapeutic alliance is also found in the professionals who have to carry out the care functions, either because of the discomfort and frustration that a person with a difficult and unpredictable evolution may generate, or because of the culturally dominant and implicit stigma that exists towards psychosis. A variant of the latter is related to what our team calls *iatro-stigma*, in reference to expert-type overprotective, self-development limiting behaviours, exercised by the staff and based on conceptions and prejudices about the unfavourable course, the presence of symptomatic and dangerous behavioural manifestations and the poor functionality of people with severe mental disorder (Díaz-Garrido et al., 2021, p. 218).

These behaviours are represented when professionals impose diagnostic labels, or promote premature admissions and disabilities, without taking into consideration the personal development and decision of the person. Valery and Prouteau (2020) point out that beliefs about biological causality in mental health constitute one of the variables most closely related to professional stigma.

Another difficulty for adequate therapeutic linkage arises from the very functioning of public mental health systems, due to the lack of stability and continuity of the same professionals throughout the person's outpatient therapeutic process, as well as the different perspectives and theoretical approach options used by them. This lack of stability and continuity in the therapeutic bond can be reduced if the people successively involved in the recovery process understand this process from a similar position. It is the professionals who have to adapt themselves during the recovery process to the person's interests, goals and values and not the person to the perspectives and theoretical understanding of each professional. From this consideration, we defend that a proposal based on acceptance and the search for valuable directions of the person must become the backbone of the intervention.

In the opposite direction, we can refer to the relationships and links that, in hospital or long-term residential resources, emerge between the users themselves and the staff. These relationships are so relevant that they come to acquire substitute functions for family ties and can be enormously harmful when they reproduce altered modes of functioning existing previously in the person's history (high expressed emotion, fusional ties...) that can lead to worsening and clinical exacerbation in people (Díaz-Garrido et al., 2021).

17.3.3 Contextual Dialogism

Open dialogue (OD) (Seikkula et al., 2001) promotes the search for a joint understanding (polyphonic) of the person's problem, with the participation of the most important people in the person's environment and all the professionals involved in the case. Dialogue seeks to harness and activate the person's own resources and their relational network, in their environment and daily life (Seikkula & Arnkill, 2016). The authors report that it is the mobilisation and quality of the social network the factors that appear to be associated with better treatment outcomes and increased chances of recovery.

The principles of OD, reinterpreted from a contextual perspective, constitute what we call *contextual dialogism* (Díaz-Garrido et al., 2021). Thus, the construction of shared meaning is understood as a process that fosters *psychological flexibility*, through the deliteralisation and the distancing of language, including hallucinations, delusions and self-stigma. In addition, dialogical interaction and the joint construction of a polyphonic narrative can contribute to the development of different *perspectives on the self.*

In its clinical application, it is crucial that the meeting with the family takes place as early as possible, as it is important to share the experience at the most distressing time, when polyphonic dialogues show the greatest potential (Seikkula & Arnkill, 2016). A fundamental rule is that all decisions and agreements regarding treatment are made consensually, in the presence of all participants, so that they are involved and responsible for them. Treatment decided unidirectionally or imposed only allows for short-term stabilisation, sometimes precarious, which makes adherence to treatment difficult.

It is important to take into consideration the special discursive difficulties that a person may present during a psychotic episode, so we recommend: respecting longer reaction and reflection times and making the necessary clarifications for understanding. From ART we seek the acceptance of different polyphonic positions, from a context that can help to disentangle the literal content of their own thoughts and emotions, encouraging psychological flexibility.

17.3.4 The Zone of Proximal Development, the Extended Therapeutic Team and FAP

The contextualisation of the Zone of Proximal Development (ZPD) (Vygotsky, 1978) allows us to understand that "the development of the person is built from verbal social interactions that are learned, reinforced in the ZPD and subsequently generalised" (Díaz-Garrido et al., 2021). The ZPD consists of the difference between a person's ability to carry out behaviours functionally adapted to the context at a given time, and that which he or she is able to achieve with the help of a more knowledgeable other (MKO), "one or more figures with a higher level of performance or functionality in a given task or domain, capable of serving as models and facilitators of contingencies through modelling and shaping procedures" (Díaz-Garrido et al., 2021).

As mentioned above, an attachment relationship can be established between the person with PTSD and any person participating in the extended therapeutic team (nursing staff, orderlies, administration staff, cleaning staff…) that is part of their usual context, and this relationship can become a powerful therapeutic tool that facilitates the approach to the ZPD under the appropriate guidance and the model of the non-therapist professional, who would become a dispenser of contingencies. This involvement of all staff in the person's treatment, with the role of models and contingency facilitators, constitutes what we call the *extended or amplified therapeutic team* (Laffite et al., 2021b) and has as its main advantage that in residential facilities and services, it is possible to influence the generalisation of behaviour in a space that constitutes the person's natural environment, through the members of the extended therapeutic team, who will constitute an extension of the therapist himself for the observation, evocation and reinforcement of the CRB...[1] The role of the team is to classify the patient's different CRBs and to specify the most appropriate consequences in each case... the therapist will be in charge of operationally describing the CRBs, the way they are evoked and their natural form of reinforcement based on the patient's values (Laffite et al., 2021b, p. 588).

This approach makes explicit the use of functional analytic therapy (FAP) (Tsai et al., 2009) as a tool for therapeutic change, for approaching the ZPD, as well as the relevance of basic training in the concepts of functional behaviour analysis and its use by the extended therapeutic team.

When the person with psychotic experiences shares spaces with others with similar experiences (e.g. attending first-person groups, mutual help groups, group psychotherapy, or mere personal relationships) they can also play the role of MKO, becoming a motivational variable bringing more strength to the model.

The differentiation by levels of cognitive/functional impairment proposed by ART allows that the difference in competence between the MKO and the observer of the behaviour to be modelled is not excessive, avoiding frustration, improving motivation and development of more effective behaviours in the person being modelled, as well as the feeling of competence, self-efficacy and worth of the person playing the role of MKO.

17.3.5 *Mindfulness in ART*

The practice of Mindfulness in psychosis produces a decrease in general stress and distress related to symptomatology (Jacobsen et al., 2020), with high acceptability (Louise et al., 2019). However, a misunderstanding of mindfulness can lead to its use as a form of distress control or avoidance. Before outlining our approach to applying mindfulness in PTSD, it is essential to present a brief overview of the classic adaptations of mindfulness practice to psychosis (Box 17.1).

Box 17.1: Guide to Basic Recommendations

Practice in small groups, between six and eight participants.

Reduce practice time (Chadwick, 2006, 2014), with a 10-min limit, rather than the traditional 40 min.

Guide of two facilitators who combine clinical experience in psychosis and mindfulness practice. This reduces the number of professionals who can apply it but ensures the safety of the practice.

(continued)

[1] CRB: Clinically Relevant Behaviour.

Box 17.1 (continued)

More frequent verbal counselling. Verbal guidance is recommended every 30–60 s. It provides an "anchoring" to the here and now that helps prevent people from getting lost in their experiences (Chadwick, 2006, 2014). Slower pace.

The therapist will guide the practice, with continuous monitoring of the person's or group's experience. Guidance may progressively fade for people with more advanced management.

In guiding the practice, psychotic sensations should be made explicit in a normalised way, without giving them a special or greater relevance than other sensations that arise and pass. This aims to subtly challenge the perceived omnipotence of voices (Chadwick & Birchwood, 1994).

Normalise the desire to block or avoid psychotic experiences, or at the other extreme, get hooked on fighting them.

Allowing oneself to take a break or stop participating at any time if necessary.

Adaptation of self-report measures. Jacobsen et al. (2011) used a visual analogue scale with "bubbles" of increasing sizes representing different degrees of stress and is easy to understand and complete, even for people with cognitive difficulties.

The subsequent dialogue will have experiential characteristics, addressed to the nature of the experience and how it is lived.

In the approach to PTSDs it is relevant to distinguish between two different types of practice: focused attention and free monitoring. Focused practices favour the process of attentional regulation, while free monitoring practices also include the change of the perspective of the self (Salgado, 2021). Therefore, these types of practices refer to different processes and skills, so they have to be proposed in a differential and gradual way according to the personal and clinical characteristics of people with psychosis.

Within focused attention, we will differentiate between: (a) general focus, aimed at facilitating observation and contact with anxiety and general discomfort, centred on breathing, the body and the senses (environment), and (b) direct focus on psychotic phenomenology and its characteristics.

Initially, we recommend the practice of exercises based on general focusing, which does not explicitly incorporate the psychotic phenomena, but the general discomfort they cause. It is important to bear in mind that kinaesthetic and somatic experiences are common in people with psychosis and are generally not explored in depth. In these cases, general focusing can become an exercise in direct focusing, which can lead to significant distress (Laffite et al., 2021a, 2022), so the presence of such experiences should be included in the exploration and caution should be exercised in the event of their possible unreported presence.

Table 17.1 Adaptations from ART for mindfulness in PTSD

General focus	Specific target	Free monitoring
Acute patients Group format Little practical experience Dissociative episodes and trauma (individual)	Individual or highly homogeneous group format More practical experience Assesses attentional deficits	Limitations Extensive practical experience No moderate or severe cognitive impairment

Therefore, general focusing exercises based on breathing, body and senses can be applied, when adapting time, use of language and considering the clinical presentation, to all people regardless of their level of cognitive impairment and are therefore suitable for use in group formats. In acute states, general focus exercises for short periods of time would also be appropriate, due to the feeling of "mental block" reported by some people due to the effect of antipsychotics (Laffite et al., 2021a, 2022).

When an adequate level of practice has been acquired, it is possible to incorporate direct focusing exercises on psychotic experiences. This practice must be adapted to each person in particular and for this, the cognitive difficulties present must be assessed, especially at the attentional level. In addition, it should be taken into account that psychotic phenomena are powerful experiences that tend to impose themselves by exerting a magnet effect, so that the person with acute symptomatology may have significant difficulties in adhering to the practice.

On the other hand, the practice known as free monitoring, which consists of a radical openness to any experience, without establishing a specific focus, has, in our opinion, the following limitations for its application in psychosis: (1) it requires significant attentional demand, which may not be appropriate for people with moderate or severe levels of cognitive impairment, (2) the magnet effect of hallucinations, (3) some psychoses involve a significant alteration of the experience of the self.

The practice of mindfulness in PTSD has enormous potential for affective and functional improvement, but it must be applied or supervised by professionals with clinical experience, adapting the exercises to the characteristics and needs of each person (Table 17.1).

17.4 Therapeutic Adaptations for Different Clinical Moments

Several authors have pointed out the need to adapt ACT for its applicability in psychosis. Pankey and Hayes (2003) recommended: (a) employing a psychoeducational and collaborative approach, (b) using simpler, more concrete and experiential interventions, (c) adapting language, metaphors and exercises, and (d) combining within each session small interventions based on acceptance, defusion, goals and action to make the link between them clear.

Morris (2019) also proposes several adaptations to facilitate understanding and recall of the intervention for people with psychosis:

1. Use and repetition of a predictable and memorable session structure
2. Use of brief mindfulness exercises, with more of a guided component
3. Use of a central metaphor as a scaffold for activities, exercises and other metaphors
4. Physicalisation of exercises and metaphors

However, not all people with PTSD need adaptations, and these should be targeted to the specific needs of each individual. ART therefore starts with an assessment of neuropsychological functions, especially the attentional, memory, executive functions and processing speed, as well as taking into account functionality (Table 17.2).

Table 17.2 ART adaptations according to neuropsychological functions

	Mild impairment >1 SD	Moderate impairment >2 SD
Attention	Slight reduction in the time of the individual sessions; they are maintained with times around the norm although their content is reduced. Use of the guiding metaphor to redirect attention.	Reduction of individual session time, with short sessions and limited content. Use of guiding metaphor to redirect attention.
Memory (working, verbal, visual)	Combine within each session a maximum of two different ACT components (acceptance, defusion, goals and action). Increased number of repetitions. Use of written or graphic elements to favour retention depending on verbal or visual memory deficits or strengths.	Individualised intervention from each of the components of ACT (acceptance, defusion, goals and action). Increased number of repetitions. Use of written or graphic elements to favour retention depending on verbal or visual memory deficits or strengths.
Executive functions (planning, etc.)	Inform about the structure of the session at the beginning of it. Encourage the making of diagrams and annotations. Reminder of the content of the previous session. Review the content of the current session before its end. Previous structure of the next session.	Inform about the structure of the session at the beginning of it. Give the information and content of the session in writing. Reminder of the content of the previous session. Review the content of the current session before the end of the session. Pre-structure of the next session.
Processing speed	Adaptation of the pace of language and presentation of content. More marked pauses to facilitate comprehension and elaboration of the discourse.	
Metacognition and social cognition	Facilitate the recognition of emotions and their discrimination. More marked communicative elements and clear and simple language.	
Abstraction	Limitation of symbolic or metaphorical load in language.	Non-inclusion of symbolic or metaphorical load in the language.

Although a broad and extensive neuropsychological assessment is always advisable, the aim of ART is to have sufficient neurocognitive information to adapt the psychotherapeutic intervention to the cognitive and functional resources of the person.

On many occasions, an extensive assessment exceeds what is necessary for our clinical objectives and represents an additional stressor for the person with PTSD. From our point of view, what is important is that the assessment and the corresponding adaptation can be carried out anywhere and by any qualified professional who has a bond with the person, trying to reduce technical and economic limitations as much as possible. This requires the choice of instruments that are accurate, easy to administer, low cost, that allows reassessment and, above all, are validated in specific populations. Among the instruments that meet these characteristics, we point out the Screening for Cognitive Impairment in Psychiatry (SCIP-S) (Pino et al., 2014).

In addition to the clinical interview and scales oriented to specific symptomatic assessment, it is recommended to complete the assessment in psychosis with a functionality scale (WHODAS 2.0, WHO, 2012), as well as to assess metacognition (MAI, Semerari et al., 2012) and social cognition (MASC, Dziobek et al., 2006).

When are adaptations made?

1. *Level without cognitive impairment or subclinical* (<1 SD, Standard Deviation). In most cases, this means a normalised level of functioning, with a level of abstraction and symbolisation that allows the person to benefit from interventions involving these factors. It is assessed whether the level of functioning is affected to any degree by the clinical features of the psychosis and, in this sense, whether the interventions are appropriate for the particular person. Interventions follow the classical ACT model together with the specificities of ART. No adaptations are made when scores <1 DT are obtained on the following neuropsychological variables: attention, memory, executive functions and processing speed.
2. *Mild cognitive impairment level* (<2 SD). This includes those persons with difficulties in attention, memory, processing speed, executive functions, cognition, perception and social awareness, emotional processing and metacognition, between 1 and 2 SD. Minimal adaptations would be made here, such as making the metaphors more concrete and a greater number of repetitions, ensuring the patient's understanding and reducing the symbolic load.
3. *Level of moderate cognitive impairment* (>2 TD). This includes people with extensive cognitive and functional difficulties. In these people, basic cognitive functions are significantly impaired, with difficulties in maintaining attention, remembering information and understanding language, with deficits in symbolisation and abstraction. Therefore, the simplification of language, the use of repetition, the use of simple metaphors where meaning is obtained in a guided and immediate way and giving priority to the use of physicalisation and support with images and objects that minimise the demands of the task are recommended. Behavioural strategies to improve autonomy will be included at this level and more intense recuperative interventions will be required.

4. *Severe and highly limiting level of impairment* (>3 TD). The person is severely cognitively limited, and the functional level is basic. At this level, rehabilitative interventions of an operant type oriented towards the reinforcement of basic and instrumental daily living skills, as well as cognitive rehabilitation, take precedence. In this line, the interventions of ART principles will be based on therapeutic skills, as well as the modelling and moulding of more functional behaviours.

In psychotherapeutic interaction, as well as in everyday life, cognitive functions can hardly be isolated, but overlap widely, so that just as the affectation of one of them is able to influence the overall performance, adaptation around one of them also has beneficial effects on the others, and therefore on the functional adaptation of the person to his or her context.

What will we adapt?

The duration of the sessions and activities is flexible in relation to the person's difficulties and the context of intervention (public or private, or acute or long-stay treatment units…), although the content of the session must have a predictable, clear and orderly structure, as Morris (2019) points out.

ART fits the psychotherapeutic *structure* proposed by Hayes and Strosahl (2004): (1) creative hopelessness, (2) control is the problem, (3) cognitive defusion, (4) self-as-context and (5) values, as well as the goals described by Wilson and Luciano (2002): clarification of values, acceptance of private events and strengthening of the self-as-context.

17.4.1 Preventive and Early Intervention

Contrary to early interventions focused on non-specific symptomatology that occurs in premorbid or prodromal periods, the ART proposal is based on the promotion of psychological flexibility and the search for values that influence risk factors and avoid stigmatisation and labelling of people who in most cases will not develop a PTSD.

It has been proposed that acceptance-directed components could be effective in attenuating stress sensitivity, as well as those commitment-directed components (values and committed action) would enhance motivated action in relation to reward (Reininghaus et al., 2019) with beneficial effects on subthreshold symptomatology (Van Aubel et al., 2020). Therefore, early interventions should be based on acceptance and the direction through values, prioritising the involvement of the person's social and family contexts, favouring the development of common interests and goals, as well as recognising and avoiding reinforcing dynamics of experiential avoidance, avoiding as far as possible the early introduction of antipsychotic drugs (Morris & Oliver, 2009).

17.4.2 Approach During Acute Symptomatology

It has been observed that during the occurrence of acute psychotic phenomena people actively seek explanations about their experiences (Drury et al., 1996). At this time the person shows an interest and motivation that facilitates the coming together and dialogue in relation to the personal experience. Taking this into consideration, the predominant interventions focused on pharmacological containment of symptomatology have a paradoxical effect that may limit the dialogue about the personal experience of psychosis if not accompanied by appropriate psychotherapeutic intervention.

Subsequently, however, the opposite effect may occur, with a strong avoidance of referring to the psychotic experience. This *sealing* (McGlashan et al., 1975) of the experience may be reinforced either by avoidance of admission or by early discharge. Therefore, for the approach and the establishment of the therapeutic alliance with the person with acute psychotic phenomena, it is important to distinguish between these two moments.

The experience of admission as a deprivation of freedom and rights, together with the lack of introspection about psychotic symptoms, may initially make psychotherapeutic intervention difficult, as it is not uncommon for people admitted involuntarily to be reluctant to participate in interventions or to be unmotivated. However, since ACT does not focus on the elimination of symptoms and on judging whether one is "mad" or "sane," or whether a hallucination or delusion is true or false, it can overcome many of the obstacles to future intervention.

Individual interventions from ACT applied in the context of hospital admission and psychosis have been shown to be effective in reducing readmission rates and symptomatology (Gaudiano & Herbert, 2006; Bach & Hayes, 2002; Bach et al., 2012, 2013). O'Donogue et al. (2018) propose that value orientation should be implemented from the beginning of the treatment, especially in involuntary admissions. Mindfulness-based interventions have been shown to be safe, highly accepted and valued by patients with psychosis in the context of admission, with low dropout rates and high follow-up (Jacobsen et al., 2020).

The recommended intervention is in line with the one described by Gaudiano et al. (2017):

1. Individual and group sessions
2. Mindfulness skills
3. Experiential exercises
4. Clarification of values and goal setting

In addition, ART proposes:

5. Dialogic-based family intervention (contextual dialogism)
6. Specific techniques for working with delusions and hallucinations
7. Inclusion of the extended therapeutic team

17.4.2.1 Individual Application

Gaudiano and Herbert (2006) noted the benefits of three short ACT sessions in the context of hospital admission. The duration will be flexible in relation to the individual's attentional capacity, with a strong emphasis on ongoing validation of the experience. The content of the sessions will depend on the specific needs of the person and the foreseeable duration of the hospital stay, and the therapist can consider the individual approach from two options:

1. Combine within each session small interventions based on the different components of ACT (acceptance, defusion, goals and action) to make the link between them clear, as suggested by Pankey and Hayes (2003).
2. Rotate the different content across sessions: values clarification, mindfulness, acceptance and cognitive defusion (Gaudiano & Herbert, 2006).

We recommend three sessions per week, with a duration of 30–45 min each, making sure that the sessions are not too long in order to be useful.

17.4.2.2 Group Application

Group sessions help to normalise and accept the psychotic experience, promoting openness to internal events as opposed to struggle and avoidance. They also promote the reduction of isolation and the development of self-compassion through peer support. They also provide an opportunity to represent metaphors experientially.

For group sessions we recommend the model of O'Donogue et al. (2018), which is closer in its characteristics to a skills workshop than to a therapeutic group.

In the context of acute symptomatology, it seems relevant to us that the group should be as homogeneous as possible in its behavioural and functional characteristics, rather than in the clinical diagnosis. Sharing how they find the practices and what they notice in the exercises will be encouraged, rather than discussing personal issues in depth. The participation of facilitators in group exercises is recommended, as it contributes to bonding and emotional support and serves as role models.

In the context of hospitalisation, closed groups of about six participants with two or three facilitators are recommended (we recommend at least one facilitator for every three participants). Four 50-min sessions are held twice a week, with no booster sessions, due to the characteristics of an acute care unit.

The format in community health tries to ensure that these groups are based on the level of impairment, adding to the four sessions of the approach a first test session and another two reinforcement sessions after a certain period.

17.4.2.3 Contextual Dialogue with the Family

ART seeks the acceptance of different polyphonic positions so that "psychotic voices become one among other voices" (Seikkula & Arnkill, 2016), in the whole relational network, while prioritising the principle of psychological flexibility.

Where emotions can be fully experienced and, in turn, deliteralised from cognition. All this approach, from a contextual perspective, from the logic maintained by the open dialogue, as the immediate principle, where the meeting with the family will take place as soon as possible.

The contextual dialogism will last about 90 min per session, trying to carry out two sessions per week, depending on the availability of the dialogic network and the situation of the person. In this context, therapists do not act from the role of expert, but are part of the dialogue at the same level, remaining open to experience and learning.

Some of Seikkula and Arnkill's (2016) recommendations are:

1. Ensure that the intervention and expression of the views of all participants take place as early as possible.
2. Speak from one's own perspective, using first-person statements.
3. Always give an adapted response ("there is nothing so terrible as not having a response").
4. Adapt the first comments to what the other person has said: repeat word by word and pauses to facilitate reflection.
5. Do not interpret or guide psychotic comments towards reality.
6. Allow enough space during the interventions of the different participants for the emotions to connect with the contents narrated.

Allowing people to talk about their psychotic experiences in a safe and facilitative context already has a positive and therapeutic effect (Freeman, 2011).

17.4.2.4 Pharmacological Treatment

The reduction of the distress generated by psychotic experiences through pharmacological treatment facilitates the discrimination of the present reinforcers and motivational function (when negative symptomatology does not predominate). This allows us to conceptualise pharmacological treatment as an establishment operation aimed at facilitating the psychotherapeutic approach.

17.4.3 Outpatient Treatment and Follow-Up in the Public or Private Sector

The approach from an outpatient monitoring device or in the field of private practice can include different intervention formats (individual, group and family), with different levels of intensity according to the characteristics and needs of each person, aimed at relapse prevention and recovery of functionality.

From this perspective, recovery is understood as the ability to accept discomfort and limitations as well as to engage in a meaningful and valuable life.

The structure of individual intervention also follows the typical phases and processes of ACT (Wilson & Luciano, 2002; Hayes and Strosahl, 2004, 2016), with the addition of adaptations of tools and strategies specific to psychosis and to each person's impairment (Díaz-Garrido et al., 2021).

The group work structure will follow the model proposed by O'Donogue et al. (2018). Particularly interesting is the inclusion by these authors of group workshops for informal carers of people with PTSD, with good results (O'Donogue et al., 2018; Jolley et al., 2020).

17.4.4 Medium and Long-Stay Facilities: Psychosocial Rehabilitation

Long-standing PTSD and/or those whose progression has not been favourable can be associated with high levels of cognitive impairment and a large loss of functionality. For this reason, specific adaptations are required in the overall functioning of rehabilitation devices.

For the development of the intervention from these devices, we suggest the following scheme:

7. Individual sessions.
8. Group sessions with a distinction based on impairment and functionality.
9. Family and multi-family interventions.
10. Workshops and activities. Occupational therapy and social integration.
11. Training and care sessions for staff.

In people with long-standing PTSD, processing speed and executive functions are particularly impaired (Kern et al., 2011; Burdick et al., 2006), so sessions will be shorter in duration, will include less content and will be specific in nature. The use of summaries and visual aids is recommended. In this way, it is useful to use a «scaffolding metaphor» to facilitate the follow-up of the session.

The higher the level of cognitive and functional impairment, the greater the relevance of interventions based on operant models and rehabilitative activities aimed at the functional recovery of basic and instrumental daily living skills, reducing the importance of psychotherapeutic interventions based on the use of language.

The care and the stress resistance of staff dealing with people with long-term psychosis can be enhanced through the practice of support and mindfulness sessions that facilitate the expression of distress, as well as the practice of the principles of acceptance, non-judgement and direction towards values from a dialogical position. The inclusion in these sessions of elements and principles identical to those of therapy users facilitates their knowledge and implementation by all staff members, which facilitates generalisation, as well as improving interpersonal relationships and communication (Laffite et al., 2021a, b).

17.5 Intervention on Hallucinations and Delusions

Although positive symptomatology is not the priority target for intervention in ART, its specific approach is important, especially at the beginning. Hallucinatory and delusional activity can be extremely distressing and have the capacity to intercept the person's attention, making it difficult for them to perform adaptive behaviours in their context and interrupting their direction towards values. Therefore, acting on this symptomatology reduces distress, facilitates the establishment of the therapeutic alliance and removes an immediate barrier to the implementation of committed actions. The initial approach to the psychotic clinic as a barrier to valuable directions, which can be understood as an establishment operation, is highly relevant since engaged action constitutes an indispensable element for the subsequent approach to negative symptomatology and functional deficits, if necessary.

In cases where positive symptomatology is present, both acute and resistant, and specific therapeutic work is required, two different types of intervention are proposed: focus on voices (on hallucinations) and spiral process (on delusions).

17.5.1 Acoustic-Verbal Hallucinations

From a contextual perspective, auditory hallucinations can be understood as attempts at experiential avoidance, with the same function of reducing discomfort as thought suppression (García-Montes & Pérez-Álvarez, 2001). According to García-Montes and Pérez-Álvarez (2005), avoidance consists of experiencing one's own thought as if it were something foreign (a voice). Although, as Corstens et al. (2014, quoted by García-Montes et al., 2021) point out, surely, hallucinatory experiences themselves do not need to always constitute an experiential avoidance, but can be a meaningful human experience.

In this way, acoustic-verbal phenomena are maintained through negative reinforcement, derived from the initial reduction of the discomfort that generates a sense of struggle and control, but which subsequently results in increased hallucinations. The content of the auditory hallucinations is usually related to highly relevant topics for the person, with whom they are therefore fused.

17.5.1.1 Voice-Focused Therapy: A Contextual View

Voice-focused therapy (Bentall et al., 1994) proposes an approach to persistent hallucinatory phenomena based on the reduction of discomfort that allows the (cognitive) reattribution and reinterpretation of the hallucinations to the person him/herself, and not to the outside, as the source of origin of the voices.

Unlike the cognitive approach, ART does not seek a reinterpretation of the voices or their control, but rather a distancing and a change in the relationship with them, so that the focus on the voices will occur in successive stages:

1. *Focusing on physical characteristics.* Full attention through the senses, including the one from the active hallucinatory phenomenology. Thus, the senses are explored one by one, paying attention to the global context perceived, accepting the variations of the voices, without judgement, in the here and now, with continued practice being necessary to acquire mastery. Material may be provided for practice at home.

This procedure will also be used for somatic or kinaesthetic hallucinations, redirecting attention again and again to noticing the sensations without judgement. The difficulty with these kind of phenomena lies in the interpretation of them, either in relation to their origin and causes, or to the feared consequences for the health or life direction.

It is extremely important to note that the anchors used to redirect attention have to be chosen by each person after repeated practice of these in individual therapy, since the therapist's guidance towards common anchors could lead the person to directly contact unsafe elements. Therefore, we recommend redirection during practice to the anchors to be done in a neutral way, directing people to their respective anchors or safe zones.

1. *Focus on the content of the voices.* Acceptance and change of relationship are sought in terms of the literalness of the voices, facilitating defusion. This practice can be generalised and physicalised through the exercise of «taking the voices for a walk» (Thomas et al., 2013). The content of the voices can be recorded during the practice in consultation with the patient's voice or with other members of the therapeutic team, so that these recordings can be used between sessions as functional exposure to the voices while doing other activities.
2. *Acceptance of distress.* Behaviour is directed towards values despite phenomenological activity, actively seeking acceptance of discomfort. Metaphors such as the "bus," the "swamp" (Wilson & Luciano, 2002) or the bicycle (Díaz-Garrido et al., 2021) can be used.
3. *Value-driven.* Modification or control of the hallucinatory experience is not sought.

17.5.2 Delusional Activity

Delusion can be understood as an "active form of experiential avoidance," through which the person not only avoids but also psychotically (re)constructs the reality they wish to achieve or eliminates the obstacles that prevent them from doing so (García-Montes & Pérez-Álvarez, 2005). Normally, the greater the relationship with the concept-self, the greater the fusion with delusion. Similarly, the greater the seniority and/or the greater the link to already established verbal rules, the greater the degree of fusion with the delusional content.

For the approach to delusional activity, it is important to take into consideration that:

4. Culture, belief system and personal history play an important role in delusional development, where elements from certain experiences acquire a special cognitive and emotional significance for the person.
5. They are fluctuating. Delusions are not usually maintained continuously or with the same degree of certainty or conviction… [and]… they do not always produce the same degree of disturbance (Tizón, 2013).
6. Delusions are multidimensional and develop along a continuum, best described by various parameters (preoccupation, frequency, intensity…) (Jackson et al., 1999).
7. The delusional experience needs to be validated, with respect and neutrality. In general, delusion is not confronted, nor is evidence or proof to the contrary presented (Chadwick et al., 1996).
8. Contextual factors may alter the function of the delusion (reassurance, therapeutic relationship…).

It is also of interest to distinguish between:

1. *Systematised delusional activity*, when it is articulated with a certain degree of coherence and plausibility, as well as with a relative order and clarity in the exposition of ideas. It usually requires preserved cognitive abilities.
2. *Non-systematised, stereotyped and impoverished delusional activity*, generally linked to deteriorating forms of psychosis.

17.5.2.1 TRF and Our Understanding of Delusional Activity

The derivation of functions with aversive feature content is particularly difficult to break (Wilson & Hayes, 1996) and generalises the experiential avoidance of the initial aversive stimulus to stimuli that are related, transforming the functions of these stimuli. It is important to note that the function of a stimulus is not an inherent quality of the stimulus itself, and that the same stimuli may have different functions, acquired through personal learning history (Törneke, 2016). From this point of view, TRF is able to explain the "generalisation" and systematisation of delusion. Thus, an element that acquires aversive characteristics through its "relational framing" with an element of special significance within the delusion, will be included in the same delusion with identical characteristics, so it will also be avoided, generating a spiral that can acquire extensive qualities, greatly restricting the person's quality of life.

Delusional activity is characterised by self-reflexive entanglement and cognitive fusion, reducing sensitivity to contingencies. As the entanglement increases, the transfer of negative emotional functions increases, with more attempts at suppression and avoidance of discomfort, which increases functional salience and results in an increase in the frequency of avoided thoughts and feelings (Pankey & Hayes, 2003). Thus, the greater the attention (hyper-reflexivity) and elaboration (structure) these thoughts acquire, the greater the centrality and fusion with the 'I-concept', becoming more aversive the closer they are to the person's values and identity. In addition to being reinforced and maintained by the avoidance of discomfort (negative reinforcement), the delusion is positively reinforced by maintaining coherence with the person's own history.

Hence, delusional activity arises from events that acquire special significance because of their relationship to the person's history and are therefore affectively charged (response conditioning) and maintained by reinforcement (operant conditioning), which implies that they are also under the control of antecedents and consequences. However, it is from TRF that we can consider how a delusional idea reaches and transforms other elements, which end up being included in the form of a plot. From this point of view, delusional activity can be related to metaphorical activity, albeit from a morbid point of view. Metaphors and delusion function by transferring characteristics from one event/stimulus to another or between networks of events and stimuli.

Delusion can be "generalised" through frames of coordination (X is the same or similar to Y), and of opposition, (X and Y are opposites). The latter is of particular relevance within paranoid delusions, with a tendency to dichotomise "good/bad, fair/unfair." Clearly, the derived relationship is not based solely on physical properties, but on arbitrary, abstract relationships relevant to the person on the basis of his or her own history. This way, a broader series of events or objects can become, either by generalisation by similarity or by derivation of arbitrary functions, discriminative antecedents of delusional activity. This would also apply conversely, so that delusion could be approached by the progressive discrimination of different events/objects and stimulus functions.

The ability to establish co-ordinating relationships is related to the ability to symbolise, which is altered in some psychoses. Also, poorer performance on tasks requiring relational responses has been reported in the presence of language difficulties (Devany et al., 1986). This suggests that cognitive impairment may hinder the ability to frame relationally and may explain the disconnection between ideas in the so-called schizophrenic (stereotyped and impoverished) delusions. Similarly, it may be hypothesised that the rehabilitation of neurocognitive functions involved in relational referral could help in the management of delusions.

Three ways of learning or establishing stimuli may be at work in a delusion:

1. The responsive, with the association of emotions and somatic sensations. Recall that responsive functions can also be established through stimulus-derived relations (Dougher et al., 1994).
2. The operant, with the maintenance of delusion through the avoidance of the discomfort, the (re)construction of reality, and the maintenance of coherence.
3. Relational, through the derivation of the functions between networks or stimuli that are related to the idea and the delusional idea(s).

According to TRF, responsive and operant stimulus functions are established in a direct way, while relational stimulus functions are established in an indirect or derived way. Although in many cases it is not possible to distinguish the way in which stimulus functions are established, as it is not possible to know the totality of the contingencies involved, the identification of one of these sources of acquisition/maintenance of delusion allows for differential interventions (direct, indirect or mixed) depending on whether they are directed at the different ways of establishing the functions referred to. In cognitive impairment, only direct derivations (non-generalised responding and operant) are addressed.

Once the derived elements have been identified, other features of these or closely related events/networks (of a positive or neutral nature for the person) can be used to extend or change the valence (transform or alter the function) of these and reduce the delusional fusion.

17.5.2.2 Deictic Frames in Delusional Activity

The delusion as a private (and rigid) event with special significance for the person has important implications for the experience of the self (defensive, avoidance, maintenance of coherence, etc.). Within the perspectives of the self, it is clear that the ego-contained self is affected in psychopathology in general, since it is the domain where fusion exerts the greatest influence and where delusional behaviours have the function of maintaining coherence with the morbid contained self.

The self as a process also finds its implication in delusional activity, and may even be closely related to hallucinatory phenomena, in which people become hyper- or hypo-conscious of the functioning of certain psychic processes, or of sensations that are not occurring, or whose automatic functioning should remain in the background. This is situated within the transdiagnostic proposal that supposes *hyperreflexivity*, or intensified self-awareness of the body itself, ceasing to be "silent," acquiring a kind of morbid objectification and becoming the object of explicit analysis (Pérez-Álvarez, 2014). Therefore, we are faced with a self as a morbid process, characteristic of somatic or kinaesthetic delusions, or of denial such as Cotard's Syndrome, in the opposite extreme.

However, the self as context provides a neutral point of stabilisation of the experience of the self for people with delusions of non-manic dimensions, non-schizophrenic characteristics and without self-affectation (ipseity). The self as a context allows the delusion to be approached in moments of greatest distress from the reestablishment of the deictic perspective (I/here/now, I feel safe and validated). The loss of deictic perspective generates enormous discomfort and can be worked on and reinforced through dialogue with Socratic characteristics, as well as with experiential exercises (observer's exercise) and metaphors (chessboard) that can be found in the work of Hayes et al. (2004, 2016).

Working with the self as a context from mindfulness is recommended with people with an adequate level of practice, through the use of anchors and safe zones specific to each person, taking into consideration the level of impairment described in the section on the application of mindfulness in ART, and the clinical specifications indicated.

17.5.2.3 Spiral Process for Delusional Activity

Spiral work is based on the deliteralisation of verbal content, instead of the work on the certainty or not of the delusion, and the psychological impact due to rule-governed behaviour, facilitating a learning shaped by direct contingencies, increasing acceptance, mindfulness and the person's behavioural repertoire, as well as compassion towards oneself and others, fostering flexible functionality to the environment. Our aim is not the elimination of delusional activity, as this fulfils a certain function for the person, the aim is to improve functionality and to ensure that the person maintains a meaningful and value-oriented life direction despite the delusional activity (Díaz-Garrido et al., 2021).

Dealing with delusions is a process in which progress and setbacks often occur. The therapist's position is aimed at facilitating, from a symmetrical and non-confrontational position, the self-exposure of the person to the delusional elements most susceptible to being addressed at each moment, through successive approximations and learning shaped by contingencies. Exposure is carried out through experiential exercises, in ACT terminology, or "reality testing" or behavioural experiments, according to cognitive-behavioural therapies, which are selected on the basis of functional criteria. Experiential exercises emphasise the relationship between behaviour and context, whereas reality testing emphasises the relationship between thought and behaviour/consequence. In this way, the person connects with the experience, discovering an alternative story that contrasts with the delusion and with the verbal rules that form the I-concept (Díaz-Garrido et al., 2021).

In cases where there is more than one delusional plot (e.g. megaloids and persecutory), or if the delusion within the same theme has been bifurcated, generalising the response to different contexts (e.g. initial conviction of damage by the local police authorities, which later expands into an international plot), we would start with the spiral process through the most recent delusion, going little by little, from the superficial to the core of the delusion in an iterative process. Our aim is not to end it, not to defeat it, as it has a history and an avoidant function within this history, but to make the person functional again in spite of it, to make him or her life full, meaningful and value-driven again.

From a contextual understanding, an exchange of subjective experiences takes place, working, encouraging and establishing a genuine, empathic and solid alliance from day one; from mimetic positions, where we join as allies, from respect and neutrality towards the delusional plot. There is no discussion, evidence or proof to the contrary that are not presented; only the patient's experience is acknowledged and validated (Chadwick et al., 1996). By mimicking (Minuchin, 1974) we allow a frank dialogue, from a common point of view, of exchange of information from non-confrontational symmetrical positions; introducing, through functional self-exposures, a new perspective less fused with the literalness of the delusion. By mimicking the delusional content, we take advantage of "opportunities" for the person to perform actions, that is, to expose him/herself, in many cases in a self-induced way, to different aspects of the delusion, based on functional criteria. In this way, the person connects with the experience, discovering an alternative story that contrasts with the delusion and that conflicts with the verbal rules that form the "I-concept." This can be done, as we have already indicated, by encouraging self-exposures, and by successive approximations, through learning shaped by contingencies. Dealing with delusions is neither quick nor easy, but a laborious and constant work, in which progress and setbacks can occur. We would advance from the periphery of the delusion, from the superficial, in a subtle way, with indirect exposure; looking for and generating "behavioural reality tests" until we reach the core of the delusion, orienting all the work towards a reconnection with values and a commitment to them.

The approach to spiral delusion is made up of a series of stages, which are applied in a flexible way according to the characteristics of the delusion and the needs of the person (Fig. 17.1). These are as follows:

1. Establishment of a genuine and strong therapeutic alliance. Mimicry.
2. Functional analysis and history.
3. "Traps" to functional self-exposure.
4. Creative hopelessness, non-control and acceptance: mindfulness exercises, metaphors and behavioural reality testing. Examples of useful exercises: paper clip box, tambourine exercise, window watcher, white bear metaphor.
5. Redirection towards values. Committed action. Identifying barriers to functional self-exposure. Bus metaphor.
6. Commitment to values. Bridge to values. Bicycle metaphor. Garden metaphor.

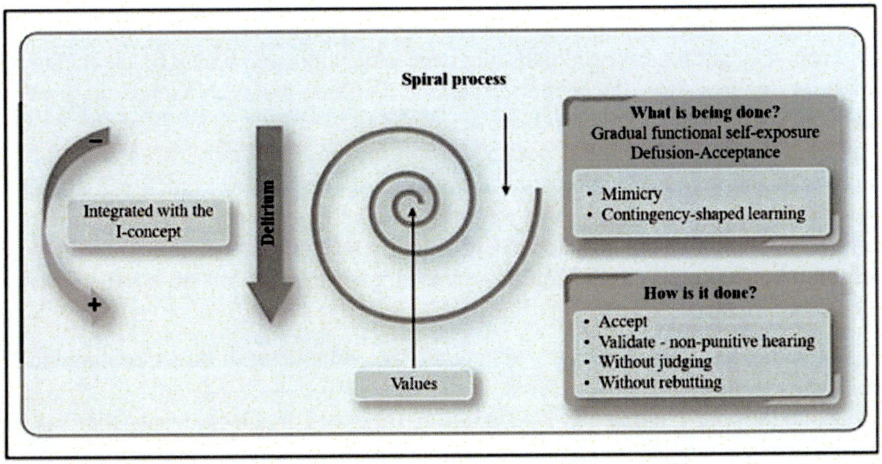

Fig. 17.1 Approach to spiral delusion. (Reproduced from Díaz-Garrido et al., 2021)

From the conceptualisation of FAP, the clinically relevant behaviours CRB1 would work on behaviours related to the delusional ideation, CRB2 to weaken the literalness of the delusion and increase the probability of a more functional response and its generalisation, and CRB3 with respect to verbalisations and awareness of the functional viability of their behaviour, validating at all times their emotions and the meaning that their delusion has for the person (Díaz-Garrido et al., 2021).

Due to the characteristics of this work, the aim of which is to make a brief approach to the new models of approaching psychosis, we will try to present the spiral process in a practical way through a brief case study.

X., a 48-year-old woman, was in the process of separating from her partner and fighting for custody of her two daughters. As part of this stressful event, her partner accused her of engaging in behaviours that he felt were not compatible with what he believed to be a "good mother," and that he would present graphic evidence of this to a judge so that she would not be granted custody of her daughters.

One morning, when he was in a coffee shop, he noticed that a girl had her mobile phone pointed at her, and he was certain that she was recording her in order to use the recording against her.

Several days later, when she was leaving her house, she noticed a dark-coloured car, which she did not recognise and which was parked in a strange way, with a person in the driver's seat. X. called the police to express her concern and her conviction that she was being watched by this vehicle. However, not only did the police not respond to the call, but a few days later a non-uniformed officer delivered a summons to her home with a complaint filed by her husband. X. immediately made the connection that the police were working for her husband, trying to take her daughters away from her, so she had an episode of disturbed behaviour for which she had to be taken to the emergency department, where her distress was reduced pharmacologically. Since then, she believes that the police have been keeping a surveillance operation on her and she has developed a great anxiety about leaving her home.

From the spiral intervention, one element to be addressed would be the inclusion of the police in a surveillance plot. In session we examined with X. the relevance of the concept of "watching/controlling/spying," and how this was in common with the different situations that had generated discomfort on her. As discussed, the derivation of functions also involves the derivation of (responsive) emotional content, which allows us to understand why stimulus functions can also be altered in different ways. Therefore, for this element, the functional analysis that will guide the type of intervention to be carried out is proposed, among some of the alternatives we point out:

1. Blocking avoidance so that it can come into contact with direct contingencies (operant, direct).
2. Blocking and altering the derivation of functions between events (derivative, indirect).

Work is based on the possibility of observing and discriminating (mindfulness), both one's own behaviour (self-discrimination) as well as and the consequences that occur in different situations. The ability to discriminate appropriately corresponds to what clinicians sometimes call reality judgement or insight. It is highly relevant that discrimination includes for the person the realisation that their behaviour is not value-directed (creative hopelessness).

Emotional distress has an impact on function derivation, generalising aversive or negative responses to other events or stimuli, so it is essential to reduce distress prior to addressing spiral delusion. The derivation of function has the capacity to extend emotional distress and trauma. Content aimed at acceptance and engaged action is included at this stage. The capacity for acceptance and valued direction interact to create a margin of tolerance that supports and allows exposure to the delusion. However, this margin of tolerance fluctuates, so that acceptance and values will be continually reintroduced throughout the process.

For an inexperienced therapist, it would be easy to attempt to address the trauma once it has been identified, however, the application of the spiral proposes the initial approach from the secondary derivations, which have an emotional valence that is not based on themselves, but on the initial traumatic event, so that the exposure to the central discomfort is produced from peripheral elements, which confers greater tolerability and greater opportunity for acceptance.

(De-literalisation, defusion) We address the derivation of functions "watch/control/spy" relevant in the case of X., through contextualisation with other functions also performed by the Security Forces "protect, regulate traffic." Cognitive and metaphorical defusion interventions aimed at decreasing language control, such as the "suggestion box" (Törneke, 2020), fit into this stage. Interventions from language allow altering the established relational framework, and even incorporating new frames of "distinction," thus contributing synergistically to the discriminative work.

Once X.'s discomfort and distress are within an acceptable range of tolerability, based on her capacity for acceptance and commitment to her values, experiential exercises (functional self-exposures) are initiated, blocking the kinds of responses corresponding to avoidance and reinforcing the committed action oriented towards personal values. Examples of some exercises such as paper clip box, tambourine exercise, observer at the window, white bear metaphor, etc. can be found in Díaz-Garrido et al. (2021).

This process is carried out in a repetitive way, spirally, for the different constituent elements of the delusion that are functionally identified.

17.6 Conclusions

The proposal of the acceptance and recovery therapy by levels (ART) is not only a model of inter- and multidisciplinary psychotherapeutic intervention but also a commitment to optimise and standardise the work in mental health services for people with psychosis spectrum disorders.

In recent years there has been an increase in the literature related to the approach to PTSD from ACT and open dialogue. This, together with other proposals that place the person at the centre of the approach and the respect for their freedom of decision, constitutes the basis for a paradigm shift in psychosis. Our aim is to continue this line of work with the ART approach, and thus bring contextual therapies closer to patients on the psychotic spectrum.

We firmly believe that the consideration of the different levels of cognitive and functional impairment, as well as the adaptation of interventions to these, open up a new perspective for the treatment, from which to make psychotherapy accessible to all people, regardless of their difficulties, and we invite the different professionals to put into practice, complete and improve this idea.

Ethical Statement This study was conducted in accordance with the Declaration of Helsinki. We obtained the patient's informed consent before publication. The patient grants her permission for her information to be published in this case report.

OR

Disclaimer Clinical cases presented in this chapter do not include real names or personal information of real persons.

References

Anda, L., Brønnick, K. K., Johannessen, J. O., Joa, I., Kroken, R. A., Johnsen, E., Rettenbacher, M., Fathian, F., & Løberg, E. M. (2019). Cognitive profile in ultra high risk for psychosis and schizophrenia: A comparison using coordinated norms. *Frontiers in Psychiatry, 10*, 695. https://doi.org/10.3389/fpsyt.2019.00695

Bach, P., & Hayes, S. C. (2002). The use of acceptance and commitment therapy to prevent the rehospitalization of psychotic patients: A randomized controlled trial. *Journal of Consulting and Clinical Psychology, 70*(5), 1129–1139. https://doi.org/10.1037//0022-006x.70.5.1129

Bach, P., Hayes, S. C., & Gallop, R. (2012). Long-term effects of brief acceptance and commitment therapy for psychosis. *Behavior Modification, 36*(2), 165–181. https://doi.org/10.1177/0145445511427193

Bach, P., Gaudiano, B. A., Hayes, S. C., & Herbert, J. D. (2013). Acceptance and commitment therapy for psychosis: Intent to treat, hospitalization outcome and mediation by believability. *Psychosis: Psychological, Social and Integrative Approaches, 5*(2), 166–174. https://doi.org/10.1080/17522439.2012.671349

Bentall, R. P., Haddock, G., & Slade, P. D. (1994). Cognitive behavior therapy for persistent auditory hallucinations: From theory to therapy. *Behavior Therapy, 25*(1), 51–66. https://doi.org/10.1016/S0005-7894(05)80145-5

Berna, F., Bennouna-Greene, M., Potheegado, J., Verry, P., Conway, M. A., & Danion, J. M. (2011). Impaired ability to give a meaning to personally significant events in patients with schizophrenia. *Consciousness and Cognition, 20*(3), 703–711. https://doi.org/10.1016/j.concog.2010.12.004

Berry, K., Palmer, T., Gregg, L., Barrowclough, C., & Lobban, F. (2018). Attachment and therapeutic alliance in psychological therapy for people with recent onset psychosis who use cannabis. *Clinical Psychology & Psychotherapy, 25*(3), 440–445. https://doi.org/10.1002/cpp.2178

Bleuler, E. (1993). *Demencia Precoz. El grupo de las esquizofrenias* (2.a ed.). Lumen [ed. Original Bleuler, E. (1911). *Dementia praecox oder Gruppe der Schizophrenien*].

Bloomfield, M., Chang, T., Woodl, M. J., Lyons, L. M., Cheng, Z., Bauer-Staeb, C., Hobbs, C., Bracke, S., Kennerley, H., Isham, L., Brewin, C., Billings, J., Greene, T., & Lewis, G. (2021).

Psychological processes mediating the association between developmental trauma and specific psychotic symptoms in adults: A systematic review and meta-analysis. *World Psychiatry: Official Journal of the World Psychiatric Association (WPA), 20*(1), 107–123. https://doi.org/10.1002/wps.20841

Burdick, K. E., Goldberg, J. F., Harrow, M., Faull, R. N., & Malhotra, A. K. (2006). Neurocognition as a stable endophenotype in bipolar disorder and schizophrenia. *The Journal of Nervous and Mental Disease, 194*(4), 255–260. https://doi.org/10.1097/01.nmd.0000207360.70337.7e

Chadwick, P. (2006). *Person-based cognitive therapy for distressing psychosis*. Wiley.

Chadwick, P. (2014). Mindfulness for psychosis. *British Journal of Psychiatry, 204*(5), 333–334. https://doi.org/10.1192/bjp.bp.113.136044

Chadwick, P., & Birchwood, M. (1994). The omnipotence of voices: A cognitive approach to auditory hallucinations. *The British Journal of Psychiatry, 164*, 190–201. https://doi.org/10.1192/bjp.164.2.190

Chadwick, P., Birchwood, M., & Trower, P. (1996). *Cognitive therapy for delusions, voices and paranoia*. Wiley.

Corstens, D., Longden, E., McCarthy-Jones, S., Waddingham, R., & Thomas, N. (2014). Emerging perspectives from the hearing voices movement: implications for research and practice. *Schizophrenia bulletin, 40*(Suppl 4), S285–S294. https://doi.org/10.1093/schbul/sbu007

Croft, J., Heron, J., Teufel, C., Cannon, M., Wolke, D., Thompson, A., Houtepen, L., & Zammit, S. (2019). Association of trauma type, age of exposure, and frequency in childhood and adolescence with psychotic experiences in early adulthood. *JAMA Psychiatry, 76*(1), 79–86. https://doi.org/10.1001/jamapsychiatry.2018.3155

Davies, G., Fowler, D., & Greenwood, K. (2017). Metacognition as a mediating variable between neurocognition and functional outcome in first episode psychosis. *Schizophrenia Bulletin, 43*(4), 824–832. https://doi.org/10.1093/schbul/sbw128

Devany, J. M., Hayes, S. C., & Nelson, R. O. (1986). Equivalence class formation in language-able and language-disabled children. *Journal of the Experimental Analysis of Behavior, 46*(3), 243–257. https://doi.org/10.1901/jeab.1986.46-243

Díaz-Garrido, J. A., Laffite, H., & Zúñiga, R. (2021). Terapia de aceptación y recuperación por niveles para la psicosis. In J. A. Díaz-Garrido, H. Laffite, & R. Zúñiga (coords), *Terapia de Aceptación y Compromiso en psicosis. Aceptación y recuperación por niveles (ART)*. Pirámide.

Dougher, M. J., Augustson, E., Markham, M. R., Greenway, D. E., & Wulfert, E. (1994). The transfer of respondent eliciting and extinction functions through stimulus equivalence classes. *Journal of the Experimental Analysis of Behavior, 62*(3), 331–351. https://doi.org/10.1901/jeab.1994.62-331

Drury, V., Birchwood, M., Cochrane, R., & Macmillan, F. (1996). Cognitive therapy and recovery from acute psychosis: A controlled trial. I. Impact on psychotic symptoms. *The British Journal of Psychiatry: The Journal of Mental Science, 169*(5), 593–601. https://doi.org/10.1192/bjp.169.5.593

Dziobek, I., Fleck, S., Kalbe, E., Rogers, K., Hassenstab, J., Brand, M., Kessler, J., Woike, J. K., Wolf, O. T., & Convit, A. (2006). Introducing MASC: A movie for the assessment of social cognition. *Journal of Autism and Developmental Disorders, 36*(5), 623–636. https://doi.org/10.1007/s10803-006-0107-0

Engen, M. J., Simonsen, C., Melle, I., Færden, A., Lyngstad, S. H., Haatveit, B., Vaskinn, A., & Ueland, T. (2019). Cognitive functioning in patients with first-episode psychosis stratified by level of negative symptoms: A 1-year follow-up study. *Psychiatry Research, 281*, 112554. https://doi.org/10.1016/j.psychres.2019.112554

Fan, F., Xiang, H., Tan, S., Yang, F., Fan, H., Guo, H., Kochunov, P., Wang, Z., Hong, L. E., & Tan, Y. (2019). Subcortical structures and cognitive dysfunction in first episode schizophrenia. *Psychiatry Research. Neuroimaging, 286*, 69–75. https://doi.org/10.1016/j.pscychresns.2019.01.003

Foody, M., Barnes-Holmes, Y., Barnes-Holmes, D., Törneke, N., Luciano, C., Stewart, I., & McEnteggart, C. (2014). RFT for clinical use: The example of metaphor. *Journal of Contextual Behavioral Science, 3*(4), 305–313. https://doi.org/10.1016/j.jcbs.2014.08.001

Freeman, D. (2011). Improving cognitive treatment for delusions. *Schizophrenia Research, 13*, 135–139. https://doi.org/10.1016/j.schres.2011.08.012

García Montes, J. M., & Pérez Álvarez, M. (2001). ACT como tratamiento de síntomas psicóticos. El caso de las alucinaciones auditivas [ACT as treatment for psychotic symptoms: The case of auditory hallucinations]. *Análisis y Modificación de Conducta, 27*(113), 455–472.

García-Montes, J. M., & Pérez-Álvarez, M. (2005). Fundamentación experimental y primeras aplicaciones clínicas de la Terapia de Aceptación y Compromiso (ACT) en el campo de los síntomas psicóticos [Experimental foundations and early clinical applications of Acceptance and Commitment Therapy in the field of psychotic disorders]. *Revista Latinoamericana de Psicología, 37*(2), 379–393.

García-Montes, J. M., Pérez-Álvarez, M., López-Ríos, F., Sánchez-Sánchez, L., & Vallina-Fernández, O. (2021). ACT aplicada a síntomas psicóticos positivos. In J. A. Díaz-Garrido, H. Laffite, & R. Zúñiga, *Terapia de aceptación y compromiso en psicosis. Aceptación y recuperación por niveles (ART)*. Pirámide.

Gaudiano, B. A., & Herbert, J. D. (2006). Acute treatment of inpatients with psychotic symptoms using Acceptance and Commitment Therapy: Pilot results. *Behaviour Research and Therapy, 44*(3), 415–437. https://doi.org/10.1016/j.brat.2005.02.007

Gaudiano, B. A., Davis, C. H., Epstein-Lubow, G., Johnson, J. E., Mueser, K. T., & Miller, I. W. (2017). Acceptance and commitment therapy for inpatients with psychosis (the REACH study): Protocol for treatment development and pilot testing. *Healthcare, 5*(2), 23. https://doi.org/10.3390/healthcare5020023

Hayes, S. C., & Strosahl, K. D. (2004). *A practical guide to acceptance and commitment therapy*. Springer.

Hayes, S. C., Barnes-Holmes, D., & Roche, B. (2001). *Relational frame theory: A post-Skinnerian account of human language and cognition*. Kluwer Academic/Plenum Publishers.

Hayes, S. C., Strosahl, K. D., & Wilson, K. G. (2016). *Acceptance and commitment therapy: The process and practice of mindful change*. Guilford Press.

Hoenig, J. (1982). Kurt Schneider and Anglophone psychiatry. *Comprehensive Psychiatry, 23*(5), 391–400. https://doi.org/10.1016/0010-440x(82)90152-3

Hoff, P. (2012). Kraepelin. Sección clínica. 1.a parte. In G. E. Berrios & R. Porter (Eds.), *Una historia de la psiquiatría clínica*. Triacastela.

Islam, M. A., Habtewold, T. D., van Es, F. D., Quee, P. J., van den Heuvel, E. R., Alizadeh, B. Z., Bruggeman, R., & GROUP Investigators. (2018). Long-term cognitive trajectories and heterogeneity in patients with schizophrenia and their unaffected siblings. *Acta Psychiatrica Scandinavica, 138*(6), 591–604. https://doi.org/10.1111/acps.12961

Jablensky, A. (2010). The diagnostic concept of schizophrenia: Its history, evolution, and future prospects. *Dialogues in Clinical Neuroscience, 12*(3), 271–287. https://doi.org/10.31887/DCNS.2010.12.3/ajablensky

Jackson, H. J., Edwards, J., Hulbert, C., & McGorry, P. D. (1999). Recovery from psychosis: Psychological interventions. In P. D. McGorry & H. Jackson (Eds.), *The recognition and management of early psychosis: A preventive approach* (pp. 265–307). Cambridge University Press.

Jacobsen, P., Morris, E., Johns, L., & Hodkinson, K. (2011). Mindfulness groups for psychosis; key issues for implementation on an inpatient unit. *Behavioural and Cognitive Psychotherapy, 39*(3), 349–353. https://doi.org/10.1017/S1352465810000639

Jacobsen, P., Peters, E., Robinson, E., & Chadwick, P. (2020). Mindfulness-based crisis interventions (MBCI) for psychosis within acute inpatient psychiatric settings: A feasibility randomised controlled trial. *BMC Psychiatry, 20*, 193. https://doi.org/10.1186/s12888-020-02608-x

Jolley, S., Johns, L. C., O'Donoghue, E., Oliver, J., Khondoker, M., Byrne, M., Butler, L., De Rosa, C., Leal, D., McGovern, J., Rasiukeviciute, B., Sim, F., & Morris, E. (2020). Group acceptance and commitment therapy for patients and caregivers in psychosis services: Feasibility of training and a preliminary randomized controlled evaluation. *The British Journal of Clinical Psychology, 59*(4), 524–551. https://doi.org/10.1111/bjc.12265

Kern, R. S., Gold, J. M., Dickinson, D., Green, M. F., Nuechterlein, K. H., Baade, L. E., Keefe, R. S., Mesholam-Gately, R. I., Seidman, L. J., Lee, C., Sugar, C. A., & Marder, S. R. (2011). The MCCB impairment profile for schizophrenia outpatients: Results from the MATRICS psychometric and standardization study. *Schizophrenia Research, 126*(1–3), 124–131. https://doi.org/10.1016/j.schres.2010.11.008

Koren, D., Seidman, L. J., Goldsmith, M., & Harvey, P. D. (2006). Real-world cognitive – And metacognitive – Dysfunction in schizophrenia: A new approach for measuring (and remediating) more "right stuff". *Schizophrenia Bulletin, 32*(2), 310–326. https://doi.org/10.1093/schbul/sbj035

Laffite, H., Díaz-Garrido, J. A., & Zúñiga, R. (2021a). Mindfulness y psicosis. *INSPIRA, Mindfulness, Compasión y Ciencia, 5*, 28–31.

Laffite, H., Zúñiga, R., & Díaz-Garrido, J. A. (2021b). Involucrando a todos. Una propuesta de aplicación de ACT y FAP en psicosis crónica. In J. Ruiz (coord.), *FACT de grupo. Integrando ACT y FAP de grupo*. Psara ediciones.

Laffite, H., Díaz-Garrido, J. A., Zúñiga, R., Martínez-Huidobro, M. F., & Hernández-Fleta, J. L. (2022). La Terapia de aceptación y recuperación por niveles para la psicosis (ART). Un modelo centrado en el contexto. En Díaz-Garrido, J. A., Zúñiga, R., Laffite, H., & Morris, E. (coords.). *Los Modelos del Cambio: Casos Clínicos en Psicosis*. Pirámide.

Langdon, R., Coltheart, M., Ward, P. B., & Catts, S. V. (2001). Mentalizing, executive planning and disengagement in schizophrenia. *Cognitive Neuropsychiatry, 6*(2), 81–108. https://doi.org/10.1080/13546800042000061

Lavin, R., Bucci, S., Varese, F., & Berry, K. (2020). The relationship between insecure attachment and paranoia in psychosis: A systematic literature review. *The British Journal of Clinical Psychology, 59*(1), 39–65. https://doi.org/10.1111/bjc.12231

Liu, D., Ji, C., Zhuo, K., Song, Z., Wang, Y., Mei, L., Zhu, D., Xiang, Q., Chen, T., Yang, Z., Zhu, G., Wang, Y., Cheung, E. F., Xiang, Y. T., Fan, X., Chan, R. C., Xu, Y., & Jiang, K. (2017). Impaired cue identification and intention retrieval underlie prospective memory deficits in patients with first-episode schizophrenia. *The Australian and New Zealand Journal of Psychiatry, 51*(3), 270–277. https://doi.org/10.1177/0004867416640097

Louise, S., Rossell, S. L., & Thomas, N. (2019). The acceptability, feasibility and potential outcomes of an individual mindfulness-based intervention for hearing voices. *Behavioural and Cognitive Psychotherapy, 47*(2), 200–216. https://doi.org/10.1017/S1352465818000425

McCurry, S. M., & Hayes, S. C. (1992). Clinical and experimental perspectives on metaphorical talk. *Clinical Psychology Review, 12*(7), 763–785. https://doi.org/10.1016/0272-7358(92)90023-2

McGlashan, T. H., Levy, S. T., & Carpenter, W. T., Jr. (1975). Integration and sealing over. Clinically distinct recovery styles from schizophrenia. *Archives of General Psychiatry, 32*(10), 1269–1272. https://doi.org/10.1001/archpsyc.1975.01760280067006

Minuchin, S. (1974). *Families & family therapy*. The President and Fellows of Harvard College.

Morris, E. (2019). Acceptance and commitment therapy. In C. Cupitt (Ed.), *CBT for psychosis: Process-orientated therapies and the third wave* (pp. 79–97). Routledge/Taylor & Francis Group.

Morris, E., & Oliver, J. (2009). ACT early: Acceptance and commitment therapy in early intervention in psychosis. *Clinical Psychology Forum, 196*, 28–31.

O'Donogue, E. K., Morris, E. M., Oliver, J. E., & Johns, L. C. (2018). *ACT for psychosis recovery: A practical manual for group-based interventions using acceptance and commitment therapy*. Context Press.

Pankey, J., & Hayes, S. C. (2003). Acceptance and commitment therapy for psychosis. *International Journal of Psychology & Psychological Therapy, 3*(2), 311–328.

Pérez-Álvarez, M. (2014). *Las terapias de tercera generación como terapias contextuales* (p. 48). Síntesis.

Pino, O., Guilera, G., Rojo, J. E., Gómez-Benito, J., & Purdon, S. E. (2014). *SCIP-S, Screening del Deterioro Cognitivo en Psiquiatría*. TEA Ediciones.

Reininghaus, U., Klippel, A., Steinhart, H., Vaessen, T., van Nierop, M., Viechtbauer, W., Batink, T., Kasanova, Z., van Aubel, E., van Winkel, R., Marcelis, M., van Amelsvoort, T., van der Gaag, M., de Haan, L., & Myin-Germeys, I. (2019). Efficacy of Acceptance and Commitment Therapy in Daily Life (ACT-DL) in early psychosis: Study protocol for a multi-centre randomized controlled trial. *Trials, 20*(1), 769. https://doi.org/10.1186/s13063-019-3912-4

Ruiz, F. J., & Luciano, C. (2015). Common physical properties among relational networks improve analogy aptness. *Journal of the Experimental Analysis of Behavior, 103*(3), 498–510. https://doi.org/10.1002/jeab.147

Salgado, C. F. (2021). Mindfulness en la persona con psicosis. In J. A. Díaz-Garrido, H. Laffite, & R. Zúñiga (Eds.), *Terapia de Aceptación y Compromiso en Psicosis: Aceptación y Recuperación por Niveles (ART)*. Pirámide.

Sass, L. A., & Parnas, J. (2003). Schizophrenia, consciousness, and the self. *Schizophrenia Bulletin, 29*(3), 427–444. https://doi.org/10.1093/oxfordjournals.schbul.a007017

Schneider, K. (1997). *Psicopatología clínica* (1.a ed.). Fundación de Archivos de Neurobiología [ed. Original: Schneider, K. (1946). *Klinische Psychopathologie*].

Seikkula, J., & Arnkill, T. (2016). *Diálogos terapéuticos en la red social*. Herder.

Seikkula, J., Alakare, B., & Aaltonen, J. (2001). Open dialogue in psychosis I: An introduction and case illustration. *Journal of Constructivist Psychology, 14*(4), 247–265. https://doi.org/10.1080/107205301750433397

Semerari, A., Cucchi, M., Dimaggio, G., Cavadini, D., Carcione, A., Battelli, V., Nicolò, G., Pedone, R., Siccardi, T., D'Angerio, S., Ronchi, P., Maffei, C., & Smeraldi, E. (2012). The development of the Metacognition Assessment interview: Instrument description, factor structure and reliability in a non-clinical sample. *Psychiatry Research, 200*(2–3), 890–895. https://doi.org/10.1016/j.psychres.2012.07.01

Shakeel, M. K., Lu, L., Woods, S. W., Perkins, D. O., & Addington, J. (2020). Neurocognitive predictors of metacognition in individuals at clinical high risk for psychosis. *Behavioural and Cognitive Psychotherapy, 48*(2), 248–252. https://doi.org/10.1017/S1352465819000328

Shattock, L., Berry, K., Degnan, A., & Edge, D. (2018). Therapeutic alliance in psychological therapy for people with schizophrenia and related psychoses: A systematic review. *Clinical Psychology & Psychotherapy, 25*(1), e60–e85. https://doi.org/10.1002/cpp.2135

Sheffield, J. M., Karcher, N. R., & Barch, D. M. (2018). Cognitive deficits in psychotic disorders: A lifespan perspective. *Neuropsychology Review, 28*(4), 509–533. https://doi.org/10.1007/s11065-018-9388-2

Shepherd, G. (1998). Developments in psychosocial rehabilitation for early psychosis. *International Clinical Psychopharmacology, 13*(Suppl 1), S53–S57. https://doi.org/10.1097/00004850-199801001-00009

Sierra, M. A., Ruiz, F. J., Flórez, C. L., Riaño Hernández, D., & Luciano, C. (2016). The role of common physical properties and augmental functions in metaphor effect. *International Journal of Psychology & Psychological Therapy, 16*(3), 265–279.

Stramecki, F., Kotowicz, K., Piotrowski, P., Beszłej, J. A., Rymaszewska, J., Samochowiec, J., Samochowiec, A., Moustafa, A. A., Jabłoński, M., Podwalski, P., Waszczuk, K., Wroński, M., & Misiak, B. (2019). Coping styles and symptomatic manifestation of first-episode psychosis: Focus on cognitive performance. *Psychiatry Research, 272*, 246–251. https://doi.org/10.1016/j.psychres.2018.12.083

Thomas, N., Morris, E. M. J., Shawyer, F., & Farhall, J. (2013). Acceptance and commitment therapy for voices. In E. M. J. Morris, L. C. Johns, & J. E. Oliver (Eds.), *Acceptance and commitment therapy and mindfulness for psychosis* (pp. 95–112). Wiley-Blackwell.

Tizón, J. (2013). *Entender las psicosis*. Herder.

Törneke, N. (2016). *Aprendiendo TMR. Una introducción a la Teoría del Marco Relacional y sus Aplicaciones Clínicas*. MICPSY publicaciones.

Törneke, N. (2020). *La metáfora en la práctica clínica. Una guía profesional para usar la ciencia del Lenguaje en Psicoterapia*. MICPSY publicaciones.

Trauelsen, A. M., Gumley, A., Jansen, J. E., Pedersen, M. B., Nielsen, H. L., Trier, C. H., Haahr, U. H., & Simonsen, E. (2016). Metacognition in first-episode psychosis and its association with positive and negative symptom profiles. *Psychiatry Research, 238*, 14–23. https://doi.org/10.1016/j.psychres.2016.02.003

Tsai, M., Kohlenberg, R. J., Kanter, J. W., Kohlenberg, B., Follette, W. C., & Callaghan, G. M. (2009). *A guide to functional analytic psychotherapy. Awareness, courage, love, and behaviorism*. Springer.

Valdivia, S., & Luciano, M. C. (2006). Una revisión de la alteración de las propiedades reforzantes de los eventos en humanos. *International Journal of Psychology and Psychological Therapy, 3*(6), 425–444.

Valery, K. M., & Prouteau, A. (2020). Schizophrenia stigma in mental health professionals and associated factors: A systematic review. *Psychiatry Research, 290*, 113068. https://doi.org/10.1016/j.psychres.2020.11306

Vallina, O. (2003). Los orígenes de la cronicidad: intervenciones iniciales en psicosis. *Boletín de la Asociación Madrileña de Rehabilitación Psicosocial, 15–16*, 15–27.

Van Aubel, E., Bakker, J. M., Batink, T., Michielse, S., Goossens, L., Lange, I., Schruers, K., Lieverse, R., Marcelis, M., Van Amelsvoort, T., Van Os, J., Wichers, M., Vaessen, T., Reininghaus, U., & Myin-Germeis, I. (2020). Blended care in the treatment of subthreshold symptoms of depression and psychosis in emerging adults: A randomised controlled trial of Acceptance and Commitment Therapy in Daily-Life (ACT-DL). *Behaviour Research and Therapy, 128*, 103592. https://doi.org/10.1016/j.brat.2020.103592

Vygotsky, L. (1978). *Pensamiento y lenguaje*. Paidós.

Wells, R., Jacomb, I., Swaminathan, V., Sundram, S., Weinberg, D., Bruggemann, J., Cropley, V., Lenroot, R. K., Pereira, A. M., Zalesky, A., Bousman, C., Pantelis, C., Weickert, C. S., & Weickert, T. W. (2020). The impact of childhood adversity on cognitive development in schizophrenia. *Schizophrenia Bulletin, 46*(1), 140–153. https://doi.org/10.1093/schbul/sbz033

World Health Organization (WHO). (2012). Measuring health and diasability: Manual for WHO disability assesment schedule (WHODAS 2.0). https://www.who.int/standards/classifications/international-classification-of-functioning-disability-and-health/who-disability-assessment-schedule

Wilson, K. G., & Hayes, S. C. (1996). Resurgence of derived stimulus relations. *Journal of the Experimental Analysis of Behavior, 66*(3), 267–281. https://doi.org/10.1901/jeab.1996.66-267

Wilson, K. G., & Luciano, M. C. (2002). *Terapia de aceptación y compromiso (ACT). Un tratamiento orientado a los valores*. Pirámide.

Chapter 18
About Hobbits, Jedi, Goddesses and Magical Energies: Clinical Cases from ART

Raquel Zúñiga, Juan Antonio Díaz-Garrido, Horus Laffite, and Maria del Rosario Cejas-Mendez

18.1 Introduction

Acceptance and recovery therapy by levels for psychosis (ART) proposes a contextual, multidimensional and interdisciplinary approach, from a stable and integrative psychotherapeutic intervention framework over time and in different forms, where the different professionals who take part with the person, either simultaneously or successively, work along the same line, taking into account the dynamic evolution of the person, their vital moment and the level of cognitive/functional deterioration they may present at any given time. The freedom of the person to decide on their treatment is the starting point of the ART approach, allowing the empowerment of the person from a secure base to choose a valuable vital direction.

It is not possible to present, or accommodate, in a single text the enormous variety of clinical and developmental manifestations of psychosis and how ART tries to adapt ideographically to them. Therefore, in this short chapter, we only intend to bring the reader, through extracts from various cases, closer to some of the possible adaptations and therapeutic adjustments in relation to the different levels of impairment, in the also different phases and evolutionary stages of psychosis.

Usually, when a clinical case or an intervention is presented, cases that represent the efficacy of a model are presented, and although they initially set out important difficulties and raise a variety of questions, in the end, they reflect a good evolution. This will not be different in our case, as the examples selected have been chosen because they meet the objectives proposed within the framework of the

R. Zúñiga (✉) · M. del Rosario Cejas-Mendez
Hospital Universitario Canarias, Santa Cruz de Tenerife, Spain
e-mail: rzuncos@gobiernodecanarias.org; mcejasme@ull.edu.es

J. A. Díaz-Garrido · H. Laffite
Hospital Universitario de Gran Canaria Doctor Negrín, Las Palmas de Gran Canaria, Spain
e-mail: jdiagarb@gobiernodecanarias.org; hlafcab@gobiernodecanarias.org

J. A. Díaz-Garrido et al. (eds.), *Psychological Interventions for Psychosis*,
https://doi.org/10.1007/978-3-031-27003-1_18

intervention. However, in psychotherapy in general, "successes" do not always occur; on the contrary, sessions are interrupted, drop-outs occur, misunderstandings occur, and we have more or less successful interventions… "Failed" interventions, which do not produce the result that the therapist expects, can be a huge source of frustration, especially in people with cognitive and functional impairment. However, what is fundamental is to understand that the interventions that we consider "failed" are part of a process (of acceptance for the therapist), in which the best strategy is to show patience and respect for the rhythm of the other person, and to persist in search of those elements (values) that may be able to get the person going again.

ART's lines of work have been previously explained, as well as its proposal for intervention in different dimensions and contexts of the person: individual, group and family (also including other significant people) and can be applicable in both private and public environments. Given the characteristics of this text, we will focus on individual intervention and we will not describe dialogic-contextual interventions, family interventions with other characteristics, or interventions in group format, since the reader can refer to the specific chapters found in this work (open dialogue and family intervention), as well as to works where these topics are developed extensively, as is the case of group intervention (see Ruiz, 2021; O'Donogue et al., 2018).

The cases presented below are real cases, however, some data have been modified to avoid their identification, likewise, some aspects of the dialogue or the description of the therapeutic process have been changed and synthesised, focusing on the most illustrative and didactic aspects of the intervention.

18.2 Prevention

The primary preventive intervention from this ART follows the ACT model, therefore, it should be directed towards the establishment of a different relationship with suffering, based on acceptance, not being rooted in literal language, awareness in the here and now and orientation towards values; which implies a different way of dealing with discomfort, as opposed to traditional interventions based on control and the search for well-being. For this, the use of psychoeducation is proposed, and above all, the development of psychological flexibility and the search for values. An example of this is the model known as Attention Focused on what is Important to the Person (ACIP –*Atención Centrada en lo Importante para la Persona* – for its acronym in Spanish) (Salgado & Mateos, 2021).

A growing number of studies demonstrate that intervention on risk factors in psychosis can reduce the intensity, improve the prognosis and even prevent a possible psychotic episode (Klippel et al., 2017; Myin-Germeys et al., 2016; Reininghaus et al., 2016). The recent formulation of ACT adapted to psychosis in daily life (ACT-DL) emphasises the role of behaviour in the concrete context (Vaessen et al., 2019) and thus the enhancement and extension of therapeutic effects to the ecological context of the person. It has been pointed out that social contact and behavioural activation are sufficient, by themselves, to generate a positive effect on subthreshold symptoms (Fledderus et al., 2012). One of the many virtues of the ACT model is its flexibility, and thus, its lack of dogmatism, which makes it applicable to the general population, to people with subthreshold symptoms and to the clinical population (van Aubel et al., 2020). In people with subthreshold psychotic symptoms (sometimes referred to as high-risk), intervention focused on improving psychological flexibility requires a period of 6–12 months, which supports continuation of ACT-DL training after the "face-to-face" therapy sessions have ended.

It has been proposed that acceptance-directed components of ACT could be effective in attenuating stress sensitivity and that commitment-directed components (values and committed action) would enhance reward-motivated action (Reininghaus et al., 2019). In addition, interventions that include members of the immediate environment can be powerful protective factors against possible episodes, relapses and/or exacerbations. From this consideration, contextualised dialogue can contribute to radical acceptance and mutual understanding in the person's natural context, through the promotion of psychological flexibility. Following this line of action, the available empirical evidence-based interventions provided by ACT and Open Dialogue, resituated and integrated with the ART model, make it a very promising intervention in the area of subthreshold psychotic symptoms, where the possible impairment of neuropsychological functions would also be taken into consideration. The latter is a factor of enormous relevance for psychotherapeutic intervention, which unfortunately has not been given sufficient attention. It should not be overlooked that there is ample evidence that cognitive deficits may be present from the premorbid stage and have a predictive capacity on the emergence of psychosis (Sheffield et al., 2018). Moreover, cognitive impairment is not only related to the course and evolution of other symptoms but is also strongly associated with difficulties in daily functioning (Green, 1996), having been identified as the most powerful predictor of the functional impact of the disorder (Heinrichs & Zakzanis, 1988), to a greater extent than positive and negative symptomatology.

Morris and Oliver (2009) propose the introduction of early intervention based on acceptance and mindfulness, linked to value-driven behavioural principles. These authors highlight:

- Learning to live in the here and now.
- Finding choices in each moment.
- Sticking to doing what is important to you.
- Observing when your mind helps you and when it does not.
- Accepting what you cannot change.
- Being compassionate with yourself.

From ART the initial objective focuses on establishing a genuine therapeutic alliance with the person and their family, limiting the impact and stigma that can be caused by the first phenomena related to the emergence of psychosis, promoting health and wellbeing through behavioural activation and values, avoiding as far as possible the early introduction of antipsychotic drugs.

18.3 Case 1: The Boy Who Hid His Smile (or the Story of Samwise Gamyee)

Sam is a young man, who is 18 years old when he comes for consultation. He has been studying Vocational Education and Training in IT. He is the first of three brothers. His parents separated when he was 7 years old, his mother was of Scandinavian origin and his father was Spanish. He grew up in shared custody, living with his mother and siblings and spending alternate weekends with his father. Sam describes his parents as very demanding, inflexible, with few social skills, but at the same time overprotective. In the family interview, there is a great deal of emotion expressed, where criticism and emotional over-involvement prevail, although they also show signs of warmth in their relationship with their son and there is a capacity for expressing positive comments.

Sam comes to the Community Mental Health Unit in the area, referred by his GP as he presents behavioural changes, isolation, insomnia and high levels of distress perceived by his family. At the Mental Health Unit, he was treated by both Clinical Psychology and Psychiatry.

On the psychopathological examination, he was conscious and globally oriented, attention problems, slightly psychomotor restlessness and intact cognition. His appearance is somewhat neglected, approachable, adequate in the consultation room and cooperative, although he seems to have a certain fear that he verbalises during the examination. Spontaneous, fluid, orderly, coherent and well-structured speech focused on the situations of high anxiety and on the clinical presentation described below. He reports depressive symptoms consisting of decrease in the intensity of emotions, anguish, apathy, anhedonia, anergy, isolation, loss of contact with peers and abandonment of activities. He denies sensory-perceptual alterations. No alterations are observed in the course of thought, but in the content, presenting ruminative ideas that are associated with great discomfort, as well as not very structured referential ideation of which he makes some criticism. Persistent mixed insomnia and diminished appetite. No self-harming ideation present. How long has it been going on?

Sam was under high stress in relation to his academic situation (he was in the middle of the exam period), against which he used strategies oriented towards control and resistance. This was compounded by family demands to maintain good grades at the end of the year, during which he experienced significant discomfort.

Sam reports that during this period of exams, he went to a meeting on the beach with several classmates. In this group, there was a girl he was attracted to, and he felt a bit nervous because he was going to be able to interact with her outside of class. He describes that, for a moment, he felt that he was being watched by the girl and when he looked back at her and smiled at her, he noticed that he was having an erection, which he experienced with great embarrassment. From then on, he began to feel anxious and to feel observed by people, thinking that they were looking at the area of his sexual organs. To this was added the fear of the idea that if he smiles at someone he could have an erection, which others would notice; he even has the idea that with a simple smile the other person could think that he is attracted to him. He is also fearful of his social environment and perceives himself as an object of mockery by his peers. This resulted in significant distress, together with a decrease in sleep and appetite, deterioration of self-care, as well as social isolation, with the abandonment of pleasant activities and a considerable decrease in academic performance.

This event appeared as the main concern in the consultation, and he repeatedly commented on it in search of reassurance, in order to calm his suffering and anguish in the presence of recurrent ego-dystonic thoughts about which he had the sensation of imposition.

Despite the commitment to a transdiagnostic model, which limits stigma and early nosological labelling, it is useful to analyse the symptoms that may be indicators of vulnerability or risk and to orient our intervention towards strengthening the psychological resources of the person. In order to be illustrative, we can see how the case presented here brings together a series of prodromal symptoms that some authors have proposed as high risk (Yung, 2003) and that, according to the DSM-5 (APA, 2014), could be labelled as Attenuated Psychosis Syndrome, a diagnosis that still requires research and validation.

As explained in "Acceptance and Commitment Therapy in Psychosis: Acceptance and Recovery Therapy by levels (ART)" (Díaz-Garrido et al., 2021b) to improve the quality of psychotherapeutic intervention, it must be adapted to the needs of the person at a given time, so it is necessary to assess the presence of cognitive and/or functional impairment. In this case, as we are dealing with a case of a few months of evolution and in which no premorbid symptoms are described, it was decided not to carry out an extensive neurocognitive assessment to evaluate the presence of impairment, obtaining normal results, where a borderline score at the attentional level stands out, which is related to the level of cognitive intrusions.

The first sessions are essential and focus on establishing a suitable therapeutic alliance, based, from our perspective, on symmetry, mimicry, empathy, congruence, validation and unconditional acceptance of the person and their experience. Our attitude has to be patient, with the intention of understanding and validating the discomfort and the desire to help the person to return to a valuable direction. With Sam, from the very beginning we were able to establish a good therapeutic relationship, for which, in addition to what was described above, we used self-disclosure, facilitating a genuine approach, as well as a frame of reference and a learning model (more information is available in the chapter "The use of Therapist Self-Disclosure in Acceptance and Commitment Therapy for Psychosis").

With Sam, we "broke the ice" in the first session by talking about his hobbies and interests, some of which he had given up. Among them he described his love for chess, which was a good opportunity to use self-disclosure and find a common bond that naturally allowed him to feel closer to the therapist, reducing the tension of the initial interview. This generated a relaxed discussion about types of openness, famous players, etc., which placed Sam in an environment in which he felt comfortable and competent, breaking the role of passive patient.

The intervention then focused on helping Sam to reconnect with aspects of his life that he considered essential and from which he had distanced himself by trying to protect himself from discomfort, through the avoidance of those situations that he anticipated as threatening. To do this, we followed the classic model of intervention proposed by ACT, starting with the generation of *creative hopelessness*.

Below are short extracts from the intervention to exemplify aspects that are considered relevant in preventive work.

Therapist: *Have you got in touch with your friends lately?*
Sam: *No, some of them have called home, but I haven't answered, I've asked my mum to say I'm not home.*
T: *I guess you still don't feel like meeting them, is that because of what you've told me?*
Sam: *Yeah (looks dejected, keeping quiet).*
Sam: *They'll be laughing at me, and when they see me they'll be laughing too, and I don't want to be embarrassed.*
T: *I understand that you feel bad when you think they're laughing at you. Were they good friends? Did you have problems with them?*
Sam: *They were good friends, I miss them...*
T: *But they laugh...*
Sam: *Yeah...*
T: *It looks like you stay in your room more and more and go out less and less.*
Sam: *Yeah... I'm not comfortable outside. Because sometimes I feel like I'm being watched.*

(At this point the aim is to generate creative hopelessness, so we avoid going into phenomena with psychotic characteristics, however striking they might seem).

T: *Does staying in your room make you feel better? Because it seems like you're trying to avoid feeling bad, but I don't know if it does.*
Sam: *I feel nervous, I don't want to worry about what people will think of me or if they're going to laugh, I'm more relaxed in my room.*
T: *And do you really get it?*
Sam: *Well, not fully. I keep wondering if they'll be talking about me or if they'll be making fun of me.*
T: *You know, this reminds me, next to this room there is another room, behind the wall. Imagine that this room is the "tranquility room" and this is the "discomfort room". As you can see, they are separated by a wall, not very thick, but made of bricks and cement. We want to go to the other side, but we have no tools, we only have our hands. To test its resistance we can give it a blow (we hit the wall with our closed hand), it sounds a bit hollow, maybe if we hit it harder we can break it (we hit the wall three times harder). How do you see the wall?*
Sam: *The same?*

T: *Exactly. And my hand hurts a bit. The thing is, I still want to be on that side. So imagine now I start punching with all my strength, punching the wall. I'm likely to hurt my hand badly, or I might even break a bone in my hand. But the wall will stay the same.*

Sam: *Even with a hole in it (laughs).*

T: *Yes (laughs). We have the need to escape from this room, from the anguish, and be on the side of the "tranquility room". The funny thing is that even though I want it so badly I'm still in the "discomfort room" and I'm hurting myself more and more.*

Sam: Nods. *Do I have to get out of my room? But I don't know how to control my moods.*

T: *I don't know how to control them either. What I do know is that by hitting the wall you're hurting yourself.*

The *metaphor of the wall* acted as a "guiding metaphor" (at the end of the chapter all the metaphors are collected) during the intervention, helping Sam to identify the moments when he again struggled with his thoughts, eventually isolating himself as a way of avoiding discomfort.

The following experiential activity was incorporated at this point in the intervention:

T: *Right now you are giving up things that are important to you for the fear that these thoughts that are so upsetting to you will appear and you won't be able to control them. It's as if you don't want them to wake up and you have to go through your life slowly, quietly. This fear has even led you to stop moving and moving forward. So that's what this exercise is all about, there (several metres away) is the table, and on it I have prepared a chessboard so that we can play a short game. If it is important for you to play this game, I want you to come to it with an extra handicap (arms and legs are wrapped with aluminium foil), use the same strategy that you are using every day, don't make noise.*

S: *It's impossible to move like that! (laughs)*

T: *it seems that trying to control not making noise doesn't allow you to move as you would like to. Maybe the impossible thing is to move without making noise.*

Sam, after about a minute of moving slowly and awkwardly because of the effect of the aluminium foil, starts to walk normally as the aluminium foil adapts to the movement.

S: *Let's play.*

T: *But that noise is still with you, won't it bother you to play?*

S: *No, I have white.*

The aluminium foil exercise has a wide applicability in the different phases of ACT (creative hopelessness, control as a problem, value orientation, willingness and commitment). The initial explanation of the exercise is metaphorical in nature and will need to be adapted to the individual's level of understanding. In Sam's case, there is no cognitive impairment, but we have nevertheless guided the metaphor and made several clarifications, limiting the interpretation and possible relational derivations. However, once the metaphors and experiential exercises have been completed, it is necessary to explore the meaning that the person has derived from them.

The main objective of the intervention with Sam was to learn to live with his feelings of discomfort, for which we initially focused on a psychoeducational orientation, normalising and giving meaning to anxiety, learning to live with it and understanding that the avoidance/escape and control of it could generate not only an increase in anxiety, but also have an impact on our internal speech, increasing the cognitive fusion of previous thoughts (low self-esteem, tendency to comparison, need to be accepted by his peers…). We worked from ACT and different dialogic-contextual family interventions were carried out. This helped to de-stigmatise the problems of the "identified patient", promoting greater psychological flexibility with respect to the problem presented by Sam on the part of the family members. Functional exposure was the guiding principle of the approach.

Throughout the intervention Sam gradually tolerated the discomfort of the idea and the feeling of having become the focus of ridicule from others, decreasing the frequency and number of avoidance behaviours. He also achieved a change in his relationship with his thoughts, being able to observe them without becoming attached to them and identifying them as just another thought (defusion). Sam returned to his usual routines and activities, integrating into the group of friends without major difficulties and initiating new activities in relation to his values.

And, like the character Samwise Gamyee, after his odyssey and journey in Lord of the Rings, he approached the girl he liked and started a relationship with her. Although this was not the aim of the intervention, as it was oriented towards changing the relationship with the discomfort, the intrusive ideas stopped occurring. During the therapeutic process, Sam never received neuroleptic treatment, only anxiolytic and hypnotic treatment to preserve sleep. He is currently asymptomatic and does not require psychiatric medication.

18.4 Approach During Acute "Symptomatology"

The acute clinical phase is a period during which people may present severe psychotic symptoms such as delusions, hallucinations, severely disorganised thoughts and behaviour. Acute symptomatology capable of requiring admission implies for the person a significant decrease in functionality and adaptation to his or her environment.

It is essential to take into account the specific and characteristic aspects that require the care and admission to the Emergency Services or Psychiatric Care and Hospitalisation Units, as they can have an enormous influence on subsequent interventions due to the fact that:

1. Both patients and relatives have described acute units as unsafe and with a negative effect on mental health, rather than promoting recovery (Schizophrenia Commission, 2012).

2. People who have been admitted report feelings of being trapped, shame, fear, stigma, as well as a sense of life defeat.
3. Trauma in care (Anthony, 1993; Frueh et al., 2005).
4. Resistance and struggle against the process entail an experience of "imprisonment".
5. Inpatients report insufficient access to psychotherapy, while psychotherapy is considered a high priority for them (Jones et al., 2010; Lelliott & Quirk, 2004).

Despite the scarce presence of psychotherapy in acute units, there are data supporting the benefits of its use from the acute phase of the illness. Recent meta-analyses indicate that cognitive behavioural therapy, metacognitive therapy and acceptance and commitment therapy are effective in hospitalised patients (Wood et al., 2020) and those brief ACT interventions during hospital admissions can help people stay out of hospital longer after discharge (Gaudiano & Herbert, 2006; Bach & Hayes, 2002). Furthermore, mindfulness-based interventions have been shown to be safe, feasible, highly accepted and valued by patients with psychosis in an inpatient setting, with low drop-out rates and high follow-up (Jacobsen et al., 2020). Data indicate a lower risk of readmission and relapse at 12 months in patients who have received mindfulness-based crisis interventions (MBCI). Moreover, available studies on open dialogue also indicate longitudinally sustained efficacy over time (Seikkula et al., 2006; Bergström et al., 2018).

Given that studies to date support the efficacy of cognitive-behavioural and contextual interventions, metacognitive interventions, mindfulness, as well as open dialogue, which are an integral part of ART, intervention from this model may be a promising approach in acute settings and in the psychiatric inpatient situation.

ART interventions in the acute inpatient setting follow the following recommendations:

- **Individual sessions.** The intervention includes experiential exercises and stories, mindfulness, values clarification and goal setting, as proposed by Gaudiano et al. (2017).
- **Group sessions.** In the context of hospitalisation, it is recommended to include group activities for all people who are frequently hospitalised. To work from ART we follow the model of O'Donogue et al. (2018) adapting it to the level of cognitive/functional impairment. This follows a skills workshop model, with about six participants and two or three facilitators. Four 50-min sessions are held twice a week. The group will be as homogeneous as possible according to their behavioural characteristics, rather than clinical diagnosis, and at a similar stage of recovery. This model of group intervention is not intended to discuss personal issues in depth, but rather to be aware of the experience and learn from it. We refer the reader to the work of Ruiz (2017, 2021; Ruiz & Ruiz, 2018) and Butler et al. (2016).
- **Dialogic-based family intervention (contextual dialogism).** We propose two weekly sessions lasting around an hour and a half.
- **Specific techniques for working with delusions and hallucinations.** Although it is not our priority objective of intervention, in some cases it is difficult to work with people who are excessively attentive and fused to their mental production, as the personal suffering is so high that it is difficult to reach them if we do not

provide them with a specific strategy, as well as the fact that on many occasions this is the central demand. Therefore, an "extra" is needed to reach the person and to promote a value-based approach and psychological flexibility. Interventions for positive symptomatology: *Contextualised Voice Focusing* and *Spiral* in delusions.

- **Coordination and case management.** Including the extended or expanded therapeutic team from horizontality with contextual dialogical principles.
- **Intervention and self-care workshops.** Aimed at all staff in the field of Mental Health nursing, to serve as a respite and to work on difficulties and/or specific problems of teamwork, iatrostigma and compassion fatigue.
- **Regular training plans on contextual principles.**

18.5 Case 2: Luke, Do. Or Do Not. There Is No Try

The case presented for the exposition of the intervention on people with acute psychotic symptomatology follows the model proposed by ART. As stated above, this model is based on the conceptualisation and approach of ACT, which will be extended by including specific techniques and adaptations.

Following the proposed intervention model, and adjusting to the characteristics of the person, as well as the time of admission and the resources present in the acute unit, the following intervention scheme was proposed:

- **Individual sessions.** Three sessions were held per week, each lasting between 30 and 45 min. Occasionally, and at the patient's request, brief interventions were carried out at times of increased distress. In the development of the sessions, the classic ACT protocol was followed, focusing on applications oriented towards: creative hopelessness, acceptance, behavioural disposition as an alternative to control and entrapment in unproductive struggle, defusion of the "I-content", orientation towards values.
- **Group sessions.** This person participated in four group sessions during the last 2 weeks of admission. A total of five people participated in this group in the context of acute hospitalisation, all of them with similar cognitive/functional functioning, adjusting the pace to the person with the greatest difficulty. The facilitators were a nurse and a nursing assistant, as well as the clinical psychologist of the unit. It was not possible to assess the specific effectiveness of the group intervention, although in the satisfaction and quality questionnaires the presence of the group activity was positively evaluated, being considered by the participants as valuable and useful for emotional management, the normalisation of discomfort and the formation of emotional bonds with other participants.
- **Dialogic-based family intervention (contextual dialogism).** Three sessions were held throughout the admission, with the participation of the parents, a close friend and a cousin, and the psychologist and the nurse referring the case on behalf of the therapeutic team. The meeting was held at the beginning of the

admission, trying to combine the principle of immediate response adapted to the limitations of the psychiatric ward of the public health service. Although in this particular case, given the availability of the person's support network and the difficulty to coordinate the person's support network timetable with the possibilities of the unit, it was not possible to comply with the periodicity recommended by the ART model of two weekly sessions. The sessions held lasted 90 min. This type of family intervention integrates the theoretical-practical formulation of open dialogue with the contextual philosophy, proposing a scenario where emotions can be experienced and deliteralised from cognition in a safe context, where acceptance and respect for the different polyphonic positions are also sought, encouraging the development of psychological flexibility. The dialogic sessions will not be presented in this chapter; for further information on how to proceed with this model, we refer the reader to the corresponding chapters of this work.

- **Specific techniques for working with delusions and hallucinations.** Throughout the time of admission, we work with contextualised voice focusing. The intervention is described below.
- **Coordination and case management.** Coordination was maintained with the Community Mental Health team and the work carried out during admission was reported at discharge for continuity on an outpatient basis. Likewise, the nurse from the local Mental Health unit attended the unit on two occasions (first and last week) as a representative of the team to accompany and liaise between units, favouring the therapeutic alliance, adherence to treatment and guaranteeing continuity of care. In addition, daily team meetings were held where individual, group and dialogic/family work was coordinated.

Luke was a 43-year-old male who at the time we met him lived with his family of origin (father and mother). He had a degree in engineering but did not work or receive any kind of income. His medical history included three involuntary psychiatric admissions, with a diagnosis of paranoid schizophrenia.

From the time he was discharged from the first admission, he went to the Community Mental Health Unit in his area, where he was treated by both psychiatry and clinical psychology. He was prescribed antipsychotic and anxiolytic treatment.

Approximately 18 years ago, after a conflict at work, he began to have the feeling of being watched by people around him, a feeling which progressively increased, and was joined by the idea that the situation was related to a conspiracy by his company to prevent him from denouncing a possible corruption scheme at international level. There were also "voices" warning him that his life was in danger: "he is watching you, he wants to kill you", "you are in danger, hide", "don't trust him". This resulted in a significant behavioural disturbance, engaging in verbal confrontation with those by whom he felt persecuted or threatened, eventually running away and hiding for days. This dynamic occurred in a similar way on several occasions over the following years. Despite the symptomatological improvement obtained during psychiatric admissions, on discharge the voices and suspicion reappeared, requiring repeated admissions over time, a phenomenon known as the "revolving door".

On a fourth admission, during the psychopathological examination, he showed himself:

Conscious and oriented in the three spheres, no attention problems, psychomotor restlessness. In the gross examination, no alteration of cognitive functions was observed. Interpretative and hostile in his treatment, with contained aggressiveness in the interview, showing little collaboration. Throughout the entire interview, he holds a book of religious character. Although he gives little information, his speech is spontaneous, fluid, coherent and well-structured. Excessively rationalising, of a morbid nature, showing himself to be vindictive and litigious. Minimising clinical symptomatology, as well as behavioural repercussions during the last few weeks. Dysphoric, with delirious mood and reactive affect. Denies sensory-perceptual alterations, although these cannot be ruled out, given that during the interview he states that he is being warned of harm to himself ("they warn me that they want to lock me up"), and what appears to be "listening" behaviour is also observed. Spontaneous verbalisation of delusions centred on the family environment ("this is because of my parents, they are bought off, they want to lock me up"), as well as references to health staff ("they coerce me to administer me drugs that make me feel bad"). Alteration in the sleep pattern that the patient minimises and does not specify. No self-harming ideation or self- or heteroaggressive intention at the present time. Impaired judgement of reality.[1]

Since Luke is being followed up in the Mental Health Unit, we know his level of cognitive functioning during the stabilisation phases. We can place him at a level of mild cognitive impairment, as he has slight difficulties with attention, memory, processing speed and executive functions. In addition, clinical observation revealed difficulties in emotional processing and social perception. At the time of admission, the alteration of cognitive functions is greater, with significant problems in maintaining attention and remembering information, on the other hand, functional capacity is practically abolished, not being able to maintain minimal self-care. The level of cognitive/functional impairment is a dynamic and changing concept, and the person's functioning may be affected by numerous factors, such as the increased severity of psychotic phenomenology, loss of stimulation and increased social isolation, treatment modifications and adjustments and even global stigma, among others. During admission, pharmacological treatment was established and modified; we will not go into a description of this as it is beyond the scope of this chapter.

Luke's admission lasted 41 days, during which he went through different phases. Initially, he was remaining most of the time in his room, defiant and suspicious, with a rationalising and vindictive discourse and a clinical foreground with ideas of harm, impressing the perceptive experience of hearing voices. In this first phase, given the level of distress, as well as the deterioration of his attentional capacity, which was fixed in psychotic phenomena, the main therapeutic objective was to

[1] In psychopathological examinations, concepts such as awareness of illness and the presence or absence of insight are often added. In addition to the complexity of describing such states, with marked discrepancies in the literature, we start from the idea that these concepts, arising from the biomedical model, are neither necessary nor relevant to a person's recovery.

provide a structured, safe and stable environment, allowing the verbalisation of his discomfort, showing closeness and unconditional acceptance.

Below are extracts from the intervention that was carried out individually during Luke's stay in the Acute Unit. It should be noted that extracts are shown here to illustrate the intervention, so it may appear that each session worked on a different experiential exercise or metaphor. However, each metaphor or exercise was usually repeated throughout the sessions, alluding to them to reinforce the work done, clarify doubts and guide the interpretations made. Thus, for example, the metaphor of the *white polar bear* was recalled every time Luke presented a new thought and ruminative verbalisations, or when he became more hermetic about his suffering we reminded him of the "*smell of the kitchen*" (full description at the end of the chapter). In addition, although it will not be described in this section, Luke participated in group sessions, where the guiding metaphor used was the one of the *bus passengers* (Hayes et al., 1999). During the individual sessions, the latter metaphor was also worked on and the intervention was oriented towards Luke's values. In relation to the use of metaphors, the recommendations proposed by Morris (2019) were followed: use of a central metaphor that would function as a scaffold, easily remembered, capable of reflecting the essence of the problems that the person describes and with repetition in the different sessions. Furthermore, as pointed out in Díaz-Garrido et al. (2021b), when applying psychotherapeutic strategies and their possible adaptations, several relevant factors should be taken into account: the person's history and context, the clinical phase in which he/she is, the psychopathology present and the level of impairment.

18.5.1 Making Contact: Working the Alliance

Within the ART model, attachment and the quality of the close, human and genuine therapeutic relationship guide the whole intervention process as psychotherapeutic principles. They are the main points around which the rest of the interventions are articulated.

This first phase lasted approximately 1 week, after which Luke began to be more communicative, both with other patients and with the ward staff. In addition, at an attentional level, he was able to remain focused on the conversations and dynamics of the ward. In this circumstance, the following meeting took place (a summary of the dialogue is made):

Therapist: *How are you Luke?*
Luke: *(he remains silent, returning a gesture of resignation and rejection).*
T: *(we remain silent for a few seconds) Do you feel like talking? I'd like to have a conversation with you and find out how this admission is going for you.*
Luke: *I don't feel like it, but I don't seem to have any other choice…*

T: *You don't have to talk to me. Part of my professional role is to help the people on this floor in any way I can. So I'd like to get to know you and see together how I can be of help to you.*

Luke: *Yeah sure, help… like forcing me to be here.*

T: *That's right, you're forced to be here and I understand that's not nice. I can imagine how I would feel in your situation and I think I would be very angry. My job is to take care of people, and I have to try to do that. That's why I propose something to you, you are going to be the one to decide whether or not to talk to me, I will come by every day and I will continue to offer it to you. If you say no, I'll respect that and I'll leave, although I have to tell you that I'd like to, because that's my intention, to help. So it's up to you to decide.*

The next day Luke is sitting talking to another user in the common recreation room. As we enter the room we position ourselves in a visible space, from which Luke can anticipate our availability. Luke initially refuses to talk and the therapist, respecting the agreement, prepares to leave the room. Just then, Luke calls out to the therapist with a smile and says "just kidding, you passed the test". Thus, Luke allows us to start the intervention, from a position of free choice that will favour active involvement and the therapeutic relationship.

Despite allowing interaction, in the first encounters, he is hermetic and uncommunicative about the reason for admission. However, he is able to communicate his discomfort at being in a situation of admission, being able to talk about other topics of interest, about which he is more relaxed. In this context, the following dialogue takes place:

Therapist: *I think you find it difficult to talk about what is going on with you.*

Luke: *What do you mean? (his expression changes and he looks annoyed).*

T: *You've been on this floor for over a week, you still haven't told me what brought you here.*

Luke: *Well, it's my personal stuff, I see no reason why I should be obliged to tell you. I'm sure you've got it there (points to the computer screen).*

T: *My colleagues left things written down when you came to the emergency room. However, there are always different points of view that can be equally valid and understandable when heard. So I'd like to hear what your point of view is.*

Luke remains hesitant without beginning to speak.

T: *I thought I'd tell you something, do you have or have you ever had a pet?*

Luke: *No, but I'd like to have a dog.*

T: *Great, then. Imagine you've already adopted a dog and one day, he has a poo and you know when he has a poo he poops all over the house, everywhere, all the time. And you know that everything stinks. You decide that night to put the feeder and the water bowl, along with his blanket for him to sleep in the kitchen and you close the door so that if he's still sick he won't poop all over the house during the night. So you go to sleep. The next morning, when you go to open the kitchen door and.... you are hit by a dreadful smell that floods your nostrils, you can almost feel it in your mouth, and a terrifying sight! Your dog has been sick to his stomach all night and has defecated all over the kitchen, everything is brown, there's nowhere to step! You carefully get the dog out and immediately close the door, knowing that you won't be back for a few hours. So you have breakfast outside. Meanwhile, in the kitchen the smell will become more and more intense, even sticking to the walls and furniture. The longer it stays closed the worse it gets. What do you plan to do?*

We use this metaphor with Luke because in our experience it is useful when the person is fearful and secretive about talking about "the symptoms", and it is applicable at any level of cognitive/functional impairment. It is also mobilising when the person is fearful of taking value-oriented action because of the barriers they foresee.

Following this intervention Luke began to refer to the thoughts that had made him so distressed, giving examples of situations where he felt he was the victim of external instigators.

From this point on, the typical ACT phases described by García-Montes and Pérez-Álvarez (2016) were followed.

18.5.2 "Creative Despair"

The aim is for the person to get in touch with the lack of success of the strategies they have repeatedly carried out to resolve their situation. The aim is to make emotional contact with the uncertainty and lack of progress towards vital goals, moving away from strategies that have produced short-term relief, but which in the long run, have worsened the real situation or have kept the subject in the vicious circle of avoidance.

Follow-up interview. Luke and the therapist already have a good therapeutic alliance, so he accepts and actively participates in the intervention.

Therapist: *How are you feeling today?*

Luke: *How am I going to feel? They take away my freedom, they force me to be here, I'm in a prison. Everyone here is crazy. I just want to go home and get on with my life. How would you be in my place?*

T: *You know, you're right. How can I not give it to you? Probably if I were in your place I would feel in a very similar way to you. In fact, sometimes I feel that way too. Let me tell you something. At the time, I had a job where I met my first partner and everything was going very well until we broke up, which made me feel terrible. Every time we met, I felt anxious, I felt self-conscious, I thought he thought badly of me... and I even considered taking a break, and even leaving it. In that situation I had two options: to quit my job so I wouldn't feel so bad, or, on the contrary, to continue working, get over the bad feeling and continue to maintain the things that mattered to me and my way of life. What would you choose if you were me?*

Luke: *Well, if you liked the job, stay in the job.*

T: *That's what I think too. There are situations that keep us trapped. Often what we do is fight them and hold on to the fight with the intention of changing them. For example, you have told me on several occasions that you are convinced that there is a plot against you, and that is why you are here involuntarily, so that you cannot fight against that plot. But you have also told me that you want to get on with your life. As I see it, you are presented with two options: to fight against your admission and the plot, where you never end up feeling good, or to move on with your life. Which one do you choose now?*

Luke is then given the "Chinese finger trap" to physicalise the unsuccessful fight. After a while of trying to free his fingers, the conversation continues.

T: *I see you haven't managed to get out of the trap. After many attempts and struggles, it seems that the finger trap has you more and more trapped. But if you notice, oddly enough, if you push your fingers slightly into the tube you have more room and can move them.*

Luke: *(testing) You're right, I feel more liberated. (laughing) That's funny.*

T: *The funny thing is that, even if you don't like it, I get the impression that in your life, with these sensations of being persecuted, of losing your freedom, the more you pull, the more you struggle to escape… the tighter the trap and the more trapped you become. And in the meantime, what have you done with your life? It's like with the finger trap, you seem to get more and more trapped, and you live less and less.*

Luke: *Seen like that, it seems like I've pretty much given up on myself. I've been doing this for so long, I haven't been able to be calm. What can I do?*

T: *I'm not sure. But fighting doesn't seem to work, just like pulling out doesn't seem to work, does it? On the other hand, doing something illogical, like wiggling your fingers inwards instead of outwards, sometimes works. Maybe doing something different from what you have done so far could give you the freedom to go back to your life. What could you do differently now?*

In the above excerpt, self-disclosure is used with the function of providing personal experiences that normalise suffering as an inherent condition of people, presenting the therapist as a human being who also suffers, which favours the therapeutic bond and models self-disclosure behaviour. Emotionally strong self-disclosures increase feelings of closeness and support (Laurenceau et al., 1998) and dispel the illusion that the world is made up of unproblematic and patient people, as well as providing normality and instilling hope (Chadwick, 2009).

As shown, given the presence of attentional and memory difficulties, it is chosen to combine dialogue with an experiential exercise. In this way, the person has a more vivid memory of the session and we have the object (the "finger trap") that we will keep present throughout the sessions as a reminder.

18.5.3 Control as a Problem

It shows the bad results of trying to control internal events. It seeks to make the person understand that there are aspects of their experience, such as emotions, thoughts, memories and sensations that are impossible to keep under control. For example, the fight against the discomfort generated by the voices by avoidance through social isolation or sensory isolation (locking oneself in a room, listening to music through headphones…), which seem to reduce the immediate aversive stimulation at a high cost, generating a rebound effect with an increase in sensory-perceptual phenomena. On the other hand, we seek acceptance, not in a passive way, but an active acceptance, far from resignation, which allows the person to focus on what is really important to them.

To work on the avoidance of thoughts and voices, we introduce the *white bear exercise* (modification of the classic exercise by Wegner et al., 1987):

Therapist: *What do you do when these thoughts come?*
Luke: *I try to distract myself, I tell myself not to think about it and to think about the positive part, that's what my family and friends also tell me.*
T: *And does it work for you?*
Luke: *No, sometimes I manage to distract myself for a while, but then they come back.*
T: *Of course, telling ourselves not to think about something never works; in fact, it doesn't work for anyone.*

Then we propose the following:

"I want you to imagine that you are a cameraman for a famous channel, we are going to record a documentary about the animal world, I will be the director and I will give you the indications about what to focus on at each moment. Imagine that we have moved to the Arctic and we are going to film a white polar bear, can you see it? Focus on the bear with your camera. Can you see where it is? Is it alone or is it accompanied by other white polar bears? What is it doing? Now let's zoom in on our white polar bear, zoom in on its face, how are the eyes of the white polar bear?; now open its jaws, how are the teeth of the white polar bear?; how is the fur of this white polar bear?; it is beautiful, but it might be better not to get too close to a white polar bear. And its paws?; they are big and strong, the white polar bear is an imposing animal. How tall is this white polar bear?

Now I want you to stop thinking about the white polar bear, you must make an effort to stop thinking about it, be careful!, don't think about the white polar bear, not even about the word bear... (After a few seconds) But if I told you not to think about it, why do you keep thinking about the white polar bear?"

At the end of this exercise, with the idea of generating greater emotional impact, we can bang on the table while saying "I don't want you to think about a polar bear…" in a firm voice, applying an attempt to *stop the thought* and demonstrating that it is impossible to control it.

Although Luke at this point presents greater attentional capacity than in previous sessions and is able to understand the exercise, it is decided to continue working on the concept of control as a problem with a physicalised exercise, so that we reinforce the function worked on according to the level of cognitive/functional impairment assessed at the time of the intervention.

18.5.4 Tambourine Exercise

Therapist: *You have told me that these thoughts that you have taken you up a lot of time, they give you anxiety and sometimes even fear. And that the voices you hear, although they are not very frequent, seem to become more present the more stressed and anxious you feel. What do you usually do when the thoughts and voices appear?*

Luke: *I get in a bad mood, I don't want to be with anyone, because I know I'm being watched and watched, I go into my room, I put my headphones on.*

T: *You try to avoid them. I would say even more, you try not to feel all that.*

Luke: *Yeah, although I think that's the way it is… I'm tired of feeling that way. I try, and I try, but I just can't do it.*

T: *I can think of something, look what I brought today.*

The therapist shows a tambourine with a string attached to it.

T: *I propose something fun, something different from what we usually do.*

Luke: *(smiles) I don't know…, come on, tell me…*

T: *I propose we tie this tambourine to your ankle and take a little walk around the office area. Don't worry, it's just you and me in this area.*

Luke puts on the tambourine and starts to walk around, making a lot of noise.

Luke: *It's uncomfortable to walk with this, it bothers me, I make a lot of noise and it's annoying, even though I try to walk slower and shuffle my feet so I don't lift the tambourine I still make a lot of noise.*

T: *What would happen if you walked faster and lifted your feet normally?*

Luke: *I would make a lot more noise, plus the tambourine would move back and forth and I might end up in front of my feet and trip.*

T: *What if there were people around, would it work to try to go slowly and shuffle so as not to attract attention?*

Luke: *It wouldn't matter, everyone would look at me, I'd make noise, and I'd walk funny. They'd laugh and think I'm stupid, they'd think I'm crazy, they'd think I'm clowning around.*

T: *I mean, it seems that despite the attempts to control the noise of the tambourine, it keeps going. It's as if you don't want to have the tambourine with you, as if you want to take it away so that it doesn't bother you. Now I want you to hold the tambourine with your hands, even if it is still tied to your foot. Walk around the room like this. How does it feel now?*

Luke: *It's less uncomfortable, it makes some noise, but not that much.*
T: *It's the same tambourine though, still tied to the foot, but it seems that instead of fighting it, you've accepted it and you're carrying it with you. Do you think you'd get other people's attention that way?*
Luke: *No, it wouldn't be so weird that way, it doesn't make so much noise.*
T: *Exactly, acceptance is not giving up, acceptance is continuing to do the things you want to do despite carrying the tambourine.*

This exercise can be adapted and done with other objects that make noise, such as a box full of paper clips, dragging it with your foot on the floor first.

18.5.5 "Cognitive Defusion"

Aimed at the person distancing himself or herself from certain cognitions. Cognitive fusion refers to excessive or inappropriate control of language that limits flexibility and the implementation of more adaptive behaviours in a particular context. In contrast, defusion seeks to create a context of deliteralisation that diminishes the regulatory nature of language and facilitates contact with ongoing events. Defusion focuses primarily on the verbal aspects of human experience and by deliteralising we weaken the functional domain of literal and evaluative rule-based response.

An ART strategy to be used when sensory-perceptual phenomenology significantly interferes with functionality is the *focus on voices*, a reformulation of the classic model of Bentall et al. (1994) in which the aim is not to control or eliminate voices but to distance and change the relationship with them.

This strategy has four stages already described in the previous chapter:

1. Mindfulness through the senses.
2. Mindfulness of thoughts (including voices). Functional exposure.
3. Acceptance of discomfort and value-directed behaviour. Metaphors such as the "bus", the "swamp" (Wilson & Luciano, 2002) or the bicycle (Díaz-Garrido et al., 2021b) are used.
4. Addressing values.

Another deliteralisation exercise that we use for cognitive defusion when working on voices with Luke is the adaptation that we propose of the exercise *Take Your Mind for a Walk* (Hayes et al., 1999; Wilson & Luciano, 2002).

Thus, we used this adaptation once he was discharged from the inpatient unit. It is noteworthy that at this point Luke is less distressed and is able to continue with the intervention on an outpatient basis; however, both delusions and auditory hallucinations remain and are a source of distress.

In relation to the level of cognitive/functional impairment, Luke has returned to the level of functioning prior to hospital admission, with a level of mild impairment (level 2).

18.5.6 Taking Voices for a Walk

After discharge, psychotherapeutic sessions continue on an outpatient basis. Luke is offered an exercise to work on the defusion of voices. Beforehand, we must know which are the most frequent and common voices of the person, as well as those that most disturb him or have interfered with his activities in the past. In this case, we suggest going for a walk around the hospital grounds (a garden area where we know we are not going to meet many people), accompanied by a nurse from the Acute Hospitalisation Unit team. Before starting the exercise, Luke is told that the therapist and the nurse will act as the voices, Luke should simply continue walking, walking wherever he prefers, but he should not interact with us. During the walk he is spoken to with phrases that refer to the usual comments of "their voices": "they are going to hurt you", "everything is a plot", "they are against you", "that person is watching you", "they have sent spies to watch you", "you'd better go home". At the end of the walk, he is reinforced for having continued the walk, despite the voices, emphasising that these voices do not have the strength to prevent the action they are doing or what they want to do.

18.5.7 "A Transcendent Sense of Self"

It aims for the person to create a flexible sense of self. It seeks to bring the person into contact with all that they experience or have experienced throughout their existence: the variety of their thoughts, sensations and emotions, to get in touch with their contextual self. In contrast, what is known as the conceptualised self or the concept self is the personal narrative and description of what one believes oneself to be. The promotion of the self as a context helps people to take perspective regarding experiences, feared and avoided until now, through metaphors, experiential exercises, mindfulness, etc. A widely used exercise in this sense is the *Chessboard Metaphor* (Hayes et al., 1999), aimed at the distinction between the contained self and the context self or the *Observer Self exercise* (Hayes et al., 1999). We can also use the metaphor of the *observer at the window*.

This exercise is useful for people who have difficulties with abstraction, as well as those who have attentional problems, since using an element that is present helps to anchor their attention and does not require the generation of a mental image.

18.5.8 Metaphor of the Observer at the Window

Therapist: *Come with me to the window, let's look at the sky. Notice how the sky takes up everything. Sometimes there are no clouds, sometimes there are lots of clouds. For example, today we found quite a lot of clouds. Let's imagine that each cloud is a thought, a memory, an emotion. That one (we point) is reminding me "I have to eat at three o'clock in the afternoon", that one brings back the memory "the day I fell out of the tree when I was ten years old", the other one tells me "my head itches", another one "I'm not having a good day today". The sky is the space where all those clouds are, and the funny thing is that the sky is always there, regardless of the number of clouds. Imagine that the sky is your mind, the space where your emotions, feelings, thoughts and memories are, and each cloud is one of these that tells you something. Who are you really?*

Luke: *I am the clouds and I am the sky.*

T: *Are you sure? I would say otherwise.*

Luke: *What would you say?*

T: *I am the one looking through the window, and I choose what to look at. Aren't you?*

18.5.9 Value Orientation

Values are vital directions, achievable through behaviour, but never finished, never completely concluded, always present as a framework for behaviour, giving meaning and purpose to behaviour (Páez et al., 2006). In people with PSD, it is common to find a personal history of high expressed emotion, recurrent invalidation, abuse, trauma and social exclusion in their environment, so they may not be clear about what their values are. In addition, they may be imbued by their psychotic experiences, through struggle, avoidance or involvement with them, which can make it difficult to reflect on their values and their own identity. In view of this, it is necessary to generate with the person a sense of advancement, an advancement oriented from the perspective of freedom, where it is the person who decides at each moment the direction he/she wants to follow, without having to justify his/her choice.

Through the *Values Questionnaire* (Wilson & Luciano, 2002) and therapeutic dialogue, we construct values with Luke, using psychoeducational explanations of what values are.

T: *Values are like walking towards the north, you can ask and they will answer you where the north is, imagine that someone tells you "the north is there on the horizon", and you can walk towards that horizon, but when you go there you realise that as you walk there is always a horizon to the north and you never end up there. The important thing is the way, but the way, always towards the north.*

Continuing with the work on value orientation, the spiral process is introduced, which was developed during several sessions. The spiral process attempts to weaken verbal evaluations and their psychological impact due to rule-governed behaviour, instead of confronting the delusion, thus facilitating learning modelled by direct contingencies, increasing acceptance, mindfulness and the person's behavioural repertoire, as well as compassion towards oneself and others, fostering a flexible functionality to the environment. Delusions not only avoid but also psychotically construct the reality they wish to achieve or the obstacles that impede it (García-Montes & Pérez-Álvarez, 2005).

The more fused the delusion is, the more integrated it is with the I-concept, and it is logical to think that the older it is and/or the more it is linked to established rules, the greater the degree of fusion with the content (Díaz-Garrido et al., 2021a). Thus, the spiral process starts with the most recent delusion, going little by little from the superficial to the core of the delusion in an iterative process. The purpose is not to end the delusion, nor to defeat it, but to recover the previous functionality interfered with by the delusional process.

Stages of the spiral process:

1. Establishment of a genuine and solid therapeutic alliance. Mimicry (the therapist accommodates the person's communication style, affective modalities, tone, rhythm, etc., including delusions).
2. Functional analysis and history.
3. "Traps" to functional self-exposure
4. Non-control and acceptance: Mindfulness exercises, metaphors and reality testing. Examples of useful exercises: Paper clip box, tambourine exercise, observer at the window, white bear metaphor.
5. Value redirection. Bus metaphor.
6. Commitment to values. Bridge to values. Bicycle metaphor. Garden metaphor.

Below we develop several extracts from the spiral process carried out with Luke over several sessions. This work is initiated when in Luke's evolution some delusional aspects interfere again with his functioning.

Luke: *I'm noticing a bit of "that" thing I was worried about. (Luke remains silent for a few minutes, showing signs of concern).*
T: *Are you anxious again, like when you were in the hospital?*
Luke: *No, it's not that. It's the feeling.... Well, you know... Although you'll think it's all in my head, just like everyone else.*
T: *The important thing is how you're feeling, how do you deny what you're feeling? Would you like to explain to me what's happening to you?*
Luke: *Well... Yeah... It's... (hesitates for a few moments). Well okay, I was just starting to go out to do my shopping at the supermarket near my house. There sits a homeless man with a big dog. At first I didn't notice anything, but I started to notice that every time I appeared he started shouting and swearing, and the dog started barking, more and more.*
T: *And what's he doing there, is he someone asking at the door of the shop?*
Luke: *It looked like that.... But I know he's there for me, to keep an eye on me. They've reactivated the surveillance system and I've detected one of their agents.*

In this first phase we see how the delusion has become stronger than in previous weeks, again diminishing Luke's functionality. The first step in order to start the spiral process and work on the delusion with the aim of regaining functionality is mimicry. Furthermore, with this we try to validate his experience and emotions, without judgement or rebuttal on the basis of a strong therapeutic alliance.

T: *I've been thinking about what you told me the other day and how this web of agents makes you isolate yourself at home and not do what you enjoy.*
Luke: *Right, so this way I avoid being controlled.*
T: *How about looking at it from the other side? It seems like they're getting total control by getting you to stay at home.*
Luke: *I hadn't thought of that.*
T: *It looks like you've hit a dead end, by staying at home to avoid being controlled they've taken complete control. It looks like we're going to have to find a way out of this situation.*
Luke: *Yes... But what can I do?*
T: *It occurs to me that, with any excuse, you can stay near the entrance of the establishment, so that you can observe this person and his dog. This may make you anxious, distressed and anxious to run away, wanting to go home. However, it is very important that you hold on because it is important for you to study this person and their dog, remember the voices on the bus... What is your destination?*

In a second phase we try to promote functionality and redirection towards values through "self-exposure traps" and different exercises, focusing on the bus metaphor exercise.

T: *I was looking forward to seeing you and hearing what data you were able to collect. How did it go?*
Luke: *Well... at first I found it hard to keep watching the homeless man, I was afraid he would notice. But I remembered about the voices on the bus and I stayed.*
T: *I'm glad you were able to accomplish your goal. And what did you observe?*
Luke: *The dog man was sometimes calm, sometimes he was kind of upset, and anyway, he wasn't always there. I noticed that when he was upset, the dog would also get upset, it would bark a lot. And I would get more nervous as the dog barked. He didn't really seem to pay much attention to me... maybe he was acting.*
T: *And how did you feel?*
Luke: *I don't really know, but after watching him for a while, I always end up doing the shopping now (laughs).*

As can be seen in this extract from the interventions, when Luke was able to feel validated and encouraged to approach his own doubts, the level of distress decreased, and he was able to return to previous activities, generalising them to other contexts, and thus regaining functionality and direction towards his values.

18.5.10 "Will and Commitment"

Its aim is for the person to head for her/his values, committing to relevant goals, directed towards something that is meaningful to her/him (and not arbitrarily chosen by others); it must be an action that moves in the context of a value, with a willingness to insist on it, despite the presence of discomfort, aversive feelings and thoughts. ACT promotes the creation of more far-reaching, value-directed, committed patterns of action. Therefore, it is essential to reinforce small steps, promoting the person's persistence and psychological flexibility in making decisions and taking actions. Working on commitment is putting the person on the path to a purposeful life, as well as working on possible relapses.

Taking advantage of the interests of the patient, a big Star Wars fan, for the development of will and commitment to values, we decided to use the phrase "do… or do not" (Yoda), so that this ended up being a recurring phrase for the patient that helped him when he felt he was losing sight of his values.

Therapist:	*You say that going to the gym has always been something you've wanted to do, and that you've felt really good when you've done it, are you going to commit to it?*
Luke:	*Well, the truth is I always think about it and want to do it, but in the end I never do it. Mainly because when I feel bad, I find it hard to go.*
T:	*So what does that mean, are you going to commit to it, or are you going to go back to avoiding your emotions and abandoning what really defines you?*
Luke:	*Well, I'll try.*
T:	*As Yoda says, "Do, or do not… There is no try".*
Luke:	*(laughs) OK, I will.*
T:	*And will you keep it up?*
Luke:	*And I'll keep it up.*

18.5.11 Case Progress

Luke was discharged from the Acute Hospitalisation Unit. He was followed up for a couple of months in this unit. The subjective assessment of the recovery and its impact on the family context was very positive, both for Luke and his parents. He was followed up by his local Mental Health Unit. The psychotic symptoms did not disappear completely, however, an important functional recovery was achieved, resuming valuable activities for him, such as learning languages or playing sports.

18.6 Outpatient Follow-Up

In this phase of clinical stabilisation and depending on the level of cognitive/functional impairment, therapeutic care should be more prolonged in time, seeking, as we have already explained in the previous chapter, a change in the person's relationship with that which causes him/her discomfort. Thus, one of the fundamental tasks of the outpatient intervention will be the prevention of relapses, as well as the recovery and restitution of functionality.

The ART interventions in the context of outpatient follow-up follow the proposed scheme with a similar structure to the therapeutic process described in acute care:

1. **Individual sessions.** We recommend individual weekly sessions at discharge and at times of partial destabilisation, even extending the frequency if necessary, following the principle of immediate response. Subsequently, sessions can be spaced out, based on the situation and needs of the person. They will flexibly follow the outline of the classic phases of ACT, taking into account the different levels of cognitive and functional impairment and their specific adaptation needs. Other interventions, such as the *spiral* or *focusing on voices*, are included.
2. **Group sessions.** The phases of ACT will be followed. Groups are recommended based on the level of impairment of the participants.
3. **Dialogical-based family intervention.** It is recommended to maintain family sessions and their support network throughout the outpatient intervention, their frequency depending on the context and their availability.
4. **Multifamily interventions and group sessions for caregivers** (see O'Donogue et al., 2018).
5. **Coordination and management of the case.** The therapeutic team of the different devices that may be involved with the person (home help devices, psychosocial rehabilitation centres, etc.) is included.

18.7 Case 3: Minerva, Goddess of Wisdom

A 58-year-old woman who lives with her family of origin (mother), does not work and receives a contributory pension. She has higher education in teaching and art history.

She first consulted a clinical psychologist more than 30 years after being diagnosed with schizophrenia. Prior to this, she had been under continuous follow-ups with various psychiatrists. She is currently being followed up by both psychiatry and clinical psychology.

Minerva presented at the age of 23 with a first psychotic episode in which delusions of persecution and harm structured around the existence of a worldwide secret organisation about which she knows too much and for which she is going to be eliminated. Added to this were auditory hallucinations in the form of voices telling her that she was in danger.

At the time of this first psychotic episode, she was involuntarily admitted to the then psychiatric hospital.

Despite numerous different pharmacological treatments, Minerva's psychotic symptomatology has remained present ever since. However, its impact has been minor, requiring admission only on a second occasion approximately 4 years ago.

Currently, Minerva presents positive delusional symptoms, although there is no longer a structured delusion, but a vague feeling that sometimes someone might want to manipulate her, harm her or bother her. However, the symptomatology of disorganisation prevails, as well as the presence of formal thought disorders. In her speech, the perseveration of certain ideas stands out, as well as incoherence, with great confusion at a semantic level, and illogicality, making associations that do not follow inductive inferences. Moreover, she uses numerous approximations of words and neologisms, which sometimes makes the discourse unintelligible. This word-abundant discourse reached verbosity at times, being poverty and empty in the content of the speech.

On a functional level, although in the first years after the first psychotic episode, Minerva was able to finish her studies and start working, she remembers doing so with great difficulty, which she attributes both to the secondary symptoms of the medication (especially sedation), and to the maintenance of the psychotic symptoms, which worsened in situations of stress or emotional discomfort.

At around the age of 30, after several medical leaves, due to the presence of behavioural and thought disorganisation, as well as affective and negative symptoms that resulted in poor functionality both at work and in daily life, she was declared permanently and totally incapacitated.

When Minerva went for her first consultation with Clinical Psychology, there was a great deterioration at a functional level, and she was no longer able to carry out basic activities of daily living independently. She requires supervision for any task and accompaniment for any management. In addition, she does not maintain any social relationship beyond her family of origin (mother and a sister).

In terms of cognitive functioning, she shows a significant deterioration, with impaired attention span, having difficulty following the thread of a conversation, watching a television or radio programme, as well as extensive problems with working memory and medium and long-term memory. This contrasts with her cultural and educational level, which could be described as high, with two university degrees and postgraduate training. In addition, her family's socio-verbal context was cultured and demanding in terms of academic achievement.

Although we cannot state the causes of this deterioration, we must bear in mind that Minerva has maintained pharmacological treatment since her twenties, both with neuroleptics and anxiolytics, having routinely combined several antipsychotic drugs at maximal doses.

Sustained high-dose antipsychotic treatment has been associated with functional organic damage and cognitive/functional impairment (Albert et al., 2019; Omachi

& Sumiyoshi, 2018; Ibi et al., 2017; Pol Yanguas, 2015; Wunderink et al., 2013; Harrow et al., 2012).

Given Minerva's current functioning we can consider her to be at a level of moderate cognitive/functional impairment (level 3) (Díaz-Garrido et al., 2021a, b). This level includes people with extensive cognitive and functional difficulties. In these individuals, basic cognitive functions are significantly impaired, with difficulties in maintaining attention, remembering information and understanding language, with deficits in symbolisation and abstraction.

Following the proposed intervention model, and adjusting to the characteristics of the person, the following intervention scheme was followed:

- **Individual sessions.** Although the general recommendation is for a weekly session, or more intense sessions depending on the case, we must always adjust to the needs and willingness of the person. In Minerva's case, she was distrustful at the beginning of the sessions and asked for them to be spaced out and limited to one a month. Subsequently, and after establishing a good therapeutic alliance, the sessions were held fortnightly.
- **Group sessions.** It has not been possible to hold group sessions.
- **Family intervention.** Minerva's family context is limited to her mother, a woman in her nineties, with whom it has not been possible to hold sessions due to her state of health. However, occasional telephone contact has been maintained at times when Minerva's symptoms have worsened, requiring her consultation to indicate management guidelines and carry out basic psychoeducation. In cases where the person is at cognitive/functional impairment levels 3–4, we do not recommend dialogue sessions, but rather the use of classic family therapy.
- **Coordination and case management.** Frequent coordination is maintained both with her psychiatrist and with the occupational therapists who care for her in an adapted leisure resource.

Given Minerva's level of impairment, the intervention recommendations proposed by Diaz-Garrido, Laffite and Zúñiga (2021b) were followed.

In this therapeutic context, given the level of cognitive/functional impairment, it was decided, following the ART model, to limit the duration of the work sessions to around 30 min, so as not to produce excessive fatigue or information saturation in the person. However, in situations where the context allowed, the remaining time above 30 min was used to improve and strengthen the therapeutic relationship through informal conversation centred on Minerva's interests.

Priority was given to the use of simple language, as well as the use of repetition of concepts, indications, recommendations, etc., to emphasise the most relevant aspects of the work session. Efforts were made not to use overly symbolic or abstract concepts. Taking into account the characteristics of Minerva's thinking and discourse (poor speech content, tendency towards circumlocutions, incoherence and loss of direction), it was necessary for the weight of the interventions in the sessions to fall on the therapist.

Regarding the use of tools such as metaphors, a very simplified guiding metaphor was used and repeated throughout the sessions to help integration. In addition, when constructing this metaphor, it was based on elements brought to the session by Minerva. For better recall and integration of the metaphor, physical elements such as visual representations were added to help extrapolate it to situations outside the consultation. In addition, very simple experiential exercises were included.

Using her taste for surrealist painting, a very small colour print of an author recognisable to Minerva was placed in the room and on the wall furthest from her field of vision. The exercise consisted of a gradual approach to the reinforcer through verbal guidance, using very simple questions about aspects of the work that Minerva cannot see from her distance. With this, she is instructed to approach it progressively until she can observe its characteristics. Subsequently, the meaning of the exercise is guided and explicitly contrasted: "in order to enjoy things that are important to us, we need to get closer to them". With this exercise, the work is guided towards increasing Minerva's level of functionality, using her values as reinforcers.

The central objective in the work with Minerva was the increase of functionality, the reinforcement of autonomy and the inclusion of her in group activities. For this purpose, mainly behavioural operant interventions developed for basic and instrumental activities of daily living were used.

Other strategies normally used in ART were either not used or were applied in a very simple way to promote functionality.

After a year of working in this line with Minerva, she has significantly increased her functionality, always guided and directed by her values. Thus, she now carries out a greater number of activities outside her home (she goes to museums and exhibition halls, goes for walks to see the different sculptures in the city's parks), she has increased her circle of relationships through her participation in adapted leisure activities (painting workshops). In addition, she is now doing some of the shopping for the home and is learning to make simple dishes.

Over time, Minerva's language skills have not changed significantly, with a slight improvement in terms of organisation and turn-taking in conversation. However, there is a greater understanding as they share terminology and have given meaning to Minerva's idiosyncratic phrases. For example, when she says "neither you are a fishmonger, nor I am a hard-boiled egg". When Minerva uses this phrase, the therapist knows, on the basis of information from successive interviews, that she is distressed because she remembers an episode with a delusional interpretation where a fishmonger criticises the fact that Minerva has not had children.

At present, the therapeutic work continues with sessions every 2 weeks. The therapeutic alliance is solid and Minerva turns to the therapist in moments of greatest discomfort, intervening immediately in brief telephone contacts (10–15 min).

They continue to work towards shared goals oriented towards functionality and the direction of her values.

18.8 Case 4: Stephen Vincent, Doctor Strange – Another Example of the Spiral Process

We develop the spiral strategy over several sessions with Doctor Strange. We will not report the whole intervention but will focus on the development of the process. Doctor Strange presented multiple delusional themes, mainly of a fantastic and referential nature. He described a belief in the use of cosmic energy through the mind with which he believed he could change the world.

Doctor Strange:	I'm not going to tell you what I think about my abilities, because I already know what you're going to tell me.
Therapist:	I'm not quite sure what you mean, do you mean the use of energy that you have told me about on occasion?
Doctor Strange:	Yes, you're going to tell me that I'm crazy and that what I think is not real, but that's because you don't have the ability. I can make a better world using energies, even if people don't see it.
DS:	How can I dare to deny what you experience? That's not my job, my job is to help you not to have such a bad time, I wouldn't dare to deny something I haven't seen or don't understand, in fact, it's not important to me whether it's true or not. What matters to me is that you suffer.

...

DS:	I want to write a book with my ideas on how to change the world and how I am going to do it with the energies, through the quantum transformation of the planet.
T:	I think it's a great idea, I think a book can guide you and direct you towards what matters to you, your values *(having worked on this concept)*.
DS:	I have a lot of ideas written down in a notebook and I'm going to use them to write the book.
T:	That's fantastic, I think that notebook can be very useful.
DS:	I have it here *(offers it to the therapist)*.

(The therapist silently reads several pages of the notebook in the presence of the Doctor Strange, observing incoherent, disorganised, persevering sentences without a logical thread, such as: "The transforming energy of the worlds", "the cosmic energy transforms the world", "the base energy to change the world", "the energy flows through me and radiates to the world").

T:	They seem to me to be very interesting ideas, now the important thing is to go through them and translate them into the work. To make a book, documentation is very important, to collect all our previous ideas in an orderly way.

...

DS: I've changed my mind, I'm not going to make a book, I'm going to write a novel.

T: I see you've changed your mind, what's the reason?

DS: I was going through the notebook and I noticed that it was… a bit chaotic… it was difficult to understand… *(it is observed at the level of non-verbal communication that he is embarrassed and hesitant).*

T: When you showed me the notebook I also saw that you had been reflecting your ideas in a somewhat disorganised way and that they were repeated. However, what is important now is not that, but the idea of your novel. What is it about?

DS: It's about two alien species, one with the power to handle quantum energies, and the other that wants to dominate the galaxy. The one that can use the energy is trying to stop them…

T: It's very interesting the plot of this novel, I encourage you to continue it.

Throughout the sessions, it was observed that Doctor Strange went from long-standing severe isolation to participating in social activities, such as sports activities, meetings with friends… He was less persevering in relation to delusion, and when he presented ideas of energies in session, he always did so in reference to his literary creation, showing less fusion with the idea, as well as less anguish when dealing with it.

18.9 Metaphors and Adaptations

18.9.1 Metaphor of the Wall

Imagine for a moment that this room you are in is your mind, now your mind is suffering, we call this room "the discomfort room". In your mind are present your memories, thoughts, sensations and emotions. Right now, there are thoughts that distress you, unpleasant sensations and emotions like anger, rage and sadness, we are in the "discomfort room". Next to this room, there is another room, behind the wall. Imagine that this room is the "tranquillity room". As you can see, a wall separates them, not very thick, but made of brick and cement. We want to pass to the other side, but we have no tools, we only have our hands. To test its resistance we can give it a blow (we hit the wall with our closed hand), it sounds a little hollow, maybe if we hit it harder we can break it (we give three more strong blows to the wall).

As you can see the wall is still the same. In fact, my hand hurts a bit. The point is that I still want to be on that side. So imagine that now I start punching with all my might, punching the wall. I'm likely to hurt my hand badly, leave my knuckles red, or if I continue perhaps bloody, or I might even break a bone in my hand. However, the wall will remain the same.

We need to escape from this room, from the anguish, and be on the side of the "tranquillity room". The funny thing is that even though I want it so badly, I'm still in the "discomfort room" and I'm hurting myself more and more. Are you going to keep hitting the wall?

Modifications

- This metaphor can be physicalised by having the person take an active part in hitting the wall together with the therapist, thus adding experiential activity.
- This metaphor could be used for patients at any stage (people who have not presented a frank psychosis and work is being done in a preventive way, in acute or chronic psychosis).
- In people with moderate/severe impairment, it is recommended to guide by adding that "there is a door in the room and we can reach it with other strategies, maybe it is better to change the strategy when things are not going well".

18.9.2 Metaphor of the Observer at the Window

Notice how the sky takes up everything, today we find few clouds. Let's imagine that each cloud is a thought, a memory, or an emotion. That one (we point) is reminding me "I have to eat at three o'clock in the afternoon", that one brings back the memory of "the day I fell out of the tree when I was ten years old", the other one tells me "my head itches", another one "I'm not having a good day today". The sky is the space where all those clouds are, and the funny thing is that the sky is always there, regardless of the number of clouds. Imagine that the sky is your mind, the space where your emotions, feelings, thoughts and memories are, and each cloud is one of these that tells you something. Who are you really? You are neither the sky, nor the clouds, nor both together, you are the one watching from the window.

Modifications

- You can accompany the exercise with drawings and physical elements such as balls of paper, etc.; this will help to understand and maintain attention in those who are more impaired.

18.9.3 Metaphor of the Road to the North

Values are like walking towards the north, you can ask and they will answer you where the north is, imagine that someone tells you "the north is there in the horizon", and you can walk towards that horizon, but when you go there you realise that as you walk there is always a horizon to the north and you never end up arriving. The important thing is the path, but the path, always to the north.

Modifications

- We can increase its impact by adding examples of "elements in the north": You want to go north, do you see the tallest building by the coast? That's where the north is. When you get there, you ask someone if you've reached the north, and they say no, get a boat and head for Europe. When you get to the south of Europe, they tell you to continue to the Scandinavian countries, and from there to the North Pole. When you get to the North Pole, right in the middle of it... An Eskimo tells you that you can continue, and that north is that way (pointing)!
- We can physicalise the metaphor, accompanying it with the use of a map to make the journey with the person.
- In cases of moderate/severe impairment the meaning of the metaphor would be guided by indicating that the values are never reached. In addition, concrete examples would be given in the case of the person.

18.9.4 White Polar Bear Metaphor

I want you to imagine that you are a cameraman for a famous TV channel, we are going to record a documentary about the animal world, I will be the director and I will give you the indications about what to focus on at each moment. Imagine that we have moved to the Arctic and we are going to film a white polar bear, can you see it? Focus on it with your camera, look closely, can you see where it is, is it alone or is it accompanied by other white polar bears, what is it doing? Now let's zoom in on our white polar bear, zoom in on its face, how are the eyes of the white polar bear?; now open its jaws, how are the teeth of the white polar bear?; how is the fur of this white polar bear?; it is beautiful, but it might be better not to get too close to a white polar bear. And its paws?; they are big and strong, the white polar bear is an imposing animal. How tall is this white polar bear?

Now I want you to stop thinking about the white polar bear, you must make an effort to stop thinking about it, be careful!, don't think about the white polar bear, not even about the word bear ... (After a few seconds) But, if I told you not to think about it, why do you keep thinking about the white polar bear?"

Modifications

- At the end of this exercise, with the idea of generating greater emotional impact, we can bang on the table while saying "I don't want you to think about a polar bear..." in a firm voice, applying an attempt to stop the thought and demonstrating that it is impossible to control it. We do not recommend the use of the punch when the person is very distressed or if we feel that the person will not tolerate it well.
- We recommend using this metaphor in people with a subclinical/mild level of impairment and not at the time of an acute psychotic episode.

18.9.5 Adaptation of Polygraph Metaphor

"Imagine you are connected to the best polygraph ever built. It is a perfect machine, the most sensitive of all. When you're connected to it, there's no way you can feel emotionally activated or anxious without the machine detecting it. Well, here's a simple task for you to do: All you have to do is stay relaxed! If you get nervous, the machine will detect it. I know you're going to try really hard, but I want to add an extra incentive, and that is that you're going to have a Magnum 44 pointing at your head [the machine has the ability to emit electric shocks]. If you stay relaxed, it won't blow your brains out, [it won't electrocute you] but if you get nervous, and we'll detect it because you're connected to that perfect machine, we're going to have to eliminate you [it will electrocute you]. So, relax!... What do you think would happen... Can you guess...? The slightest hint of anxiety would be terrible. You, naturally, would be thinking, "Oh, my God! I'm getting nervous! They're going to shoot me! Bang! [It's going to electrocute me!] Could it be otherwise?"

Modifications

- The introduction in the imagination of people suffering from some kind of psychosis of elements of high lethality such as the gun, can lead to an increase in autolytic ideation and discomfort, so we suggest modifying the metaphor of the polygraph, introducing as a consequence the electrical action derived from the machine itself, due to the simplicity of this association, so the result of the anxiety will not be a shot from a gun, but a painful cramp. Before introducing this metaphor, it is recommended to rule out somatic symptomatology or phenomena of bodily influence (example of the assumption of cosmic energies).

18.9.6 Hole for Families with High Expressed Emotion or Conveying Ambivalent Messages

Imagine life as a field full of holes, of all sizes, some are simple dips or ruts and others are very deep holes. In life we all start with a blindfold over our eyes, we don't know what will happen on our next step. When it comes to crossing the field, each person has their own qualities and over time they perfect others, some are faster, others have better reflexes, others jump more..., which can help to depend on the depth of the hole into which they fall. Sometimes we rely on the help of those closest to us. Let's imagine that your relative has fallen into a deep hole, from which he alone is not managing to get out.

Modifications

You are trying to help him/her in the following way:

- **In case of families with high expressed emotion.** "You are reaching out to him, but before you help him up you are saying: "you'll see when you climb up", "you fell down because you were clumsy", "I told you so".

- **In the case of families with contradictory or ambivalent messages.** "While your relative is making an enormous effort to climb up the walls of the hole blindfolded, and is waiting for directions on where to lean on, each one of you is telling him to step in a different place, confusing him, with the risk that he/she may fall down again".

18.9.7 Metaphor of the Bridge to Values

You are in front of a wide and deep river, its waters vary according to different times, seasons and events; they can be slow, clear and calm waters, or they can become a strong flood due to the rains. Imagine that on the other side of the river is what matters most to you. To cross the river you have to build a bridge, we all have to build our own bridge, but each of us accumulates different resources and support over time to build it. Sometimes, due to the circumstances, the bridge may not be firm and solid enough to withstand the river when its waters are turbulent and it may sway under the current's blows. Of course, one can fall off the bridge and sink in the swirling waters, then one can decide to go with the flow, or struggle to get one's head above water, and to return to rebuild the bridge to what one cares about. You know those waters, and now you are here. My question is: are you willing to keep building the bridge?

Modifications

- If the concept of the bridge is an object of discomfort in the patient's life history, we can change it to a boat.
- Support with graphic material or construction sheets.
- The metaphor can be represented and physicalised through various exercises in the consultation room to facilitate understanding and to increase emotional contact.

18.9.8 Metaphor of the Bicycle on the Way to Values

You are about to start the race of your life, a bicycle race. There are no medals, no cups, nobody wins, but the important thing is to reach the end. All the participants have already chosen theirs and there is only one left, which you will have to take in order to take part in the race of life. When the riders set off you realise that almost all the bikes are road bikes, they are designed for long distances and for running fast, very fast. Your bike is not the same, it's a mountain bike, but it's the bike you've been given, it's heavier and to go fast you have to make more effort. From the beginning of the race you're at the back of the pack and you're struggling to keep up the pace. With each pedal stroke your strength weakens, you sweat and pant, but you see that your fellow riders are hardly suffering at all, they are comfortable, relaxed and even have the energy to talk to each other! Little by little, you lose the pace, the bunch is gaining more and more metres on you, until you can barely see them in the distance and fatigue and listlessness take over. But you know that this is the race of life, and whatever happens you must continue. Luck allies itself with you. A red light has stopped the peloton and the cyclists are resting, lying down and sitting on the ground. You catch up with your strength at the limit. You want to get off your bike and end the race now. You know it's not a fair race, but you also know that now they're stopped, and you're stopped, you're back at the same starting point and you know that the race is different for everyone, and you also know that the important thing is to get to the end and that you still don't know where the rest of the way is going to go. What are you going to do? Drop out?

Modifications

- Figures can be used to represent the cyclists.
- An alternative could be to carry rucksacks of different weights on a walk.
- This exercise could also be useful in group therapy by applying it through experiential exercises where a difficult race is represented and where everyone has their own obstacles.

18.9.9 Metaphor of the Dog in the Kitchen That Defecates

Imagine you have a dog and 1 day, which is very common, he has a poo and you know that when he has a poo he poops all over the house, anywhere and at any time. And you know that everything stinks. You decide that night to put the feeder and water bowl, along with his blanket for him to sleep in the kitchen and you close the door so that if he's still sick he will not poop all over the house during the night. So you go to sleep. The next morning, you go to open the kitchen door and.... you are struck by a dreadful smell that floods your nostrils, you can almost feel it in your mouth, and a terrifying sight! Your dog has been sick to his stomach all night and has defecated all over the kitchen, everything is brown, there's nowhere to step! You carefully take the dog out and immediately close the door, knowing that you won't be back for a few hours. So you have breakfast outside. Meanwhile, in the kitchen the smell will become more and more intense, even sticking to the walls and furniture. The longer it stays closed the worse it will get - what do you plan to do?

Modifications

- This metaphor connects easily with the emotions of repulsion and disgust, which makes it easy to be understood by even moderately/severely impaired patients. However, we recommend modifying to guide further reflection, including clarifying the meaning of the metaphor.

Indications

- This intervention is especially recommended in acute patients or when there are difficulties in talking about symptoms.
- It is also mobilising when the person is afraid to take value-oriented actions because of the barriers they foresee.

Table 18.1 summarizes adaptations of techniques and therapeutic aspects by levels.

Table 18.1 Adaptation of techniques and therapeutic aspects by levels

Clinical situation/ modifications	Acute	Stable without impairment	Stable, slight impairment	Stable, moderate impairment	Stable, severe impairment
Time.	Sessions of limited length.	Standard sessions in due time and form.	Sessions close to the norm, with less content.	Short sessions.	Short, informal sessions.
Features	Observe attentional deficits and level of distress associated with the presence of positive psychotic symptoms. Presence of positive symptomatology and disorganisation is a priority.	Consider possible difficulties in social cognition and social perception. Positive symptomatology is not present or attenuated and does not interfere. Predominant negative symptomatology.	Observe impairment present and in which cognitive aspects there are greater for the adaptation of interventions. Positive symptomatology is not present or attenuated and does not interfere. Predominant negative symptomatology.	The patient may have generalised impairment. Support from physical and visual elements to guide speech. Awkwardness in social interaction, needing guidance and feedback. Predominance of negative symptomatology.	Great cognitive impairment. Use of physical and visual elements during conversation. Tendency towards social isolation or behavioural disinhibition. Predominance of negative symptomatology.
Type of language used	Be extremely careful with language elaboration to avoid interpretations by the patient. Avoid prolonged silences and use paraphrases	Usual. Be careful with interpretative aspects. Avoid prolonged silences.	Little use of symbolism. Attention to language comprehension. Speak slowly, allowing time for comprehension but without prolonged silences.	Simple language, use of repetition, no use of symbolism. Lead in exercises and metaphors. Usually, carry the weight of the conversation.	More repetition, simple, no use of symbolism, not very elaborate. Conversation guided by the therapist.
Paradoxes	No.	Yes.	Yes, guided.	No.	No.

Clinical situation/ modifications	Acute	Stable without impairment	Stable, slight impairment	Stable, moderate impairment	Stable, severe impairment
Mindfulness	Short sessions, more use of anchoring and verbal guidance.	Short sessions. To advance very gradually in time. Primarily informal practice. After guidance in the first practices, autonomy can be achieved.	Short sessions. Progress very gradually. Prioritise simple informal practice. Increase the number of guided rehearsals prior to autonomy.	Patient may have difficulty following practice, and short sessions. Use physically focused practice with guidance present.	Use very short sessions, always guided. Generalisation is not present. Look for alternatives such as yoga or tai chi.
Spiral	Abbreviated, distress-oriented spiral. Delusion may give way only slightly, doubt is sought to be initiated.	Complete spiral. The entire process can be carried out.	Use of the spiral technique, with slower progress. Functional self-exposures.	Elements of the spiral can be used, but the complete development is not carried out.	No spiral.
Functional recovery	Direction towards values.	Direction towards values.	Direction towards values.	IADL and value-based behavioural activation, simple actions.	IADL. Actions towards values are very simple actions.

(continued)

Table 18.1 (continued)

Clinical situation/ modifications	Acute	Stable without impairment	Stable, slight impairment	Stable, moderate impairment	Stable, severe impairment
Metaphors	Metaphors related to awareness of discomfort and difficulties in general. Guidance and clarification throughout the metaphor. The meaning that the person gives to the metaphor is explicitly contrasted. Avoid symbolism and clarify meaning through guidance. Use of fewer metaphors. Daily monitoring of the meaning given to the metaphor.	Metaphors directed towards specific problems and discomfort.	Metaphors directed towards the specific problem and discomfort. Guidance and clarification throughout the metaphor. In case of difficulty physicalise the metaphor. Use of physical elements as a way of keeping the metaphor in mind.	Preference for physicalisation of metaphors and experiential exercises, with avoidance of symbolisation in the most severe cases. Guidance and clarifications throughout the metaphor. As deterioration progresses, more explanatory predominance and physical guidance. The meaning that the person gives to the metaphor is explicitly contrasted.	Assess individual capacity for the use of physicalised metaphors.
Dialogism	Yes. Introduce as soon as possible.	Yes.	Yes.	No. Use of classical family therapy.	No. Use of classical family therapy.

Disclaimer Clinical cases presented in this chapter do not include real names or personal information of real persons.

References

Albert, N., Randers, L., Allott, K., Jensen, H. D., Melau, M., Hjorthøj, C., & Nordentoft, M. (2019). Cognitive functioning following discontinuation of antipsychotic medication. A naturalistic sub-group analysis from the OPUS II trial. *Psychological Medicine, 49*(7), 1138–1147. https://doi.org/10.1017/S0033291718001836

American Psychiatric Association. (2014). *Manual diagnóstico y estadístico de los trastornos mentales, DSM-5*. Editorial Médica Panamericana.

Anthony, W. A. (1993). Recovery from mental illness: The guiding vision of the mental health service system in the 1990s. *Psychosocial Rehabilitation Journal, 16*(4), 11–23. https://doi.org/10.1037/h0095655

Bach, P., & Hayes, S. C. (2002). The use of acceptance and commitment therapy to prevent the rehospitalization of psychotic patients: A randomized controlled trial. *Journal of Consulting and Clinical Psychology, 70*(5), 1129–1139. https://doi.org/10.1037//0022006x.70.5.1129

Bentall, R. P., Haddock, G., & Slade, P. D. (1994). Cognitive behavior therapy for persistent auditory hallucinations: From theory to therapy. *Behavior Therapy, 25*, 51–66. https://doi.org/10.1016/S00057894(05)80145-5

Bergström, T., Seikkula, J., Alakare, B., Mäki, P., Köngäs-Saviaro, P., Taskila, J. J., Tolvanen, A., & Aaltonen, J. (2018). The family-oriented open dialogue approach in the treatment of first-episode psychosis: Nineteen-year outcomes. *Psychiatry Research, 270*, 168–175. https://doi.org/10.1016/j.psychres.2018.09.039

Butler, L., Jhons, L., Byrne, M., Joseph, C., O'Donoghue, E., Jolley, S., Morris, E., & Oliver, J. (2016). Running acceptance and commitment therapy groups for psychosis in community settings. *Journal of Contextual Behavioral Science, 5*, 33–38. https://doi.org/10.1016/j.jcbs.2015.12.001

Chadwick, P. (2009). *Terapia Cognitiva basada en la persona para la psicosis perturbadora*. Fundación para la investigación y tratamiento de la esquizofrenia y otras psicosis. [edición original, Chadwick, P. (2006) Person-based cognitive therapy for distressing psychosis].

Díaz-Garrido, J. A., Laffite, H., & Zúñiga, R. (2021a). ACT en psicosis. In J. A. Díaz-Garrido, H. Laffite, & R. Zúñiga (Eds.), *Terapia de Aceptación y Compromiso en psicosis. Aceptación y Recuperación por niveles (ART)* (p. XX). Pirámide.

Díaz-Garrido, J. A., Laffite, H., & Zúñiga, R. (2021b). Terapia de aceptación y recuperación por niveles para la psicosis (ART). In J. A. Díaz-Garrido, H. Laffite, & R. Zúñiga (Eds.), *Terapia de Aceptación y Compromiso en psicosis. Aceptación y Recuperación por niveles (ART)* (p. XX). Pirámide.

Fledderus, M., Bohlmeijer, E. T., Pieterse, M. E., & Schreurs, K. M. G. (2012). Acceptance and commitment therapy as guided self-help for psychological distress and positive mental health: A randomized controlled trial. *Psychological Medicine, 42*(3), 485–495. https://doi.org/10.1017/S0033291711001206

Frueh, B. C., Knapp, R. G., Cusack, K. J., Grubaugh, A. L., Sauvageot, J. A., Cousins, V. C., Yim, E., Robins, C. S., Monnier, J., & Hiers, T. G. (2005). Patients' reports of traumatic or harmful experiences within the psychiatric setting. *Psychiatric services (Washington, D.C.), 56*(9), 1123–1133. https://doi.org/10.1176/appi.ps.56.9.1123

García-Montes, J. M., & Pérez-Álvarez, M. (2005). Fundamentación experimental y primeras aplicaciones clínicas de la terapia de aceptación y compromiso (ACT) en el campo de los síntomas psicóticos. *Revista Latinoamericana de Psicología, 37*(2), 379–393.

García-Montes, J. M., & Pérez-Álvarez, M. (2016). Terapia de Aceptación y Compromiso aplicada a la esquizofrenia. Estado actual y direcciones futuras. *Análisis y Modificación de Conducta, 42*(165–166), 99–119. https://doi.org/10.33776/amc.v42i165-66.2796

Gaudiano, B. A., & Herbert, J. D. (2006). Acute treatment of inpatients with psychotic symptoms using acceptance and commitment therapy: Pilot results. *Behaviour Research and Therapy, 44*(3), 415–437. https://doi.org/10.1016/j.brat.2005.02.007

Gaudiano, B. A., Davis, C. H., Epstein-Lubow, G., Johnson, J. E., Mueser, K. T., & Miller, I. W. (2017). Acceptance and commitment therapy for inpatients with psychosis (the REACH study): Protocol for treatment development and pilot testing. *Healthcare (Basel, Switzerland), 5*(2), 23. https://doi.org/10.3390/healthcare5020023

Green, M. F. (1996). What are the functional consequences of neurocognitive deficits in schizophrenia? *The American Journal of Psychiatry, 153*(3), 321–330. https://doi.org/10.1176/ajp.153.3.321

Harrow, M., Jobe, T. H., & Faull, R. N. (2012). Do all schizophrenia patients need antipsychotic treatment continuously throughout their lifetime? A 20-year longitudinal study. *Psychological Medicine, 42*(10), 2145–2155. https://doi.org/10.1017/S0033291712000220

Hayes, S. C., Stronshal, K. D., & Wilson, K. G. (1999). *Acceptance and commitment therapy: An experiential approach to behavior change*. Guildford Press.

Heinrichs, R. W., & Zakzanis, K. K. (1988). Neurocognitive deficit in schizophrenia: A quantitative review of the evidence. *Neuropsychology, 12*, 426–445. https://doi.org/10.1037//0894-4105.12.3.426

Ibi, D., de la Fuente Revenga, M., Kezunovic, N., Muguruza, C., Saunders, J. M., Gaitonde, S. A., Moreno, J. L., Ijaz, M. K., Santosh, V., Kozlenkov, A., Holloway, T., Seto, J., García-Bea, A., Kurita, M., Mosley, G. E., Jiang, Y., Christoffel, D. J., Callado, L. F., Russo, S. J., Dracheva, S., et al. (2017). Antipsychotic-induced Hdac2 transcription via NF-κB leads to synaptic and cognitive side effects. *Nature Neuroscience, 20*(9), 1247–1259. https://doi.org/10.1038/nn.4616

Jacobsen, P., Peters, E., Robinson, E., & Chadwick, P. (2020). Mindfulness-based crisis interventions (MBCI) for psychosis within acute inpatient psychiatric settings; a feasibility randomised controlled trial. *BMC Psychiatry, 20*(1), 193. https://doi.org/10.1186/s12888-020-02608-x

Jones, J., Nolan, P., Bowers, L., Simpson, A., Whittington, R., Hackney, D., & Bhui, K. (2010). Psychiatric wards: Places of safety? *Journal of Psychiatric and Mental Health Nursing, 17*(2), 124–130. https://doi.org/10.1111/j.1365-2850.2009.01482.x

Klippel, A., Myin-Germeys, I., Chavez-Baldini, U., Preacher, K. J., Kempton, M., Valmaggia, L., Calem, M., So, S., Beards, S., Hubbard, K., Gayer-Anderson, C., Onyejiaka, A., Wichers, M., McGuire, P., Murray, R., Garety, P., van Os, J., Wykes, T., Morgan, C., & Reininghaus, U. (2017). Modeling the interplay between psychological processes and adverse, stressful contexts and experiences in pathways to psychosis: An experience sampling study. *Schizophrenia Bulletin, 43*(2), 302–315. https://doi.org/10.1093/schbul/sbw185

Laurenceau, J. P., Barrett, L. F., & Pietromonaco, P. R. (1998). Intimacy as an interpersonal process: The importance of self-disclosure, partner disclosure, and perceived partner responsiveness in interpersonal exchanges. *Journal of Personality and Social Psychology, 74*(5), 1238–1251. https://doi.org/10.1037//0022-3514.74.5.1238

Lelliott, P., & Quirk, A. (2004). What is life like on acute psychiatric wards? *Current Opinion in Psychiatry, 17*(4), 297–301. https://doi.org/10.1097/01.yco.0000133833.49790.53

Morris, E. (2019). Acceptance and commitment therapy. In C. Cupitt (Ed.), *CBT for psychosis: Process-orientated therapies and the third wave* (pp. 79–97). Routledge Taylor & Francis Group.

Morris, E., & Oliver, J. (2009). ACT early: Acceptance and commitment therapy in early intervention in psychosis. *Clinical Psychology Forum, 196*, 28–31.

Myin-Germeys, I., Klippel, A., Steinhart, H., & Reininghaus, U. (2016). Ecological momentary interventions in psychiatry. *Current Opinion in Psychiatry, 29*(4), 258–263. https://doi.org/10.1097/YCO.0000000000000255

O'Donogue, E. K., Morris, E. M., Oliver, J. E., & Johns, L. C. (2018). *ACT for psychosis recovery: A practical manual for group-based interventions using acceptance and commitment therapy*. Context Press.

Omachi, Y., & Sumiyoshi, T. (2018). Dose reduction/discontinuation of antipsychotic drugs in psychosis: Effect on cognition and functional outcomes. *Frontiers in Psychiatry, 9*, 447. https://doi.org/10.3389/fpsyt.2018.00447

Páez, M., Gutiérrez, O., Valdivia, S., & Luciano, C. (2006). Terapia de Aceptación y Compromiso (ACT) y la importancia de los valores personales en el contexto de la terapia psicológica. *International Journal of Psychology and Psychological Therapy, 6*(1), 1–20. Disponible en: https://www.redalyc.org/articulo.oa?id=56060101

Pol Yanguas, E. (2015). Antipsicóticos para la esquizofrenia. Paradigma de los medicamentos psiquiátricos. *Salud Colectiva, 11*(1), 115–128. https://doi.org/10.18294/sc.2015.410

Reininghaus, U., Depp, C. A., & Myin-Germeys, I. (2016). Ecological interventionist causal models in psychosis: Targeting psychological mechanisms in daily life. *Schizophrenia Bulletin, 42*(2), 264–269. https://doi.org/10.1093/schbul/sbv193

Reininghaus, U., Klippel, A., Steinhart, H., Vaessen, T., van Nierop, M., Viechtbauer, W., Batink, T., Kasanova, Z., van Aubel, E., van Winkel, R., Marcelis, M., van Amelsvoort, T., van der Gaag, M., de Haan, L., & Myin-Germeys, I. (2019). Efficacy of acceptance and commitment therapy in daily life (ACT-DL) in early psychosis: Study protocol for a multi-Centre randomized controlled trial. *Trials, 20*(1), 769. https://doi.org/10.1186/s13063-019-3912-4

Ruiz, J. J. (2017). *Terapia de aceptación y compromiso de grupo. Basada en la Teoría del marco relacional y el socioconductismo*. Editorial Lulú.

Ruiz, J. J. (2021). ACT de grupo para personas con experiencias psicóticas. In J. A. Díaz-Garrido, H. Laffite, & R. Zúñiga (Eds.), *Terapia de Aceptación y Compromiso en psicosis. Aceptación y Recuperación por niveles (ART)*. Pirámide.

Ruiz, J. J., & Ruiz, I. (2018). *Psicoterapia analítica funcional de grupos*. Edual.

Salgado, C. F., & Mateos, M. (2021). La prevención de casos de psicosis ¿es posible? Propuesta de un modelo atencional basado en lo importante para la persona. In J. A. Díaz-Garrido, H. Laffite, & R. Zúñiga (Eds.), *Terapia de Aceptación y Compromiso en psicosis. Aceptación y Recuperación por niveles (ART)*. Pirámide.

Schizophrenia Commission. (2012). *The abandoned illness: A report from the schizophrenia Commision*. Rethink Mentall Illness. https://www.rethink.org/media/2637/the-abandoned-illness-final.pdf

Seikkula, J., Aaltonen, J., Alakare, B., Haarakangas, K., Keränen, J., & Lehtinen, K. (2006). Five-year experience of first-episode nonaffective psychosis in open-dialogue approach: Treatment principles, follow-up outcomes, and two case studies. *Psychotherapy Research, 16*, 214–228. https://doi.org/10.1080/10503300500268490

Sheffield, J. M., Karcher, N. R., & Barch, D. M. (2018). Cognitive deficits in psychotic disorders: A lifespan perspective. *Neuropsychology Review, 28*, 509–533.

Vaessen, T., Steinhart, H., Batink, T., Klippel, A., van Nierop, M., Reininghaus, U., & Myin-Germeys, I. (2019). ACT in daily life in early psychosis: An ecological momentary intervention approach. *Psychosis, 11*(2), 93–104. https://doi.org/10.1080/17522439.2019.1578401

van Aubel, E., Bakker, J. M., Batink, T., Michielse, S., Goossens, L., Lange, I., Schruers, K., Lieverse, R., Marcelis, M., van Amelsvoort, T., van Os, J., Wichers, M., Vaessen, T., Reininghaus, U., & Myin-Germeis, I. (2020). Blended care in the treatment of subthreshold symptoms of depression and psychosis in emerging adults: A randomised controlled trial of acceptance and commitment therapy in daily-life (ACT-DL). *Behaviour Research and Therapy, 128*, 103592. https://doi.org/10.1016/j.brat.2020.103592

Wegner, D. M., Schneider, D. J., Carter, S. R., & White, T. L. (1987). Paradoxical effects of thought suppression. *Journal of Personality and Social Psychology, 53*(1), 5–13. https://doi.org/10.1037//0022-3514.53.1.5

Wilson, K. G., & Luciano, M. C. (2002). *Terapia de Aceptación y Compromiso (ACT). Un tratamiento orientado a los valores*. Pirámide.

Wood, L., Williams, C., Billings, J., & Johnson, S. (2020). A systematic review and meta-analysis of cognitive behavioural informed psychological interventions for psychiatric inpatients with psychosis. *Schizophrenia Research, 222*, 133–144. https://doi.org/10.1016/j.schres.2020.03.041

Wunderink, L., Nieboer, R. M., Wiersma, D., Sytema, S., & Nienhuis, F. J. (2013). Recovery in remitted first-episode psychosis at 7 years of follow-up of an early dose reduction/discontinuation or maintenance treatment strategy: Long-term follow-up of a 2-year randomized clinical trial. *JAMA Psychiatry, 70*(9), 913–920. https://doi.org/10.1001/jamapsychiatry.2013.19

Yung, A. R. (2003). Commentary: The schizophrenia prodrome: A high-risk concept. *Schizophrenia Bulletin, 29*(4), 859–865.

Chapter 19
Psychosocial Rehabilitation: An ART Approach – Clinical Cases

María Francisca Martínez-Huidobro, Hiurma Gil-Santiago, María Jesús Peña-Pérez, Virginia Martín-Santana, and José Luis Hernández-Fleta

19.1 Introduction

The leveled Acceptance and Recovery Therapy for psychosis (ART), based on the principles and philosophy of Acceptance and Commitment Therapy (ACT), addresses the limitations of other psychotherapeutic models in the treatment of Psychotic Spectrum Disorders (PSD). It places the affected person at the centre of their rehabilitative process, empowering them and adapting itself not only to their individual needs but also to their expectations of quality of life, demystifying the cultural ideal of happiness and encouraging the recognition and acceptance of their own personal history. It is a form of care focused on the person, on the interaction, on the understanding of experiences in the biographical context, on a recovery of the sense of self and on giving back the horizon of life to the person (Pérez Álvarez et al., 2011).

One of its main goals is to ensure the continuity of care for people with PSD from a biopsychosocial approach and an interdisciplinary perspective, which is not always easily achievable for the intervening team, due, in some cases, to the disparity of intrateam professional criteria and/or the fragmentation of the socio-health system itself, hindering the fluidity of communication. It is proposed as a humanistic model, focused on functionality, with the aim of taking advantage of the synergies of the interventions made by the different professionals participating within the therapy with the common objective of supporting the person so they can achieve the fullest, freest and most satisfactory life possible.

M. F. Martínez-Huidobro (✉) · H. Gil-Santiago · M. J. Peña-Pérez · J. L. Hernández-Fleta
Hospital Universitario de Gran Canaria Doctor Negrín, Las Palmas de Gran Canaria, Spain

V. Martín-Santana
Complejo Hospitalario Universitario Insular – Materno Infantil,
Las Palmas de Gran Canaria, Spain

J. A. Díaz-Garrido et al. (eds.), *Psychological Interventions for Psychosis*,
https://doi.org/10.1007/978-3-031-27003-1_19

The three clinical cases presented in this chapter comprise real clinical situations that we have faced in the context of psychosocial rehabilitation. The diversity of both clinical and social influencing factors makes it necessary to formulate each case, in which hypotheses of the origin and maintenance of the problems are considered. This subsequently allows for individualized planning of the intervention. ART provides innovative elements of its own and permits its complementation with interventions based on other models to adapt the processes, techniques and strategies to each particular case.

19.2 First Case: In the Right Direction – Addressing Behavioural Disorganisation in Psychosis

First Hand Experience *"I have not had an easy life. Some of the experiences that I have had, especially during my childhood, have left a mark on me. Hearing voices insulting me or feeling that everyone is against me, without understanding what was happening to me, has been hard. Fortunately, my mother and my sister have always supported me, although sometimes, when I was not well, it was difficult for me to acknowledge it and I have even thought they were against me as well. But deep down, I know that they love me and that they do what is best for me. I would not have been able to get through this without my mother. Professionals' support has also been very important. I know that I have not always made things easy for them and I apologise. Their closeness, understanding and availability have been fundamental for me to get better. They helped me to better understand what is happening to me and to find ways to relieve the suffering. Thanks to this, I have been able to escape from a chaotic life and to focus on things that are important to me in life and that help me live better. I thank all those who have been by my side for their patience and dedication".*

19.2.1 Introduction

Assertive Community Treatment, developed by Leonard Stein and Mary Ann Test in Wisconsin (USA), is a way of structuring care for people with Severe Mental Disorders (SMD) that focuses its field of action on the closest environment of the patient (Stein et al., 1975). The flexibility in care, its adaptation to the particular circumstances of the patient, and the members' availability and accessibility to attend and deal with possible incidents and unforeseen events are other principles of this model.

Assertive Community Treatment focuses on taking care of people with SMD with a high level of clinical severity that significantly affects the patient and/or their environment, who usually present a high level of dysfunctionality and who, in addition, lack of consistent support figures to help them get out of the situation in which they find themselves. Following Martínez-Huidobro and Herrera (2021), in the daily clinical practice of this treatment's teams, we observe that users can be divided in different clinical profiles, according to the following factors:

- Social situation
- Degree of impairment and dysfunctionality
- Level of behavioural disorganisation and alteration
- Subjective perception of the need for support

According to these authors, if we take these factors into account, we can classify the profile of users into four groups:

1. User with predominance of social exclusion
2. Users with predominance of impairment and dysfunctionality
3. Users with predominance of behavioural disorganisation and alteration
4. Users with predominance of anosognosia (Martínez & Herrera, 2021)

Below we present the clinical case of a patient with predominance of disorganisation and behavioural alteration who is being followed-up by an Assertive Community Treatment Team (ACTT), approached from a contextual perspective, and based on the principles of ACT and Functional Analytical Psychotherapy (FAP), as well as some of those proposed by layered ART (Díaz-Garrido et al., 2021).

19.2.2 Clinical Functional Description

19.2.2.1 Clinical Case

Patricia is a 26-year-old woman diagnosed with paranoid schizophrenia since the age of 18, with numerous admissions to the acute psychiatric hospitalisation unit. She has been legally incapacitated for about 4 years, with her mother being her legal guardian. She has a history of serious self-harm attempts in the context of psychotic decompensation and associated depressive symptoms. She has had multiple partners throughout her life and tends to maintain short, unstable relationships. She was admitted to the medium-stay unit for 6 months. When she was discharged, she was followed up by the ACTT and referred to a day centre for psychosocial rehabilitation activities. Follow-up visits at the user's home are carried out twice a week, while she attends the day centre three times a week. Patricia lives with her mother, but they do not have a good relationship since the patient has difficulties in complying with the rules of cohabitation and tends to present frequent behavioural alterations. In general, Patricia has low tolerance for frustration and a tendency to overwhelm in stressful situations that she does not know how to manage. In this context, she tends to present disorganised behaviours. Within the clinical dimensions recognised in PSD, one of the dimensions that has not received much attention is disorganised behaviour, despite the fact that it generates significant functional impairment. In this dimension we can find, among others, formal thought disorders, disorganised and bizarre conduct, as well as inappropriate affect. In Patricia's case, we observe how in moments of instability, thinking becomes disordered, which is expressed through a maniac, lax and even disintegrated discourse, and which hinders coherent and logical reasoning that allows planning behaviours oriented towards specific goals. In turn, affect also loses internal consistency and its relationship with direct contingencies, so that inappropriate affect is presented, which does not seem to be in accordance with the circumstance. All this leads to Patricia's conducts being chaotic, erratic and without a clear purpose. These behaviours usually occur abruptly, in relation to stressors and generate alarm and overwhelm in her environment, especially in the figure of her mother. The last presents high expressed emotion, which at the same time is a source of stress for Patricia, thus generating a vicious circle. The duration of these periods of disorganisation is variable (from hours to days) and often depends on how soon she can count on some form of support (usually psychotherapeutic or psychopharmacological intervention).

19.2.2.2 Formulation from a Functional Analytical Psychotherapy Approach

The following is a brief formulation of the case from the perspective of FAP, an approach in which the therapeutic relation itself takes on primary importance as the main working tool. Verbal dialogue constitutes the basic interaction, and the therapist acts as social reinforcer (by being natural, emphatic and by allowing intimacy) (Kaholokula et al., 2013). One of the great advantages of working with the FAP approach in an ACTT is that it allows all members of the team involved in the case to have a clear outline of what the patient's main problems are, as well as the goals of the treatment, understanding the relationship between the behaviours that come up in the follow-up interviews and their generalisation to the person's daily life. In a relatively simple way, FAP allows all professionals to work on the same line, to use the same reinforcers and to evaluate from time to time as a team both the objectives and their achievement.

The therapeutic process in FAP is fundamentally based on what the client does and say in the clinical session itself. These behaviours have been named as Clinically Relevant Behaviours (CRB): CRB1 are the client's problems that occur during the sessions, which the therapy must try to diminish; while CRB2 are the client's behaviours that are considered improvements that happen during the session.

We will briefly review the main aspects to be considered from the FAP approach for the formulation of Patricia's case.

(a) *Daily Life Problems*

- Difficulties in communication with her mother and little collaboration in household chores, which leads to frequent conflicts between them.
- Low tolerance to frustration, with escape responses to emotional discomfort. In the face of arguments in the family context, Patricia responds by escaping

from home, frequenting marginal environments and exposing herself to various risky situations (consumption of toxic substances, promiscuity, etc.).
- Difficulty in keeping daily schedules and routines.
- Irregular intake of psychopharmacological medication.

(b) *Problems in the Session (CRB1)*

- Passive attitude towards the recovery process. She is extremely complacent, responding affirmatively to the therapeutic tasks and objectives proposed, but showing superficial commitment, as in general she does not make an effort or carry out concrete actions to comply with what has been agreed.
- Tendency to minimise behavioural alterations, frequently presenting and external locus of control, blaming the environment and the circumstances.
- Difficulty in developing intimate relationships.
- Difficulty in identifying and expressing her internal events.

(c) *Cognitive Concepts that Interfere with Therapy*

Since Patricia's discourse tends to be induced, sparse and rather superficial, it is not easy to determine, at first, which cognitive concepts interfere with therapy. Even so, the belief that she is a "victim of the disease" and that she does not have an active role in the evolution and development of her own life and future stands out particularly.

(d) *Daily Life Goals*

- Improve communication with her mother and reduce conflicts.
- Collaborate in household chores.
- Reduce avoidance/escape behaviour and increase tolerance in stressful situations.
- Comply with the schedules established with her mother for arriving home, and in case of going out, give an account of where and with whom she is, so as not to generate an alarm in the intra-family environment.
- Create routines and schedules to be able to get up early and attend the day centre for activities focused on psychosocial rehabilitation.
- Reduce the consumption of toxic substances.
- Avoid risky sexual behaviour. Use contraceptive and barrier methods to avoid unwanted pregnancies and the spread of sexually transmitted diseases.
- Improve adherence to psychopharmacological treatment.

(e) *Objectives in the Session (CRB2)*

- Increase the frequency of the verbalisation of mental and emotional processes.
- Increase the number and frequency of assertive statements, making direct requests about one need's and wishes; recognise when she does not agree with any of the proposals made in therapy and be able to introduce her own criteria and negotiate with the therapists regarding the objectives to be achieved during the approach.
- Clarify values and promote concrete value-oriented actions.
- Improve the ability to foresee the potential consequences of her actions.
- Increase involvement and active commitment in her therapeutical and recovery process.

19.2.2.3 Functional Analysis

In the profile of patients in whom behavioural alterations and disorganisation predominate, such as with Patricia, functional analysis of conduct is particularly useful, as it allows professionals and the patient to understand problematic behaviours in terms of the interaction between the environmental variables and those of the person themselves, in order to be able to influence these variables to modify these behaviours (Martínez-Huidobro & Herrera, 2021).

When carrying out the functional analysis in PSD, it is essential to take into consideration the existence of possible difficulties at a cognitive level. Patricia presents attentional and working memory deficits, which is why it is necessary to simplify the functional analysis. Some adaptations to keep in mind when preparing this analysis together with patients with cognitive impairment are (a) not to use technical terms, (b) use a chain analysis instead of organizing the elements under the three-term contingency and (c) the number of elements included should be relative to the working memory capacity.

As it can be observed in the conducted formulation based on the FAP perspective, Patricia has multiple problems both in her daily life and in the session itself. This means that various functional analyses of the case can be carried out if we want to break down and try to understand each of the patient's behaviours in different contexts. However, a maintenance hypothesis is proposed based on the negative reinforcement paradigm of the escaping/avoidance response type, which attempts to relate some of the daily problems to the difficulties that exhibited during the session. Description of prototypical situation: Patricia was at home with her mother during a therapeutic leave and her mother criticises her for spending the whole morning in bed without doing any housework. Patricia feels anger, distress and impotence, she thinks everyone is against her, that no one loves her and that she can no longer bear the situation, so she leaves the house amidst unintelligible shouting and slamming the door.

What is the problematic behaviour? The one to be analysed was that of escaping/running away from home and from the psychotherapeutic session itself, as a response to unpleasant internal events.

What precedes this conduct? It can be understood that the antecedent of the problematic behaviour in the described situation is the argument with her mother (interpersonal stressor) and the unpleasant internal events (thoughts, emotions and sensations), which from Patricia's reinforcement history have acquired a discriminative stimulus function. Patricia's escape responses tend to occur in interpersonal contexts that involve participation and bonding in intimate relationships. It is crucial to consider that context and conduct have a bidirectional relationship.

And what are the consequences of such conduct? The short-term consequence of the problematic behaviour, the escaping, is the relief of discomfort. However, this brings some other problems, since during this escaping, Patricia tends to frequent marginal environments, consume toxic substances, engage in risky sexual behaviour, abandon her medication and expose herself to other risky situations. In turn, this generates discomfort and emotional overwhelm in her mother, resulting in higher levels of expressed emotion and the subsequent conflict between them. The hypothesis formulated following the functional analysis of the escaping/running away response type states that this behaviour is maintained through the reduction of emotional distress, with negative reinforcement as a function.

And how does the functional analysis of this problematic behaviour relate to the problems that appear during the session? (Figure 19.1). The escaping behaviour that usually occurred in the family context in response to emotional distress had also occurred in therapy context, since Patricia abruptly stood up and left the shouting in two occasions. During the sessions, a poor ability to perceive her own psychological events is continuously observed. It is likely that this difficulty in observing and describing what is happening to her on a cognitive and emotional level, which occurs during the session, also happens in her daily life, for example, during arguments with her mother. Since she is not able to tolerate such discomfort, she tends to escape from aversive situations.

19.2.2.4 Evaluation

Following ART's proposal, in order to plan and tailor the intervention to the person's needs, it is necessary to take into consideration whether there is cognitive or functional impairment, and if so, to what degree. The patient was referred to the neuropsychology unit for a cognitive functioning assessment. The results are shown below:

Used Tests and Psychometric Results
Qualitative Results

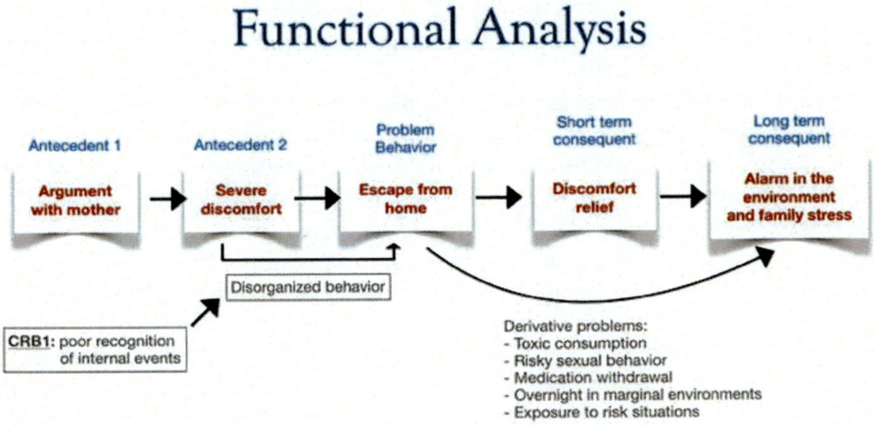

Fig 19.1 Functional analysis

The results obtained show:

- At the attentional level, the patient obtains pathological results.
- The same occurs in visuoconstruction, with results that are considered pathological. In visuorientation and perception (gnosia), the results are established as average.
- Working memory shows low but not pathological results. There is difficulty in learning, with impaired capacity for information storage (pathological).
- Executive functions measured through the capacity for response inhibition show pathological results. Alternating attention shows low but no pathological results.
- Language is affected at the level of phonological fluency, not semantic fluency (the lower limit).
- Functionality has not been ascertained.

19.2.2.5 Psychotherapeutic Intervention

From FAP's point of view, what the client does both inside and outside the consultation room is directly related, so that, by working on the objectives in the session, they would be generalised and would also be applicable to the "daily life goals."

In this case, the escape behaviour that usually occurs in the family context in response to the emotional distress had also occurred within the therapeutic context, where, on two previous occasions, Patricia had got up abruptly and left the room screaming.

In this case, the limited ability to observe and describe her own internal events results in the disruptive appearance of disorganised behavioural disturbances in everyday life. Therefore, we tried to help Patricia increase her capacity to observe and discriminate her own internal events, as well as to understand their relationship with her conduct in different contexts, reducing her disorganised behaviour and its negative consequences. The main tool used in therapy to move from CRB1 to CRB2, as proposed by FAP, is the therapeutic relationship itself, with the therapist using their own reaction as a possible natural contingent reinforcer to Patricia's conduct.

Hence, one of the ways of increasing the recognition and expression of emotions involves the modelling and reinforcement that take place during the session. Thus, the therapist has the role of evoking Patricia's emotional response to encourage and reinforce discrimination (tacting), as well as sharing her own emotional reactions in the therapy setting, in a way that models intimate behaviours. Continuous feedback and clarification of the therapist's own emotional response is of enormous importance in the treatment of schizophrenia, as the tendency to interpret facial expressions representing neutral emotions as negative has been described.

The generalisation of CRB2 can be facilitated if it is systematically reinforced by the members of the *extended therapeutic team*, "who will constitute an extension of the therapist for observation, evocation and reinforcement of CRBs". As an example, we will discuss its application within the present case: Patricia, when she is distressed, starts to wander around the hospital ward and makes continuous demands to the staff to provide her with certain tools (tobacco, toiletries and especially medication). These repeated demands generate stress in the staff, who end up using punitive responses that increase Patricia's distress and discomfort, with greater behavioural and emotional instability.

A broader outlook at the function of the conduct allows us to understand that Patricia's demands were attention-seeking and constituted a form of dysfunctional communication. Through the joint understanding of the patient's conduct by the extended therapeutic team and the application of consequences contingent on the "real" function of the behaviour by all members, it is easier to get an increased emotional expression and the establishment of bonds of intimacy, as well as their generalisation. This way, the "disguised authorities" were extinguished, while facilitating the implementation of the alternative conduct, emotional expression and direct request of needs, which was reinforced in the form of active listening by team members.

Regarding the discrimination of internal events (sensations, thoughts and emotions), mindfulness was also implemented, intending to facilitate the distancing from the literal content (cognitive defusion) and increase the window of tolerance to discomfort. Cognitive defusion interventions are especially useful in patients with a predominance of impulsivity, given the difficulty in distinguishing between external events and their own thoughts, which conditions an imminent reaction to the subjective experience felt at that moment (Martínez-Huidobro & Herrera, 2021). We therefore work in gradually weakening the control that internal events exert over behaviour. For example, Patricia was able to understand that her feelings and thoughts of "imminent harm and catastrophe" associated with the intense discomfort she felt when arguing with her mother were more a response to her own inner world than to external events.

The mindfulness activity lasted for five minutes during individual sessions, with verbal guidance (that faded progressively) redirecting Patricia to *environmental sounds* as anchors every sixty seconds initially. Mindfulness was also included in other group activities, in which the duration was increased to ten minutes. This reduction and adjustment of the duration of mindfulness-based exercises responds to Chadwick's proposals (2009) in relation to psychosis, but above all to the need to adapt the intervention to the patient's attentional difficulties. In psychosis, it is important that the anchors are chosen by the patients, especially when there is sensory-perceptual phenomenology, since if the symptomatology is not adequately explored, the therapist's guidance towards generic anchors can lead the person to have psychotic experiences directly. In Patricia's case, no hallucinatory or delusional symptoms were present during the intervention.

Continuous work in the functional analysis of problematic behaviours makes it easier for the person to become aware of the sequence that leads and maintains dysfunctional behaviour. It facilitates the observation and discrimination of internal events and conduct, promotes the ability to anticipate consequences, and the understanding of the relationship between the different variables, thus easing the implementation of alternative conducts that are more context-adaptive (reinforcing).

Furthermore, the joint performance of the functional analysis favours an active involvement in the recovery process and strengthens the therapeutic alliance.

The behavioural alterations of this patient profile often lead to a high degree of alarm in their immediate environment, therefore, working with the people around them, training them in the recognition and management of their own emotions and facilitating the understanding of how their behaviour/response can influence the patient can be of great help (Martínez & Herrera, 2021). Two types of approaches were carried out in the family setting:

(a) Contextual dialogic intervention. During one of the patient's escapes, after being found by the police and returned to her home, part of the therapeutic team (psychiatrist, nurse and social worker) went to her home and carried out an intervention in situ, with the presence of her social support network (her mother and a very close friend), where the point of view of the different parties about Patricia's current situation was presented and decisions were taken jointly regarding a therapeutic plan.
(b) Psychoeducational intervention, where in addition to emotional recognition and management, aspects such as high expressed emotion and functional analysis were addressed. This helped Patricia's mother to understand her role in the events and how she could also influence them with some behavioural modifications. For example, by decreasing criticism and expressing emotion during conversations with her daughter. In addition, work was done on the use of explicit and direct wish requests and expression of needs, as this also difficulted family communication.

Values orientation was another fundamental pillar in the intervention, due to the fact that for long periods of time, they had been living a chaotic, precarious life without a clear orientation because of their life circumstances. The process consisted basically in a clarification of values at first (family, friends, academic training, work and sport) through the Values Questionnaire of Wilson and Luciano (2019), and then to start taking concrete steps that were translated into actions oriented towards these values. Emphasis was placed on the difference between "wanting" to do something and "having the will" to do it. It was necessary to use experiential exercises to make the interventions more concrete, given that the patient has some difficulty in abstract thinking, like many psychotic patients with neurocognitive impairment (Reininghaus et al., 2019). The introduction of metaphors and experiential exercises is important as it involves biographical elements in the memory, thus facilitating recall. It is also important to take into consideration that episodic memory is generally preserved in psychosis, and that deficits are found in semantic memory. Thus, for example, we applied the experiential exercise of the glass of water with Patricia, in which, at first, she was asked to walk from one side of the room to another with a glass full of water in her hand, without spilling a drop. Patricia tried to do it with great difficulty and could not practically take a step without spilling water, so she was unable to move forward. Secondly, she was told to try to focus on getting to the other side of the room, without paying much attention to whether or not water spills out of the glass. This way, Patricia was able to make the functional equivalence between the stalemate of focusing on avoiding spilling water and her personal situation of actively trying to avoid discomfort, yet still being able to move forward.

According to the neuropsychological assessment carried out, Patricia presented neurocognitive impairment in some neuropsychological areas, for which a series of adaptations were made in the interventions following ART (Díaz-Garrido et al., 2021). In general, attention difficulties require a reduction in consultation time, continuous repetition of the elements throughout the sessions, with a slower pace of presentation, using verbal and written summaries. The sessions focused on psychotherapeutic aspects and had a duration of 35 minutes, due to the difficulties in maintaining attention, and with a frequency of twice a week, so that Patricia would have enough space and time to assimilate the content. Individual sessions were structured as follows:

- Five minutes for mindfulness exercises to work on the observation and description of body sensations and emotions.
- Five minutes to remember the content of the previous session. An outline of the previous session is provided, and the amnesic evocation is addressed, giving clues in case of difficulty, to facilitate recognition. The elements remembered or recognised are written down by Patricia on the diagram provided.
- Ten minutes for the elaboration and comprehension of the functional analysis adapted to the cognitive capacities of the patient.
- Ten minutes on value orientation and agreement on the implementation of specific valued-oriented actions. Likewise, sessions were focused on a specific topic, avoiding addressing several topics at the same time, due to the difficulties detected in response inhibition. In addition, if at any time Patricia's discourse was more maniac or disperse, she was redirected as many times as necessary to focus her attention. A single experiential exercise (the one with the glass of water) was used as a guide for the whole process, so that by performing it repeatedly, Patricia could internalise its functional equivalence in her daily life. Similarly, instead of resorting to multiple metaphors, which could have been overwhelming and even confusing for Patricia, a single guiding metaphor was used, in this case, the "Storm Metaphor" proposed by Díaz-Garrido et al. (2021).
- The last five minutes are devoted to reviewing and elaborating an outline of the content covered to facilitate recall of the session.

Throughout the process, the therapeutical bond was the fundamental pillar of each intervention, and the adaptative behaviours were successively reinforced and moulded. It should be noted that given that ACT provides a holistic approach, in addition to these spaces dedicated to psychotherapy, other spaces were also dedicated to social-community aspects and rehabilitative activities (accompaniment to shopping, financial management, supervision of personal hygiene, etc.).

After a period of intensive work based on the assertive community approach and the contextual principals and some of the adaptation proposed by ART, the patient has made significant progress in her recovery process, which mainly translates into an improvement in her psychosocial functioning and quality of life. She has been able to understand the dynamics underpinning her behaviours through the

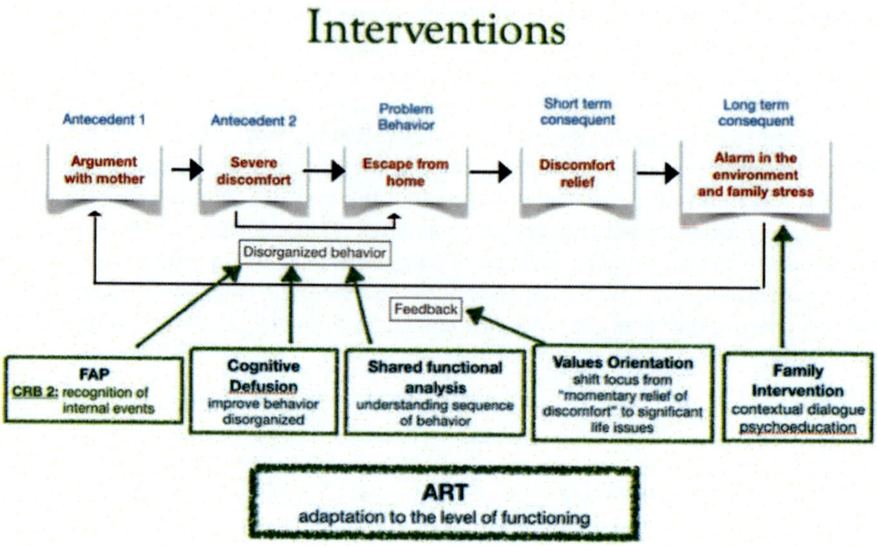

Fig 19.2 Interventions

functional analysis carried out jointly with the professionals. As stated in the everyday objectives proposed since the formulation of FAP, Patricia has improved her communication with her mother and conflicts between them have been significantly reduced. Even when differences of opinion or any other type of problem arise, the patient can manage her emotions better, to distance herself from them and dysfunctional behaviours such as escaping from home have been reduced. Consequently, the rest of the problematic behaviours have also been reduced. At present, there is greater collaboration in household chores, she has established routines and schedules, has substantially reduced her consumption of toxic substances, and has improved her adherence to psychopharmacological treatment. Attendance at the day centre has been regular, and her activities are being oriented towards her next academic training in the field of hairdressing and cosmetics. She spends quality time with her family and friends and engages in healthy leisure activities to direct her life IN THE RIGHT DIRECTION, while having the support of professionals and significant people in her life in this process.

Figure 19.2 shows a review of the intervention.

19.3 Case 2: Moving Forward in a More Calmly, Safely Way

First-Hand Experience *"I started to feel bad in high school, with my schoolmates I felt like a misfit, invisible, as if I did not exist. Sometimes, I did things to make myself visible. I could not study, I wanted to leave. I was lost and disoriented. Later*

I started going to a meditation centre where they gave talks about mental connection and destiny. I have experienced a lot of emotional instability, anguish, and psychosis. My main supports in life are my family and mental health professionals and I want to highlight how much they have helped me. My experience has been hard, but I have come a long way by communicating with them and accepting reality. Accepting the treatment and trusting the team has been fundamental. I have now stabilized, and I have a calm life. I feel more peace and self-confidence. The work in the unit and in day centres has been so positive for my psychosocial rehabilitation. I feel recovered: I am active, and I have some projects, like getting my driving license or studying something for the future".

19.3.1 Clinical Case

Luis is a 26-year-old, single and childless, with basic education and no work experience, that lives with his mother and sister. He grew up and spent part of his childhood in Colombia, homeland of his father's family, without incidents, although with hard experiences. At the age of 4, he moved to Gran Canaria with his mother and sister due to insecurity in the country. His father died at that time.

At the age of thirteen, he started to be seen by mental health services due to family and school problems. When he was 19, he went to the emergency department for behavioural disturbances in his family home. He presented cognitive distortions, and paranoid ideas of harm and felt that his thoughts were being controlled by someone else: he was perplexed and suspicious, with unmotivated laughter and probable hallucinations. He was first admitted to acute care and diagnosed with paranoid schizophrenia. When his positive symptoms subsided and he was discharged, he continued his follow-up with psychiatry, clinical psychology, nursing and social work professionals in the outpatient mental health unit.

In the following years, he went several times to the emergency department and had other acute admissions, sometimes presenting grandiose and mystical delusions, frequently intense anguish, significant obsessive symptomatology and suicidal ideation. Given his negative symptomatology and Luis' request for help to organize his time, he was referred to the Day Centre for Psychosocial Rehabilitation (DCPR), which he attended several times a week for years.

At the age of 25, he attempted suicide in the context of intense psychotic distress, and he was hospitalized following several fractures and admitted for the fourth time in acute care.

When discharged, Luis was transferred to the Medium Stay Unit (MSU), a clinical and intensive rehabilitation unit. Initially, the pharmacological treatment comprising antipsychotics, antidepressants and anxiolytics had been adjusted and multidisciplinary interventions had been carried out, involving the participation in nursing activities and occupational therapy. After some improvement, family permission was tried, which was long due to COVID regulations. This required an early return to the MSU and again to acute care due to high anguish with new suicide attempts and risk of committing suicide.

After the last discharge from acute care, the psychotherapeutic approach based on ART begins.

19.3.2 Clinical Formulation

Luis' main identified problems are described below:

(a) *Symptoms, expression of intense discomfort:*

Affective symptoms are related to inflexible avoidance (Van Os & Kapur, 2009). Luis presented some depressive symptoms, which are associated with increased relapse, suicidal behaviour (McGinty et al., 2018) and interpersonal problems (Vallina et al., 2019). Luis described depressive ruminative thoughts about feeling trapped by his problems, hopeless about the future, with no realistic current goals and having difficulty enjoying free time. He expressed significant frustration for not being a policeman or civil guard as he wished, for not having been able to continue his studies and he felt also guilty for "not having improved earlier". Luis frequently presented anxiety, which plays an important role in threatening interpretations and the maintenance of delusions (Freeman, 2016). He was particularly anxious about some interpersonal situations, about his own emotional distress resulting from the fear of experiencing a psychotic crisis, and about new situations such as "getting back to normality" and dealing with the community outside the hospital.

Positive psychotic symptomatology. Auditory-verbal hallucinations persisted. These are paranoid interpretations which, together with overvalued mystical ideas, occupied his attention daily, mentally dialoguing with them. As Chadwick and Birchwood (1995) describe positive hallucinations during a stage of little meaningful activity cause him to respond with involvement, which has made Luis' social life difficult. Unpleasant hallucinations generated him anger or confusion, tending to fight them through action. For example, in a crowded shopping centre, he heard former high schoolmates threatening him. This made him angry, and he changed his behaviour, becoming "more arrogant, as if prepared for a possible fight".

As precipitating factors for Luis' emotional distress, we found situations that entailed a high demand on his cognitive and/or emotional resources, such as emotionally charged social interactions, a high level of environmental stimulation (complex external stimulation) or the experience of ego-dystonic mental content (complex internal stimulation), which is difficult to understand and cope.

(b) *Deficits or limitations in his behavioural repertoire:*

Difficulty in developing information and identifying own and other people's emotions. This can be explained to a large extent by deficits in basic cognition (Dickinson et al., 2004) and social cognition.

Tendency towards rigid rationalization. Luis tended to solve all problems with rigid rationalization, thinking about them and trying to find an explanation, which led him to ruminate about experiences both from distant and recent past. He was very attentive to his mental contents (thoughts, emotions, psychotic symptoms) and he judged them, getting caught it vicious circles that generated significant distress and isolation. The excessive self-reflection to fight against one's own experiences difficult the situation (Sellers et al., 2017) and feedback into the control-focused attention and lack of social involvement (Pérez-Álvarez, 2008).

Poor development of skills to tolerate and/or manage distress, partly conditioned by deficits and lack of learning experiences in his difficult past.

Avoidance of situations perceived as stressful and *hyper-reflexivity* (transdiagnostic phenomena) was very prominent in Luis and played a role both in the maintenance of emotional distress and its symptomatic expression and in the maintenance of the deficits, reducing the learning opportunities and experiences.

(c) *Significant problems in his psychosocial functioning, influenced by the limitations and symptoms experienced:*

Self or aggressive behavioural alterations at times of high distress. This affected family dynamics. There was an environment of emotional tension. His family expressed intense fear of new suicide attempts and, in general, of the loss of control.

Isolation, with loss of social network outside the family of origin and desire to have it.

Lack of value-directed actions. He carried out few meaningful activities, which made him feel "lost".

(d) *As predisposing factors* to the symptomatic expression of his intense emotional distress and limitations in his behavioural repertoire, the following are considered:

Biography with traumatic experiences in early stages, such as the suicide of his father, the experience of loneliness, rejection in adolescence and school dropout. This had led Luis to a personal narrative very focused on death and the absence of his father, as well as his social inadaptation in the adolescence. He presented marked emotions that were difficult to manage regarding his main family figures: a certain envy and guilt in relation to his sister, intense anger towards his father and moderate anger towards his mother and maternal grandfather because, as adult reference figures, "they could not help me" (they could not avoid his intense suffering and the development of the psychosis) either due to a perception of excessive control or the lack of it.

Consumpsion of cannabis and alcohol at an important stage for the development of his personality and relationships with others.

Family culture with a tendency towards self-control and complex communication, sometimes deviant or with a tendency towards abstract, mystic contents, which in Luis' case generated confusion and fusion with mental contents.

Figure 19.3 summarizes the formulations of the described problems and related factors.

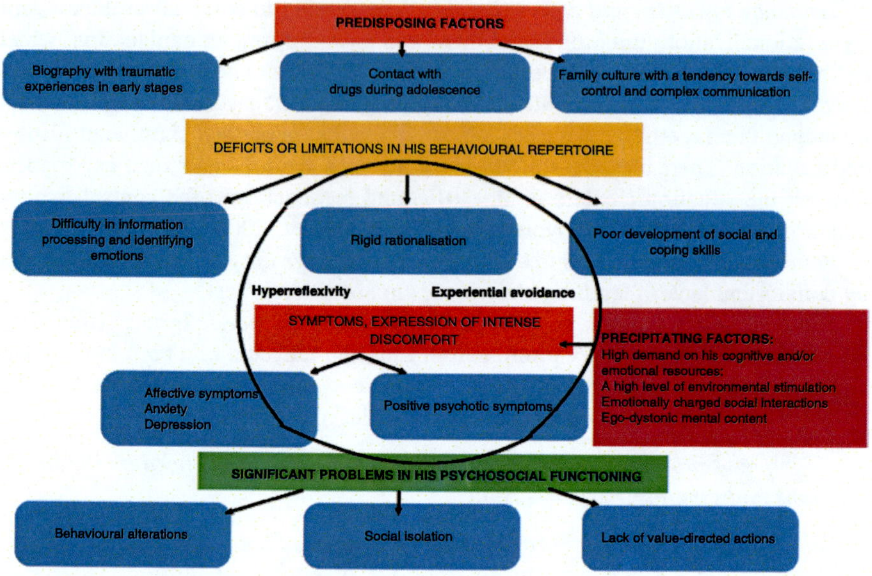

Fig 19.3 Formulations of the described problems and related factors

19.3.3 Intervention and Progress

The work with Luis has been aimed at improving his well-being and life-satisfaction. For this purpose, we have tried to reduce his hyper-reflexivity and avoidance and we have intervened specifically in the different levels of problems he presented: in his psychosocial functioning, in his emotional distress and in his limitations (promoting rehabilitation and development of skills), helping him to modulate the effect of predisposing and precipitating factors.

Luis has been treated using ART (Díaz-Garrido et al., 2021). A fundamental aspect is that the model understands the therapeutic relationship based on humanistic values, such as unconditional acceptance, empathy and authenticity and also understands human behaviour in a global and holistic way, as a part of a unique story. It uses a transdiagnostic approach, avoiding a focus on reductionist stigmatising labels.

Other outlined principles of ART model that were especially useful in planning Luis' intervention include the following:

- Multidimensionality, guarantees the continuity of care through different dimensions and contexts of the person: integration into normalized community activities and coherent integration of elements from other models, such as the empty-chair technique from Gestalt orientation (Martín, 2007). The use of contextual dialogism maintained both with the professionals of the different departments involved, in order to consider the vision that each one contributed to the case, and especially with the family, stands out. The family's approach to difficult experiences and

current dynamics made it possible to listen to the different voices and perspectives of each person, achieving a certain systemic psychological flexibility. For example, in a family meeting, his mother affirmed that "it is the first time that I feel that we are three, three different people", redefining a new position of the family members and thus marking the identification of an important change.
- Interdisciplinarity, highlights the important of the work of the extended therapeutic team in which, in addition to psychiatrists, clinical psychologists and nurses, there are also nursing assistants, occupational therapists, social workers, social integrators, etc. Their work has favoured his learning of various instrumental activities, his perseverance, and his implementation in community contexts.
- Adaptation to the cognitive and functional impairment level, for which, in addition to the clinical interview and observation, specific scales were administered, resulting in an assessment of "mild impairment", which implied slight adaptations in the interventions (such as sessions with less content, informal mindfulness practice and the use of clarifications and physical elements in some metaphors).

Before starting, it is essential to highlight the *strengths and resources* of Luis and his family, because their contribution has made it possible to move forward in his recovery process. These include the following:

- High motivation to feel better and desire to get involved. He wanted professional help and put his trust in it. Professionals who previously treated Luis also played a part in this motivation, which constituted a helpful experience for him.
- Luis' prosocial values such as respect for others, solidarity and humility.
- Personal values such as honesty, responsibility, desire to improve, perseverance and determination.
- Well-preserved autonomous functioning.
- Tendency towards introspection, which favoured a good level of psychotherapeutic work.
- Involved family, highly resilient, having faced traumatic experiences, oriented to the development of its members and to encourage their own responsibility and autonomy.
- Having basic needs covered, with accommodation in the family housing and financial availability, which made it possible to participate in community activities that required costs.

Interventions have taken place in the flexible ACT phases described by García Montes and Pérez-Álvarez (2016):

(a) *Creative hopelessness* to contact with the need for change, with the difficulty to move towards vital goals with the strategies used so far. Luis attributed his difficulty in achieving his current goals to his father's suicide. This narrative, which in short term was used as a strategy to soothe the contact with his problems and his lack of committed action, in long term kept him in the vicious circle of avoidance, remaining trapped in his mind. During the sessions, we discussed what Luis needed and demanded about his past experiences, but we also encouraged him to focus his attention on the present and on the future, on his current life and what he was doing in it. He became aware of the fact that the previous narrative extremely focused on his hard past was not helping him to feel better and was not useful to move forward to where he wanted to be.

(b) *Control as a problem*, promoting the understanding that internal events cannot be controlled and that avoidance strategies such as hyperactivity or isolation have a high cost.

Luis had tried to control unpleasant emotions such as sadness, fear, or boredom by organizing free time in a very structured way to avoid discomfort. The control and scheduling of activities made it hard to enjoy leisure and free time in a relaxed way, experiencing it as "dangerous unproductivity".

We tried to foster greater understanding and acceptance of his mental states.

Different emotions, including the unpleasant ones, were normalized, and the need to accept the inevitability of some degree of suffering in human beings was raised. Both at the individual and group level, within the Social Cognition and Interaction Training (SCIT) (Roberts et al., 2009), emotions were treated as human, universal and functional, without pathologizing them. He participated in the SCIT carried out in the unit, contextualized. Metacognition was addressed in an interactive way, in which patients had the opportunity to share personal experiences of social situations, encouraging group identification of emotions, emerging and alternative thoughts, as well as congruent values and actions. Participation in the group provided both elements for the continuous evaluation of his cognitive and psychosocial functioning, and conditions favouring psychological flexibility. Luis was able to talk about his emotions, understanding them as shared human experiences, for which identification with peers and some self-revelation were important (Chadwick, 2009).

To help Luis identify, understand and respond to his emotions with greater awareness, we functionally analysed the most salient recent emotional experiences, encouraging him to name them, identify in which situation (internal or external) they had arisen and how he responded. It was extremely important that he became aware of the transitory nature of emotions. We tried out some mindfulness exercises and encouraged non-formal practice, which involved the adoption of an attentional focus in the present activity and an observer attitude of his mental contents without becoming confused by them. Focused attention was especially promoted, both in moments of wellbeing and in those in which the discomfort just disappears, to raise awareness and personal narrative about them. Luis was able to recognize the emotions and distance himself from them, so that, being less overwhelmed, he could feel freer to take what he needed and try to address it. He stopped talking in general, non-specific terms such as "I experienced suffering yesterday" to specify "I was angry when I was talked like that" or "I was bored, but I joined in playing parchesi with others and I got better".

Luis was looking to feel in control of several areas in his life. It was a matter of gradually fostering greater self-confidence and acceptance of some uncertainty in the future. Key was his growing capacity to focus his attention on the present reality and the dialogue in which he was also experiencing his ability to tolerate unresolved doubts. Today, Luis can set future-oriented goals more calmly: "I'm interested in this right now…but we will see".

(c) *Cognitive defusion* to promote the distancing from certain mental contents in which he was trapped, limiting his functioning. We worked on changing the relationship with different mental contents, such as some mystical overvalued ideas that directed his attention and action towards focusing on auditory hallucinations. We deeply conversed about telepathy and mental connection, some beliefs he took from a potential sect that he frequented for months. He found some alternative interpretations that explained his experiences without causing him confusion and isolation. We differentiated these beliefs from others that belong to a spiritual dimension (beliefs in the intangible: the soul, God and the experience of prayer), taking care of important values for him, which also transmitted security, tranquility and transcendent meaning to his existence.

A change in the relationship with psychotic experiences was promoted, encouraging mental flexibility. Specifically, paranoid interpretations were addressed as possible hypotheses instead of convictions, favouring the generation of alternatives and the evaluation of the degree of certainty given to them. The work carried out in the SCIT group and the individual sessions in which personal situations were analysed were useful for this purpose. For example, sometimes when he went home on leave, he thought that his mother could know everything he was doing. When asked about this, he described specific situations in which he wanted to hide something (which was objectively conspicuous) and his mother suspected what was going on. We asked about the occasions in which he informed his mother of what he had done or was planning to do, without her having the slightest idea beforehand, which was the most common. He began to understand that this happened occasionally, due to objective signs, which differed from his mother being able to know "everything" he did. Gradually, Luis increased his ability to interpret many interpersonal situations in different ways.

Regarding the change in relationship with his hallucinations, Luis talked about their characteristics and contents. The understanding of symptoms as being linked to his biography was promoted. Luis was able to recognize desires and fears in the content of the voices and these could be considered and addressed from a value-directed action. For example, he heard a neighbour say "you are mine" while her image came frequently to his mind. He interpreted that she wanted to be his partner, which was an obstacle for him to pay attention to other girls, as he did not want to be unfaithful to her. Through therapeutic work, he became aware that it was him who wanted to have a partner and that he had found that neighbour attractive. Another example was that he heard his schoolmates tell him "Let's fix this". At times he experienced it as a threat and tried to show himself as superior or as an authority figure who establishes order, sometimes even believing that he was a policeman. At other times, he could interpret it as a reconciliation request made by people from his past. Luis became aware that it was him who wanted to make up for his experience of relationships with peers, which had been difficult in the past.

He realized that he spent a lot of time talking internally with the voices, thinking about them and changing his behaviour accordingly. He decided to try to spend as little time as possible on them to direct his energies to his goals.

Luis was astonished as he came to understand more about his mental functioning and the fact that sometimes his fears and desires could be perceived in this way. Most importantly, as his relationship with his hallucinations changed, he was able to experience them without feeling anguish or limiting his behaviour.

(d) *"A transcendent sense of self"* (Hayes & Strosahl, 2004) to foster a sense of himself in touch with what he had experienced throughout his existence.

Luis also sought a sense of control with a closed definition of himself, which made it difficult to access new experiences, especially in a social context. In order to favour a more flexible sense of self, sometimes, when he provided rigid adjectives about his way of being, after validating the experiences on which he relied, other experiences were provided that made him consider that the opposite adjectives were also applicable, fostering a more dialectical perspective of himself. For example, when Luis said, "I am shy, reserved, because…", we added "Yes, although yesterday you gave a presentation in front of several people".

In order to encourage a more integrated sense of self, we jointly reviewed his biography. He needed to work more on his difficult adolescence and early youth, when he experienced intense anguish, and social maladjustment and learned that his father's death had been a suicide. More experiential exercises were helpful and adapted (Morris, 2019) by describing them in advance and stating the objective, respecting his needs and pace. Particularly necessary was the work related to his father, where the empty-chair technique was important, so that unresolved issues and emotions could be addressed. At first, he expressed intense anger at his father, and he accused him of abandonment, of having caused him and his family suffering and blaming him for practically all his problems in life. Then he began to ask himself questions and to consider the enormous difficulty in coping with the suffering he probably experienced. Gradually, he began to express some compassion for him, while also differentiating himself from this father: "I would not have done it. You have to try to solve things and let yourself be helped too". Subsequently, he spoke about this very occasionally and more calmly, saying that he was more aware of it and without it being the centre of his discourse.

(e) *Value orientation*

Luis wanted to maintain a good relationship with his family, have a quiet life, open up to some new social relationships, do sports, continue studying or working, and feel proud of himself. We supported him in identifying and committing to these goals.

This is fundamental in the recovery process, as proposed by Le Boutillier et al. (2011) with the acronym CHIME: Connectedness with other human beings; Hope with choices and actions committed to life; flexible Identity, able to observe if mental contents are useful; Meaning, giving meaning and dignity to all experiences, including the painful ones; Empowerment, acting based on values rather than fears.

Luis admission in a unit that tries to function as a therapeutic community, together with his continuity in the Day Centre for Psychosocial Rehabilitation, his home leaves and group work fostered the identification, empathy and connection with others. The process of recognizing himself and giving meaning to different experiences favoured his personal identity, to the point where he voluntarily exposes his first-hand experience in front of others, as he did in the "Patient's Classroom" (a space in the General Hospital aimed at promoting patients' knowledge and proactivity in their treatment process). Personal and shared recognition of his achievements, as well as meaningful short-term goals, have fostered a hopeful outlook. The identification of values and his own choices to move towards them make him aware of his capacity of self-direction, feeling more protagonist in his life and more satisfied with himself.

(f) *"Willingness and commitment"* to address and commit to goals relevant to him despite discomfort.

He decided to attend the "Digital Competences" course at a school near his home, even though he felt ambivalent at the beginning and preferred to avoid attending. Nevertheless, he kept going even if he faced some uncomfortable situations during the course. He feels satisfied with the experience he shared with his peers and with his certified learning. Luis continues to attend the DCPR three times a week. At first, he felt that the previous one was very related to a stage of great psychopathological instability and suffering. His ability to identify and communicate the problem and propose a solution was validated and strengthened. He now attends a new centre. He has agreed with professionals on the activities that are meaningful to him: sport, English and debates.

Family relationships are of great value to him, he focuses on taking care of them and respecting himself. He expresses his needs more assertively and manages disagreements more calmly. He collaborates with his mother and his sister in household chores. He also goes with them on family outings and shares pleasant moments with them, such as watching series with his sister, with whom the relationship has grown closer. He enjoys simple things like walking his dog every day.

For Luis, studies and sport are important and he has been analysing the level at which he wants and can participate in these activities in different spaces. For example, as he has always liked martial arts, he decided to sign up for some classes at a gymnasium, attending for several weeks even though he found them hard.

He thinks it would suit him well to work and is gradually opening to different options. For this reason, he has recently been referred to the Employment Support Program and is being counselled.

19.3.4 Conclusion

The ART model brings together very valuable elements for therapeutic work with people with psychosis due to its humanity, subjectivity, ethics, knowledge and research, making it a model that accepts complexity and diversity, that integrates elements from other orientations with coherence and flexibility and is directed towards people's recovery, beyond symptomatic remission.

19.4 Case 3: Recovering a Meaningful Life

First Hand Experience *"I am willing to introduce myself: my name is Carmen. Maybe my story will help other people that have gone through experiences like mine, or to better understand what it is like to live with a diagnosis like mine in a hospital for some many years. I often wonder "Why me?" I have tried to be strong, but it has not been easy. I remember that my childhood was normal. I think I was a happy child, with a comfortable life, with no big complications. My parents worked outside home, my sibling and I went to school, and we all got along well. When I got to high school, things started to change I felt alone, it was difficult for me to connect with others, I was not one of the "popular girls". They started to behave in a very cruel way towards me, they insulted me saying "You are so ugly, you are horrible". I was not able to ask for help, to talk to my family about what was happening to me. I lived in isolation and shame. When I got to the university it was even worst, they continued insulting me...and I broke down. That's when I made my first suicide attempt. At that time, I had already asked for help, but it did not help me, they did not give me any answers. That is when treatments and admissions started. I believe I have improved over the years thanks to the constant support of my family. I think that if I died tomorrow, I would not have done much, but now I want to do other things to fill my life. The relationship with my family is still good, although I have always clashed a lot with my mother. In the last few months, I have noticed that she is calmer, I think my siblings have something to do with it. She does not get so upset about anything anymore. I try not to clash with her so much, I do not like arguing with her. I consider my family as my strength; I would not have been able keep moving forward on without them. Other things that have helped me to be more stable is my desire to move forward in life, to recover and to prosper. Now I go to language lessons, and I would like that to help me find a job. I like teaching and libraries. The illness has robbed me of a lot of things and although I am better, things are still complicated. People still talk to me when I walk down the street, but I am now able to do things that were unthinkable before. I could not go out alone, go into a shop. They insulted me over the loudspeaker, they shouted at me. During this year, the Hearing Voices Group experience has helped me a lot, I have felt supported, and I have been able to talk about what was happening to me. At the beginning, I did not believe that other people were going through the same things as me, or with the same intensity. But yes, and we have supported each other a lot. I wish I could get out of the hospital and live in a supervised flat, with support. Find friends. I always wanted to have friends, but I did not know how. For a long time, I was looking for people's attention. I would like not to hear voices, not to be shouted at in the street, but I think I could still live out of here. The last time I was at home, I could hear my* *neighbours constantly criticising me, but I kept doing my own thing, on the computer...and I ignored them".*

19.4.1 Personal History and Appearance of the Problem

Carmen, the pseudonym proposed by the protagonist, is a woman in her forties. Much of her life has been marked by great suffering and years of hospitalisation in medium and long-stay units. She is the youngest of five siblings and has a good relationship with her widowed mother and her siblings, despite the years she has been hospitalised.

She reports having had a normal development during her childhood and pre-adolescence. In adolescence, she began to experience difficulties with her peers. During this time, she began to be bullied by a group of schoolmates, which made her become more reserved and to tend to isolate herself. For some months, she attends a private psychologist who helps her to cope during this stage. She enrolled at the University to study philology, but during the first year of her career (at the age of 19), her first episode takes place and is admitted to the Acute Unit of the Hospital. When she was discharged, already diagnosed with paranoid schizophrenia, she was referred to a Mental Health Unit.

Since then, the evolution has been slow and with a very poor response to psychopharmaceuticals. She displays a very intense symptomatology, in the form of voices (from her neighbours) insulting her or "talking to each other" about aspects of her intimacy. She reacted to this experience with an intense anguish and desperation, which led to two self-harming attempts. Admissions to the Short Stay Unit (SSU) or private centres followed one after another. She was treated with Electroconvulsive Therapy in some of these episodes without significant improvement.

Due to the poor response to treatment, the severity of the symptoms, the level of suffering and the family's difficulties in managing the problem at home, Carmen is referred to an MSU, where she remained for 2 years. She achieved a certain degree of stability, but a significant positive symptomatology persisted, so she is referred to the Clinical and Rehabilitation Unit, where she has remained since 2015.

Currently, Carmen continues to experience delusions of harm and paranoid ideation, phenomena related to the course and content of thought, such as mind reading or mental blocks. She feels invaded by voices (generally from TV or radio) that talk about her. For this reason, she avoids watching TV, listening to music, etc., which are activities she used to enjoy in the past. On the other hand, she is a woman with cultural inquisitiveness, who likes languages (as long as she is not feeling anxious) and who lives her hospital stay with a lot of frustration. She is very selective with people and does not make friends easily. She has never had a partner or significant friendships. Her relationship with the staff is ambivalent and has caused significant problems. She reacts and refers towards some of the staff with defensive and hostile behaviour relatively frequently.

Looking into the future is unlikely that she returns home due to her mother's age. She is a candidate for the alternative or residential accommodation program as she needs some supervision. She raises the need for discharge very frequently but finds it difficult to get involved in drawing up a realistic plan that would lead her to take steps towards discharge. She continuously complains about "the bad luck she has had for not being able to live a normal life like her siblings".

19.4.2 Intervention

The intervention that is carried out tries to apply ACT within the context of psychotic symptoms. There is great deal of evidence of its use among this complex spectrum that generates so much suffering in people who suffer from it (García-Montes & Pérez-Álvarez, 2016). In this case, the aim is to help Carmen reconsider the unsuccessful fight against the symptoms that have accompanied her since her early adult life and to explore new paths that bring her closer to what she wants to achieve despite them. In the same way, the aim is to deepen the experience of positive symptomatology as active form of experiential avoidance, to increase competences that allow to integrate these events in a less incapacitating way and to increase her coping capacity. "Experiential avoidance" is the phenomenon that occurs when a person is unable to have contact with private experiences and strives to decrease the frequency of contact with the contexts that causes them. It is a behavioural mechanism that can be apparently effective in short term but can become chronic, limiting the person's life. Delusional symptomatology could be considered an active, highly elaborated form of experiential avoidance in which the person not only avoids but also tries to build the reality they wish to achieve or the insurmountable obstacles that would justify not having achieved it (García-Montes & Pérez-Álvarez, 2005).

The contribution made by ART is of great value as an intervention model that focuses on changing the relationship with what disturbs us (Díaz-Garrido et al., 2021). The principles of the model (contextual, multidimensional, transdiagnostic, interdisciplinary and adapted to the level of impairment and functionality of the person) fit with an intervention that tries to adapt to Carmen's needs, reality and context.

Third-generation therapies bring a new and revolutionary perspective on the relationship with internal events. Unlike second-generation therapies, which look at understanding and changing cognitions, the contextual approach seeks to improve the relationship with them, developing tolerance to that which causes suffering, without trying to actively change it. This new outlook does not have to imply an absolutist and definitive separation between cognitive and contextual therapies. In fact, a good therapist must be able to use the therapeutical tools that are needed for each case and at each specific moment, whether they are grounded in cognitive, behavioural or any other model, as long as they make sense and maintain internal coherence within the therapeutic process of each patient. It could be said that second and third-generation therapies opt for different paths but arrive to a similar destination. That is to say, in second-generation therapies, through a series of interventions, it is sought that those irrational thoughts or beliefs that cause the suffering are replaced by less harmful ones, for example, the thought "I am worthless" can be replaced by "I am valuable". Third-generation therapies do not opt for a direct change, as this could be counterproductive and generate an exhausting and unsuccessful inner struggle, and therefore they propose a process of observation, acceptance and distancing, which will progressively generate a change in the person's relationship with their internal events. In short, second and third-generation therapies do not have to confront each other, and their principles can be complementary and have similar objectives. Their joint use, adapted to each case, can enrich the intervention.

In Carmen's case, not only the contextual principles have been followed, but we have also tried to generate a collaborative style based on Motivational Interviewing (MI) (Miller & Rollnick, 2015). Although it is an approach that emerged in the early 1990s from the field of addictions, in recent years it has been extended to other areas related to education, health or penal mediation, in those contexts in which the aim is to strengthen the person's motivation and commitment to change. The word "change" may at first seem counterproductive in the context of third-generation therapies. However, in the spirit of both MI and the contextual approach a balance is advocated between "acceptance and change" or, in the word of ACT itself, between "acceptance and commitment to action towards values". The therapist, therefore, becomes a guide who helps the patient to maintain this balance and to adapt flexibly to the direct contingencies of the moment. The aim is not, however, to find the mechanism of cognitive change that MI promulgates, but to provide a communicative style that facilitates this collaborative work and respects the person's values.

Finally, the group element is introduced with the implementation of a "Group of Unusual Experiences", following the *Hearing Voices* model proposed by Romme and Escher (2005), which can also help to understand the experience of symptoms in a less limiting, more normalised way and together with a group of residents who have lived with the symptoms for a long time. In this sense, the combination of the group element as a source of support and reference seems appropriate to maintain motivation and find other spaces to achieve the therapeutical goals set.

Another important aim of the intervention was to help her to increase her emotional regulation and decrease the hostile reactions that occurred with some frequency with the staff in the unit. As a result of these psychotic experiences, there was a repetitive pattern of self-referentiality to which she tended to defend herself with anger in certain situations and with certain people. Along the therapeutic process, it was possible to explore some aspects of her autobiography in which she had experienced situations of humiliation by schoolmates and to which she had reacted with avoidance and isolation. In current situations, she tended to justify herself by arguing that she would "never let herself be humiliated again", and she was angry in some moments which reminded her to painful situations she had experienced before.

Initially, the aim was to generate an experience of creative hopelessness, making her realise the cost of avoidance and how limiting it was in terms of taking steps towards her recovery. The metaphor of "feeding the dog" was used in many sessions as a common thread. As she tried to increase the number of activities she wanted to do, there was a tendency to feel overwhelmed by discomfort and to maintain a very chronic pattern of avoidance. The metaphor helped to understand the importance of continuing to move forward despite the symptomatology.

In the same way, it is a matter of clarifying goals and desires and providing means to try to achieve them, minimising the impact that psychosis has had on her so far. Values work is fundamental in ACT. These are defined as global, desired and verbally constructed life directions that are present as a vital horizon and that give actions a direction and purpose (Wilson & Luciano, 2019). In this case, this element is crucial since the impact that Carmen's pathology has in her life, as well as the dynamics of a long-term admission without a clearly established end, facilitate resignation and the role of "passive patient" who can do little to reverse the situation.

The clarification of values was addressed through exercises that help to find concreteness in her life goals. Despite chronicity, she maintains interests and the desire to continue building a more productive life, as well as being discharged from the unit. During some sessions, a narrative assessment of values (Wilson & Luciano, 2019) was carried out to explore vital areas such as family, friendship, education, or autonomy, and to discover concrete steps that could be taken in each of them. The elaboration of different cards where she expressed a goal (continue my career, improve my health, get discharged, improve relations with my family or have more friends) was used as a support. These cards were displayed on the wall of the office where the sessions were normally held and were reread to make them more concrete or to increase her commitment to them.

It is of great value to understand the psychotic symptomatology that she presents in terms of the psychological inflexibility that leads Carmen to experience and re-experience life circumstances in a limited way due to the experiential avoidance, lack of clarity in her values, literality in her private experiences or resignation to her suffering. The exercises proposed in the course of therapy are intended to help her to recognise the futility of trying to control her symptoms and to understand the great vital cost of allowing herself to be permanently driven by these internal experiences. The aim is to address hyper-reflexivity (reducing the so present self-referential reflective processes) by distancing herself and increasing her diminished sense of self, involving herself in areas of personal activity that are relevant to her. For a long time, when Carmen felt distressed and invaded, she tended to become emotionally overwhelmed and to manifest very significant distress that led her to remain in her room, free of stimuli, limiting her participation in activities and to increase the intake of medication to relieve her discomfort at those moments. In a way, we could affirm that the setting of the unit also tried to exert some control over the symptoms, taking away her capacity to act on them. The possibility of accompanying these situations in another way was raised, encouraging her to continue doing what she had committed to do and offering strategies to minimise the intensity of the episodes.

Another important goal in the process was the reflection on symptom control. To create a distance from language, the exercise "Mind walk" was introduced. While walking around the compound gardens, she was constantly told things that had to do with her internal dialogues or messages from the voices ("they want to humiliate you", "they laugh at you", "they think you will not get what you want"), to which Carmen reacted with discomfort and tried to argue. These exercises enabled a greater connection and understanding of what was happening to her and to talk in greater depth about the experience of the voices, as well as validating the experience of suffering sustained for so many years, especially in her adolescence.

Establishing a separation between the contextual and contained "Self" is a complex aspect in which we continue to intervene. Carmen remains very fused to the symptomatology experienced in these years. Her "Self" is closely linked to the verbal contents and, although she expresses her desire to be "understood and taken seriously" by her close referents, she tends to show herself to others through her symptoms and more negative life events. Many of the verbalisations she makes have to do with continual complaints about her experiences, about "not being able to have a normal life like her siblings", about her "bad luck". In this sense, it is often necessary to invite her to focus on the present moment. The exercise "Observing herself" at different moments in her life was proposed. Another frequently used exercise consisted of asking her to express her complaint in a comical way, which helped to reduce tension and break the loop that limited us from continuing with the work to be done.

The commitment to the chosen direction continues to be addressed despite the difficulties. One exercise that proved very helpful was to imagine the goals in front of her and to move forward with a blindfold over her eyes. In a second instance, she had to move forward with the blindfold under her arm. It helped her to value the importance of continuing to move forward despite everything we carry on our backs, but in a way that limits us as little as possible.

19.4.3 Progress and Results

The aim of this intervention has mainly been focused on trying to get Carmen to accept those symptoms that were distressing her and from which she was trying to escape without success, as well as encouraging her not to remain paralysed and to move towards goals that were valuable to her.

The intervention has offered the possibility to expand the knowledge and practice of ACT, while at the same time integrating this with other elements of great value for promoting change. ACT seeks to create the required conditions for the person to appreciate the paradox of their behaviour, to realise that what they are doing is in the opposite direction to what they really want to achieve, and seeks to enhance clinical interactions that allow the patient to become fully aware of the flow of private events, so that they notice them and can plan their actions according to what their values demand at that moment rather than acting according to the literalness of private events (Hayes et al., 2015). In this sense, together with the tools that ACT provides (metaphors, paradoxes, or experiential exercises), we have opted for a collaborative intervention style that emanates from MI. It focuses fundamentally on the processes of change, trying to activate the person's own motivation and resources so that they become the protagonist of this process and increase their capacity to commit themselves to get where they want. MI can enrich the practice of ACT in that it situates the clinician as a figure who guides the process, without forcing it, through reflective listening, constant attention to ambivalences that may arise and avoiding falling into the traps of the expert, the label or judgement. In short, it is about intervening from a respectful stance that aims to generate a dynamic of change and hope, which understands the dilemmas and helps the person to be the one who resolves them. ART enriches the intervention and broadens the focus so that the person's reality, capacity and functionality are taken into account.

The results of the intervention, in general, show a clinical improvement and encourage the continuation of the line of work initiated. At present, Carmen carries out valuable actions within the community on a daily basis: she attends an Official Language School where she studies German and English, she goes for walks, goes shopping and runs errands independently and spends the weekends at her family home. At the moment, the renunciations that have accompanied her for so many years are no longer there, and she continues to take action despite the hallucinatory experiences she continues to have. Relationships with staff have significantly improved, with no conflicts and being able to resolve everyday situations with greater serenity. The changes observed throughout the intervention have been maintained, although we continue to work along these lines.

The application of ACT opens up a promising path: despite the severity and chronicity, we can set goals and move forward within a framework in which people are the protagonists of their stories and continue to have goals and values that help them to keep moving forward as far as they consider. It also challenges the professionals who accompany them in the process: the need to not conform and to continue to look for alternatives to suffering, to maintain a hopeful outlook and to try to ensure that, despite everything, life continues to have a meaning, since as Ortega y Gasset said, "life takes on meaning when we make of it an aspiration to renounce nothing".

19.5 Conclusions

The recent increase of publications related to the care of people with PSD grounded in the philosophy and principles of ACT and other therapies that place the person at the centre of their rehabilitation process highlight the need for a paradigm shift in the treatment of psychosis, where the primacy of positive symptomatology gives way to addressing the negative one and the cognitive impairment. The assessment of the level of cognitive and functional impairment and the design of techniques and interventions adapted to achieve individualized rehabilitative goals that reduce disability and the deterioration in the affected person's quality of life should be the main objective for a progressive change of perspective when approaching the person affected by PSD. ART is a contextual model, with ACT principles, which follows a transdiagnostic approach, avoiding reductionist and stigmatising labels; interdisciplinary, in the broad sense of the word, including not only specialized health professionals but also social workers, social integrators, auxiliary staff, etc.; multidimensional, guaranteeing continuity of care in the different areas of the person's life (individual, familiar and community, through inclusive interventions); integrative, incorporating its own elements and contextualizing those coming from other approaches, adapting the intensity of the interventions to the clinical and functional needs of the individual with PSD at different times of life.

This chapter illustrates the therapeutic and rehabilitative process, based on ART, of three people diagnosed with psychosis, which was carried out within the public healthcare system. It highlights the feasibility and usefulness of ART in the comprehensive treatment of people with PSD within the public system, as well as the subjective satisfaction reported by the people treated in their recovery process. We hope it contributes to the deepening and extension of framework based on knowledge and centred on the person.

Disclaimer Clinical cases presented in this chapter do not include real names or personal information of real persons.

References

Chadwick, P. (2009). *Terapia cognitiva basada en la persona para la psicosis perturbadora*. Fundación para la investigación y tratamiento de la esquizofrenia y otras psicosis (edición original, Chadwick, P. (2006). *Person-based cognitive therapy for distressing psychosis*).

Chadwick, P., & Birchwood, M. (1995). The omnipotence of voices. II: The Beliefs About Voices Questionnaire (BAVQ). *The British Journal of Psychiatry: The Journal of Mental Science, 166*(6), 773–776.

Díaz-Garrido, J. A., Laffite, H., & Zuñiga, R. (2021). Terapia de aceptación y recuperación por niveles para la psicosis. In J. A. Díaz-Garrido, H. Laffite, & R. Zuñiga (coords.), *Terapia de aceptación y compromiso en psicosis. Aceptación y recuperación por niveles*. Ediciones Pirámide.

Dickinson, D., Ianone, V. N., Wild, C. M., & Gold, J. M. (2004). General and specific cognitive deficits in schizophrenia. *Biological Psychiatry, 55*(8), 826–833.

Freeman, D. (2016). Persecutory delusions: A cognitive perspective on understanding and treatment. *Lancet Psychiatry, 3*(7), 685–692.

García-Montes, J. M., & Pérez, M. (2005). Fundamentación experimental y primeras aplicaciones clínicas de la Terapia de Aceptación y Compromiso (ACT) en el campo de los síntomas psicóticos. *Revista Latinoamericana de Psicología, 37*(2), 379–393.

García-Montes, J. M., & Pérez, M. (2016). Terapia de Aceptación y Compromiso aplicada a la esquizofrenia. Estado actual y direcciones futuras. *Análisis y modificación de conducta, 42*(165–166), 99–119.

Hayes, S. C., & Strosahl, K. D. (2004). *A practical guide to acceptance and commitment therapy*. Springer.

Hayes, S., Stroshal, K., & Wilson, K. (2015). *Terapia de Aceptación y Compromiso. Proceso y práctica del cambio consciente*. Desclée de Brouwer.
Kaholokula, J. K., Godoy, A., O'Brien, W. H., Haynes, S. N., & Gavino, A. (2013). Análisis funcional en evaluación conductual y formulación de casos clínicos. *Clínica y Salud, 24*(2), 117–127. https://doi.org/10.5093/cl2013a13
Le Boutillier, C., Leamy, M., Bird, V. J., Davidson, L., Williams, J., & Slade, M. (2011). What does recovery mean in practice? A qualitative analysis of international recovery-oriented practice guidance. *Psychiatric Services, 62*(12), 1470–1476.
Martín, A. (2007). *Manual práctico de psicoterapia Gestalt*. Desclée de Brower.
Martínez-Huidobro, M. F., & Herrera, J. (2021). A pie de calle. In J. Díaz-Garrido, H. Laffite, & R. Zúñiga (coords.), *Terapia de Aceptación y Compromiso en Psicosis*. Pirámide.
McGinty, J. S., Haque, M., & Upthegrove, R. (2018). Depression during first episode Psychosis and subsequent suicide risk: A systematic review and metaanalysis of longitudinal studies. *Schizophrenia Research, 195*, 58–66.
Miller, W., & Rollnick, S. (2015). *La Entrevista Motivacional*. Paidós.
Morris, E. M. J. (2019). Acceptance and commitment therapy. In C. Cupitt (Ed.), *CBT for psychosis: Process-orientated therapies and the third wave* (pp. 79–97). Routledge Taylor & Francis Group.
Pérez-Alvarez, M. (2008). Hyperreflexivity as a condition of mental disorder: A clinical and historical perspective. *Psicothema, 20*(2), 181–187.
Pérez-Álvarez, M., García-Montes, J. M., Vallina-Fernández, O., Perona-Garcelán, S., & Cuevas-Yust, C. (2011). New life for schizophrenia psychotherapy in the light of phenomenology. *Clinical Psychology and Psychotherapy, 18*(3), 187–201.
Reininghaus, U., Klippel, A., Steinhart, H., Vaessen, T., Van Nierop, M., Viechtbauer, W., Batink, T., Kasanova, Z., Van Aubel, E., Van Winkel, R., Marcelis, M., Van Amelsvoort, T., Van Der Gaag, M., De Haan, L., & Myin-Germeys, I. (2019). Efficacy of acceptance and commitment therapy in daily life (ACT-DL) in early psychosis: Study protocol for a multicentre randomized controlled trial. *Trials, 20*(1). https://doi.org/10.1186/s13063-019-3912-4
Roberts, D. L., Penn, D. L., & Combs, D. R. (2009). *Entrenamiento en Interacción y Cognición Social (EICS)*. Manual de Tratamiento.
Romme, M., & Escher, S. (2005). *Dando sentido a las Voces. Guía para los profesionales de la salud mental que trabajan con personas que escuchan voces*. Fundación para la Investigación y el Tratamiento de la Esquizofrenia y otras psicosis.
Sellers, R., Wells, A., & Morrison, A. P. (2017). Are experiences of psychosis associated with unhelpful metacognitive coping strategies? A systematic review of the evidence. *Clinical Psychology and Psychotherapy, 25*(1), 31–49. https://doi.org/10.1002/cpp.2132
Stein, L. I., Test, M. A., & Marx, A. J. (1975). Alternative to the hospital: A controlled study. *American Journal of Psychiatry, 132*(5), 517–522.
Vallina, O., Pérez-Álvarez, M., Fernández, M. P., & García-Montes, J. M. (2019). Terapias contextuales para la psicosis. In E. Fonseca (coord.), *Tratamientos psicológicos para la psicosis* (pp. 453–510). Pirámide.
Van Os, J., & Kapur, S. (2009). Schizophrenia. *Lancet, 374*(9690), 635–645.
Wilson, K., & Luciano, M. C. (2019). *Terapia de Aceptación y Compromiso. Un tratamiento conductual orientado a los valores*. Pirámide.

Chapter 20
The "Incluyete" (*Get Involved*) Program: A Socio-educational Experience for Social Inclusion in Mental Health

Adolfo J. Cangas, Eduardo Sánchez, Manuel López de Lemus, and Andrés López-Pardo

20.1 Introduction

In recent years, there have been increasingly more approaches based on interventions far removed from the traditional medical model, in which special emphasis is placed on the needs, barriers, aspirations, and goals of the individual. Although treatment of schizophrenia has classically focused more on controlling symptoms, research has found that it features constraints and requires a more holistic understanding of the patient (Vallina Fernández et al., 2014).

Hence, it is necessary to promote perspectives aimed at developing a life plan for people diagnosed with mental problems in which social integration plays a crucial role (Stanghellini & Ballerini, 2007, 2011). For example, it is especially important to end the social isolation common among many people with psychopathological problems, brought on by both the typical characteristics of such disorders and the stigma and self-stigma that are unfortunately very common in these situations (Çapar & Kavak, 2019; Corrigan et al., 2012; Or et al., 2013). Thus, by facilitating interactions with the rest of the population, it is possible to help these individuals truly lead a fulfilling life structured upon values (Cangas & Martín-Murcia, 2021).

A. J. Cangas (✉)
University of Almería, Almería, Spain
e-mail: ajcangas@ual.es

E. Sánchez
Get Involved Program, Almería, Spain

M. L. de Lemus
Torrecardenas University Hospital, Almería, Spain

A. López-Pardo
Andalusian Public Foundation for the Social Integration of People with Mental Illness (FAISEM), Seville, Spain

J. A. Díaz-Garrido et al. (eds.), *Psychological Interventions for Psychosis*,
https://doi.org/10.1007/978-3-031-27003-1_20

A necessary measure to begin approaching these objectives is for people who have experienced their own mental health problems to assume an increasingly more active role in their recovery. Opportunities for such interaction could be found in mutual support groups, interventions promoting horizontal relationships with healthcare professionals, and participation in inclusive programs favoring the true integration of all of those taking part (WHO, 2021).

Similarly, it is increasingly evident that cultural, artistic, and sports activities are a good tool for promoting the participation and social inclusion of all people. For example, the WHO, after reviewing 900 articles on this subject, confirmed the benefits provided by utilizing activities related to art and culture in mental health treatments (WHO, 2019).

In addition, numerous investigations in this field observe that physical activity and sport not only favor improved health among the participants but also quality of life and better coping skills for psychopathological problems, such as difficulties related to depression or stress (Arsović et al., 2020; Kandola et al., 2019; Ramos-Sanchez et al., 2021; Schuch et al., 2016). Furthermore, in relation to severe mental disorders, such activities can aid in improving both positive and negative symptoms (Firth et al., 2015; Mullor et al., 2020).

Physical activity and sports can therefore serve as an ideal complement to standard clinical treatment prescribed within mental health services. It was with these goals in mind that the program called "Inclúyete" (*Get Involved*) was founded 5 years ago in Almeria – a program whose main features are described below.

20.2 Socio-educational Experience in Mental Health: The *Inclúyete* Program

The *Inclúyete* program is an initiative that started at the University of Almeria, in collaboration with the Public Foundation for the Social Integration of People with Mental Disorders (FAISEM), the Mental Health Clinical Management Unit at the University Hospital of Torrecardenas and the Mental Health Advocacy Board of Almeria (which unites various associations and healthcare entities working in the province of Almeria). The objective is, on one hand, to promote the social inclusion of individuals with severe mental disorders and, on the other, reduce social stigma toward people with mental health problems. To this end, several workshop programs are in operation which shares the following characteristics:

1. Participation in the program is open to anyone, both people who have experienced their own mental health problems and students and average citizens interested in the subject matter of the workshop. The proportion of attendees is normally two-thirds individuals with mental health problems, while the remainder is composed of people from different backgrounds. However, this proportion obviously may vary depending on course demand. In any case, it is essential that participation not only be limited to mental health patients and that the other

people taking part assume more than merely the role of "volunteers"; instead, they should join because they are genuinely interested in the subject of the activity itself. For this purpose, as will be explained further, efforts are made to present original and appealing workshops for all people.

2. It is essential that the school or learning center collaborating in the program both guarantee a reasonable number of students (university, high school, or bachelorette age) and facilitate the dynamic atmosphere young people tend to provide. It is worth bearing in mind that stigma among students and professionals is similar to that of the general population (Navarro Gómez & Triguero Ramos, 2019), which means that working with students is also important when attempting to reduce stigma. In our case, we actively collaborate with the University of Almeria, which is where the courses are organized and a considerable number of professors, grantees, and students from this institution participate.
3. Requisites for joining a group are not based on any diagnostic criteria (information that is not requested). Instead, attendees can simply participate because they take interest or find utility in the workshop. Moreover, no previous academic requisites (degrees or certifications) are necessary to take part in the experience.
4. Participation in the workshops is free. Cost is not an obstacle as attendees are not charged at all for enrollment. The program is funded by the Public Foundation for the Social Integration of People with Mental Disorders (FAISEM) and receives some financial contribution from the University of Almeria, as well as from other institutions interested in collaborating in the experience (such as the Almeria Council and the Town Hall of Almeria).
5. It is essential that the workshop teachers be highly motivated and possess a high-level recognition in their respective fields, so as to offer the best learning experience possible to all the group participants. What is more, the close involvement of the teachers, who in many cases have never had any prior contact with aspects related to mental health, leads to them becoming outspoken champions of the program. As a result, through their example, they help to greatly reduce social stigma towards people with mental health problems.
6. Individuals that have mental health problems and those with knowledge on the subject are supported so they may assume the role of course teachers or teaching collaborators. Such is the case of the literary expression workshop, as will be detailed later.
7. Workshops are held at public spaces around the city and enjoy the collaboration of public institutions and cultural, artistic, and sports initiatives throughout the province. The collaboration of institutions that can offer venues, personnel, or resources (e.g., museums, sports grounds, or artistic groups) for carrying out the activities helps to promote the program in two ways: Firstly, by maximizing the number of participants and citizen involvement; and secondly, aiding in "normalize" the experience.
8. Activities are sought out which are highly motivating for the participants. With this aim, novel and stimulating activities are regularly introduced, for which

there is little possibility of previous experience, making them interesting to all participants.

9. A respectful, cooperative, and inclusive environment is created among the members of the group. Whichever their background, participants are all treated equality, promoting a spirit of collaboration, allowing each individual to contribute their knowledge, abilities, and experience, whilst appreciating and respecting the learning speed of each person.
10. The workshops promote practical activities and culminate with a final group exhibition and diploma ceremony. Although the workshops are predominantly practical in nature, a portion of the activity, generally the introduction, is based on theory. In this way, the activities are more dynamic and promote interaction among all the participants. A key objective is finishing the learning process with some kind of joint collaboration, in which all or most of the members can participate, such as competing in a sporting event or presenting works to the public (e.g., an exhibition, a book publication). Similarly, having concluded the workshop, certificates for active involvement are presented, an aspect which is considered of vital importance as it is a recognition of the effort and commitment made by each participant in the course.

In its 5 years of existence, the program has been quite active and has organized approximately twenty activities. A complete list of these can be seen on the program's blog (http://incluyete.blog), as well as on its social network platforms (i.e., Instagram, Twitter, and Facebook). The most notable among them are detailed below.

Nautical sports. Almeria – the city where the program takes place – is located on the Mediterranean coast. Thus, from the outset of the program, it seemed logical that activities related to nautical sports would be ideal for several reasons: physical activity can be performed outdoors; many of the participants would otherwise have difficulty accessing such sports; the activities are highly stimulating, generally producing feelings of wellbeing, relaxation, and pleasure, and can be easily adapted to any person. In this respect, workshops carried out include sailing, kayaking, paddle surfing, and, most recently, dragon boat.

Animal-assisted physical activity. Many people may have difficulty interacting with other people despite being very caring and open with animals. In this regard, it has been observed that activities with dogs are quite interesting as they produce pleasant feelings and reduce stress (Hoy-Gerlach et al., 2022), while also fostering the sense of responsibility required when looking after animals. This workshop is held in an environment where the animals facilitate pleasant interactions among the group. Therapy dogs from the Almeria Animal Shelter are used (which are available for adoption), along with those of the participants. Basic canine training exercises are carried out, as well as games and general animal care.

Radio and podcasts. Radio is an ideal format for giving a voice to many people who generally do not have the same opportunities to be heard socially, making it a perfect communication tool. Currently, there are a number of successful radio programs around the world that focus on mental health, such as *Radio La Colifata* and *Radio Nikosia*, among others. In our case, the program *Inclúyete Radio* broadcasts from the University of Almeria on a weekly basis, and the participants determine what subjects will be discussed (which always deal with mental health), how to organize the sections of the program, which guests will be invited to be interviewed, and so on. The episodes of the podcast are available on Spotify and Ivoox.

Physical training (athletics). It is well known that physical activity provides benefits for personal well-being and health. The program Inclúyete boasts the privilege of collaborating with the World Masters Athletics Champion Emilia Paunica, who trains participants twice a week and whose coaching has led many individuals to participate in popular races and championship events, among other achievements.

Literary expression. Writing is a format for participants to express their emotions, concerns, and interests. This workshop seeks to encourage artistic expression through creation and group reading of short stories written by the workshop participants. The section Personal Experience will delve further into the details of this activity.

Art and emotions. Art is an ideal medium for dealing with many emotions. This form of expression is promoted through the study of different artistic periods and the creation of various works of art. The workshop has addressed different artistic epochs and styles, such as prehistoric art, Roman art, Muslim art, and Barroque art. Most notably, in 2019, the participants organized an exhibition in the Museum of Almeria with works they had produced which were open to the public for 2 months.

Pickleball. This last activity is a racquet sport which is popular in various countries (e.g.; the USA), although it is still relativity unknown in Spain. It is an ideal sport for any individual, independent of their age or physical condition, and its rules allow all players to actively participate in the game, making it inclusive and a lot of fun.

With regard to the results of the experience, the complete Inclúyete program has still not been evaluated. Here, we have mainly focused on evaluating the sports workshops. More specifically, regarding the physical activity program, it has been observed that all participants with mental health problems maintain high attendance (more than 80% after 1 year). Furthermore, statistically significant improvements in negative symptomology were achieved, as well as changes in positive symptomology and an improvement in functional autonomy (Mullor et al., 2020). In addition, the sports program has aided in improving different physical variables (e.g., weight, adiposity, etc.), which also tend to be serious problems among this population (Mullor et al., 2017, 2019).

These changes were particularly evident among the people who regularly participated in the program (in at least 50% of the sessions). However, it was also observed that when the program ended, these improvements were lost, highlighting the need for the continuity of the program over time in order for the results to be maintained (Mullor et al., 2020).

20.3 Personal Experience

This section describes the personal experience of participants in the literary expression workshop, organized by a person with his own experience in mental health and who had already collaborated in previous literary activities. Three editions of this course have been held, and although the activity was interrupted in 2020 due to the COVID-19 pandemic, we hope it will once again be available when the situation has improved.

In the literary expression classes students composed and read the poems and short stories they wrote together, participated in improvisational and creative theater, and performed micro plays. A portion of their written works was submitted to different literary contests. In addition, participants produced short biographies of their favorite authors, of which short extracts were read before the group. Similarly, in commemoration of World Book Day, the students performed a chain reading of various works and exchanged books. What is more, two students, along with the course teacher, participated in the Almeria Council's radio program.

In this sense, the objectives established in this workshop, in keeping with the underlining philosophy of the Inclúyete program, were the following:

- Favor social inclusion of individuals who have experienced mental health problems through training and contact with students.
- Reduce stigma among students towards people with mental health problems.
- Reduce self-stigma among mental health patients.
- Favor interpersonal relationships.
- Promote leisure activities and various pastimes.
- Promote inclusive activities in public spaces.
- Promote creativity.
- Develop interest in literature.
- Favor the empowering of individuals coping with mental health problems.

To evaluate the objectives, focus groups were organized to obtain subjective assessments and a satisfaction survey was also carried out. The attendance for the literary workshop was over 75% for enrolled students. The experience helped the participants to either begin, continue or once again find their interest in narrative, poetry or theater, and favor new social relationships. As for the university students, it was an opportunity to meet people with severe mental health problems and change many of the stigmatizing preconceptions they held prior.

As for the interviews and satisfaction surveys, the participants expressed high satisfaction levels, increased interest in literature, more productive use of free time, as well as decreased stigma and self-stigma, which generated subjective perceptions of greater social inclusion and empowerment.

Some of the quantitative results from the surveys, which were conducted anonymously, were the following (with scores on a scale from 1 to 10):

Level of satisfaction with the course: 8.72.
Level of satisfaction with the teacher: 9.2.

Level of organization of the course: 8.
Connection with personal interests: 8.9.
Fulfillment of expectations: 8.72.

Some of the positive aspects of the course cited by the participants, which summarize the dynamic of the course itself include: "Atmosphere of camaraderie, tolerance, and understanding", "I was encouraged to write and develop my creativity", and "Meeting and interacting first-hand with people who are stigmatized, and also having fun with them". The keywords used by the students to define the course were Share, Participatory/Inclusive, Oasis, Fraternal, and Discovery.

The idea to create this workshop arose precisely from the opportunity to work with Eduardo Sánchez, who was a patient receiving treatment at the hospital's mental health facilities. This person expressed great interest in literature, had already participated in previous literary activities, wrote short stories to submit to various literary contests, and was a member of an association and a group of people that promoted reading and writing. Ultimately, this person became the teacher of the literary expression workshop.

Several of the short stories written in the workshop were published in a book (Various Authors, 2019). In addition, the teacher was part of a committee and participated in the edition of another book for a short story contest organized by FAISEM during the confinement period in Spain, whose title is *Relatos contra el Coronavirus* [translation: *Short Stories against the Coronavirus*]. Finally, the students were also able to attend the book presentation of *Toros de Sangre* (Sánchez, 2019), written by Eduardo Sánchez himself.

The following is the teacher's impression of the most positive aspects and highlights of the experience:

The idea emerged as an opportunity to carry out a cultural activity in Almeria within the field of literature and writing. I had never led a workshop of this kind, so it was new for me. Three editions have been held, and I feel highly motivated because I've continued to prepare and improve myself to lead the course the best I can. At the same time, I'm fulfilled by the students' desire to learn. We all get better with each class. The atmosphere and the creative process are phenomenal. The students create their own texts and made contributions to Inclúyete libremente, a book we edited to compile their short stories and poetry. Each student writes according to their own style, which is the most important point – the endeavor of delving into their creativity and presenting their point of view, telling stories that convey emotions to readers. To dare to venture beyond the manual and theory presented in the course.

Achieving the objectives of the Inclúyete Program is challenging, ensuring the integration of the mental health patients at all levels. This workshop invites everyone to expose their creative soul and experience enriching accomplishments, such as overcoming insecurity of expressing emotions, speaking in public to present one's writings and taking advantage of the exchange of ideas to simply have a good time. It is highly motivating to observe students surpassing themselves and remembering what those first steps as a writer are like. In addition, the workshop is supported with parallel activities, our celebration of Book Day and the organization of a literary contest, which served as an example for FAISEM.

The workshop continues to grow through the Inclúyete Program, with the support of the University of Almeria and other collaborators. This project has been consolidated thanks to everyone's effort and dedication. We hope to continue with this cultural initiative next term, and at no charge to anyone interested. Just like a great wine, we aspire to get better as time goes on.

This experience also helped Eduardo's recovery process. The therapy team in charge of his treatment remark that his cognitive abilities have improved, especially his attention and concentration, he functions better as an individual and socially, he has developed social skills and expanded his social support system, he feels more accepted socially, his family relationships have improved, he deals with stressful situations better, his self-esteem and resilience have grown stronger while his sense of self-stigma has decreased. Similarly, Eduardo feels more empowered, which has allowed him to develop a life plan. He has been able to leave a supervised-living home and rent his own accommodation with a roommate. He has started a training path aimed at helping him to find a job, and dedicates his leisure time to what he most enjoys – literature.

20.4 Conclusions

Having presented the basic principles of the program, the workshops, the personal experience with the literary expression program, and the results, the utility of these types of experiences are quite evident. The program ventures beyond simply carrying out "entertainment activities". Instead, it aims to become an additional part of the participants' specific interests and contribute to the promotion of active participation, to generating new interests and life projects, and to improving the quality of life of all the participants.

The program features certain components that we consider to be essential and also different from other types of experiences. For example, we consider the involvement of the university community to be crucial, both to stimulate the dynamics of the activities the participants carry out and also for the experience's utility in reducing stigma among young people, not to mention that it facilitates future research in the field (Mullor et al., 2019).

Similarly, it is essential that the activities themselves be appealing for all the participants. The intention is not for people from the general public to participate as if they were performing some kind of volunteer service (which in itself would be extremely positive), but rather to genuinely want to participate for the learning experience that can provide the impact on their lives which the activity promises. For this reason, it is vital that the workshops be appealing and/or original and the professionals that teach the courses have experience in the field and be highly motivated and devoted to the activities.

The fact that the program is open to any citizen also seems fundamental. In this regard, the goal is to generate new horizontal relationships, open to new interests shared with a group, which creates more personal interest and awareness of the everyday problems of other people.

Similarly, whenever possible, it is important that people with mental health problems acquire a more active role in the experience, as teachers if possible. This aspect is essential for these individuals for the sense of fulfillment born of the opportunity to teach and have a unifying experience which, in turn, favors greater self-worth and, therefore, a decrease in self-stigma.

In the same line, as it is an appealing socio-educational program, it contributes by motivating some individuals to also engage in future learning, such as finishing academic studies or enrolling in a more specialized course. We also consider this aspect of equal importance precisely because mental health problems tend to emerge during adolescence, when many people drop out of school and are likely never to return. Taking part in an enjoyable socio-educational experience allows some individuals to reconsider these options.

In addition, it is essential to promote active leisure activities among this population. Offering new opportunities to participate in artistic and sport activities or to take up past interests are opportunities to discover new stimuli in sociocultural activities, which is a key aspect of personal well-being and social recovery (Iwasaki et al., 2010). Similarly, the experience makes it possible to meet new classmates, thereby expanding the social circle of the participants, and not only among people with mental health problems.

Furthermore, there is the benefit of promoting social responsibility, which is taught, for example, through caring for animals and gathering and organizing sports materials. What is more, participants can emulate their classmates who act as role models to others, which is a natural way of promoting social inclusion. What is more, the activities are held in normal public spaces throughout the city, which is another aspect of the program's social nature.

Finally, the empowerment of the participants in the activities is vital. Not only can anyone join the activities, but everyone collaborates and cooperates insofar as they are capable. This aspect favors enjoyment in the activities and the feeling of self-worth within the group, which is of key importance.

Closely related to the above-mentioned aspects is the reduction of stigma. In fact, it has been demonstrated that the best way to decrease stigma is by fostering contact, as specifically set out by the principles established by Allport in the mid-twentieth century (Allport et al., 1954), which are:

- Prolonged engagement over time.
- Cooperative activities.
- Activities among people or groups of similar status or station.
- Proportional numbers of members within the groups.
- Contact in a variety of situations and social contexts.
- Contact with people who are representative of the group.

Inclúyete seeks to precisely promote these principles. What is more, likewise, we believe the experience can contribute to reduce self-stigma. In fact, in a similar initiative carried out in Madrid, specifically in a 5-on-5 football league of 13 mental health teams, it was verified that there was a statistically significant reduction in self-stigma among the participants (Moraleda et al., 2019).

Similarly, in order for the program to have an effect on reducing stigma, it is necessary that the information disseminated on mental health problems be related more to biographical aspects, such as adverse circumstances and suffering, rather than approach them as the manifestation of a supposedly biological origin (Longdon & Read, 2017). Although medical discourse is widespread in our society and among people with their own problems with mental health, which leads many of them to consider themselves "mentally ill", the activities like those described in this program, when engaged in daily, manage to focus interest on personal difficulties and biological aspects, among others, which ultimately helps others to view these factors from a more personal and empathetic perspective. Moreover, in many cases, we can identify with some of the experiences shared by the participants, which is an important component of normalizing the circumstances of others and allowing all group members to realize that similar or related situations can happen to everyone.

For these reasons, we believe the program favors social inclusion and the reduction of stigma and self-stigma, making it an ideal and necessary complement to the psychological support that people receive from various clinical sources. Figure 20.1 presents a graphic representation of the benefits that we consider the program offers.

Nonetheless, in order for the results of such programs to successfully endure, there must be sustained continuity over time. When activities cease, a large portion of the effects is subsequently lost, as some studies have observed (Mullor et al., 2020). To ensure this does not occur, along with the conviction of numerous

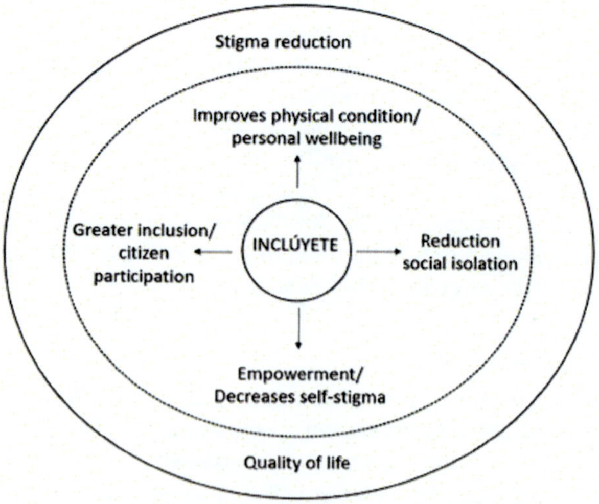

Fig. 20.1 Benefits of the Inclúyete program

professionals and organizers that the program is of great utility, it is necessary to seek out the involvement of various entities to be able to guarantee stable funding.

Looking into the future, we also believe it is important to intensify the involvement of different social entities that can help disseminate information and favor the engagement of more participants in the experience, such as people that have not yet established contact with healthcare services, as well as the general public. Furthermore, we believe it is important to expand the program to other regions of Spain. In doing so, its influence can be expanded and the effects of all the workshops can be further evaluated.FundingThis publication is part of the I+D+i PY20_00232 project, financed by the Agencia Andaluza del Conocimiento (*Andalusian Agency for Knowledge*) – the Consejería de Transformación Económica, Industria, Conocimiento y Universidades de la Junta de Andalucía (*Andalusian Regional Government's Ministry of Economic Transformation, Industry, Knowledge and Universities*).

References

Allport, G. W., Clark, K., & Pettigrew, T. (1954). *The nature of prejudice*. Allison-Wesley.

Arsović, N., Đurović, R., & Rakočević, R. (2020). *Influence of physical and sports activity on mental health* (Series: Physical education and sport) (pp. 559–568). Facta Universitatis. https://doi.org/10.22190/FUPES190413050A

Cangas, A. J., & Martín-Murcia, F. (2021). Valores y psicosis. In J. A. Díaz, H. Laffite, & R. Zúñiga (Eds.), *Terapia de Aceptación y Compromiso en Psicosis, Aceptación y recuperación por niveles (ART)* (pp. 473–484). Pirámide.

Çapar, M., & Kavak, F. (2019). Effect of internalized stigma on functional recovery in patients with schizophrenia. *Perspectives in Psychiatric Care, 55*, 103–111. https://doi.org/10.1111/ppc.1230

Corrigan, P. W., Powell, K. J., & Rüsch, N. (2012). How does stigma affect work in people with serious mental illnesses? *Psychiatric Rehabilitation Journal, 35*, 381. https://doi.org/10.1037/h0094497

Firth, J., Cotter, J., Elliott, R., French, P., & Yung, A. R. (2015). A systematic review and meta-analysis of exercise interventions in schizophrenia patients. *Psychological Medicine, 45*, 1343–1361. https://doi.org/10.1017/S0033291714003110

Hoy-Gerlach, J., Vincent, A., Scheuermann, B., & Ojha, M. (2022). Exploring Benefits of Emotional Support Animals (ESAs): A Longitudinal Pilot Study with Adults with Serious Mental Illness (SMI). *Human-Animal Interaction Bulletin, 10*, 1–19.

Iwasaki, Y., Coyle, C. P., & Shank, J. W. (2010). Leisure as a context for active living, recovery, health and life quality for persons with mental illness in a global context. *Health Promotion International, 25*, 483–494. https://doi.org/10.1093/heapro/daq037

Kandola, A., Ashdown-Franks, G., Hendrikse, J., Sabiston, C. M., & Stubbs, B. (2019). Physical activity and depression: Towards understanding the antidepressant mechanisms of physical activity. *Neuroscience & Biobehavioral Reviews, 107*, 525–539. https://doi.org/10.1016/j.neubiorev.2019.09.04

Longdon, E., & Read, J. (2017). People with problems, not patients with illnesses: Using psychosocial frameworks to reduce the stigma of psychosis. *The Israel Journal of Psychiatry and Related Sciences, 54*, 24–28. PMID: 28857755.

Moraleda, A., Galán, D., & Cangas, A. J. (2019). Reducing self-stigma in people with severe mental illness participating in a regular football league: An exploratory study. *International Journal of Environmental Research of Public Health, 16*, 3599. https://doi.org/10.3390/ijerph16193599

Mullor, D., Gallego, J., Cangas, A. J., Aguilar-Parra, J. M., Valenzuela, L., Mateu, J. M., & López-Pardo, A. (2017). Efectividad de un programa de actividad física en personas con trastorno mental grave. *Revista Internacional de Medicina y Ciencias de la Actividad Física y el Deporte, 17*, 507–521. https://doi.org/10.15366/rimcafd2017.67.008

Mullor, D., Cangas, A. J., Gallego, J., Aguilar, J. M., Rosado, A., & López, A. (2019). A longitudinal study about the impact of an inclusive sports program in people with diagnosis of schizophrenia. *Psychosis – Psychological Social and Integrative Approaches, 11*, 75–84. https://doi.org/10.1080/17522439.2018.1559873

Mullor, D., Cangas, A. J., Gallego, J., Trigueros, R., & López, A. (2020). Impacto psicológico y social de un programa de deporte inclusivo entre estudiantes y personas con trastorno mental grave. *Revista de Psicología del Deporte, 29*, 5–15.

Navarro Gómez, N., & Triguero Ramos, R. (2019). Estigma en los profesionales de la Salud Mental: una revisión sistemática. *Psychology, Society & Education, 11*, 253–266. https://doi.org/10.25115/psye.v10i1.2268

Or, S. E. B., Hasson-Ohayon, I., Feingold, D., Vahab, K., Amiaz, R., Weiser, M., & Lysaker, P. H. (2013). Meaning in life, insight and self-stigma among people with severe mental illness. *Comprehensive Psychiatry, 54*, 195–200. https://doi.org/10.1016/j.comppsych.2012.07.011

Ramos-Sanchez, C. P., Schuch, F. B., Seedat, S., Louw, Q. A., Stubbs, B., Rosenbaum, S., & Vancampfort, D. (2021). The anxiolytic effects of exercise for people with anxiety and related disorders: An update of the available meta-analytic evidence. *Psychiatry Research, 302*, 114046. https://doi.org/10.1016/j.psychres.2021.114046

Sánchez, E. (2019). *Toros de sangre*. Available in Amazon: https://www.amazon.es/Toros-Sangre-Eduardo-S%C3%A1nchez-Fern%C3%A1ndez/dp/1799090248

Schuch, F. B., Vancampfort, D., Richards, J., Rosenbaum, S., Ward, P. B., & Stubbs, B. (2016). Exercise as a treatment for depression: A meta-analysis adjusting for publication bias. *Journal of Psychiatric Research, 77*, 42–51. https://doi.org/10.1016/j.jpsychires.2016.02.023

Stanghellini, G., & Ballerini, M. (2007). Values in persons with schizophrenia. *Schizophrenia Bulletin, 33*, 131–141. https://doi.org/10.1093/schbul/sbl036

Stanghellini, G., & Ballerini, M. (2011). What is it like to be a person with Schizophrenia in the social world? A first-person perspective study on Schizophrenic Dissociality–part 2: Methodological issues and empirical findings. *Psychopathology, 44*, 183–192. https://doi.org/10.1159/000322638

Vallina Fernández, O., Pérez Álvarez, M., Fernández Iglesias, P., Soto Balbuena, C., Perona Garcelán, S. F., & García Montes, J. M. (2014). Person-based contextual therapy applied to a complex case of schizophrenia. *Psicothema, 26*, 299–307. https://doi.org/10.7334/psicothema2013.247

Various Authors. (2019). *Inclúyete libremente*. Available in Amazon: https://www.amazon.es/Incl%C3%BAyete-Libre-mente-Varios-Autores/dp/1076092098

World Health Organization. (2019). *What is the evidence on the role of the arts in improving health and Well-being? A scoping review*. World Health Organization. Regional Office for Europe.

World Health Organization. (2021). *Guidance on community mental health services: Promoting person-centred and rights-based approaches*. Descargado de. https://apps.who.int/iris/bitstream/handle/10665/341648/9789240025707-eng.pdf?sequence=1

Chapter 21
Attention Centred on What Is Important for the Person (ACIP) Approach to a First-Episode Psychosis (FEP)

Carlos Francisco Salgado-Pascual

21.1 Introduction

This chapter aims to set out the practical approach and psychological support for a person after a first psychotic episode, from the perspective of Attention centred on what is Important for the Person (ACIP). The aim is to exemplify prevention from the point of view of depathologisation, destigmatisation and empowerment of the person so that, in these circumstances, they do not turn away from what gives meaning to their lives.

It is not about curing any pathology or making the person stop being psychotic by embarking on a tenacious struggle to avoid a certain label and/or diagnosis. The aim is to train them, through unconditional acceptance, to take charge of what is under their control and to move towards the kind of life they want to live or the kind of person they want to be.

Traditionally, prevention in the field of psychosis has been limited to secondary and tertiary prevention (OMS, 2005). In this sense, the objective is to reduce prevalence through early detection and treatment, on the one hand, and to minimise disability and relapses, on the other. Historically, these objectives have been associated with the use of diagnostic tests and the application of labels and interventions aimed at raising awareness of the disease. However, these reinforce stigma, undervalue the person and do not take their diversity into account, and consequently engender a feeling of social exclusion.

It is important, therefore, to raise concerns about the impact that the diagnosis of mental illness and the specific label of psychosis generate in people and how the response from a professional will make a difference to their relationship with the symptomatology. All these elements can be of great assistance in empathising with

C. F. Salgado-Pascual (✉)
Psychology Center PsicACT, European University Miguel de Cervantes, Valladolid, Spain
e-mail: csalgado@cop.es

J. A. Díaz-Garrido et al. (eds.), *Psychological Interventions for Psychosis*,
https://doi.org/10.1007/978-3-031-27003-1_21

and providing support to the person diagnosed as mentally ill, from their condition as a person rather than as a sick person.

Professional practice in the field of mental health has allowed me to refer to three aspects that I would like to highlight below for their value in contextualising and giving added meaning to the support proposal presented in this chapter.

Firstly, when faced with the term "mentally ill" (or a similar label), this has a huge impact on the person in many different ways. Expressions include, "strange", "aggressive", "disabled", "lonely", "useless", "incapable", "murderer", "criminal", and "mad". From this frame of reference, the reader can easily understand how diagnosis and labelling are not neutral and can signal the start of a hard journey. A journey characterised by the emission of topographically different behaviours, the common function of which is to fight against all this as a way of safeguarding integrity and dignity. This struggle sometimes distances the person from what matters to him/her and, paradoxically, brings him/her even closer to the diagnosis and the label (Salgado & Mateos, 2021).

Secondly, it is relevant to highlight that one of the most widespread practices to help the treatment (mainly psychopharmacological) of people diagnosed with psychosis has been the work on "illness awareness" through psychoeducational strategies. But if we bear in mind, as we have outlined in the previous paragraph, that the awareness of being mentally ill is not something neutral, but has an enormous negative connotation, it is easy to foresee that this practice means placing the person close to the edge of the abyss of exclusion.

Ultimately, the person diagnosed as mentally ill is undoubtedly a fighter, even though their struggle has the paradoxical effect of moving them away from the life that matters to them. Nor can there be any doubt that society is doing its best to remove the stigma of mental illness, but as we have argued above there is a certain incoherence between this process of de-stigmatisation and the insistence on an automatic model that persists in the awareness of illness as a prerequisite for an adequate approach from such a perspective.

Finally, in third place, we could question the differentiation between chronic mental disorder and chronified mental disorder: to what extent is psychosis a chronic disorder per se, or does it become chronic to the extent that we are unable to deal with it in a suitable and pragmatic way? To what extent can the response we give to mental illness be part of the chronification itself? This argument may seem far from scientific, but it is worth exploring the possibility that, from a functional perspective of human behaviour, the well-intentioned response aimed at symptom reduction and/or compensation for disability may form part of the problem.

All these insights from professional practice prompt us to take a fresh look at and trust in new ways of dealing with human suffering. Alternative ways that do not put the focus on repairing something that is considered pathological, but rather specialised support centred on what happens to the person, where the symptomatology has a history and is understandable only in that historical context (Alanen et al., 1991; Lehtinen et al., 1999; Pérez-Álvarez et al., 2008). In short, it is a matter of focusing on what is a meaningful life for the person (what is important), highlighting, on the one hand, what makes him/her unique (his/her essence and identity as a person) and, on the other, what binds him/her with the rest of humanity (his/her vulnerability).

A multitude of classical orientations has moved along the same lines, such as Humanism (Rogers, 1981), Logotherapy or, more recently, Acceptance and Commitment Therapy (ACT) as focusing on the person's values (Hayes et al., 2012) and its evolution towards the attentional ACIP model, which will be discussed in the following section.

Psychosocial Rehabilitation is also a model that takes the focus away from symptomatic control and shifts it towards the person's interests, although their interventions (social, psychological and service level interventions) have generated very inconclusive results that are unlikely to improve social functioning (Pérez Álvarez et al., 2003). There are several reasons that may explain these data, but what seems to be common to all of them is that, although the frame of reference is based on the interests of the person, the focus on skills training and the provision of support, the methods used do not really move away from the predominant medical model in which the emphasis is still placed on the symptom instead of guiding the work towards what is important to the person (Salgado, 2011).

Many voices now advocate a paradigm shift as to how we care for people. This has given rise to a new way of doing things. This process is called ACIP and can be summarised as follows:

Need to perceive the person as valuable, having dreams and values and the right to live a meaningful life.
Need to follow a constructive paradigm.
Need to develop support mechanisms that focus on interests and on what matters.
Need to integrate the applied field with the advances of basic research.
Need to empower the person in the face of personal circumstances.

For further development of these needs, see Salgado and Mateos (2021).

In this particular case, an attentional model is presented that is aimed at prevention by sharing the goal of reducing the possibility of disability and chronification after a first psychotic break. The intervention balances, on the one hand, early care and support through increasing protective factors in the person and, on the other hand, prevents stigmatisation and enhances a sense of belonging.

21.2 Attention Centred on What Is Important for the Person (ACIP)

The ACIP model is a contextual-functional approach to the care and support of people in a situation or at risk of vulnerability, both in a social and health context.

The development of ACIP has taken into account, on the one hand, the advances arising from experimentation in recent years on the nature of private events and their relationship with human behaviour and, on the other hand, the conclusions emerging from the context applied in different areas of people care (e.g. mental health,

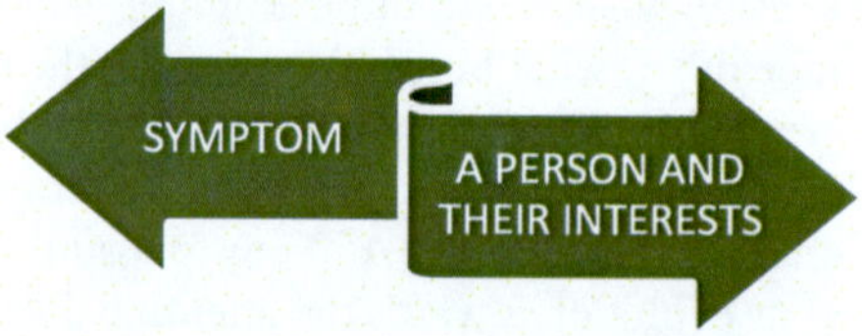

Fig. 21.1 Moving the focus of attention from the symptom to the person and their interests

early care and care for people with disabilities). All of these areas, in one way or another, advocate a paradigm shift in care by moving the focus of attention from the symptom to the person and their interests (see Fig. 21.1).

In the acronym of Attention centred on what is Important for the Person (ACIP) the "P" and the "C" also maintain the processes of "acceptance" and "commitment" derived from Acceptance and Commitment Therapy (ACT) and the definition of psychological flexibility (Hayes et al., 2006; Hayes & Strosahl, 2004; Luciano et al., 2004). Therefore, in the methodology derived from ACIP, alternative ways of implementing the processes involved in ACT will be found with a special initial emphasis on working with personal values (what is important to the person). In addition, the reader will be able to identify principles and procedures from other contextual models such as Client-Centred Therapy (Rogers, 1981) and Functional Analytic Psychotherapy (FAP-Kohlenberg & Tsai, 1991) among others.

ACIP is defined as "a constructive model that dignifies the person and takes into account what research has shown to be a source of importance for most human beings, but also what makes them a person, their identity, their essence, interests and values, while training them to take control of their actions in order to take steps in the valued direction". (Salgado and Mateos, 2021).

This definition highlights several of the essential elements of the model, which will be presented as basic pillars to be built explicitly or implicitly through the relationship between the professional and the person. Thus, it takes into account the part of the person that connects them with other human beings, such as shared vulnerability, and also what makes them unique, their essence, their value as a human beings and what matters to them based on what they like and are passionate about and also based on what makes them suffer. In the same way, the definition highlights the concept of training, as a way of taking into consideration the person and not his or her condition of being ill. It works on those skills that will enhance the protective factors and help the person to build a meaningful life under any circumstances.

With regard to the approach to and support for people diagnosed with psychosis, ACIP is aimed at the real empowerment of the person in terms of what they think and feel in order to increase their protective factors when moving in a meaningful direction. Thus, without forgetting the other objectives of prevention, such as reducing the duration and severity, as well as reducing the impact of the symptomatology on the person so that it does not prevent them from living a meaningful life.

As mentioned above, the philosophical frame of reference for ACIP is Functional-Contextualism. It follows, on the one hand, that we cannot explain behaviour without knowing the context in which it occurs and, on the other hand, that a functional approach to behaviour puts us in the best position to support people.

From this perspective, it can be affirmed that the way the therapist reacts to the behaviour of the person with psychosis will make a difference in two very significant ways: Firstly, because their response shapes the way in which the person relates to the symptomatology when it is present, and this will turn out to be of great importance in the case of productive symptomatology, as we will see in the case study below; and secondly, but not less important, because this interaction will lead to the construction of a context formed by six basic pillars that support the model: de-pathologisation, dignity, shared vulnerability, construction, real empowerment and social connection. For a more extensive description of the basic pillars, see Salgado and Mateos (2021).

These basic pillars are established through meaningful conversations that are characterised by honesty, genuineness, closeness, trust and attachment. The professional engages in interactions that make the person feel that they are not alone. This is done through a horizontal relationship of unconditional acceptance where vulnerability is allowed and where it is made clear, implicitly or explicitly, that the person is not broken. Trust is enhanced through the validation of what the person feels and thinks, taking the perspective of what the professional may consider to be better or worse, and always focusing on the direction that sets the compass of what is important to the person.

In short, the professional reflects unconditional acceptance and promotes inclusion through meaningful interactions, which involve being genuine, and other-centred, making them feel heard, that they are not alone and that they matter to us.

How does the way the therapist interacts with the person with psychosis make a difference; how do we build the building blocks in people with a high level of cognitive fusion and literal following of what their thoughts and beliefs labelled as psychotic say; how do we promote de-pathologisation in people who have been diagnosed with psychosis or who are going through a first outbreak; how do we promote de-pathologisation in people who have been diagnosed with psychosis or who are going through a first outbreak; how can we empower the person in a real way, so that they are above their thought and feeling and take action to control of what matters to them; how can we put training in different ways of relating to their psychotic thoughts to support their values?

The development of this case study aims to respond to the above questions, through the presentation of the design and procedures adhered to for a person diagnosed with psychosis (first outbreak). It is not intended to be a development that follows the canons of a case study, but rather a reliable description of the steps that were developed during the support process from a contextual-functional perspective. The reader will perceive the linear development of the intervention, with different intervention periods that may not fit perfectly into any one model.

Therefore, what follows is a descriptive analysis of the intervention from the perspective of Attention centred on what is Important for the Person (ACIP). It aims to provide a practical approach to such an attentional model, even if this departs from an orthodox exposition of traditional case studies.

21.3 Case Study

21.3.1 Description

M is a young woman (21 years old) who comes in for a consultation. She has been referred by her psychiatrist because of an initial suspicion of dissociative behaviour, due to the fact that one day, she got on a bus from her home town and appeared in another town 50 km away without having a clear awareness of what had brought her there. In that moment of confusion, she nervously called her parents, claiming that she had no idea what she was doing there. Following this episode, her parents accompanied her to a psychiatric clinic. M was given psychopharmacological treatment (low-dose Risperidone and Lorazepam) and refused hospital admission. After several days at home, her parents report finding her very nervous, very susceptible to everything; when she goes out in the street, she is very restless and attentive to everything, she says she is being chased, she does not stop to talk to anyone, and at home, if there are visitors, she goes to a place of her own. One day, at lunchtime, she came across as very nervous and irritable and saying strange things, which led to her being admitted for 5 days and diagnosed with a brief psychotic disorder with a serious trigger in an objective and subjective situation of stress. On discharge, it was decided to go for a psychology consultation in addition to the check-ups with her usual psychiatrist.

Once in session, M is approachable, but, on the other hand, she speaks very fast, laughs without motivation, jumps from one topic to another to the point of seeming incoherent, making it very difficult to gain a clear understanding of what she is experiencing.

She says strange things, such as “I am John Lennon”; “they want to kidnap me, I walk down the road and there is always a white van chasing me, but my parents don’t believe me”; “I am a person very marked by the separation of my parents”; “I am the daughter of the Tsar of Russia”, “in the street they call me Sandy”, “I am a model and I appear in many magazines”, “there are bats in the waiting room, can you hear them?”

21.3.2 Background

Some of the information gathered through interviews with the parents is presented below.

At the time of the consultation, M is a university student, achieving good results. She has spent a year studying in Portugal on an Erasmus scholarship and previously in the United States learning English.

Several years ago, due to the conflictive separation of her parents, she consulted psychiatry for the first time due to an anxious–depressive syndrome that was treated pharmacologically and from which she recovered within a few weeks. The post-separation situation was highly conflictual as M found herself at the centre of enormous pressure from both parents. Her mother has also gone through depression with anxiety symptoms.

The parents report in the first interviews that currently, M does not like other people visiting her home. When the family is there, she goes somewhere else, and when they go for a walk, they cannot stop to chat with anyone as she quickly wants to leave. They describe situations in which she is very angry and irascible with them, verbalising: "you are all in cahoots", "there is a plot against me" and other ideas of persecution.

The ACIP stresses the importance of knowing what is important to the person, and doing so based on what they like, what they are passionate about and what they are good at doing, and also on what makes them suffer. Although in the first interviews with M, it was not possible to talk about this, as is explained more extensively in the part dedicated to the intervention this information was provided by the parents.

In this sense, they point out that M has always been a very introverted girl; she does not go out much, nor does she have many friends. They point out that she is keen on movies and fashion. It is also important to M to help others, and she loves travelling, learning and practising other languages.

On the other hand, they share the information that M has always been very nervous about studying and has put a lot of pressure on herself. This seems to reflect that education and career are areas that are important to her.

21.3.3 Intervention

The description of the intervention will follow a temporal thread (see Fig. 21.3) with the aim of facilitating the understanding of the ACIP adjustment.

As mentioned above, the aim of the ACIP attentional model is to bring out what is important in order to support the person in taking actions under the influence of this unlimited source of motivation (values). Some of what was important to M was verbalised by her parents during the first sessions, which were aimed at getting to know the current situation, but also at getting to know the essence and identity of M. This last objective was initially hindered by the presence of symptomatology, in which M was hooked.

21.3.3.1 First Interviews: Attention to the Present Moment and Construction of Basic Pillars

The ACIP process starts with conversations based on the person's interests and values, making them feel that they are unique, singular and have value by the mere fact that they are born (basic pillar of dignity). These interactions are characterised by naturalness, closeness, and the validation of what the person thinks and feels and the allowed presence of vulnerability. The aim is to bring out what is important to the person through his or her life story. It is not a biographical history, but a deep understanding of the essence of the person. It is important to get to know what emerges as significant, initially on the basis of what the person likes, is passionate about and is good at, and later on the basis of what makes him/her suffer.

Due to the presence of productive symptomatology in those first moments that interfered with the emergence of what was important, the first interactions were aimed at training, on the one hand, focusing the attention on the present moment, taking perspective of what was present in those moments and directing attention to what was significant. On the other hand, the therapist's reaction to these private events was used as a way to build the pillars of depathologisation, dignity, shared vulnerability and real empowerment.

Below is a dialogue from the first sessions that exemplifies this:

During the conversation, M is angry with her father, with whom she has always been on good terms. She talks very fast, insults him for putting pressure on her studies and jumps from one topic to another. At one point, M remarks, without any connection, that she "hears bats in the waiting room":

T: Tell me M., are you listening to them now while you are talking to me?

M: Yes, can't you hear them?

T: No, I don't hear them. It must be complicated to listen to that now. It would be important for me to be able to experience in some way what you are perceiving. Could you tell me what the sound is like, what you are hearing? As if I could go inside you and experience what you are experiencing. It's very important to me.

M: I hear them fluttering and screaming.

T: Very good. Now I invite you to focus your attention on those sounds. Please, tell me what they sound like so that I can know what we are talking about, are they high-pitched or low-pitched?

M: They are high-pitched, like screams.

T: Very good, do you hear them far away or close?

M: Now far away, like coming from the waiting room, out there.

T: Ok M. Now, notice there's you and there's the sound, there's that screaming and/or fluttering. Notice that here is M (pointing to her) and there are the sounds (pointing outside). Notice that there is a part of you that is perceiving them.

T: Are they continuous sounds or do they stop from time to time?

M: Continuous.

T: If you could write on a piece of paper what you hear, what would it be like? What would you put?

M: It would be like "gri, griii" and the fluttering would be "rrrr" (trying to make the continuous "r" sound).

T: Could you write it here? (Taking a piece of paper).

M: (writing on the paper).

T: Where is M right now?

M: Here, on the sofa.

T: Where is the sound now?

M: There, on the paper (pointing to the paper).

T: Notice that you are here (pointing to M) and the sound is there (pointing to the paper). Notice that there is a part of you that is being observant of the sound written on the paper.

T: What other things can you hear right now?

M: Your voice...and the sound of footsteps in the hallway (at that moment people were passing in the corridor).

And while this verbalisation is taking place, a calmer tone of voice is observed and M's verbalisations are slowing down.

Several aspects can be observed in this interaction. Firstly, the therapist is using deictic and hierarchical cues (Gil-Luciano et al., 2017; López-López and Luciano, 2017; Luciano, 2016) with the aim of bringing the person to the present moment, helping her to differentiate from her private events, to take perspective on them and to support her in not getting hooked on literalism, as well as to be able to look at other elements of the conversation that are related to what matters to her. Secondly, this way of responding by the therapist to the private events that characterise M's productive symptomatology allowed for the construction of some of the basic pillars of ACIP. A response in which the therapist makes M see that these thoughts and feelings are private events that can be paid attention to, observed and seen for what they are and not for what they say, and that their presence does not imply that the person has something inside him/her that is broken or malfunctioning and, therefore, there is no imperative need to get rid of them, hide them or avoid them. In other words, this type of interaction makes it possible to build, little by little, the pillar of depathologisation, dignity and shared vulnerability.

Conversations like the one illustrated above took place during five more sessions in relation to many other issues that arose (see below) and in which M felt trapped, for example: "Everyone is against me, there is a plot", "why won't they leave me alone", "they have destroyed my life", "a white van is chasing me", "they want to hurt me because I am famous", "my grandmother is not dead, I saw her the other day at dinner with my family".

Finally, all this made it possible to work with multiple private events (productive symptomatology) so that, through the therapist's reactions and responses to these private events, she was shaping and training a different way of relating to them so that she was not trapped in their literalness and could direct her attention to what was important. In this way, the pillar of M's real empowerment was built, managing the deictic, hierarchical and functional cues of behavioural regulation in multiple interactions.

21.3.3.2 Bringing Out the Important Issue

Following the previous five sessions, and for a further 5 months, M attends weekly individual sessions.

Once the speed and intensity of the thoughts had decreased with the help of medication, and M began to relate to these private events with a little more perspective and equanimity, the phase aimed at getting to know and bringing out what was important to M could begin, with the objective that this would become a source of influence for taking actions in coherence with a meaningful life.

In this phase, it is important to empathise and to bear in mind that going through experiences such as those M went through has a great impact on people and their meaningful lives.

Although it is true that M, after the first five sessions, showed significant improvement in these symptoms, from that moment on, feelings emerged derived from the break with what had been her life until then (university classes and studies, friendships, travel, etc.). These feelings stemmed from her admission to hospital, the subsequent diagnosis of a psychiatric disorder and also from the side effects of the medication. In this sense, we cannot forget that stopping the mind in its tracks stops the delusions, but it also halts and slows down other types of thinking activity. M starts to feel that she is not able to think clearly, her head feels dull and slow, she is unable to concentrate on anything, and discouragement, anxiety and fear of it happening again lead to the emergence of a feeling of "being overwhelmed" at not being able to resume the activities she used to participate in. Faced with this type of symptom, M spent a lot of time lying down, went for walks and carried out other types of behaviour in order to be relaxed and calm.

Paradoxically, this way of reacting in coherence with what she thinks and feels at that moment does not allow the person to glimpse a return to her meaningful life, increasing her discouragement and anxiety.

This is the precise moment when attention is focused on bringing out what is important to M, with the aim of providing a renewed source of motivation and a functionality that will contribute to the subsequent what she thinks and feels.

It is advisable, in order to adjust to the ACIP attentional model and to move away from an excessive focus on problems or on the fight against symptomatology, to use close interactions aimed at getting to know the person's life story. These are quality, genuine, close conversations, where vulnerability is validated and allowed and with the aim of discovering the essence and identity of the person. In short, the aim is to get to know the person with warmth and acceptance and without judgement, bringing out what is important in those actions or situations that trap them or make them suffer, and moving away from the mere description of activities.

In this sense, in conversations based on what is important, it is not the specific questions that are asked that are relevant, but the essence and the spirit that emerges from them and that should characterise a style centred on what matters (Salgado, 2019).

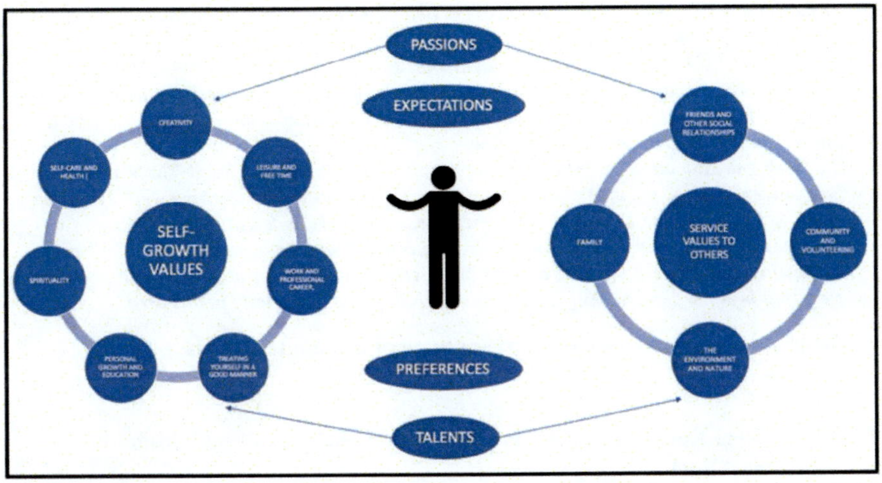

Fig. 21.2 Representation of the emergence of self-growth values and service values to others from what the person likes, is passionate about and is good at (Salgado, 2019). (Based on McKay et al., 2010)

In bringing out the key values, the distinction between values of self-growth and values of service to others proposed by McKay et al. (2010) has been chosen as a framework.

The ACIP outlines the importance of starting by focusing attention on what matters to the person, on what she likes, is passionate about and is good at, rather than initially getting into what is a problem and makes the person suffer. In Fig. 21.2, the reader can observe the distinction between the two sets of values, emphasising the central figure of the person and adding his or her passions, preferences and talents that make up activities and/or actions from which the important emerge and are therefore hierarchically related to the value dimensions.

What emerged from these conversations aimed at bringing out what is important to M. is set out below:

> *M says (and this is also confirmed by her parents) that she likes to help other people very much, she is always there for friends or for anyone in need. She helps and supports as much as possible foreign students who stay at her home. She also likes movies and reading, she likes to get into the characters. She enjoys reading and watching films about important personalities from history, but also from other fields such as fashion, music,* etc. *She is interested in the lives of people who have managed to contribute to society through what they do.*
>
> *She is also passionate about fashion and especially about being able to see things that she can then make herself. She feels satisfaction doing it and seeing a final result that she has created herself. Related to all this, she likes to look good physically and take care of her health.*
>
> *As for her leisure time, one of her favourite activities is travelling. When she travels, she loves getting to know other cultures, other ways of life and is the feeling of being part of a very wide world. During her travels, she can also cultivate one of the qualities she is best at: languages. It is easy for her to study different languages and she enjoys practising them.*

As before, she is able to increase her sense of belonging (this is one of the sources of importance for most people).

M explicitly highlights family as an important area of value. She would like to be remembered as a "noble person who has always been there when needed". In the family area, she also highlights that she would like to fulfil the role of a mother, to be a reference for her children and an example to follow.

Work and education are also very important to M. On the one hand, she wants to be independent and, on the other, to be a professional person who does her job well. This area never fails to motivate M, but at the same time, as already stated at the beginning of this point, it is a major source of discomfort due to the break with her academic life. The burden of the diagnosis of mental illness and the negative symptomatology present turned into barriers that kept her from moving in a meaningful direction, especially in this area.

Table 21.1 summarises the central aspects of these interactions.

21.3.3.3 Real Empowerment: Train to Be Above What You Think and Feel

Once what was important had emerged, and continuing with the weekly sessions, work began on *setting goals* connected to what was important. The idea is that M, under the intrinsic motivation of values, establishes small steps in a significant direction. As was to be expected, when it came to taking these actions with the aim of returning to her former life, barriers appeared in the form of thoughts and feelings. *Training in defusion skills* was proposed as a means of support. The purpose was to learn to relate to such unpleasant private events in a different way and to ensure that they did not have the impact they previously had on M's life.

ACIP places special emphasis on the fact that this *training* (not treatment) aims to build a meaningful life. The purpose is to give the training a function, connecting it to the type of life that the person wants to live, allowing the person to incorporate these tools to prevent discomfort.

In summary, the sessions held over the following months were aimed at providing multiple interactions, in which M was trained in different ways to relate to her more complicated private events, so that she could be on top of it all, be in control and take action depending on what was important.

M's most significant private events were present as she tried to incorporate them into her daily life. M reported that when reading, watching TV or going to the

Table 21.1 Summary table of what matters

My values of self-growth	My talents	My passions	My service values to others
Work and training (professionalism) Self-care and health creativity (making my Own clothes, autonomy) Travelling (getting to know other cultures)	Languages	The cinema Fashion Dressmaking and sewing Reading Travelling	The family Children Helping others (contributing)

cinema, she found it difficult to pay attention and from the morning onwards she felt very discouraged, which was of particular concern to her. She used to sleep for long periods of time and when she found that everything was very difficult and felt that going back to school was a long way off, she became depressed and often cried.

This work, called *real empowerment* of the person (Salgado & Mateos, 2021), was carried out by making private unpleasant events present in the session itself and through classic exercises with closed eyes, defusion and attention to the present moment enriched with deictic, hierarchical and behavioural regulation function cues (Gil-Luciano et al., 2017; López-López & Luciano, 2017; Luciano 2016).

In summary, this training consisted of integrating the following three phases in the eyes-closed exercises:

1. Trying to put M in the perspective of an observer of her private events, with special emphasis on differentiating between the person and her inner experience.

   Examples: *"See who is having that thought now", "notice that there is that feeling and there is you", "notice that one thing is the feeling and another is you", "see if you can put that thought on the table, as if you can write it down and put it on the table, and notice the space between the thought and you. And notice that you are the one who can perceive it".*
2. Fostering a hierarchical (or rather an inclusive) relationship between private events and her.

   Examples: *"Where are you noticing what you're sensing, where in your body? If it had a shape, what shape would it have? and so on with other characteristics that allow you to physicalise the person's inner experience" (after this physicalisation exercise you are given a silhouette of a human body to draw inside you)" "notice that there is a part of you that is observing what you are thinking and feeling" "notice that you are bigger than what you are experiencing", "see if you can go around the boundaries of what you are noticing, make a small hole of one centimetre and breathe over it as if you could wrap your breath around it".*
3. Empowering the person through multiple practices in which she notices who is able to exercise control over actions. It is not only about experiencing, from the depths of the heart, who she wants to be in charge in her life (herself or her private events) but, after working on changing the relationship with what she thinks and feels, she notices that she is the one who can choose to move her arms and legs. In short, it is about her being above what she thinks and feels and taking control of what she really controls, her actions, in order to build and move in a meaningful direction.

   Ultimately, the purpose is that, after training in framing her private events in deictic and inclusive frameworks with respect to oneself, together with what is important in the present, she connects with the unlimited source of motivation to take control of her actions, cultivating and watering, step by step, the qualities and/or the imprint that she wants to enhance in her life.

   Examples: "What invites you to do what you feel...? And what do you choose?" *"Noticing that you are bigger than what you think and feel, if it were important for you to get up out of your chair and get going, who could do it better, you or your thoughts and feelings? Ok, do it."*

In addition to the above aspects, the interactions during those months were aimed at working on other relevant aspects of the qualities of inner experience and how M related to it all. In short, M was trained to be in the present moment, to deal with the transience of thoughts and feelings, to relate to the mind as a counsellor that can be listened to or not, and all with the aim of motivating acceptance to live in accordance with her interests.

A more specific focus on the training procedure is beyond the scope of this chapter. For more details see Salgado and Mateos (2021).

Throughout this time, M was developing proposals in the form of small objectives in the direction she valued. These were put into action with the use of the tools trained during the sessions. In addition, we worked with the family to generate a constructive and depathologising context, as they had a high level of anxiety and concern for their daughter's future, reacting in a manner that sometimes influenced M in the same way.

Descriptively, the result of this phase was an increase in activities in a significant direction. Among the proposed actions and objectives, M undertook were reading, going to the cinema on several occasions and travelling with her father as a way of nurturing her interests.

In order to resume her education and become the professional she wanted to be, she started going to the library to study. And she also started going to the gym as a way of nurturing her self-care.

Another notable milestone during these months is that she was attending follow-up consultations in the psychiatry service, and her psychiatrist considered it relevant to reduce the medication, on the one hand, because of the small progress M was showing, and on the other hand, because some of the side effects interfered with her commitments, such as lack of concentration when studying and when reading.

21.3.3.4 Day Care Service

Despite making significant progress towards what was important to her, M continued to struggle with what the diagnosis of mental illness meant and with the unpleasant feelings that arose when she was working towards her commitments. She pointed out that, although she went to the library and to the cinema, she had a lot of difficulty concentrating, she found it hard to get out of bed, she felt very flat, she still did not feel she was ready to go to class (although she had already enrolled) and sit exams as she had a lot of trouble remembering information.

All these barriers made it difficult for M to move towards what mattered to her. In response, she proposed to go to the day care service for more intensive training in situations similar to real life. This service consisted of attending 3 days a week (for 3 h each day) for group sessions and specific work on those tasks in which she had greater difficulties, such as studying.

She attended for 3 months during which training was intensified in the same aspects as those mentioned in the previous point, but in this case in real situations.

For example, she would initially do group training sessions on cognitive defusion skills, and then move on to sessions in which the important issues were brought to the surface in order not to lose contact with that source of motivation before training with private events. At these times, she would go to the centre's library where she would either read or study (whatever she chose) while distractions would appear sporadically. These distractions could come from someone trying to talk her out of her study, or a professional throwing small balls of paper at her as thoughts or feelings that came to her unintentionally and demanded her attention. Her task at that moment was to become aware of it, to notice what the distracting event was inviting her to do, and under the influence of what was important – her studies and her future professionalism – to carry on or return to reading or studying.

This work was implemented for approximately 3 months. She subsequently attended follow-up sessions on the objectives and actions she had proposed and carried out.

Finally, it should be noted, along the same lines as mentioned in previous points, that M's progress also made it possible to reduce her antipsychotic medication as much as possible, stopping it completely in January.

21.3.3.5 Follow-Up

Among the advances in her vital functioning over the subsequent months of follow-up, the following were noted: she intends to go to class and does so every day, she revisits the subjects and enters them into the computer, in January she begins to sit exams, she visits the library in the mornings and attends class in the afternoons, she writes a paper and presents it in class, all of which helps her grow in her studies and prepares her for a professional career.

Furthermore, she signs up for a photography course, still attends the gym 2 days a week and travels with her father on several occasions. She verbalises that this is not enough for her. As she likes languages very much and cannot travel as much as she would like, from time to time she joins English conversation groups that meet in cafés in the city.

From then on, the follow-up sessions are held less frequently, initially once every 2 months and then every 3 months for the next year.

And finally, during this time, the following goals connected with what matters to her stand out: *she manages to finish her degree, she continues to go to the gym for self-care, she continues to enjoy reading, she is going to take an Italian course abroad during the summer and now she wants to pass her driving test as a way of increasing her autonomy. In terms of leisure, she has met up with a few friends, but not in large groups, stating that she has never been an excessively open person.*

Nevertheless, the unpleasant thoughts and feelings associated with the whole situation that M has been through have not disappeared. She says that she still finds it hard to concentrate, she is sometimes nervous, she is afraid of everything to do with exams and now that she has finished her degree, she is uncomfortable with the

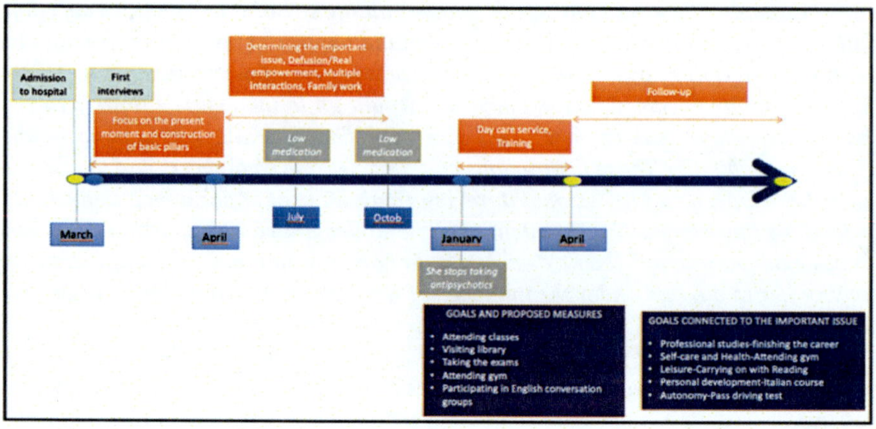

Fig. 21.3 Temporary process of intervention

uncertainty of whether or not to take the entrance exams. But none of this has the impact on her that it used to (Fig. 21.3).

21.4 Conclusions

We began the chapter by highlighting three aspects that emerged from professional practice with people diagnosed with psychosis. Firstly, the huge burden of being diagnosed with an illness that has the prefix "mental". Secondly, how an excessive focus on the awareness of illness emphasised and made this burden even heavier. And thirdly, the possibility emerged that mental disorders could become chronic because we are not able to deal with them in an adequate way. All of this leads to an enormous isolation and sense of exclusion from society for the person diagnosed with psychosis.

ACIP is an attentional model that takes into account these three aspects and their consequences, building through interactions based on what is important for the person, the pillars of de-pathologisation, dignity, shared vulnerability, real empowerment and social connection. These pillars will constitute a healthy context that will sustain the person, making what is important and valued (instead of the illness) the focus of the intervention.

In this chapter we have tried to exemplify the support process for a person with a first psychotic outbreak under the perspective of the ACIP, showing it as a depathologising care and close process, where vulnerability is allowed and with the purpose of training (not treating) the person to acquire the skills to rise above what he thinks and feels. We can state that it is a form of prevention, but that it wants to go further. It not only aims to reduce disability and prevent relapses but also steers the situation away from becoming chronic. Moreover, it allows the person to build a meaningful life.

From this process we would like to highlight the following points:

- It is key to emphasise the importance, on the one hand, of knowing the context (both close and historical) in which behaviours occur and, on the other hand, of the functional (not topographical) approach to the explanation of behaviours, as a way of putting ourselves in the best position to support the person.
- ACIP has proven to be a supportive intervention or process – as we like to call it – that provides the technical tools for the person to live the life they want to live. In this sense, it places special emphasis on ensuring that these tools are not used to serve the same avoidance function as other problem behaviours that take the person away from what is important.
- The sessions were not aimed at solving problems and/or fighting with their symptomatology, but at accompanying and supporting through training, the construction of a valuable life for M.
- Derived from the above, it is important to note that the final objective was not for M to achieve defusion but to give this defusion the function of being a tool that allows the person to get in touch with what is important.
- Another relevant aspect worth investigating in future is that the presence of values from the beginning of the intervention seems to provide an unlimited source of motivation to move in a meaningful direction. This fact may cast doubt on the necessary presence of the creative hopelessness process as a motivational element. Getting the person to take actions governed by the intrinsic positive reinforcement of what is important has obvious advantages over taking different actions as a consequence of the awareness of the paradoxical effect of one's own avoidance behaviour. This is not to say that they are mutually exclusive, but it can give us a clue as to the importance of starting the intervention (whenever possible) in line with what is important.
- Following on from the above, it can be seen how the focus was always on values, being the source of motivation for M to take actions connected with these values, despite the burden of the diagnosis of mental illness and private events, which had a negative effect.

We can conclude, therefore, that the intervention has succeeded in increasing M's protective factors through training so that the symptomatology has less of an impact on her actions and life.

Psychological interventions in psychosocial rehabilitation have traditionally been criticised on the grounds that their effectiveness was only limited to the skills trained, but with a poor impact on the person's social functioning. In this sense, the intervention presented by the ACIP has achieved improvements in M's social functioning, translating itself into actions that she carried out in line with what was important. In short, she tried to fulfil objectives that were aligned with her values, increasing both her objective and subjective social performance, despite the existence of unpleasant private events.

We cannot end this presentation without highlighting an aspect that was present in the intervention, although it was not intentionally sought. We refer to the importance of coordination between the psychiatric service and the psychological work. And we are not referring to the fact that positive coordination meetings were held (in fact, such meetings never took place), but rather that both the psychiatrist and, in this case, ourselves, took a joint approach to the intervention, which was important for M. Due to her age, the psychiatric service was very clear from the beginning that the objective was to support her inclusion in a meaningful life. To this end, as progress was observed in her protective factors and skills training, the medication was gradually decreased, despite taking into account the fact that the side effects of withdrawal interfered with some of those essential actions that M had set herself.

In conclusion, we can say that a de-pathologising and validating process, which emphasises the emergence of what is important from the beginning and uses the person's training to support this, produces adequate results in social functioning and prevents chronification.

Disclaimer Clinical cases presented in this chapter do not include real names or personal information of real persons.

References

Alanen, Y. O., Lehtinen, K., Räkköläinen, V., & Aaltonen, J. (1991). Need-adapted treatment of new schizophrenic patients: Experiences and results of the Turku Project. *Acta Psychiatrica Scandinavica*. https://doi.org/10.1111/j.1600-0447.1991.tb05557.x

Gil-Luciano, B., Ruiz, F. J., Valdivia-Salas, S., & Suárez-Falcón, J. C. (2017). Promoting psychological flexibility on tolerance tasks: Framing behavior through deictic/hierarchical relations and specifying augmental functions. *Psychological Record*. https://doi.org/10.1007/s40732-016-0200-5

Hayes, S., & Strosahl, K. D. (2004). *A practical guide to acceptance and commitment therapy*. https://doi.org/10.1007/978-0-387-23369-7.

Hayes, S. C., Luoma, J. B., Bond, F. W., Masuda, A., & Lillis, J. (2006). Acceptance and commitment therapy: Model, processes and outcomes. *Behaviour Research and Therapy*. https://doi.org/10.1016/j.brat.2005.06.006

Hayes, S. C., Strosahl, K. D., & Wilson, K. G. (2012). Acceptance and commitment therapy: The process and practice of mindful change. In *Acceptance and commitment therapy The process and practice of mindful change* (2nd ed.). The Guilford Press.

Kohlenberg, R. J., & Tsai, M. (1991). KİTAP Functional analytic psychotherapy: Creating intense and curative therapeutic relationships. In *Functional analytic psychotherapy: Creating intense and curative therapeutic relationships*. https://doi.org/10.1007/978-0-387-70855-3.

Lehtinen, V., Alanen, Y. O., Aaltonen, J., Lehtinen, K., & Räkköläinen, V. (1999). Family intervention as an essential part of the treatment of new schizophrenic patients: Experiences from Finland. *Italian Journal of Psychiatry and Behavioural Sciences*.

López-López, J. C., & Luciano, C. (2017). An experimental analysis of defusion interactions based on deictic and hierarchical framings and their impact on cognitive performance. *Psychological Record*. https://doi.org/10.1007/s40732-017-0250-3

Luciano, C. (2016). Evolución de ACT. *Análisis y Modificación de Conducta*. https://doi.org/10.33776/amc.v42i165-66.2791

Luciano Soriano, C., Rodriguez Valverde, M., & Gutiérrez Martínez, O. (2004). A proposal for synthesizing verbal contexts in experiential avoidance disorder and acceptance and commitment therapy. *International Journal of Psychology and Psychological Therapy*.

McKay, M., Forsyth, J. P., & Eifert, G. H. (2010). *Your life on purpose: How to find whatmatters & create the life you want*. New Harbinger Publications.

Organización Mundial de la Salud (OMS). (2005). *Prevención de los Trastornos Mentales: Intervenciones Efectivas y Opciones Políticas*. Organización Mundial de La Salud, Ginebra.

Pérez Álvarez, M., Fernández Hermida, J. R., Fernández Rodríguez, C., & Amigo Vázquez, I. (2003). *Guía de tratamientos psicològicos eficaces I. Adultos*. Pirámide.

Pérez-Álvarez, M., García-Montes, J. M., Perona-Garcelán, S., & Vallina-Fernández, O. (2008). Changing relationship with voices: New therapeutic perspectives for treating hallucinations. *Clinical Psychology and Psychotherapy*. https://doi.org/10.1002/cpp.563

Rogers, C. R. (1981). Psicoterapia centrada en el cliente: Práctica, implicaciones y teoría. In *Biblioteca de Psiquiatría, Psicopatología y Psicosomática; Serie mayor*.

Salgado, C. F. (2011). *Comparación de dos protocolos de intervención basados en la Terapia de Aceptación y Compromiso y en Mindfulness, en personas con Trastorno Mental Crónico*. Tesis Doctoral no publicada. Universidad de Almería.

Salgado, C. F. (2019). *Guía para la activación del proyecto de vida para la inclusión social*. Junta de Castilla y León. Gerencia de Servicios Sociales.

Salgado, C. F, & Mateos, M. (2021). La prevención de casos de psicosis ¿es posible?. Propuesta de un modelo atencional basado en lo importante para la persona. In E. Pirámide (Ed.), *Terapia de Aceptación y Compromiso en Psicosis. Aceptación y recuperación por niveles (ART)* (p. 11). Pirámide. Capítulo.

Chapter 22
An Approximation to a Relational Approach for Psychosis: Functional Analytic Psychotherapy (FAP)

María Marín-Vila, Carmen Ortiz-Fune, and Jonathan W. Kanter

22.1 Introduction

Different studies have documented the importance of interpersonal factors in the genesis of psychotic spectrum disorders (PSD), highlighting the impact of traumatic relational experiences at an early age (e.g., Fernández-León et al., 2020; Mørkved et al., 2018). Under this framework, different psychotherapeutic models have emerged to emphasize the relational processes which take place in the context of therapy; for example, some models describe these exchanges as emotionally corrective experiences. Functional analytic psychotherapy (FAP; Kohlenberg & Tsai, 1991; Tsai et al., 2009) is an example of this type of approach. In parallel, the psychotherapeutic potential of community resources (Fernández & Ballesteros Pérez, 2017; Rodríguez, 2005; Saiz Galdós & Chévez, 2009) in the treatment of PSD has been highlighted as these contexts provide opportunities to learn new skills in a more "natural" and deeply relational context (Ortiz-Fune & Marín-Vila, 2021).

In this chapter, the use of FAP in a case of an adolescent with psychotic symptoms will be presented. The intervention was carried out in an adolescent day hospital (ADH) within the Spanish National Health Care System. Therapeutic work on this unit is guided by the philosophy of the therapeutic community approach (Jones, 1963). First, a brief presentation of the importance of interpersonal factors in psychosis will be given. Second, these factors will be linked to an introduction to the

M. Marín-Vila (✉)
Puerta de Hierro-Majadahonda University Hospital, Madrid, Spain
e-mail: mmvila@salud.madrid.org

C. Ortiz-Fune
University Assistance Complex of Salamanca, Salamanca, Spain

J. W. Kanter
University of Washington, Seattle, WA, USA
e-mail: jonkan@uw.edu

J. A. Díaz-Garrido et al. (eds.), *Psychological Interventions for Psychosis*,
https://doi.org/10.1007/978-3-031-27003-1_22

fundamental principles of FAP. Next, the main characteristics of the adolescent day hospital will be described to contextualize the details of the intervention in this specific healthcare context. Then, in the central section of the chapter, the clinical case will be presented, highlighting the most relevant points of the intervention that was implemented. Finally, different recommendations, advantages, and limitations of the use of FAP in the psychological treatment of psychosis will be discussed.

22.1.1 Psychosis and Interpersonal Variables

Given our social nature, interactions with others are essential to our development. This is a fundamental fact which starts perinatally and continues throughout life. Our physical and psychological well-being are compromised when we lack social connections (Cohen, 2004; Holt-Lunstad et al., 2010; House et al., 1988), as feelings of belongingness (Leary & Cox, 2008) and contexts for learning interpersonal field skills across different relational domains are necessary for survival (Bugental, 2000). Classic theoretical models, such as Attachment Theory (Bowlby, 1988), provide hypotheses about how early interpersonal relationships influence our interpersonal behavior patterns throughout life, including learning rules for cognitive and emotional reactions that guide behavior.

It has been observed that a large majority of patients with psychotic symptoms report traumatic events in childhood, especially interpersonal trauma (e.g., maltreatment and sexual abuse) (Mørkved et al., 2018). In addition, histories of trauma are associated with indicators of worse clinical outcomes, such as greater severity and persistence of psychotic symptoms, as well as poorer adherence to treatment (Kreyenbuhl et al., 2009; Trotta et al., 2015; Varese et al., 2012). Consistent with these findings, a higher prevalence of insecure attachment styles has also been observed in people diagnosed with schizophrenia compared to people without this diagnosis (Carr et al., 2018). These traumatic interpersonal histories could explain, at least in part, some of the difficulties that these patients present in terms of adherence to treatment. A high percentage of these patients have difficulties establishing stable therapeutic alliances and this is a risk factor for relapse (Shattock et al., 2017).

In fact, the therapeutic alliance plays a fundamental role in the treatment of patients with psychosis. For example, a strong therapeutic alliance has been associated with fewer hospitalizations and the reduction in medication use (Priebe et al., 2010). Likewise, additional factors closely linked to the psychotherapeutic process and the therapeutic relationship are central when working with serious mental illness. These factors include consistency in the intervention process, validation of the patient, motivation, metacognition processes, and monitoring changes via feedback (Livesley et al., 2016).

Different psychotherapeutic models for psychosis share an emphasis on interpersonal factors and have emphasized the importance of intervening on early relationships and social interactions. For example, systemic therapy models have stated the association between psychotic symptoms and specific intrafamily interaction patterns, such as high levels of expressed emotionality (Brown et al., 1972). Contextual-behavioral models similarly have pointed out that developing the foundational capacity to distinguish one's self and one's needs and feelings from others, including accurately identifying one's feelings and other private events, are themselves relational processes that are necessary for mental health (Kanter et al., 2001). Likewise, attachment models emphasize the importance of developing in interaction with adults who provide secure versus disorganized or insecure attachments for these foundational capacities to develop normally (Valdivia-Salas, 2016).

As described above, these abilities seem to be deficient with individuals with psychosis. In this sense, learning these skills in the context of a safe and predictable therapeutic relationship could be essential, providing a different relational model from the one experienced at an early age. This potentially could help the person to develop a more integrated self, which ideally would be under private control (Kanter et al., 2001; Kohlenberg & Tsai, 1991; McHugh et al., 2019).

22.1.2 *Functional Analytic Psychotherapy*

Functional analytic psychotherapy, a psychotherapeutic intervention framed in contextual-behavioral science (CBS; Hayes et al., 2012), emphasizes the therapeutic relationship as a mechanism for improving interpersonal skills (Kanter et al., 2017). In general, contextual-behavioral science approaches to psychotherapy (also called third-wave cognitive-behavioral psychotherapies; Hayes, 2004) aim to develop skills so that, even in the presence of symptoms, patients can build lives with meaning, based on what is important to them (Salgado Pascual & Mateos García, 2021). These psychotherapies differ from their predecessors (first- and second-wave cognitive-behavioral psychotherapies) in that the main objective is not the elimination of or reduction in signs and symptoms of particular disorders, but rather the promotion of alternative behavioral regulation patterns in the presence of those symptoms. To achieve this purpose, a description of behaviors based on their function rather than on their topography—in other words, functional analysis—is particularly relevant (Pérez-Álvarez, 2006). In addition, CBS approaches presume a phenomenological approach to mental health problems. This means placing the person at the center of the psychotherapeutic process and promoting a first-person narrative, within a marked idiographic philosophy.

During the psychotherapeutic work, the patient's experience and the analysis of behavior in context and in the present moment stand out. In this sense, "techniques" remain in the background; the process is central. Furthermore, from this perspective, the therapist does not act as an "expert" who teaches the patient techniques or skills, but rather as a person whose behavior is understood in terms of the same learning principles and whose life is equally influenced by the sociocultural context.

In FAP, functional analysis is used to understand the interactions between therapist and patient in session. FAP assumes that much in-session behavior is functionally equivalent to the behavior that occurs outside of the therapeutic context (in "real life"). This analysis is the starting point to identify clinically relevant behaviors (CRB).

First, the therapist identifies patients' CRB1s, which are those behaviors that appear in the session and which are related to patients' difficulties in their daily lives (that is to say, which are problematic). For example, for a patient with problems self-regulating when feeling angry, CRB1s may include raising the tone of voice in an inappropriate way in response to the therapist. On the other hand, the goal of FAP is to promote CRB2s. Those are behaviors that are conceptualized as improvements within the session. For example, the previous patient would learn to regulate the tone of voice in session when talking about an anger-generating conflict. Finally, the therapist also aims to develop CRB3, which are patients' functional descriptions of their own behavior. For example, the previous patient would be able to describe in session that he has realized that he tends to yell every time the therapist talks about an issue that makes him angry, and that the relationship is improved when he can regulate his expression.

Likewise, the FAP therapist also understands that his or her own behaviors are important to the process of the therapeutic relationship, and these behaviors are also a target of analysis during the intervention. In FAP, these behaviors are called T1 and T2, and they represent the equivalent for the clinician of CRB1 and CRB2, respectively. For example, a therapist who is insecure in his daily life might be hesitant to set a limit to a patient who is disrespectful (T1). After potential work in personal supervision, the therapist may be able to show more assertive behaviors when facing this patient (T2).

To carry out the psychotherapeutic process, FAP distinguishes five rules that can guide the clinician during the intervention. These guidelines are not static or rigid but rather represent general guidelines that make salient specific processes that the therapist must keep in mind during psychotherapy. The rules described in FAP are: (1) observe CRBs; (2) evoke CRB2s; (3) reinforce CRB2s naturally; (4) identify the effects on the patient of the therapist's attempts at reinforcement; and (5) provide functional interpretations of behavior (Kohlenberg & Tsai, 1991).

FAP has been used to treat many different mental health problems, although its relevance has been highlighted and the empirical support strongest for those cases in which interpersonal difficulties are in the foreground (Ferro-García et al., 2009; Kanter et al., 2017). There is growing evidence for the application and clinical use of FAP in patients with psychosis. For example, Dykstra et al. (2010) present a broad description of the use of the five FAP rules when working with patients with psychotic symptoms. Ortiz-Fune and Marín-Vila (2021) describe how FAP may promote and cultivate the therapeutic relationship in different therapeutic contexts for the treatment of psychosis, with emphasis on its application in community and clinical contexts outside of hospitals. Working with adolescents, Díaz de Neira Hernando et al. (2021) described the use of FAP, combined with acceptance and commitment therapy (ACT), in a group format in a brief hospitalization inpatient unit, highlighting its value in improving relational problems with patients with serious mental disorders. Furthermore, in a controlled study developed by Sengupta and Singh (2021), the impact of an intervention based on FAP was assessed in patients with schizophrenia. The results show a reduction in positive symptoms and general psychopathology, as well as an improvement in coping patterns, motivational and psychosocial aspects, and cohesion with the family.

Based on these earlier findings, recent developments in FAP have proposed and tested a model of close relationships that provides a common language for identifying CRB1s and CRB2s in appropriate patients (Maitland et al., 2017; Kanter et al., 2020; Marín-Vila et al., 2020). This model summarizes and integrates the vast scientific literature on relationships within a CBS perspective that frames targets as functionally defined behaviors. Although an in-depth description of this model is beyond the scope of this chapter, throughout the presentation of the clinical case some of its key points are highlighted, so further reading is recommended.

22.1.3 Adolescent Day Hospital

Adolescent day hospitals (ADH) are intensive treatment facilities for patients with severe problems that cause functional impairment. These units provide a specific, multidisciplinary, and intensive approach to support adolescents' success in their natural social interaction contexts, such as schools and families (Villero et al., 2016). An ADH is a clinical resource that occupies the space between hospitalization and outpatient therapy.

One of the most frequently used psychotherapeutic settings in ADH has been the therapeutic community (e.g., Buiza Aguado et al., 2014; Figuera, 2019; Karterud et al., 1992; Villero et al., 2016). Seminal descriptions of this intervention model are attributed to Jones (1963), who described these contexts as intensive resources which promote coexistence and connection between patients and the therapeutic team. This context tries to reproduce "daily life" in order to favor the emergence of roles similar to those which patients play outside the therapeutic context. This provides multiple opportunities to intervene in a "here and now" setting. The coexistence and the relational features that emerge within this frame make the therapeutic community a "social system" in which all members influence each other (Alcamí, 1992). The clinical setting acts as an "extended family" (García-Badaracco, 1990). In this sense, the therapeutic community involves the intervention of a multidisciplinary team which considers all individuals in the context, not only the therapeutic team, as a part of the intervention (e.g., administrative staff).

A day hospital includes multiple healthcare scenarios and therapeutic contents, such as programs that seek to reduce acute symptoms and resolve the crisis, treatments for patients with severe symptoms who do not respond to outpatient treatments, and rehabilitation programs to prevent chronicity and functional deterioration. However, in general, a primary function of day hospitals is to provide group treatments which highlight social connections, listening, and coexistence. This facilitates the development of relational capacities and corrective emotional experiences. In this sense, the interpersonal relationships that appear in the context of the intervention are understood as psychotherapeutic experiences themselves. It is important to accompany and support the patient not only during structured therapeutic activities but also in interactions during more "informal" settings (e.g., arrival at the day hospital, breaks, and farewells). Every moment in which there is a possible personal interaction is important.

The intense relational experience that emerges in the context of these clinical resources involves multiple intervention opportunities for therapists and also reveals the vulnerabilities of clinicians and work teams. For example, unstructured or informal group interventions, the coexistence with different patient profiles, and the difficulties when coordinating with a multidisciplinary work team can be quite challenging. Likewise, working with trauma and related interpersonal problems, which are typically central for patients with serious mental disorders, can stir a host of emotional reactions in therapists, depending on their own histories and coping mechanisms. In this sense, therapists' personal backgrounds play a relevant role in their interaction with patients and workmates. Personal and work team supervision are essential in addressing possible T1s and barriers to intervention.

22.2 Clinical Case

22.2.1 Case Presentation

Miguel is a 16-year-old adolescent referred to the ADH from the Brief Hospitalization Unit (BHU), where he had been hospitalized for 20 days after a suicide attempt in the context of a psychotic episode. He tried to hang himself with a belt at home, but it broke. His parents found him and, very scared, decided to take him to the hospital where it was decided to admit him to the BHU.

Miguel is an only child and lives with his parents, Antonio and Rosa. He has no personal or family history of previous follow-ups in mental health. His parents are originally from Colombia and decided to move to Spain when Miguel's mother was pregnant. Miguel's father disclosed to have had problems with alcohol for many years, although he currently reported abstinence. The adolescent's mother avoided delving into her personal history, although she recognized that she has had a "very complicated childhood." When they were asked about the reasons for moving to Spain, they explained that Miguel's father, due to his problems with alcohol, had conflicts with "dangerous people." Fearing that they might harm his family, especially considering his wife's recent pregnancy, they decided to change their lives and move to another country. Miguel's maternal grandparents had been living in Spain for some time and they thought it would be a good idea "to start over in a place where no one knew them." However, during their first years in Spain, the family acknowledged that they tended to avoid social situations for the fear that "someone would find them." Regarding family dynamics, in general, it is a very close family, with rigid limits toward other people.

22.2.1.1 Personal and Psychosocial Development

Miguel's parents described him as a child with a normative development, but with problems in his interactions with others. This was due to his shyness and his difficulties to integrate in social situations. Later, during the treatment in the ADH, they would recognize that this fact could be related to the few opportunities they had given Miguel to interact with people outside the family because of their fear to be found. In this same sense, it seemed that Miguel has grown up with the idea that "the world is dangerous" and that, in his parents' own words, "you always have to be careful with what you say." On the other hand, Miguel's parents commented that he has always been a "very anxious child" and "very interested in paranormal matters," an aspect that he shares with his father, who admitted being a very "mystical" person.

Despite his difficulties in relating, Miguel's parents said that the first years of school passed normally at both the relational and the academic level. Miguel used to have some friends and seemed to be integrated in his class. However, 3 years before the suicide attempt, his parents changed their jobs and they moved to a different city. This involved a change of school and social environment for Miguel. In addition, the family started to live independently. Until then, they had lived with Miguel's maternal grandparents, with whom the patient had a strong connection. These changes involved a loss of social support for the entire family.

Miguel experienced many difficulties adapting to his new life. For some years, he suffered bullying at the school. He was insulted and physically assaulted by some of his classmates. During these years, his suffering was unnoticed by adults. Miguel talked about it for the first time during his stay at the BHU but showed little emotional impact.

His parents explained that, during the previous years, they had noticed a progressive tendency to isolation in Miguel, noticing that he gradually started to spend more time locked in his room. They were surprised about this fact, but they minimized it by framing this behavior in terms of Miguel's personality and his difficulties in relating. In the same way, they said that Miguel had been gradually neglecting habits in terms of hygiene, feeding, and sleeping. When the family dynamics were explored, it seemed that Miguel's parents also showed difficulties to maintain basic self-care habits, with no clear schedules and routines at home.

The few personal interactions that Miguel had before the suicide attempt took place through the Internet, where he used to spend most of the time playing videogames online with strangers. He kept some friends but preferred to talk with them by using social media rather than doing so face to face. He said that he was feeling more and more emotionally disconnected from them, showing affective indifference. Also, considering his parent's speech, it was inferred that there were difficulties with family communication patterns, presenting two opposite poles between the total absence of communication and the emission of confusing messages, such as alluding to the risks of communicating outside the family without specifying exactly what the anticipated danger was. Likewise, the parents expressed that they had tried to establish channels of communication with their son, taking an interest in Miguel's state of mind and his interests. However, the patient referred to feeling invalidated every time he had expressed verbalizations about himself regarding what he felt, wanted, or thought.

22.2.1.2 Admission to the BHU

At the beginning of the admission, Miguel was mostly silent, without wanting to delve into the reasons for his suicide attempt. He seemed very suspicious of the BHU staff, apparently showing little emotional resonance about what happened. After a few weeks, when he managed to bond with the unit's psychiatrist, he explained that a kind of entity, "The Dark Evil," had ordered him to make the suicide attempt. After this, he began to explain that he had written a self-edited book in which he tells a complex story about "The Dark Evil." The story is that this character wants to destroy the world and humans "because they are bad and only cause misfortune." Miguel explained that he has been devising this story for at least 3 years, coinciding with the beginning of the time of changes for the family. Miguel stated "not feeling identified with human beings" and expressed rejection of them, in the same way that "The Dark Evil" expresses. Likewise, he explained that this character "was a good person," but that "he had suffered a lot" and that this had made him a "villain." Delving deeper into the story, Miguel told the psychiatrist that "The Dark Evil" has an army of robots to help him in his mission and that his first objective will be to destroy the school. However, he pointed out that, in this school, there is a group of students who will organize themselves to "combat the evil," turning the whole story around this fight. Also, during his stay at the BHU, Miguel reported that he was able to control the doors of the BHU with his mind. Moreover, he thought that both other patients and professionals can hear what he thinks, presenting high suspicion.

In his speech, Miguel mixed elements of reality with fantasy, since sometimes he spoke about the story in an exclusively literary way, while in other occasions he alluded to the fact that "he is The Dark Evil," without making a clear distinction between reality and his imagination, and with a marked fusion of identity. Miguel has green hair, like "The Dark Evil" in the story, and he has the character's name tattooed on one of his wrists. However, at many other times, he identified with the "leader" of the group of the school students who are supposedly going to fight him. As it can be seen, the content of the story presented by Miguel seemed to be full of biographical meanings.

The psychiatrist of the BHU decided to investigate more aspects of the story, so Miguel asked his parents to bring to him in the hospital a folder with numerous drafts of the story. These documents were accompanied by illustrations made by Miguel himself, in which many drawings of "The Dark Evil" and his army of robots appeared. Texts described a complex network of characters and substories related to the main one. The information was disconnected and extremely disorganized, so it was very difficult to identify a clear plot line. However, Miguel seemed to explain the story in a highly structured way, with many details.

The patient's parents, in one of the interviews with the BHU psychiatrist, alluded to the fact that some of their son's schoolmates had alerted them that, in the weeks before the suicide attempt, Miguel had published alarming content on social media, alternating incomprehensible messages with others in which he threatened to harm people at the school. When they were asked about the story of "The Dark Evil," they said that most of the conversations with their son tended to revolve around this topic and the writing of his book, but that they had not given it much importance. They thought it was an exclusively literary interest, alluding to his "fantasy" personality. However, they did recognize that, at times, Miguel's excessively restrictive interest in this topic "irritated them."

As it can be seen, Miguel had grown up in an environment in which a reserved, excessively cautious, and inhibited attitude was reinforced by his main attachment figures. On the one hand, the behavior of his parents could be understood as a coherent and adaptive response to the stressful events they had experienced (e.g., perception of danger in their country). There is a clear turning point in Miguel's story that takes place with the move to a different city and the loss of relevant social connections (maternal grandparents and friends from his previous school). The tendency to isolate in the family nucleus, the probable accentuation of rigid limits, the problematic patterns of communication and lack of emotional validation, as well as the experience of real danger and harm in the school, may have contributed to the development of psychotic symptomatology. This was revealed through the story of "The Dark Evil."

22.2.2 *Psychotherapeutic Intervention at the Adolescent Day Hospital*

22.2.2.1 Establishment of the Therapeutic Relationship and Beginning of the Process

Approximately 1 week after being discharged from the hospital, Miguel attended the initial assessment at the ADH accompanied by his parents. He had received the diagnosis of "Psychotic Disorder Not Otherwise Specified" and had started psychopharmacological treatment (antidepressant and antipsychotic) at low doses.

On the first day at ADH, the whole family was cooperative with the initial evaluation, although they seemed distrustful of the process. They showed difficulties when delving into themselves and seemed more comfortable when more trivial aspects were addressed (CRB1). In addition, Miguel's parents showed very critical speech toward his son, which revealed great difficulty in being able to understand the patient's problems. They verbalized thoughts such as "he is very lazy...," "he should be studying...," or "that story about him and the book is nonsense...." They showed reluctance to talk about the suicide attempt, as well as tended to be sparing in words and anxious when the professional tried to find out about his family history. At these moments, they tended to change the topic or divert the conversation, again toward criticism of Miguel. The only aspects they managed to share about themselves were their values regarding work and resilience. Both parents described themselves as people who "have overcome numerous obstacles in their lives thanks to their effort."

In relation to the treatment, at the beginning of the process, the parents seemed to clearly reject actively participating at the ADH, although they did not state that explicitly. They showed a kind of confusing interaction that was quite similar to the one verbalized by Miguel when he explained how his parents usually communicate with him. For example, when they were invited to attend the group therapy for parents, they were initially very cooperative, but after that they tended to list multiple excuses for not attending, and they never started the intervention. Likewise, when they accompanied the patient to the ADH facilities, they avoided waiting for him in the waiting room accompanied by other parents, so they said goodbye to him on a street near the hospital. Miguel, in the initial interviews, commented that his parents "did not trust the hospital" and that they had warned him to "be careful" with the information provided so that "people did not treat him like a crazy person." From the beginning of the process, Miguel complained several times about this fact. Later in the treatment, he managed to express sadness about the fact that his parents did not want to participate in the intervention. As mentioned above, this attitude toward treatment was similar to the behavior his parents displayed in other contexts in which they had to expose themselves socially. All the behaviors described above would constitute examples of behaviors whose function is to avoid discomfort (e.g., fear of being harmed in social contexts) and were categorized, from a clinical point of view, as CRB1s.

In the first interview with Miguel, the story of "The Dark Evil" comprised his entire speech, making it difficult for the therapist to redirect the conversation to other topics. In fact, he expressed complaints about being misunderstood by his social context regarding how important his story was to him ("they tell me I'm always talking about this... they don't understand..."). When trying to address other possible areas, Miguel had a clear difficulty being able to maintain fluid and coherent speech. Reciprocal exchanges in conversation were also rare. His speech about himself was not spontaneous and was only limited to answering the interviewer's questions, with a tendency to redirect his answers toward the story of his book. Later in the course of the treatment, Miguel revealed that not showing interest in others made him feel safer, since he felt that these kinds of conversations were more likely to lead to more personal questions, which he tended to avoid. For example, at the beginning of the treatment, when he was asked about aspects about himself or his family, he tended to verbalize expressions such as "I don't know" or "I can't remember," with the clear objective of not deepening into the conversation.

From the FAP perspective, it is important to highlight the need for continuous functional analysis in order to be able to conceptualize the patient's behaviors as CRB1s or CRB2s. This depends on various contextual factors that the clinician must evaluate in detail. In this sense, talking about the story of "The Dark Evil" could be conceptualized as both a CRB1 and a CRB2 depending on the moment of the psychotherapeutic process. For example, Miguel beginning to talk about his history at the BHU could be considered as a CRB2, if we understand it as an alternative behavior to the distrustful and inhibited attitude previously observed. However, at other times of the process, it could be categorized as a CRB1 as it represented a barrier to the establishment of a reciprocal interaction. From other perspectives, and especially from models focused on the elimination of clinical symptoms, this behavior would always be considered problematic and, therefore, the role of the therapist would be to prevent it from emerging. These topographical approaches run the risk of missing the adaptive functions of symptomatology, such as the emotional and symbolic expression of suffering.

During the initial interview, Miguel carried his self-published book with him, and he avoided leaving it on the table. He shared that "having The Dark Evil with him made him feel good," without managing to be more specific with that verbalization, although professionals interpreted it as an element that made him feel safe. In line with this, Miguel's difficulty in being able to identify and express his emotions was clear, as he used to get stuck when he was explicitly asked about emotional aspects. At other times, he tended to use terms that did not seem to match his nonverbal behavior. In this sense, he showed great difficulty expressing some specific emotions, such as anger. For example, he frequently used the expression "I am bored," when on some occasions, regarding his speech and his facial expression, it was clear that he was quite angry. He had emotional distance to himself and to the professionals. Although he was really collaborative with the process, he used to act in a way that was "automated" or "robotic."

Regarding the start of treatment in the ADH, Miguel showed agreement, although he did not identify therapeutic objectives or needs in the foreground. Addressing expectations regarding peer interaction in the context of the ADH activities, he showed no interest or concerns about it, expressing that he believed that he "had no empathy."

Miguel's difficulties in identifying both emotions and life goals, as well as the limitations in his emotional expression, could be categorized as CRB1s to be addressed in the context of treatment. It should be noted that, in Miguel's family context, there had not been enough opportunities to train these skills, and even attempts at expression that arose naturally in childhood and adolescence had been punished. Therefore, it was established as the priority objective to convert the therapeutic environment into a safe context that facilitated emotional expression and bonding. In this sense, the use of the FAP rules was especially helpful, as well as some guidelines which have been recently published to generate relational and therapeutic contexts of intimacy (Kanter et al., 2020; Marín-Vila et al., 2020).

In order to facilitate the feeling of safety in the psychotherapeutic setting, the professionals focused the initial interventions on talking precisely about what made Miguel feel safe: "The Dark Evil." In this sense, in Miguel's own words, this character exemplified and symbolized everything "he was not and wanted to be." That is to say, the character was a "determined, strong" person who could face people who had hurt him. Something similar happened when he identified with the figure of the leader, who projected Miguel's wishes to opt for a certain role within the group. It also exemplified the fight against someone who causes harm. To facilitate this initial bonding process, Miguel was invited to share his texts and drawings. He was also asked to describe the process of creating the stories, which were listened to with attention and curiosity. For example, Miguel's main therapist read his book, marked significant pages, and brought the document to sessions to discuss with Miguel in detail. The adolescent was surprised, expressing with emotion that it "made him feel good that someone was interested in his story." These interactions in the context of the therapeutic relationship were an opportunity to establish functional equivalences. They were also useful to carry out different interventions which were alternative responses to the ones that Miguel had received from his natural context when he showed his stories.

Perhaps, some professionals may be concerned about reinforcing symptoms when carrying out interventions such as those described above. Likewise, it must be considered that Miguel's excessive focus on his delusional speech was specifically problematic in his daily context. However, it was considered that this starting point, focused on what was important to Miguel and made him feel safe, could facilitate, in a second moment of the treatment, addressing the problematic symptomatology more easily. Listening to Miguel's story could mean, functionally, paying attention to his expression of suffering.

In this same sense, allowing Miguel to express himself freely, regardless of the content of his messages, was considered as a strategy which had the aim of evoking and reinforcing expressions of the self. This provided, from a functional point of view, a different experience than what was provided by his early attachment figures (Kohlenberg & Tsai, 1991). Being able to respond to his verbalizations in an authentic, curious, and accepting way was an emotionally corrective experience for Miguel. The main goal was giving him a different relational experience: expressing himself in front of other people who did not punish his suffering, but rather showed a genuine interest in him.

Parallel to the individual intervention, active listening and acceptance of Miguel's speech, whatever its content, was integrated within the group therapy context. The priority objective was that he could feel heard, reinforcing any verbalization in the group interactions, despite his restricted speech being a CRB1 to be potentially modified, as mentioned above. In this sense, some situations inevitably arose in which other patients verbalized invalidating expressions such as "how boring you are… you're always talking about the same thing..." or "you always talk about very strange things...." These situations, which were functionally equivalent to those that Miguel experienced with his parents and other adolescents outside the ADH, were progressively worked on bidirectionally. When Miguel gained more distance from his psychotic symptomatology, he was able to become more aware of the impact of his speech on others (CRB2). In this same context, some of the other patients were also able to learn to modulate in a more appropriate way how they provided negative feedback to others, including Miguel.

At the beginning of the treatment, a safe therapeutic context was also established when working with the family. Given their reluctance to go personally to the ADH facilities, progressive participation was facilitated through alternatives that seemed less "threatening" to them, such as telephone contacts and, later, individual interviews. In these interactions, the possible barriers to treatment were gradually addressed, trying to discriminate with the parents their fears and concerns, as well as the explicit elements that provided them security in the therapeutic interaction, contextualizing all these variables in their personal and family history.

After the main objective of establishing the therapeutic alliance with Miguel and his family, identification and expression of emotions were proposed as secondary objectives for all members, as well as the creation of a shared and collaborative narrative about the history of stressful life events and the appearance of the symptomatology. Likewise, multidisciplinary work was done in order to establish basic life habits and routines at home to promote functional recovery. These objectives were related to personal values and the search for a life with meaning for the whole family.

22.2.2.2 Evolution

This section describes the evolution of Miguel and his parents in terms of the objectives set, highlighting the approach to the function of the delusional symptoms in relation to the family and personal history of the patient.

Following the principles of FAP, interpersonal issues were worked on in a specific and detailed manner in the therapeutic context (individual and group). The main aim was to generalize the changes to Miguel's daily life. In this sense, throughout the treatment, interpersonal contexts were created to observe and evoke CRBs (Rules 1 and 2), naturally reinforce the improvements of Miguel and his parents (Rule 3), and functionally interpret the behaviors with the objective of generalizing the changes (Rule 5). The professionals continuously explored the impact of their own behaviors on Miguel and his parents through the explanation and assessment of the psychotherapeutic process (Rule 4).

At the individual level, the professionals worked with Miguel on the identification, understanding, and distancing of psychotic symptomatology, framing its appearance within his biographical history, especially in relation to the different traumatic events, of which he was able to begin to speak in a clearer way. Progressively, Miguel was able to frame delusional symptoms as personal coping responses to intense suffering, attributing his own personal meaning to them. As he began to talk about this traumatic content, Miguel's speech gradually became clearer and less intertwined with the story of "The Dark Evil," which gradually faded into the background in the clinical interviews. This gave way to being able to talk about day-to-day conflicts, such as his difficulties with peers or communication with his parents. That is to say, the story of "The Dark Evil" was progressively acquiring an exclusively literary meaning separate from the life story of Miguel, who took center stage in the sessions. In a very symbolic conversation with his main therapist, Miguel left his book on the table and verbalized: "I can be here with you while my book is on the table. It is not acting anymore as a barrier between us. I don't need it anymore." From that moment on, Miguel began to go to the ADH without his book, which he left at home (CRB2).

This defusion between Miguel and "The Dark Evil" was instantiated through different behaviors. For example, symbolically, it should be noted that he dyed his hair back to his natural color. Progressively, he showed greater capacity for emotional identification and expression, which occurred in parallel with a strengthening of his self-identification, with a greater number of responses under private control. As will be illustrated later in a clinical conversation between Miguel and his therapist, numerous therapeutic encounters took place in which successive approximations of behaviors responsive to the moment (e.g., expressions about himself) were reinforced.

In the individual interventions, Miguel gradually became more confident, sharing more opinions and concerns with the professionals and other patients of the ADH (e.g., little communication with his parents). In this sense, his speech became more spontaneous and with a greater number of emotional nuances. It also became more congruent with his nonverbal expression. The verbalization of desires, thoughts, and emotions was encouraged in Miguel. Deep work on identifying and exploring aspects of his own identity was also done. Likewise, the performance of roles appropriate to his developmental stage was promoted, such as the search for vocational objectives.

At the interpersonal level, a positive development was also observed, both with his family and with other adolescents in his natural context. As Miguel began to feel more secure, thanks to the work carried out in the first phase of bonding, he was progressively more involved in the coexistence of the therapeutic community, establishing significant relationships with other colleagues and being able to work explicitly on some challenging areas (e.g., explaining anger to a peer, clarifying with others some situations that generated suspicion). This, like other contents, was worked on in parallel with work on the patient's interpersonal relationships outside the therapeutic context, so that the changes could be generalized.

To exemplify the latter, below is an excerpt from a conversation between Miguel and his main therapist in which a situation of interpersonal conflict was addressed due to the professional's delay in meeting with him. Note that this conversation took place later in the treatment, and Miguel was more able to identify some internal mental states, as well as to participate in relational exchanges with his therapist.

Therapist (T)	Hello Miguel, I am very sorry for the delay in meeting with you. I've had a mishap. How did it make you feel that we started the session later than usual?
Miguel (M)	I don't know, don't worry *(with a visibly angry tone, without maintaining eye contact)*. After a long silence, he adds: "I don't want to talk now… I don't know… I'm bored."
(T)	I feel that you are more silent than other days. I also notice that you are somewhat angry. I perceive it in your tone of voice and in the fact that you are more distant from me. I think it's normal that you are upset about what happened. I know how important punctuality is to you. However, I also know how difficult it is for you to say that you are angry. Sometimes it's hard for me too. I can't find the words to express it or I don't want to make the other person feel bad.
(M)	I don't know... well, it has bothered me a little... but don't worry…

(T) I understand and I'm very sorry. Next time I'll try to be more punctual or ask someone to let you know if I'm going to be too late. What do you think? Do you have anything else in mind that I could do?

(M) Ok, that would be fine, although I understand that you may have setbacks...

(T) Ok, I will try to do what we agreed. Thank you for understanding that these situations can occur in my work. However, it really helps me to know that these kinds of things don't make you feel good and that they are important to you. Given that, I'll take them even more into account. You were saying that you didn't want to talk and that you were bored. Is that right?

(M) Well… no… I think I was actually angry, but I didn't know how to tell you. I guess I'm afraid to tell you because I don't want you to get mad at me and, because of that, you don't want to see me anymore.

(T) I think I understand what you're saying...some situations are going through my mind in which I've felt something similar. The fact that you told me that you were angry really helps me understand you better. At first, I was noticing that you were more distant. How does it make you feel that I tell you this?

(M) Well... the truth... I'm glad that now you can understand me better.

(T) Miguel, I don't know if what just happened in the interaction with me is similar to what you were telling me the other day about your parents? You told me that sometimes, when you are angry with them, you tend to tell them that "you are bored."

(M) Yes… I tend to do so. I don't know… they don't understand me in those situations.

(T) Yes, regarding what you told me before, I understand that feeling misunderstood must cause you a lot of suffering. You were resisting telling me what you were thinking because of the fear of my reaction. Is that what also happens with your parents?

(M) Yes, that's right. And that makes me feel even more angry.

(T) It seems normal to me. You must feel a lot of helplessness in those situations. Were you also feeling angry before, when you felt that you couldn't really tell me what was happening to you?

(M) Yes, it was making me very angry.

(T) What do you think would have happened today, if instead of sharing that you were angry, you had insisted on saying that you were bored?

(M) Maybe you wouldn't have understood what was happening to me either.

(T) Yes, perhaps it would have been difficult for me to understand the situation and I wasn't able to find a solution. I felt somewhat confused. When you told me that you were really angry, I felt that the situation was clearer and that I could help you better. Do you think something similar could happen to your parents?

As it can be seen in the dialogue between Miguel and the therapist, she helps the patient to identify and express vulnerable emotional states in a safe context, in which all verbalizations are encouraged. This reinforcement is done not only through the validation of emotional experiences, but also through the self-disclosures of the therapist, which allows the normalization of private events and helps the patient to be able to connect to their internal experiences through hypotheses about them. Also, gradually, the therapist helps Miguel so that he can draw parallels between what happened in the session and other situations that occur in his daily life, in this case, in the interaction with his parents. These types of strategies were carried out continuously, taking advantage of the many formal and informal contexts of interaction offered by coexistence within the ADH.

Regarding Miguel's family, his parents gradually became more linked and committed to the treatment. Parallel to the approach carried out with the patient, after establishing a safe psychotherapeutic context, deep work was done with his parents in order to help them to understand the core of their son's problems, as well as the barriers in the family communication. These limitations were framed in terms of the upbringing they had experienced and their own attachment backgrounds. In this sense, the work on values with parents is especially interesting, following some strategies proposed by acceptance and commitment therapy (ACT) (Díaz de Neira Hernando et al., 2016). Miguel's parents began to go to group therapy for parents, where they presented similar progress to their son's. Initially, they tended to remain in the background, with little spontaneous participation and discourse fundamentally centered on their son (CRB1). Progressively, both demonstrated more and more ties to the group and shared more intimate details with the rest of the families.

The main objective of the group therapy for parents is working not only on more effective educational guidelines, but also, and very especially, on their barriers in the parenting process. In this sense, work with the parents usually is from an experiential point of view. It is useful to conduct different exercises that seek to explore their own personal history. In line with this, for example, working in small groups or in pairs and responding to evocative questions can be helpful to work on their own biographical histories and analyze their potential impact on their role as parents (e.g., "When you had a fear or concern in your childhood, who or what helped you calm down?" "If you could change one thing about the way you were raised, what would it be?" "If today you could give advice to the child you were, what would it be?").

This work with the family was carried out through interviews with the parents and through family sessions with Miguel in which the communication between the members in the "here and now" was explicitly addressed. It was helpful to establish functional equivalences between some of the CRB1s observed in interaction with the ADH and the natural context. During the course of treatment, positive changes in family communication were observed, resulting in clearer, more fluid, and reciprocal exchanges. These changes occurred in parallel to those that were being made in the therapeutic context.

22.2.2.3 Psychotherapeutic Termination

After approximately 1 year of treatment, and taking into account the positive progress of both the patient and the family, discharge from the ADH began to be gradually considered. At this point in the treatment, Miguel had been able to frame the appearance of the psychotic symptomatology in the context of different life events experienced and had made substantial emotional and interpersonal improvements. He also had more structure in terms of routines and schedules. In this sense, functional recovery strategies were worked on with him, which included occupational activities outside the therapeutic context, as well as a vocational plan, which consisted of looking for academic options for the following year. On the other hand, his psychiatrist at the ADH had been reducing psychopharmacological treatment throughout the intervention, and Miguel was currently stable without taking any medication.

Intrafamily communication continued to be more fluid, and members were able to talk about conflicts or problematic situations more explicitly, without the continuous guidance of professionals.

In the words of some authors (Tsai et al., 2017), the process of psychotherapeutic termination is especially important and must be addressed explicitly, if possible, from the very beginning of treatment. Although this process, especially after achieving therapeutic goals, can evoke pride in patients and therapists, it can also raise numerous barriers and fears for both, especially after intensive and prolonged treatment. For example, it is common for many patients to experience fear of being discharged, and private events associated with previous situations of abandonment or feelings of helplessness could be reactivated. In this sense, it is especially important to be able to help the patient to identify and express these concerns, not only with the objective to support him or her but also with the aim of potentially working on these private events as another therapeutic target on which functional equivalences can be made. Understanding psychotherapeutic termination as another part of the treatment process can provide opportunities for intervention, as well as give patients an emotionally corrective experience in which they could feel that, perhaps for the first time in their life, they can "say goodbye" to someone in a good manner. Likewise, it is important that the professionals analyze their own T1s and T2s when finishing the psychotherapeutic process. The therapist's self-disclosures at this point in treatment, if they are functionally appropriate, can be especially helpful in facilitating a relationally meaningful termination.

In this context, specific work was carried out with Miguel to make a progressive farewell to both the therapeutic community and his main therapist, with whom he had generated a close bond. In the same way that it is done with other patients in the ADH, Miguel was given control in the process, so that he could decide how he wanted to say goodbye. For example, he was asked to choose if he wanted to gradually stop going to ADH and which days in particular he wanted to go to treatment. To give another example, he was asked to organize a farewell activity with other patients and the staff. This moment was also used to continue working with him on decision making and autonomy, issues with which he presented difficulties at the beginning of treatment.

The individual termination process was carried out in parallel with Miguel's parents' farewells. In this sense, it is important, when working with families, not to underestimate the impact that the end of treatment has for all members. In this context, multiple CRB1s from relatives may emerge that also have to be contextualized in their own biographical histories. Issues such as the fear of losing care and help, concerns regarding the beginning of a new stage or, even, resistance to the patient's improvement due to what it implies about family dynamics must be taken into account in this moment of the intervention.

Finally, it is interesting to describe the process of Miguel's and his main therapist's farewell. A shared narrative was made about the psychotherapeutic process, in which both the therapist and Miguel shared not only the progress, barriers, and challenges perceived during the treatment, but also the relational process that had taken place between them throughout the intervention. In this sense, some exercises such as those described in Tsai et al. (2017), who propose the writing of a letter to end the psychotherapeutic process, can be really useful. In this case, and given the symbolism of writing for this patient, it made special sense to be able to carry out an exercise of this type. The therapist asked Miguel to write a letter in which he had the opportunity to describe his experience during the treatment and his relationship with the professional, while the therapist, on her end, carried out the same action describing her experiences. The fact of receiving a physical letter can symbolically facilitate the grief process for the end of treatment and serve as a kind of transitional object in which the therapist continues to be "present" in the person's life. During this process, it was interesting to hear Miguel's verbalizations that alluded to the meaning of writing for him: "The other day, while I was writing this to you, I thought that now I enjoy doing it. I used to write the story because I needed it to survive… but it wasn't entirely me… it was mostly 'The Dark Evil,' who was also me, but only a part of me. Now I really feel like it's me, finally, writing about me."

22.3 Conclusions

This chapter has described the use of FAP in a case of an adolescent with psychotic symptoms who was treated in the context of an ADH. The intervention carried out reveals several relevant aspects to formulate new proposals for intervention in psychosis.

In the first place, as different authors have indicated (Mørkved et al., 2018; Vila-Badia et al., 2022), the case presentation reveals the importance of attachment and relational issues in the genesis of problems in the psychotic spectrum. These issues have implications for understanding symptomatology (Van den Berg et al., 2022), as well as for intervention. In this sense, it seems important to be able to focus psychotherapeutic approaches on interpersonal issues that go beyond the traditional interventions focused on the elimination of symptoms, and that usually have relegated to the background both the function of symptomatology and the relationship variables that can influence the development and maintenance of patient suffering. Under this prism, approaches such as the one proposed by FAP can facilitate explicit relational work, generating an interpersonal context that allows the patient with psychosis to go deep into his or her suffering within the framework of an emotionally corrective experience.

On the other hand, the case presentation highlights the usefulness of community-based approaches that favor multiple opportunities for personal interaction to intervene in the "here and now" on the relational processes, not only with the patient but also with their immediate relational context. This implies an approach to psychosis that decentralizes the focus on the patient and their symptoms and extends to their most immediate relational context, which includes not only their relatives but also the professionals who care for them, as well as the community institution in which the therapeutic work is framed. In this sense, it should be noted that the institutional values and policies, which on many occasions limit the autonomy of the patient (Sashidharan & Saraceno, 2017) and under which the professional must carry out their professional practice, are relevant factors to consider for the establishment of the therapeutic relationship, because of the impact on both the patient and the professional. It is advisable to be able to address and explain the implications of this type of context with patients, without underestimating the relational impact they have on the person. Consistent with this, it has been observed that the possibility of making choices and to allow the patient to have some control of the process, even in small ways (e.g., being able to decide whether to turn off or not the light in the BHU room), maintains the therapeutic alliance, even though the healthcare context is coercive (Da Costa et al., 2020). The relevance of discussing expectations about therapy or facilitating a collaborative process in terms of tasks is essential to build a good psychotherapeutic relationship with patients with psychosis (Shattock et al., 2017). All these therapeutic strategies could be functionally conceptualized as elements that provide safety to the patient, assuming a first step when establishing an intimate relationship (Marín-Vila et al., 2020).

The establishment of a significant therapeutic bond implies a genuine interest in the way in which patients express their suffering, actively involving the professionals who care for them in the interpersonal relationship established within the framework of the therapy. This presents opportunities for intervention, but also challenges for clinicians, whose barriers may inevitably emerge as they become intensely involved in the therapeutic alliance. In fact, some studies have described therapists' experiences of high intensity when working with patients with psychosis, such as discomfort and distress (Martindale, 2017; Saayman, 2018). These private events can generate avoidance behaviors in therapists (T1) that could make it difficult to establish a bond. Likewise, there are other variables, such as the way in which the professional understands the psychotic symptomatology or the clinician's own attachment style, which can influence the establishment of the therapeutic relationship. On the other hand, other factors, such as the stigma associated with psychosis, from which professionals are not exempt, are variables whose impact on the therapeutic relationship should be analyzed due to their potential impact on the process (Shattock et al., 2017).

Similarly, it should be noted that a better alliance has been found when therapists are perceived as genuine, empathetic, and trustworthy, pointing out that these characteristics could be especially relevant in patients who present suspicion or refer to experiences of prejudice (Shattock et al., 2017). In this sense, given the relationship between the attachment style and the therapeutic relationship, it is essential for the professional to act in opposition to the dysfunctional bonds that the patient has experienced in his or her biographical history, establishing a safe relationship in which the person can go deeper into the suffering (Bowlby, 1988; Tyrrell et al., 1999), as can be observed in the case presented in this chapter.

The issues described above highlight the importance of supervision, self-awareness, and training in interpersonal skills as a way to care for the patients and the therapists themselves. In fact, it seems that psychological flexibility and certain interpersonal patterns that favor social connection could reduce the risk of suffering from burnout in mental health professionals (Ortiz-Fune et al., 2020). In this sense, within the frame of contextual behavioral therapies, and more specifically in FAP, professionals are encouraged to work on their own difficulties from a direct and experiential point of view with the aim of being able to identify their boundaries in the therapeutic process (Kanter et al., 2013; Tsai et al., 2009). Future lines of research could analyze in detail the therapist–patient dyad in the framework of work with psychosis to analyze the processes and private events that arise in the context of this therapeutic relationship.

Finally, it is important to highlight some limitations that FAP presents with respect to the generalization of the results. As with other pathologies in which this approach has been used, the marked idiographic nature of this psychotherapy has limited the results of research, since most studies are limited to the description of clinical cases. Although this individualization of the psychotherapeutic process implies advantages from the clinical point of view, it seems essential to be able to go deeper in the study of transversal processes common to the establishment of intimate relationships, as has been proposed by some authors (Maitland et al., 2017; Kanter et al., 2020; Marín-Vila et al., 2020). Undoubtedly, because FAP, like other more recent models, is based on the therapeutic relationship as a context to promote change at the interpersonal level, the therapeutic process is an issue that requires a specific and detailed analysis. This contrasts with other classic models that focus more on the evaluation of the techniques used and on the evaluation of the change in symptoms.

Despite the limitations previously described, the recent experiences resulting from the use of FAP with people with psychosis (Dykstra et al., 2010; Ortiz-Fune & Marín-Vila, 2021; Sengupta & Singh, 2021), as well as the growing empirical evidence on the importance of relational aspects in the genesis and treatment of this problem, could be a starting point to continue delving into this type of approach with the aim of overcoming the limitations of traditional biomedical models.

Disclaimer Clinical cases presented in this chapter do not include real names or personal information of real persons.

References

Alcamí, M. (1992). *Eficacia del Hospital de Día psiquiátrico infantil*. Tesis doctoral UCM.

Bowlby, J. (1988). *A secure base: Parent-child attachment and healthy human development*. Basic Books.

Brown, G. W., Birley, J. L. T., & Wing, J. K. (1972). Influence of family life on the course of schizophrenic disorders: A replication. *British Journal of Psychiatry, 121*, 241–258. https://doi.org/10.1192/bjp.121.3.241

Bugental, D. B. (2000). Acquisition of the algorithms of social life: A domain-based approach. *Psychological Bulletin, 126*(2), 187–219. https://doi.org/10.1037/0033-2909.126.2.187

Buiza Aguado, C., Uría Rivera, T., Serrano Coello de Portugal, A., Ahijado Guzmán, Z., Delfa Álvarez, A., Frigolet Mayo, P., Ortega Rojo, E., & Rubio Plana, A. (2014). El Hospital de Día-Centro Educativo Terapéutico Pradera de San Isidro. Un dispositivo para el tratamiento intensivo de trastornos mentales graves en niños y adolescentes. *Pediatría atención primaria, 16*(61), 19–32. https://doi.org/10.4321/S1139-76322014000100004

Carr, S. C., Hardy, A., & Fornells-Ambrojo, M. (2018). Relationship between attachment style and symptom severity across the psychosis spectrum: A meta-analysis. *Clinical Psychology Review, 59*, 145–158. https://doi.org/10.1016/j.cpr.2017.12.001

Cohen, S. (2004). Social relationships and health. *American Psychologist, 59*(8), 676–684. https://doi.org/10.1037/0003-066X.59.8.676

Da Costa, H., Martin, B., & Franck, N. (2020). Determinants of therapeutic alliance with people with psychotic disorders: A systematic literature review. *The Journal of Nervous and Mental Disease, 208*(4), 329–339. https://doi.org/10.1097/NMD.0000000000001125

Díaz de Neira Hernando, M., Vidal Mariño, C., González Rueda, S., & Gutiérrez Recacha, P. (2016). Aportaciones de la Terapia de Aceptación y Compromiso al trabajo con madres y padres de niñas y niños atendidos en salud mental: Experiencias de la intervención grupal. *Revista de psicoterapia, 27*(104), 149–165. https://doi.org/10.33898/rdp.v27i104.115

Díaz de Neira Hernando, M., Marín, M., & Martínez, L. M. (2021). Intervención psicoterapéutica grupal en una Unidad de Hospitalización Breve de Adolescentes desde las terapias contextuales. *Revista de la Asociación Española de Neuropsiquiatría, 41*(139), 67–87. https://doi.org/10.4321/s0211-57352021000100005

Dykstra, T. A., Shontz, K. A., Indovina, C. V., & Moran, D. J. (2010). The application of FAP to persons with serious mental illness. In J. Kanter, M. Tsai, & R. Kohlenberg (Eds.), *The practice of functional analytic psychotherapy* (pp. 205–224). Springer.

Fernández, P., & Ballesteros Pérez, F. (2017). La rehabilitación psicosocial de personas con trastorno mental. Un modelo para la recuperación e integración comunitaria. *Edupsykė, Revista de psicología y educación, 16*(1), 15–36. https://journals.ucjc.edu/EDU/article/view/4080

Fernández-León, S., Rodríguez-Testal, J. F., Gutiérrez-López, M. L., & Senín-Calderón, C. (2020). Interpersonal violence and psychotic-like experiences: The mediation of ideas of reference, childhood memories, and dissociation. *International Journal of Environmental Research and Public Health, 17*(12). https://doi.org/10.3390/ijerph17124587

Ferro-García, R., Valero-Aguayo, L., & Lopez-Bermudez, M. A. (2009). The conceptualization of clinical cases from functional analytic psychotherapy. *Papeles del psicólogo, 30*, 255–264. http://www.cop.es/colegiados/GR00777

Figuera, D. (2019). Una experiencia de hospital de día basada en el apego y focalizada en los vínculos. *Revista de la Asociación Española de Neuropsiquiatría, 39*(136), 239–258. https://doi.org/10.4321/s0211-57352019000200013

García-Badaracco, J. E. (1990). *Comunidad terapéutica psicoanalítica de estructura multifamiliar*. Tecnipublicaciones.

Hayes, S. C. (2004). Acceptance and commitment therapy, relational frame theory, and the third wave of behavioral and cognitive therapies. *Behavior Therapy, 35*(4), 639–665. https://doi.org/10.1016/S0005-7894(04)80013-3

Hayes, S. C., Barnes-Holmes, D., & Wilson, K. G. (2012). Contextual behavioral science: Creating a science more adequate to the challenge of the human condition. *Journal of Contextual Behavioral Science, 1*(1–2), 1–16. https://doi.org/10.1016/j.jcbs.2012.09.004

Holt-Lunstad, J., Smith, T. B., & Layton, B. (2010). Social relationships and mortality: A meta-analysis. *PLoS Medicine, 7*(7), e1000316. https://doi.org/10.1371/journal.pmed.1000316

House, J. S., Landis, K. R., & Umberson, D. (1988). Social relationships and health. *Science, 241*(4865), 540–545. https://doi.org/10.1126/science.3399889

Jones, M. (1963). *Beyond the therapeutic community: Social learning and social psychiatry*. Yale University Press.

Kanter, J. W., Parker, C. R., & Kohlenberg, R. J. (2001). Finding the self: A behavioral measure and its clinical implications. *Psychotherapy: Theory, Research, Practice, Training, 38*(2), 198–211. https://doi.org/10.1037/0033-3204.38.2.198

Kanter, J. W., Tsai, M., Holman, G., & Koerner, K. (2013). Preliminary data from a randomized pilot study of web-based functional analytic psychotherapy therapist training. *Psychotherapy: Theory, Research, Practice, Training, 50*, 248–255. https://doi.org/10.1037/a0029814

Kanter, J. W., Manbeck, K., Kuczynski, A. M., Maitland, D. W. M., Villas-Bôas, A., & Reyes, M. (2017). A comprehensive review of research on functional analytic psychotherapy. *Clinical Psychology Review, 58*, 141–156. https://doi.org/10.1016/j.cpr.2017.09.010

Kanter, J. W., Kuczynski, A. M., Manbeck, K. E., Corey, M. D., & Wallace, E. E. (2020). An integrative contextual behavioral model of intimate relations. *Journal of Contextual Behavioral Science, 18*, 75–91. https://doi.org/10.1016/j.jcbs.2020.09.001

Karterud, S., Vaglum, S., Friis, S., Irion, T., Johns, S., & Vaglum, P. (1992). Day hospital therapeutic community treatment for patients with personality disorders. An empirical evaluation of the containment function. *The Journal of Nervous and Mental Disease, 180*(4), 238–243. https://doi.org/10.1097/00005053-199204000-00005

Kohlenberg, R. J., & Tsai, M. (1991). *Functional analytic psychotherapy: A guide for creating intense and curative therapeutic relationship*. Plenum.

Kreyenbuhl, J., Nossel, I. R., & Dixon, L. B. (2009). Disengagement from mental health treatment among individuals with schizophrenia and strategies for facilitating connections to care: A review of the literature. *Schizophrenia Bulletin, 35*(4), 696–703. https://doi.org/10.1093/schbul/sbp046

Leary, M. R., & Cox, C. B. (2008). Belongingness motivation: A mainspring of social action. In J. Y. Shah & W. L. Gardner (Eds.), *Handbook of motivation science* (pp. 27–40). Guilford Press.

Livesley, W. J., Dimaggio, G., & Clarkin, J. F. (2016). *Integrated treatment for personality disorder. A modular approach*. Guilford Press.

Maitland, D. W., Kanter, J. W., Manbeck, K. E., & Kuczynski, A. M. (2017). Relationship science informed clinically relevant behaviors in functional analytic psychotherapy: The awareness, courage, and love model. *Journal of Contextual Behavioral Science, 6*(4), 347–359. https://doi.org/10.1016/j.jcbs.2017.07.002

Marín-Vila, M., Ortíz-Fune, C., & Kanter, J. W. (2020). Modelo conductual-contextual de las relaciones íntimas: aplicabilidad en psicoterapia. *International Journal of Psychology and Psychological Therapy, 20*(3), 373–394. https://www.ijpsy.com/volumen20/num3/558/modelo-conductual-contextual-de-las-relaciones-ES.pdf

Martindale, B. (2017). A psychoanalytic contribution to understanding the lack of professional involvement in psychotherapeutic work with families where there is psychosis. *British Journal of Psychotherapy, 33*(2), 224–238. https://doi.org/10.1111/bjp.12290

McHugh, L., Stewart, I., & Almada, P. (2019). *A contextual behavioral guide to the self: Theory and practice*. New Harbinger.

Mørkved, N., Winje, D., Dovran, A., Arefjord, K., Johnsen, E., Kroken, R. A., Anda-Ågotnes, L. G., Thimm, J. C., Sinkeviciute, I., Rettenbacher, M., & Løberg, E. M. (2018). Childhood trauma in schizophrenia spectrum disorders as compared to substance abuse disorders. *Psychiatry Research, 261*, 481–487. https://doi.org/10.1016/j.psychres.2018.01.011

Ortiz-Fune, C., & Marín-Vila, M. (2021). La relación terapéutica en psicosis desde las terapias contextuales. In J. A. Díaz Garrido, H. Leffite Cabrera, & R. Zúñiga Costa (Eds.), *Terapia de aceptación y compromiso en psicosis. Aceptación y recuperación por niveles* (pp. 485–503). Pirámide.

Ortiz-Fune, C., Kanter, J. W., & Arias, M. F. (2020). Burnout in mental health professionals: The roles of psychological flexibility, awareness, courage, and love. *Clínica y Salud, 31*(2), 85–90. https://doi.org/10.5093/clysa2020a8

Pérez-Álvarez, M. (2006). La terapia de conducta de tercera generación. *EduPsykhé, 5*(2), 159–172. https://journals.ucjc.edu/EDU/article/view/3781

Priebe, S., Reininghaus, U., McCabe, R., Burns, T., Eklund, M., Hansson, L., Junghan, U., Kallert, T., Van Nieuwenhuizen, C., Ruggeri, M., Slade, M., & Wang, D. (2010). Factors influencing subjective quality of life in patients with schizophrenia and other mental disorders: A pooled analysis. *Schizophrenia Research, 121*(1–3), 251–258. https://doi.org/10.1016/j.schres.2009.12.020

Rodríguez, A. (2005). *Plan de Atención Social a personas con enfermedad mental grave y crónica (2003–2007)* (Subdirección General de asistencia técnica y coordinación de planes para personas con discapacidad). Consejería de Familia y Asuntos Sociales de la Comunidad de Madrid.

Saayman, N. (2018). Psychoanalytic psychotherapists' experiences of disturbance in response to working with psychosis. *Psychosis, 10*(4), 329–339. https://doi.org/10.1080/17522439.2018.1534879

Saiz Galdós, J., & Chévez, A. (2009). La Intervención Socio-Comunitaria en Sujetos con Trastorno Mental Grave y Crónico: Modelos Teóricos y Consideraciones Prácticas. *Psychosocial Intervention, 18*(1), 75–88. https://scielo.isciii.es/pdf/inter/v18n1/v18n1a09.pdf

Salgado Pascual, C. F., & Mateos García, M. (2021). La prevención de casos de psicosis ¿es posible? Propuesta de un modelo atencional basado en lo importante para la persona. In J. A. Díaz Garrido, H. Leffite Cabrera, & R. Zúñiga Costa (Eds.), *Terapia de aceptación y compromiso en psicosis. Aceptación y recuperación por niveles* (pp. 313–334). Pirámide.

Sashidharan, S. P., & Saraceno, B. (2017). Is psychiatry becoming more coercive? *BMJ, 357*, j2904. https://doi.org/10.1136/bmj.j2904

Sengupta, U., & Singh, A. R. (2021). Application of functional analytic psychotherapy to manage schizophrenia. *Industrial Psychiatry Journal, 30*(1), 55–61. https://doi.org/10.4103/ipj.ipj_10_20

Shattock, L., Berry, K., Degnan, A., & Edge, D. (2017). Therapeutic alliance in psychological therapy for people with schizophrenia and related psychoses: A systematic review. *Clinical Psychology & Psychotherapy, 25*(1), e60. https://doi.org/10.1002/cpp.2135

Trotta, A., Murray, R. M., & Fisher, H. L. (2015). The impact of childhood adversity on the persistence of psychotic symptoms: A systematic review and meta-analysis. *Psychological Medicine, 45*(12), 2481–2498. https://doi.org/10.1017/S0033291715000574

Tsai, M., Kohlenberg, R. J., Kanter, J. W., Kohlenberg, B., Follette, W. C., & Callaghan, G. M. (2009). *A guide to functional analytic psychotherapy. Awareness, courage, love, and behaviorism*. Springer.

Tsai, M., Gustafsson, T., Kanter, J., Plummer Loudon, M., & Kohlenberg, R. J. (2017). Saying good goodbyes to your clients: A functional analytic psychotherapy (FAP) perspective. *Psychotherapy (Chicago, Ill.), 54*(1), 22–28. https://doi.org/10.1037/pst0000091

Tyrrell, C. L., Dozier, M., Teague, G. B., & Fallot, R. D. (1999). Effective treatment relationships for persons with serious psychiatric disorders: The importance of attachment states of mind. *Journal of Consulting and Clinical Psychology, 67*(5), 725–733. https://doi.org/10.1037//0022-006x.67.5.725

Valdivia-Salas, S. (2016). Ontogénesis del "yo" y distorsiones de la identidad. *Boletín de estudios de filosofía y cultura Manual Mindán, 11*.

Van den Berg, D., Tolmeijer, E., Jongeneel, A., Staring, A., Palstra, E., Van der Gaag, M., & Hardy, A. (2022). Voice phenomenology as a mirror of the past. *Psychological Medicine*, 1–9. https://doi.org/10.1017/S0033291721004955

Varese, F., Smeets, F., Drukker, M., Lieverse, R., Lataster, T., Viechtbauer, W., Read, J., van Os, J., & Bentall, R. P. (2012). Childhood adversities increase the risk of psychosis: A meta-analysis of patient-control, prospective- and cross-sectional cohort studies. *Schizophrenia Bulletin, 38*(4), 661–671. https://doi.org/10.1093/schbul/sbs050

Vila-Badia, R., Del Cacho, N., Butjosa, A., Serra Arumí, C., Esteban Santjusto, M., Abella, M., Cuevas-Esteban, J., Morelló, G., Pardo, M., Muñoz-Samons, D., Group PROFEP, & Usall, J. (2022). Prevalence and types of childhood trauma in first episode psychosis patients. Relation with clinical onset variables. *Journal of psychiatric research, 146*, 102–108. https://doi.org/10.1016/j.jpsychires.2021.12.033

Villero, S., Fuertes, P., León, L., Rodríguez, E., Sánchez-Carpintero, A., & Jiménez, A. M. (2016). Evaluación del Hospital de Día Infanto Juvenil. *Cuadernos de psiquiatría y psicoterapia del niño y del adolescente, 61*, 17–33. https://www.sepypna.com/revista-sepypna/articulos/evaluacion-hospital-dia-infanto-juvenil/

Chapter 23
Dialectical Behavior Therapy (DBT)-Informed Interventions for Psychosis

Maggie Mullen

Dialectical behavior therapy (DBT) is an evidence-based treatment for people struggling with severe emotion dysregulation. Developed initially to treat those diagnosed with borderline personality disorder who commonly experience psychotic symptoms, research over the years has demonstrated its efficacy for a wide range of issues including suicidal thoughts and suicide attempts, nonsuicidal self-injurious behaviors, problematic substance use, depression, bipolar disorder, posttraumatic stress disorder (PTSD), and eating disorders (Niemantsverdriet et al., 2017; Harley et al., 2008; Harned et al., 2014; Hill et al., 2011; Mehlum et al., 2016; van den Bosch et al., 2002; Van Dijk et al., 2013). These issues are commonly co-occurring among people diagnosed with psychotic spectrum disorders (PSD), and yet it is still uncommon for clinicians to offer DBT to these clients to cope with the emotion dysregulation they experience.

This gap between evidence and practice is only one symptom of a more general problem–the social and clinical stigmatization and neglect of people with PSD. People with psychosis face massive barriers to employment and housing, and experience disproportionately high rates of suicide, self-harm, substance use, trauma, institutionalization, and incarceration (Hor & Taylor, 2010; Schizophrenia Commission, 2012; Dallel et al., 2018; Güney et al., 2020). And until recently, the mental health field has mostly overlooked people with PSD. For example, the majority of psychotherapy research trials exclude people who experience psychosis. This is nonsensical because the same types of delusional beliefs occur in other diagnoses, but we do not exclude them from treatment so aggressively. Consider eating disorders, where people experience distorted beliefs about their bodies to the point that they are willing to risk significant health issues, or depression, where people experience distorted beliefs about their self-worth often to the point of wanting to harm themselves.

M. Mullen (✉)
Oakland, CA, USA

J. A. Díaz-Garrido et al. (eds.), *Psychological Interventions for Psychosis*,
https://doi.org/10.1007/978-3-031-27003-1_23

The result is an overemphasis on medication as the primary treatment for psychosis even though psychotherapy is unequivocally effective for PSD. And although medications can be crucial for many people, they often come with harsh side effects that impact quality of life and physical health, and thus result in poor medication adherence that leads to further stigmatization of people with PSD.

For a long time, clinicians and researchers assumed people experiencing psychosis did not experience emotions in the same way as other people because they did not express them through their body language or affect (Kring & Moran, 2008). It is now widely known though that this is untrue, people with PSD commonly struggle with emotion dysregulation and negative or challenging emotions are consistently associated with an increase in paranoid thinking and a predictor of paranoid episodes for this population (Lawlor et al., 2020). The literature on emotion dysregulation in people with PSD is robust, including 25 current studies: 10 cross-sectional, 14 experimental, and 1 meta-analysis (Ludwig et al., 2019). This means that offering treatments such as DBT skills that interrupt and prevent dysregulation is an important component of treatment.

People with PSD often get caught in a vicious cycle where their strong emotions make it more likely their challenging psychotic experiences will worsen, and their psychosis tend to cause their emotions to escalate. For example, a client might share that he is feeling sad and irritated because he got into a fight with a friend. As a result of this increase in emotions, he then experiences more symptoms like hearing suspicious voices saying to him, "you can't trust anyone." In turn, the voices may now make him feel afraid in addition to his initial feelings of sadness and irritation. This cycle can continue, increasing his suspicious thoughts and fearful emotions and ends with him screaming and punching a wall. This is where DBT comes in as a treatment modality: It provides skills for the client to break the cycle of emotion dysregulation.

23.1 Goals of DBT

DBT is *not* a suicide prevention program, as is commonly assumed. It is not focused on keeping clients alive only to have a miserable life. Instead, application of DBT to people with PSD aims to help clients build a life that is worth staying alive for. Each client's life worth living looks unique because it is specifically embedded in their cultural viewpoints, personal goals, and value system. The job of providers is to help clients get there. This perspective of building a meaningful life is critical for people with PSD, who are often discouraged from pursuing their goals as the result of antiquated ideas about the likelihood of recovery for people with severe and persistent mental health issues.

The second goal of DBT is dialectical synthesis, meaning helping clients learn to think in a more balanced way rather than going to extremes and then acting on those beliefs. Put another way, finding what is left out in a client's thinking. This goal is essential for people with PSD who deal with distorted and distressing thoughts that can cause increased anxiety.

In this chapter, I will explore how DBT skills and principles can be used to meet the needs of people experiencing PSD. Because research on DBT as a primary treatment for psychosis is still emerging, I will be discussing DBT-informed treatment rather than strict adherence to the full DBT model, which involves weekly individual therapy and skills class, a consultation team, and phone coaching. The main principles and skills of DBT were set out in Dr. Marsha Linehan's seminal DBT text from 1993, which stated: "In the research demonstrating the efficacy of DBT, patients were screened for active psychosis and organic mental disorders. For a non-research-oriented application of DBT, such screening would be needed only to the degree that significant cognitive impairments such as inability to attend to or grasp skill concepts would prevent patients from benefiting from the skills training" (p.440). DBT strategies reduce emotion dysregulation, including the behaviors clients perform in an attempt to cope with it, such as suicidal ideation, suicide attempts, drug use, and nonsuicidal self-injurious behaviors. The case example I will present utilizes primarily DBT skills and principles while occasionally weaving in other effective psychotherapies for PSD such as CBT for psychosis, prolonged exposure for PTSD, and exposure and response prevention for social anxiety.

23.2 Case Example

I will present "Laila" to demonstrate how I use DBT-informed treatment when working with someone with a PSD. Laila and I worked together for 11 months in an outpatient psychiatry department within a health maintenance organization in the United States. We met weekly for individual therapy, and she also attended my weekly DBT-informed skills group for people experiencing psychosis. In this group, she learned Dr. Linehan's foundational DBT skills class curriculum in a format where each skill and concept was broken down to be easier to grasp and more relevant to the experiences of people with PSD.

To make DBT more accessible to this population, clinicians must ensure that what is offered is concrete, simple, and free of psychological jargon. They also need to ensure the suggestions are accessible, meaning free and easy-to-use options because people with PSD are disproportionately on fixed incomes and likely to experience housing insecurity (Ayano et al., 2019). Lastly, a DBT-informed approach must integrate the reality of societal stigma faced by clients. An environment of stigma, discrimination, and often, violence, shapes their experience. Effective therapy must consider the factors that reinforce or punish certain behaviors clients perform.

For example, I often suggest to my clients that they communicate directly with their voices if distress tolerance options are not working for them. Because of the way others might judge them for doing so, however, we also must discuss the pros and cons of speaking aloud to their voices because of the potential for negative consequences of appearing to talk to themselves.

23.2.1 Overview

Laila (she/her) is a 28-year-old, bisexual, African-American, cisgender woman. She lives in a multigenerational household with her grandparents, sister, and cousins in California. For the last several years, she has worked part-time as a library assistant at the local public library. She has a partner and their relationship is up and down. Outside of work, Laila spends her time taking dance classes and playing video games. While her mental health struggle is significant, she maintains a good sense of humor.

Laila experienced symptoms of anxiety and depression throughout her teenage years but never received any mental health treatment. After her first psychiatric hospitalization at age 20 when she was experiencing command hallucinations telling her to harm herself, distressing beliefs that someone had implanted a chip in her brain, and impairing suspicious thoughts, she was diagnosed with schizophrenia. While Laila reported no known family history of psychosis, she did note an aunt who had never sought treatment but was always considered "pretty crazy and erratic." Laila has since been hospitalized multiple times due to her psychotic symptoms and suicide attempts. She regularly self-harms by cutting herself and smokes marijuana when she is stressed. She was most recently diagnosed with PTSD from childhood sexual abuse and worsened by the trauma associated with events leading up to one of her hospitalizations.

Laila often arrived at our appointments sharing situations that had occurred throughout the week. For example:

Laila reported that she recently became upset (emotionally dysregulated) at work after receiving critical feedback on her performance from her manager. On her way home from work, she heard voices (auditory hallucinations) saying critical things to her, such as "you're such an idiot, you don't deserve to live." In an effort to calm down, she smoked a joint. When Laila eventually arrived home, she experienced suspicious thoughts when her grandmother asked what was wrong and offered to help. Laila reported getting overwhelmed by these thoughts telling her not to trust her grandmother. She became upset and immediately self-harmed by cutting her leg in an effort to release the intense emotions she was feeling. She began to feel shame and isolated herself in her room for the next 36 hours, resulting in her missing work the next day.

Laila showed up to our session that day and had her head hung low, avoiding eye contact with me. She told me that she was worried she had made her situation at work worse by not showing up the next day. I started by validating Laila's honesty and noted that she seemed ashamed of her actions based on her body language. She agreed and said she regretted her decision and noted that "it all happened so fast." In DBT, we strive to balance two seemingly opposite but co-occurring needs:

acceptance and change. Before I could work on helping Laila change, I needed to start by using acceptance strategies, starting with validation.

23.2.2 Validation

I find it is easy to validate people's experience with psychosis. However, both mental health professionals and families often ask me how to validate because they are worried about reinforcing someone's distressing belief (what we formerly referred to as "delusions"). What I typically tell them is to start by validating their client's emotions, which acknowledges their struggle and ensures they feel heard. People with psychosis are often invalidated when they name their suspicious thoughts by others saying to them "that's not real" or "you're crazy." This completely disregards the fact that these experiences are very real to people with psychosis.

I encourage therapists and also loved ones to engage with people experiencing psychosis by validating their emotions first and foremost. For example, I said to Laila "of course you feel scared when you think your family is after you; I would feel that way too." And then ask curious, nonjudgmental questions like "what do the voices say?" and "what makes you worry?" Taking this approach does not mean you agree with their belief but instead you are trying to understand their experience and perspective.

In DBT, we talk about six levels of validation (Linehan, 1997). The first level is perhaps the most straightforward which involves simply being present and paying attention. In level one, you give that person your full attention and show you are listening. That means when I meet with Laila, I make eye contact and nod my head occasionally to show I am listening. Level two is reflecting back what you heard. When Laila explained what happened the day before, I could reflect back by saying, "you got overwhelmed after getting difficult feedback at work and things snowballed from there." The first two levels of validation are commonly used among mental health providers regardless of their therapeutic orientation.

Level three is to put yourself in your client's shoes and imagine the emotions and thoughts they might be experiencing. In this case, I would say to Laila, "I imagine that you were feeling scared when you started having those suspicious thoughts, is that right?" Make sure to include a similar question after to check for accuracy, and ensure you understand their experience.

Level four is to validate based on your client's history. Since I had been working with Laila for a few weeks at this point, I might say to her, "given your history of being discriminated against by your employers both for being Black and having a mental health issue, no wonder that meeting with your manager would make you feel overwhelmed." I was reminding her that her reaction makes sense in her individual historical and cultural context. In contrast, level five involves validating based exclusively on the current circumstances and sharing that the client's behavior makes sense given what happened. I said to Laila, "it makes sense that you'd feel upset after hearing critical voices."

Lastly, level six is radical genuineness which is an essential stylistic component of DBT. Radical genuineness involves communicating as you would with someone who is an equal rather than treating them as a patient. In Laila's case I told her, "I would want to escape too if I was hearing voices saying those cruel things to me that you heard!" Level six offers the strongest validation of the six levels, as the higher you move up the levels the more intensely validating the statement (Linehan, 1997). Keep in mind that all interventions we provide should be culturally responsive, so make sure to adjust your validating statements to reflect your and your client's cultural communication styles. In DBT, providers are taught to be their authentic selves and use irreverence or humor in our relationship with clients. In this case, I might both validate Laila and also joke that her day sounds like it was "very shitty."

23.2.3 Behavioral Chain Analysis

After validating Laila's honesty with me, I helped her think through what she could do differently in the future to ensure a more effective outcome with fewer negative consequences. Every time Laila arrived at a session reporting she had engaged in self-harm, we would start our session with a behavioral chain analysis (Linehan, 2015). This tool helps clients understand the factors that led up to an ineffective behavior by examining the preceding emotions, thoughts, behaviors, and physical sensations, see Fig. 23.1 for illustration. The function of a behavioral chain analysis is to get a clearer picture of what exactly happened as well as the consequences of the problem behavior, and then to conduct a solutions analysis to brainstorm ways that your client can intervene more effectively in future situations (Linehan, 2015, p.143). This is not meant to shame your client for doing something ineffective, but instead to help them understand how to be more skillful and behave in a way that results in a more desirable outcome. Once we have a lay of the land, we could figure out where Laila can be more effective in the future.

I started by asking Laila to identify any vulnerability factors that would have increased her likelihood of experiencing emotion dysregulation that day. Vulnerability factors are the influences that make us more likely to feel emotionally overwhelmed. Examples include when you have not gotten enough sleep, are feeling hungry, have existing stressors, are using or withdrawing from drugs or alcohol, or being in physical pain. These elements decreased Laila's capacity to manage her emotions and also made it more likely her symptoms of psychosis would flare up.

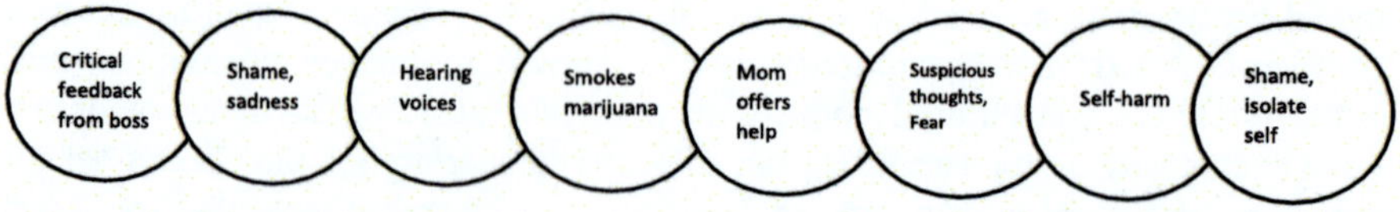

Fig. 23.1 Behavioral chain analysis

Laila observed that she noticed increased anxiety the previous few days and that she accidentally missed her medication dose that morning.

Next, we went through the events of what happened, including identifying the thoughts, emotions, behaviors, and physical sensations she experienced along the way. We started from the prompting event, in this case receiving critical feedback from her manager, and identified each of the links in the chain that led up to her self-harming. This included identifying the thoughts she had that day (e.g., "I'm such an idiot") after the meeting with her manager that resulted in intense shame and sadness, the experience of hearing louder and more bothersome voices that distracted her at work, and the ineffective behaviors she performed in an attempt to cope such as smoking marijuana, which ultimately triggered her suspicious thoughts. We then examined how each of these links impacted each other.

Once we had a clear, detailed picture of what happened, Laila and I focused on solutions analysis. This involves reviewing the chain analysis to identify where Laila could be more skillful in the future to prevent her from getting to the point of self-harming and subsequently self-isolating and missing work.

Initially when Laila and I started meeting, she needed a lot of coaching to identify moments in which she could more skillfully intervene in the future. She found it difficult to identify when she needed to ask for support from others, and would get overwhelmed by emotions and unable to choose which skills to use when experiencing distressing voices. Over the course of 3 months, Laila developed a clearer awareness of the typical cycle she would experience where her stress would increase her emotions, her emotions would increase her symptoms, and so on. By month four, she was able to readily ask for help from her loved ones, use distress tolerance skills such as distraction or self-soothing, and practice emotion regulation skills.

Around this time, Laila learned how to do a behavioral chain analysis herself and would bring it into our sessions following instances of self-harm. The first time this happened, Laila walked into my office saying, "Don't even think about asking me for one of those stupid chains, I already did it!" which gave us both a good laugh and the opportunity for me to praise her skillful behavior, which served as positive reinforcement for Laila. Keep in mind that not all people are reinforced by praise so clinicians need to identify the most effective reinforcers for their individual clients. This can include creative options such as bringing in your client's favorite food to celebrate their victories or even spending the last 5 min of session discussing an unrelated topic of their choosing, such as a favorite television show or hobby.

For the solutions analysis, Laila and I identified the points in this sequence of events where she could have been more effective. I always started a solutions analysis by asking where Laila had already tried to be skillful to understand her attempts at a different outcome. In this case, she shared that she tried to calm down by smoking marijuana. What Laila could also point out though is that marijuana often made her feel more suspicious which typically activated her psychotic symptoms. The function of her behavior in that case was an attempt at self-soothing that unfortunately was not successful. Laila and I would then identify what else might be helpful instead.

Because Laila was having a strong emotional reaction to the feedback from her manager, we started with what she might have been able to do after the meeting to manage her increasing emotions of shame and sadness. Laila noted that starting with distress tolerance might have been helpful since she was in *emotion mind*, meaning her thoughts were driven entirely by her emotions over facts or reason. This state of mind is in contrast to *reasonable mind*, where thinking is exclusively focused on facts and reason and emotion is ignored. DBT aims to help clients find balance in their thinking by finding *wise mind*, where both emotion and reason are valued (Linehan, 2015).

In Laila's case, she identified wanting to use temperature change and progressive muscle relaxation (PMR) immediately after the meeting to try to calm herself down. Temperature change involves simulating the mammalian dive reflex, where your heart rate slows down when your face is immersed in cold water (Linehan, 2015). We discussed ways to make this skill accessible while at work by keeping an ice pack in the freezer that she could readily put on her face while bending over and holding her breath for a brief period. PMR is the practice of tensing one muscle group at a time followed by a release of that tension in an effort to relax your body. Laila indicated that she could do this while in her office at work while listening to a PMR recording from YouTube on her phone.

When Laila recognized that smoking marijuana was not a successful self-soothing method after she began hearing distressing voices, we explored other strategies she could try instead such as urge surfing, distracting herself with videos on her phone, and putting in earplugs. Laila also wanted to be more skillful when her mom offered her help, so we looked at interpersonal effectiveness strategies that could be helpful such as about how to make a skillful request for help or to be left alone temporarily. In an effort to avoid self-harm when she was feeling overwhelmed, I encouraged Laila to make a pros and cons list of whether it would be effective in the long term to engage in this behavior. A solutions analysis allowed Laila to reflect on a difficult situation with a new perspective and identify how she could be more skillful in future situations (see Fig. 23.2).

Each week, Laila was learning new tools in the group session that she could use to navigate her overwhelming emotions. These skills were based on the four modules of DBT: mindfulness, distress tolerance, emotion regulation, and interpersonal effectiveness.

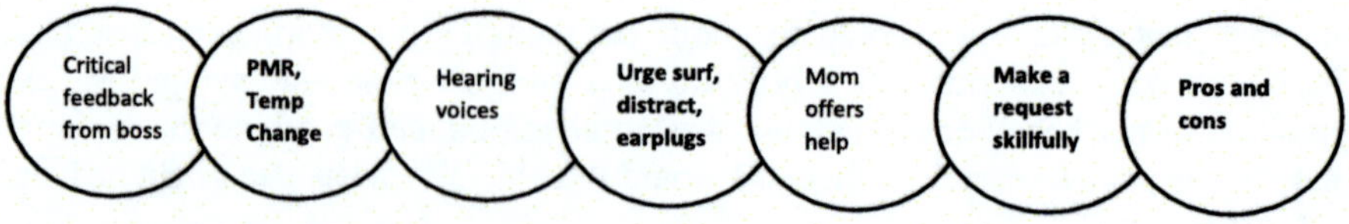

Fig. 23.2 Solutions analysis

23.2.4 Mindfulness

Mindfulness is a foundational approach in DBT. Mindfulness is at the core of all other skills and interventions because we first need to be aware of what is going on for ourselves internally as well as in our external surroundings in order to consider how to handle a situation. For example, Laila first needed to notice she was feeling anger at an 8 (out of 10) level so that she could decide she needed to use skills to deescalate her emotions.

Mindfulness is about taking an in-the-moment, nonjudgmental approach to the world where you are focused on just one thing at a time. Mindfulness is one of the first skills I taught to Laila. Research demonstrates that mindfulness can help people with PSD reduce their depressive symptoms, manage the distress that results from their symptoms by using an acceptance-based approach, and improve negative symptoms (Aust & Bradshaw, 2017; Jansen et al., 2020). General rules for practicing mindfulness with people with psychosis are choosing a shorter duration, providing more verbal guidance than silent time, and including specific mention of psychotic symptoms in a way that is normalizing during the guidance (Chadwick, 2014).

When I worked with Laila I started with mindfulness activities that were approximately 1–2 min in total, based on what she could tolerate that day based on her symptoms. During the mindfulness practice, I would help her focus on her breath, pausing only briefly before providing more guidance to keep her focused. I would mention things like, "If you notice yourself being distracted by distressing thoughts or voices, try to gently bring your attention back to your breath." On days when Laila had trouble focusing inwardly because of overwhelming voices or intrusive thoughts, I would ask her to observe and describe items in her external environment instead. Laila would practice these kinds of mindfulness activities for homework each week to build a regular mindfulness practice.

In addition to specific mindfulness activities, I taught Laila about the principles of mindfulness that can be brought into any activity she is engaged in, such as brushing her teeth, walking the dog, or riding the bus. DBT explains mindfulness principles as the *What* and *How* skills of mindfulness, referring to the skills of what you are doing when you practice mindfulness and how you are doing it. The What skills include observing your experience using all five senses, describing what you notice with words, and participating by throwing yourself fully into whatever you are doing. The How skills include taking a nonjudgmental stance, doing one thing at a time, and focusing on what is effective (Linehan, 2015). I would regularly encourage Laila to practice the principles of mindfulness to notice what was coming up for her when she felt emotionally overwhelmed. By the end of our time together, Laila developed a regular daily mindfulness practice of 5–10 min of guided meditation.

23.2.5 Distress Tolerance

Along with mindfulness, distress tolerance skills were among the first tools I offered to Laila at the start of treatment. Distress tolerance skills manage crises and ultimately help us get through a difficult situation without doing something to make it worse. Examples include distraction, self-soothing with your five senses, changing your physical state, doing a pros and cons list, and urge surfing. As with any skill offered to people experiencing psychosis, distress tolerance skills need to be concrete and accessible. Because of limitations on her income due to working part-time, I ensured that any options I offered Laila were cheap or free, such as going for a walk in the park, talking with a friend on the phone, drinking tea, or using temperature change.

After Laila was able to successfully utilize mindfulness to notice when her emotions felt overwhelming or her urges to engage in problem behaviors were high, I taught her to employ distress tolerance skills to get through those moments of heightened emotion without engaging in self-harm or marijuana use. I started by helping Laila identify what kind of distress tolerance skills she was already practicing as I find most of the clients I work with already engaged in some form of skillful distraction or self-soothing without necessarily calling it that. We found she would sometimes distract herself with a game on her phone or self-soothe by eating her favorite foods when she felt stressed, but she was not yet using these skills with much regularity or awareness. The key to our work was then to help Laila intentionally use these skills in moments of strong emotion as well as to offer her more options so she had many tools in her toolbox.

For instance, when Laila felt the urge to smoke marijuana to deal with intrusive thoughts, I helped her think through what skills she could practice and problem solve around barriers that would get in the way to using them. Laila was a particularly big fan of skills to change her physical state such as temperature change, exercise, and PMR as she felt they worked quickly. Once she noticed the urge to use marijuana went down, she could then deal with the prompting issue–intrusive thoughts–and identify strategies to manage them.

Distress tolerance skills are acceptance-based, meaning they are meant to be used to get through the moment without acting on urges but do not change the current problem (Linehan, 2015). This means that once a client has utilized distress tolerance skills to get back to a place where they can think more clearly, they may need to use other skills from the other modules of DBT to deal with the original problem. In Laila's example, once her emotions felt more in control, she needed to strategize around ways to reduce the intensity of her intrusive thoughts. With coaching, she was able to utilize mindfulness to simply notice her thoughts rather than engaging with them. In addition, she noticed a pattern where her intrusive thoughts tended to be worse when she had not slept well, so she then worked on emotion regulation strategies related to reducing this emotional vulnerability and improving her sleep.

23.2.6 Emotion Regulation

Emotion regulation is another core module of DBT. People who struggle with emotion dysregulation tend to experience their feelings as overwhelming or even explosive. As a result, they may go to great lengths to avoid feeling them. Laila was no exception. She would come into sessions in the beginning of treatment recounting how she would feel completely flooded with anger and shame when her partner said something invalidating to her. She would work hard to suppress her emotions, but without having effective skills to manage them, she would turn to self-harm to release her pain. Emotion regulation strategies work to change existing emotions, reduce the frequency of challenging emotions, and increase pleasurable emotions.

Early in treatment, I introduced emotion regulation strategies that focus on reducing the number of challenging emotions Laila experienced, such as sadness, anger, shame, guilt, envy, or jealousy, and increasing the pleasurable ones, such as happiness, joy, or excitement. Laila and I began by discussing strategies to reduce emotional vulnerabilities such as taking care of her health, developing healthy sleep habits, eating regular meals, and taking her medication as prescribed. In particular, we looked at DBT strategies related to reducing rumination, which was one factor that made it difficult for her to sleep at night. We also problem solved ways to increase her likelihood of taking her medication regularly, such as getting a pill organizer and setting a daily alarm. Laila also noticed that she tended to have more severe psychotic symptoms just before she menstruated, so we identified ways she could manage these. Interventions included scheduling more relaxation during this time, being compassionate and nonjudgmental toward herself, and an evaluation by her gynecologist, who recommended Laila start an oral contraceptive to help with mood fluctuation.

Through evaluation of her daily activities, I learned that Laila was not engaging in almost any pleasurable activities or hobbies. We explored interests that she was willing to engage in that might increase her enjoyable emotions such as dancing to music, spending time with friends, and eating food she loves. Because she often did not notice whether an activity brought her pleasure, I instructed her to do a mood rating before, during, and after each activity so she could assess whether it was in fact helpful. For people with PSD, feeling motivated to engage in activities can be a challenge, so this rating gave her data she could remind herself of in the future. The function behind increasing pleasurable emotions was twofold: One was to tip the scale so Laila experienced more pleasurable emotions than challenging ones; the second was to help her build a life worth living that was intentionally filled with experiences she chooses and enjoys.

Laila and I examined her values to explore what her life worth living looked like. Laila identified her core values as community, integrity, self-determination, creativity, humor, and love. From here, I helped her determine how to use these values to guide her behavior and bigger goals, because when she did so, it increased her pleasurable emotions as well as her sense of self-respect. Laila was particularly excited to set goals of living outside her family's home, getting a dog, improving her relationship with her partner, and going back to school.

Laila regularly experienced suspicious thoughts (e.g., "the government is controlling my thoughts") that would distract her from her activities and increase her emotion dysregulation. When these thoughts arose, I taught her to use the strategy of checking the facts to determine whether her emotions and thoughts made sense based on the current situation. When she noticed her emotions did not fit the facts of the situation because they were unjustified, she would engage in opposite action, meaning doing the opposite of whatever her emotion was telling her to do. In the case of unjustified fear or "paranoia," Laila would approach the situation in spite of her urge to avoid or run away from it.

For people who experience psychosis, checking the facts can be more challenging because they have difficulty differentiating their individual psychotic experiences from others' shared reality. When this came up for Laila, I encouraged her to adopt the perspectives of the people she trusts by asking them to weigh in on the situation. Thus, Laila would ask her grandmother and partner for their interpretation of the situation and then use this information to decide how to proceed.

23.2.7 *Interpersonal Effectiveness*

Interpersonal effectiveness, the fourth and final module in DBT, is focused on learning to be a more effective communicator who can ask for what they want, say "no," and make and maintain relationships.

Having loved ones and a strong social support network is an essential part of many people's life worth living, yet not everyone knows how to build and maintain relationships. Many people with PSD experienced their first psychotic episode during their teens and twenties, a developmentally critical time for refining relationship skills. As a result of the demand to focus their time and energy on their mental health, many people experiencing psychosis do not develop those crucial communication and relationship skills. People experiencing psychosis may also face a number of specific barriers to being effective communicators such as co-occurring social anxiety disorder (SAD), PTSD, negative symptoms, and suspicious thoughts. It is essential to screen for these issues and then adapt the intervention strategies to incorporate these specific issues.

At least 14.9% of people with schizophrenia, for example, meet criteria for SAD, and some research suggests that people with co-occurring schizophrenia and SAD have more lifetime suicide attempts (and specifically more lethal attempts), increased substance use problems, and overall lower quality of life (Achim et al., 2011; Pallanti et al., 2004). Laila met criteria for SAD, so we utilized exposure principles to address this problem by utilizing an exposure hierarchy of feared tasks she could engage in to create new learning that challenged her worries about social engagement.

Additionally, Laila and I role-played different scenarios in our sessions where she utilized DBT's interpersonal effectiveness scripts such as asking for what you want and saying no using DEARMAN, keeping the relationship with GIVE, and maintaining your self-respect utilizing FAST to practice what she might say to others (Linehan, 2015). We also practiced skills specific to making friends and ending unhealthy relationships. After spending time adapting these skills to her cultural communication style, I gave Laila homework assignments to practice these skills throughout the week. Initially, she used her therapy support group as a place to practice these communication skills, and then eventually integrated them into the rest of her life. By the end of our time together, Laila developed a regular routine of identifying when she needed help and then asking for it from her trusted loved ones. She also began building and maintaining friendships after a long period of social isolation.

In addition to SAD, PTSD is common among people with PSD given the number of traumatic experiences people with PSD typically experience such as childhood abuse, homelessness, hospitalization, and incarceration. A recent systematic review of 38 studies found a range of prevalence of co-occurring PTSD of 0–55%, with 30 studies finding a prevalence of 10% or greater (Dallel et al., 2018). Laila met criteria for PTSD, including having regular nightmares, flashbacks, and beliefs about the world being unsafe as well as engaging in avoidance behavior. After life-threatening behaviors are eliminated in stage 1 of DBT treatment, stage 2 involves treating PTSD for clients who meet criteria utilizing DBT-Prolonged Exposure (DBT-PE) therapy. After Laila's psychosis was brought to a more manageable place with the help of DBT-informed treatment, psychotropic medication, and family education and support, she was able to engage in a full course of DBT-PE to treat her PTSD.

23.2.8 Outcomes

After 11 months in treatment, Laila could more effectively manage her emotions as represented by her Difficulties in Emotion Regulation Scale (DERS) score moving from a 108 to a 45. She had avoided engaging in any life-threatening behaviors such as self-harm or suicide attempts in 8 months, and readily used distress tolerance and emotion regulation skills when feeling emotionally overwhelmed. She also implemented a daily mindfulness practice that she had maintained for the last 5 months of our time together. Her work in DBT-PE brought her initial Posttraumatic Stress Disorder Checklist (PCL-5) score down from a 64 to a 28, indicating she no longer met criteria for PTSD.

Laila described her time in DBT-informed treatment as a period of both great difficulty and great success, as she was pushed to work hard, be consistent with her self-care, and be less judgmental toward herself and her symptoms. Laila continued to experience psychotic symptoms throughout our treatment together but she described them as more manageable than before as a result of psychotherapy and medication management. For example, Laila reported being able to hear voices but not having them run her life anymore as a result of her ability to now communicate with them directly and compassionately. She also noted taking a more acceptance-based approach to her symptoms overall so that she could experience distressing or suspicious thoughts without such a strong level of agitation and fear in response to them. She also increased her adherence to her medication by coming to a place of radical acceptance on the role of medication and by creating a more balanced life in which she sought to minimize stress and increase self-care. Laila even made a video for her future self describing why staying on her medications, getting adequate sleep, and taking care of herself were critical to her stability in case she doubted it in the future.

23.3 Conclusion

Emotion dysregulation is a common experience among people with psychotic spectrum disorders. Without proper attention, dysregulation can exacerbate psychotic symptoms and make pursuing a life worth living even more difficult. Dialectical behavior therapy–informed treatment offers the opportunity for people with PSD to become more mindful as they simultaneously work on improving interpersonal relationships, tolerating distress, and regulating intense emotions. Laila's case demonstrates how DBT skills and principles can be used to meet the needs of people experiencing psychosis.

Disclaimer Clinical cases presented in this chapter do not include real names or personal information of real persons.

References

Achim, A. M., Maziade, M., Raymond, E., Olivier, D., Mérette, C., & Roy, M. A. (2011). How prevalent are anxiety disorders in schizophrenia? A meta-analysis and critical review on a significant association. *Schizophrenia Bulletin, 37*(4), 811–821.

Aust, J., & Bradshaw, T. (2017). Mindfulness interventions for psychosis: A systematic review of the literature. *Journal of Psychiatric and Mental Health Nursing, 24*, 69–83.

Ayano, G., Tesfaw, G., & Shumet, S. (2019). The prevalence of schizophrenia and other psychotic disorders among homeless people: A systematic review and meta-analysis. *BMC Psychiatry, 19*, 370.

Chadwick, P. (2014). Mindfulness for psychosis. *British Journal of Psychiatry, 204*, 333–334.

Dallel, S., Cancel, A., & Fakra, E. (2018). Prevalence of posttraumatic stress disorder in schizophrenia Spectrum disorders: A systematic review. *Neuropsychiatry, 8*(3), 1027–1037.

Güney, E., Alnıak, İ., & Erkıran, M. (2020). Predicting factors for non-suicidal self-injury in patients with schizophrenia spectrum disorders and the role of substance use. *Asian Journal of Psychiatry, 52*, 102068.

Harley, R., Sprich, S., Safren, S., Jacobo, M., & Fava, M. (2008). Adaptation of dialectical behavior therapy skills training group for treatment-resistant depression. *Journal of Nervous and Mental Disease, 196*(2), 136–143.

Harned, M. S., Korslund, K. E., & Linehan, M. M. (2014). A pilot randomized controlled trial of dialectical behavior therapy with and without the dialectical behavior therapy prolonged exposure protocol for suicidal and self-injuring women with borderline personality disorder and PTSD. *Behaviour Research and Therapy, 55*(1), 7–17.

Hill, D. M., Craighead, L. W., & Safer, D. L. (2011). Appetite-focused dialectical behavior therapy for the treatment of binge eating with purging: A preliminary trial. *International Journal of Eating Disorders, 44*(3), 249–261.

Hor, K., & Taylor, M. (2010). Suicide and schizophrenia: A systematic review of rates and risk factors. *Journal of Psychopharmacology, 24*(4 Suppl), 81–90.

Jansen, J. E., Gleeson, J., Bendall, S., Rice, S., & Alvarez-Jimenez, M. (2020). Acceptance- and mindfulness-based interventions for persons with psychosis: A systematic review and meta-analysis. *Schizophrenia Research, 215*, 25–37.

Kring, A. M., & Moran, E. K. (2008). Emotional response deficits in schizophrenia: Insights from affective science. *Schizophrenia Bulletin, 34*(5), 819–834.

Lawlor, C., Hepworth, C., Smallwood, J., Carter, B., & Jolley, S. (2020). Self-reported emotion regulation difficulties in people with psychosis compared with non-clinical controls: A systematic literature review. *Clinical Psychology & Psychotherapy, 27*(2), 107–135.

Linehan, M. (1997). Validation and psychotherapy. In A. C. Bohart & L. S. Greenberg (Eds.), *Empathy reconsidered: New directions in psychotherapy* (pp. 353–392). American Psychological Association.

Linehan, M. (2015). *DBT skills training manual* (2nd ed.). Guilford Press.

Ludwig, L., Werner, D., & Lincoln, T. M. (2019). The relevance of cognitive emotion regulation to psychotic symptoms – A systematic review and meta-analysis. *Clinical Psychology Review, 72*, 101746.

Mehlum, L., Ramberg, M., Tørmoen, A. J., Haga, E., Diep, L. M., Stanley, B. H., Miller, A. L., Sund, A. M., & Grøholt, B. (2016). Dialectical behavior therapy compared with enhanced usual care for adolescents with repeated suicidal and self-harming behavior: Outcomes over a one-year follow-up. *Journal of the American Academy of Child & Adolescent Psychiatry, 55*(4), 295–300.

Niemantsverdriet, M., Slotema, C. W., Blom, J. D., Franken, I. H., Hoek, H. W., Sommer, I., & van der Gaag, M. (2017). Hallucinations in borderline personality disorder: Prevalence, characteristics and associations with comorbid symptoms and disorders. *Scientific Reports, 7*(1), 13920.

Pallanti, S., Quercioli, L., & Hollander, E. (2004). Social anxiety in outpatients with schizophrenia: A relevant cause of disability. *The American Journal of Psychiatry, 161*(1), 53–58.

Schizophrenia Commission. (2012). *The abandoned illness: A report from the schizophrenia commission*. Rethink Mental Illness.

van den Bosch, L. M. C., Verheul, R., Schippers, G. M., & van den Brink, W. (2002). Dialectical behavior therapy of borderline patients with and without substance use problems: Implementation and long-term effects. *Addictive Behaviors, 27*(6), 911–923.

Van Dijk, S., Jeffrey, J., & Katz, M. R. (2013). A randomized, controlled, pilot study of dialectical behavior therapy skills in a psychoeducational Group for Individuals with bipolar disorder. *Journal of Affective Disorders, 145*(3), 386–393.

Chapter 24
Personality or Psychosis, a Complex Binomial

Fernando Rodriguez-Otero, Tamara del Pino Medina-Dorta, Karen Codana-Alcántara, Casimiro Cabrera-Abreu, Miguel Acosta-Ojeda, and Jose Luís Hernández-Fleta

The clinical case presented in this chapter is commonly encountered at the clinic of any psychiatrist. The available nosological systems and the reality of clinical work are often incompatible or, at the very least, do not appear to adjust to the reality of any clinician who works with patients, as it is with our case. This clinical case is another example of the complexities of the term psychosis, further, of the intertwined tapestry constituted by personality and psychosis. Perhaps, as has been proposed by some psychiatrists and psychologists, it is time to abandon the category psychosis in search for another one more in tune with our clinical realities (Bentall, 2006; Read et al., 2013).

24.1 Ana's Case

We met Ana 4 years ago. She was referred to our clinic by a relative who happened to be a colleague. At the time, she was 21 years old and had been admitted four times to a psychiatric ward. The first admission took place when she was 18 years

F. Rodriguez-Otero (✉) · M. Acosta-Ojeda · J. L. Hernández-Fleta
Hospital Universitario de Gran Canaria Doctor Negrín, Las Palmas de Gran Canaria, Spain
e-mail: joseluis.hernandezfleta@ulpgc.es

T. del Pino Medina-Dorta
Complejo Hospitalario Universitario Insular Materno Infantil, Las Palmas de Gran Canaria, Spain

K. Codana-Alcántara
Complejo Hospitalario Universitario Materno Infantil, Las Palmas de Gran Canaria, Spain

C. Cabrera-Abreu
University Department of Psychiatry, Queen's University, Kingston, ON, Canada
e-mail: cabrerac@queensu.ca

J. A. Díaz-Garrido et al. (eds.), *Psychological Interventions for Psychosis*,
https://doi.org/10.1007/978-3-031-27003-1_24

old. There was nothing new about her presentation up until then. She had received several diagnoses including the following: borderline personality disorder, transient psychotic episodes, psychotic episode secondary to substances, bipolar disorder with psychotic symptoms, and last, but not least, schizoaffective disorder. Unbeknownst to her, Ana exemplified the anomalies of our current taxonomies, depicting why we still have an interrater kappa coefficient that would not be accepted by any of the other specialties in medicine (Chnura Kraemer et al., 2002). For our first interview, we used the classical format of the psychiatric interview.

24.1.1 From the Psychiatric Interview to the Transdiagnostic Model

Ana attended her first visit accompanied by a relative. She had red hair and her physical complexion was robust, corresponding to the pyknic-cyclothymic body typology described by Kretschmer and Sagarra (1959). There was a predominance of transversal circular measurements, low height, short and thick neck, small but wide hands, with an overall tendency to obesity. She was dressed in a long flowery gown. After a short introduction, I asked her relative to leave the office. The first few questions were dedicated to knowing the scope of her problems, what understanding she had of them, and what treatment expectations she had. She said that she had had problems since her adolescence. Her parents had divorced around that time. She gave a history of bullying at school. She described herself as an introverted person who could change into the devil if she felt attacked. She did not talk much about her childhood, she had very few memories, and the ones she had were somewhat turbulent. Her mother gained custody of her after their separation. She described her mother as an emotionally distant person with difficulties dealing with emotions who had invalidated them constantly if anyone at the household dared to express them. She also described her as a rational and pragmatic person, with a tendency to minimize stressful events and cataloging them as "nonsense." She did not have many memories about her father. The separation was a complicated one in which she lost contact with her father. She regained it afterwards, but at the time she felt that his role in her life was irrelevant. She had vivid memories of her parents arguing constantly over the phone.

When she was 14 years old, she started lacerating her wrists to calm herself down in the face of family conflicts. She reported continuous arguments between her parents due to the divorce. She experienced thoughts of abandonment and feelings of rage, which led to the consumption of cannabis when she was 15 years old. It was also a way to connect and feel accepted by her peers. She noticed that she used cannabis as a tool to escape. After a short while, she was smoking four joints per day. She also reported a history of being sexually abused by a boy whilst at high school: "I never told anybody, they would think I was lying, and I was ashamed to share it" (verbatim). She reported becoming sexually promiscuous around that time. She never shared this information at home.

The presence of feelings of abandonment, the problematic impulsivity she displayed, and her difficulties regulating her emotions were suggestive of a budding borderline personality disorder. However, and despite Ana's clear narrative, she then went on to say that when she was 18 years old, there was a drastic change. When asked what she meant by this, she said that she started hearing female voices in her head telling her she was a whore, a slut, and that occasionally commented on her actions and activities; further, the said voices gave her orders. I asked her if she knew where the voices came from. She angrily answered that she did not know but that the voices had ruined her life. She stopped going out and started arguing with her parents. She angrily punched the wall on several occasions and yelled that she wanted to be left alone. During this first interview, Ana manifested clear disturbances in the content of her thoughts, in which she described thinking her family wanted to hurt her. The presence of abnormal perceptions and clear disturbance of the content of her thoughts made me shift my diagnostic impression to the realm of the psychoses and more specifically to the diagnosis of schizophrenia. I requested several blood tests, which were all normal. She also had a CT scan of her head, which was normal too. In her family history, it is worth highlighting a maternal grandaunt who was admitted to a local psychiatric hospital and died there.

The reader can conclude that we are facing a patient who suffers from a personality pathology in whom, after a while, there is a clear disturbance of reality-testing followed by auditory hallucinations, meeting the criteria of the first-rank symptoms of Schneider (1997), with a previous history of trauma. The question that arose was the following: How can we approach therapeutically a constellation of problems ranging from personality pathology to psychosis without forgetting the role of traumatic events?

24.1.2 Personality and Psychosis, Together or Separate?

Alvan Fienstein (1970) coined the term comorbidity to describe the emergence of another clinical entity in the course of an established illness without an implied relationship of causality, but what happens in the case of a patient with schizophrenia and personality problems? There is a dearth of studies regarding this issue and they follow two approaches: on the one hand, we have the classical perspective of authors such as Kraepelin or Bleuler (1993), in which psychosis is a process that destroys the personality of the patient; on the other hand, psychosis starts during the second decade of life of an individual who has previously expressed a few traits that can be understood as a permanent disposition or inclination to behave in a determined way across different situations. The relationship between psychosis and personality becomes more complex (Hansson et al., 2001).

Among the different questions that our case generates, we should also think about the place of temperament in this interplay of several components. For example, if we use Cloninger's model (Mansueto et al., 2018), patients with psychosis would have a lower score in sensation-seeking, higher in harm-avoidance, and lower again in persistence (which is intimately connected with social avoidance); they will also display negative symptoms inherent to the stable phases of their illness. From the perspective of their character, it is expected to find lower scores in self-direction (immaturity, fragility, and failure in the principle of internal organization) and cooperativity (socially intolerant, not very helpful, and destructive behaviors) in comparison to normal subjects. In our case and in using Cloninger's model, these expected findings were not endorsed, suggesting that the relationship between psychosis and personality is quite complex.

Widiger and Smith (2008) proposes three types of relationship between personality and psychopathology: first, a pathoplastic relationship in which personality and psychopathology are affected; second, a "range" or continuum relationship where, for example, a compulsive personality could be understood as a maladaptive variant of conscientiousness in the Five Factors model, which in the case of psychosis would correspond to a continuum from the schizotypal personality to schizophrenia; and finally, the etiological relationship of personality on psychopathology, such as the case of schizophrenia, in which neuroticism would always be an etiological factor across several psychopathologies. In the case of our patient, the question would be how her personality traits are related to the presence of disturbances in the course and content of her thoughts and if there is a clinical practical model with a view to help her. Be that as it may, there is an added complication to the personality versus psychopathology scenario; I am referring to the presence of a history of trauma. There are many studies connecting the presence of psychotic symptoms with trauma, although a unidirectional causal relationship has been established (Morrison et al., 2003). Besides, it is known that the adherence of these patients and their bonding with the service is not so intense (Lecomte et al., 2008).

24.1.3 Eureka! The Transdiagnostic Models

The need to establish a therapeutic model capable to help Ana was peremptory. It is conceivable to think that Ana's problems go beyond a few labels on axes I and II, hence her problems would require a transdiagnostic perspective. If we were to do this, we could classify Ana's problems in three distinct spheres:

1. Identity problems: In her case, there are problems in the creation of the "I," "I" that has been created after experiencing abandonment and trauma. Her experiences are manifested in the form of delusional ideas and auditory hallucinations.
2. Emotional dysregulation: The absence of tools to regulate her emotions amplifies her problems; if she is not able to regulate her emotions, she will not be able to be effective in her interpersonal relationships.
3. Experience avoidance: In Ana's case, the presence of voices caused a great deal of anxiety, which in turn would lead her to avoid people for weeks and months.

We initially consider dialectical behavioral therapy (DBT) for patients with schizophrenia as outlined in the textbook of Kaplan and Sadock (2018). Our therapeutic gesture was confirmed when we were able to access the *Manual of Dialectical Behavioral Therapy* for patients with schizophrenia of Mullen and Turkington (2021). It is well known that dialectical behavioral therapy is the most used and largest evidence treatment model in the treatment of personality disorders. It was developed by Marsha Linehan (1994), who posited that the problems of the patients resulted from emotional dysregulation with a biological substrate and from the presence of an invalidating environment. The treatment consists of several modules: individual therapy, skills group, telephone coaching, and supervision. In our case, we were familiar with Linehan's model since all the patients attending our service join the skills group. It was decided to include Ana in a skills group of dialectical behavior therapy regardless of her diagnosis. We will now explain the steps we followed with Ana and how was the model applied.

24.1.4 Dialectical Behavior Therapy in Ana's Case

After a few in-depth interviews and establishing that Ana's reality judgment was not intact, we thought it was appropriate to offer her therapy through the public health care system and at the Program for Patients with Personality Disorders regardless of the DSM diagnoses. We wanted to help her using the dialectical behavior therapy model (DBT-M or DBT).

Ana's problems were not very different from the problems of the other patients who attended our service. A multidisciplinary team meeting took place in which the referral of Ana was believed to be an interesting one. Based on the DBT-M on Ana's case, we were able to identify problems of interpersonal effectiveness, problems coping with intolerable emotions, problems to be in the here and now, and problems in the emotional regulation.

24.1.5 First Interviews

Even though Ana had been previously assessed in the private sector, she was interviewed again following the principles of the DBT-M. She was presented with the following problems:

1. For her to accept and stop avoidant behaviors caused by her voices and the content of her thoughts, she would work on basic mindfulness skills.
2. For her to tolerate powerful emotions, distress, and cope with self-harm, she would work on basic distress management skills, where she would have to build a survival kit as a strategy to manage critical situations.

3. For her to improve interpersonal relationships, we proposed a module of interpersonal effectiveness to achieve relationships based on respect.
4. For her to control her anger and cope with fear and all the emotions connected with her psychotic experiences and the family dynamics, we proposed a module dedicated to learning skills to regulate her emotions.

Several basic principles were applied during every interview and during the time she attended the treatment program:

1. Every patient does as well as they can.
2. Every patient wants to improve.
3. Patients need to commit harder and become motivated with change.
4. Patients are not the cause of all their problems, but they have to solve them.
5. Their lives are unbearable as they are living them.
6. Patients ought to learn new behaviors across every context.
7. Patients do not fail; therapists and therapy do.

It is a therapy based on the effectiveness of the therapist, where therapists are as supportive as they can, where validation strategies and the use of dialectic are at the central axis of every approach, and where all principles of behavior are universal and compassion is nuclear, always with a supervising team to avoid burn-out.

24.1.6 First DBT Interviews

The first time that Ana attended our program, we completed an individual interview based on the DBT program that we follow at our service. The following aspects were dealt with:

1. Clarifying goals.
2. Establishing which are the problematic behaviors.
3. Placing those behaviors in the context of the DBT-M.
4. Getting the patient's commitment to keep himself/herself alive and the need to change.
5. Presentation of the skills group, the 24-h rule, the rule of the four sessions, the daily register, and the development of a crisis plan.

Every and each of Ana's problems was contextualized in the DBT-M. In every interview, we used the strategies for change, and we repeated a question we use in every session: Do we understand that you wish to change in the face of the suffering you are experiencing? This question is obviously answered affirmatively by every patient. We go on to explain that we have a good treatment that meets their needs but that it has an inconvenience. To this, the patients ask what that inconvenience is. We then tell them that the only way to change is by learning new skills, such that we teach them, and patients must go on and practice them, but if they think they cannot change or it is not a good time to attempt a change they then can wait. This provocative use of language (Boggiano & Gagliesi, 2018) is also part of the model. The purpose of doing this is to clarify from the outset the strategies of acceptance and change throughout the whole treatment. After three pretreatment interviews, we allowed Ana to join the skills group of DBT.

24.1.7 *Skills Group*

Treatment started with Ana joining the skills group. Concerning the skills group, it is accepted that this module is efficacious in the treatment of problematic behaviors although the ideal therapeutic approach is to complete the whole treatment program. In a public health system, the skills group would allow to treat 10 patients per week for 2 h, who could benefit from an effective part of the whole treatment program of DBT. In this first part of the treatment, we would tackle issues ranging from behavioral lack of control to achieving control of behavioral stability. We will now describe how each part of the group of skills was achieved individually and in the group context.

24.1.8 *Basic Mindfulness Skills*

The adaptation of Buddhist practices to the western context has led to its incorporation in many psychotherapeutic models. Of the many definitions, the one by Kabat-Zinn (2004) summarizes well the whole purpose of our program: "a form of consciousness in which attention is focused on the present moment, without judging what is perceived and with an attitude of acceptance and care." The actual effect of mindfulness on psychosis is possibly related to a change in the perspective of the "I" (Shapiro et al., 2006). There are others who mention a mechanism of decentering (Safran & Segal, 1996). In general, current research posits three interacting elements as mechanisms associated with the improvement that follows mindfulness: an improvement of the attentional control and a better capacity to regulate emotions and to generate changes in the self-awareness or capacity of decentering (Hervas et al., 2016). Concerning the scientific evidence, the available meta-analysis (Jansen et al., 2020) shows a reduction in the number of admissions to hospital and of the symptomatology in general.

When using DBT, all the groups start and finish with the practice of mindfulness. Mindfulness itself is an independent module. This module includes two general elements: what to do and how to do it.

What to do skills:

- Describe.
- Observe.
- Participate.

In patients with psychosis where auditory hallucinations can predominate, we would highlight experiential avoidance; we can assert that when the voices are treated as invasive elements, there is worse result, with an increase in self-isolation, a poorer social functioning, and feelings of loneliness (Pérez-Álvarez et al., 2008).

Mindfulness invites you to observe and describe these experiences with the mind of a beginner without being snared by them. The patient is invited to get close to them, to let us know how they are, if they are strident or deep voices, if they hear them close or far away… In the case of Ana, she could hear them in her head and inside her thorax; they were shrill and female. Throughout the treatment, we were allowed to talk to them and after a while she was able to accept them. Ana was invited to participate actively in the group setting. This was initially very difficult, and we started with simple exercises such as building a phrase in which each of us would say a word or would count numbers and every time the number 5 came up or one of its multiples, patients were asked to say a color. We would keep this counting until we were able to reach number 30.

As reported above, in the second module of mindfulness skills, we covered the how to do it. Here we would do things dispassionately, without judging and accepting.

How to do skills:

- Nonjudgmentally.
- Focus on a single task at a time (one mindfully).
- Effectively.

The first skill, no judging, is based on the separation of opinion from fact, acknowledging what helps and what hurts, not judging for the mere sake of judging. To do this, we use a bell that is rung every time patients feel they are judgmental or they are judged. In Ana's case, a nonjudgmental attitude was important to help her solve the family dynamics; this, aided by the skills of observation and description, allowed her a clear improvement in her relationship with her family. The next skill is based on focusing on a single task at a time; for example, if we are eating, we only eat. In Ana's case, focusing on a single task forced her to participate in the activity at hand without shifting to her voices and thoughts. Whilst attending our program, Ana was able to join a course to gain meaningful employment and was able to complete this activity. Last but not least, the effectiveness skill invited the patient to focus on what works, to adapt to a situation avoiding the "what ifs" and to have clear goals. In Ana's case, this transpired on her capacity to finish the course to gain meaningful employment.

In general, all these basic mindfulness skills are used during and throughout the whole program. They introduce patients to acceptance and to center their efforts on the here and now. Here we should highlight the concept of the wise mind. Anyone who has worked with a DBT model knows that this concept is clearly understood by every patient. Whilst in therapy, we always ask the patient what your wise mind is telling you as opposed to your other two minds, the emotional mind and the rational mind. We know that we are in wise mind state when we can understand different perspectives, when we do not dwell on the "what ifs." The wise mind takes you to a mentalizing perspective, which allows you to reflect about yourself and about others. Linehan defines the wise mind thus: "finding within ourselves the inherent wisdom of each person" (Linehan, 1993).

In the case of Ana, she understood the concept of the wise mind and she would repeat "I asked my wise mind" when trying to solve her conflicts.

24.1.9 Distress Tolerance Skills

Ana had spent her adolescence self-lacerating, and when she started our program, it was usual for her to punch the wall when arguing with her father or when she felt invalidated. Her emotional dysregulation was prominent and led my colleagues to diagnose borderline personality disorder. From a transdiagnostic model, DBT would be directed to treat her emotional dysregulation.

The strategy is based on two principles: first, accepting that pain is part of life, which is a key concept of DBT and takes us to "radical acceptance." Ana had to stop fighting with the voices and to accept them. Furthermore, for her painful history of trauma including sexual abuse, she needed to use the same concept. The second part of this module consists of survival strategies to deal with crises, which are:

1. Stop.
2. TIPP – temperature, intense exercise, paced breathing and paired muscle relaxation.
3. Distraction with the strategy of the wise mind.
4. Relaxation with the five senses and movement.
5. Improving the moment.

The patients are invited to create a survival kit with the skills they have learned; the goal is to be able to use them. We provide them with a card similar in size to the Spanish National Identity card (the size of a conventional credit card) they can carry with them. In Ana's case, her survival kit consisted of the following:

1. Stop: This skill consists of stopping an action, taking a breath from a critical situation, and being able to observe it and to proceed using the wise mind. When we explained this skill to Ana, she told us that she always started with the "P" meaning that the first thing she did was to "Proceed." In time, this skill was her favorite one when dealing with a crisis.
2. Reflecting on pros and cons: This skill consists in preparing a list with the pros and cons of tolerating or not tolerating the distress caused by a critical situation and to also weigh the pros and cons in the long term.
3. Improving the moment: Ana was able to create an imaginary place where she felt safe; she chose the image of one of the beaches of Gran Canaria, finding herself naked and lying down on the sand whilst listening to the murmur of the waves and feeling the pleasant sea breeze.

4. Distraction using the strategy of the wise mind: She chose to complete mental puzzles in her mind.
5. Relaxation with the five senses and movement: Here she would listen to rap music and eat an ice cream while walking by the beach.
6. TIPP: She would reduce the temperature of her face splashing herself with cold water.

24.1.10 Emotion Regulation Skills

The effort to regulate the emotions is a complex one involving the regulation of positive and negative emotions (Gross, 1998). The objectives of the module dedicated to the regulation of emotions include the following:

1. Identify and label emotions.
2. Decrease the frequency of undesirable emotions.
3. Reduce emotional suffering.
4. Decrease emotional vulnerability.

In patients with auditory hallucinations, emotional regulation becomes a complex task. Manfred, Eugen Bleuler's son, considered that the affective problems were at the core of schizophrenia. He used the term emotional dysfunction as an important part of the process of recovery (Palma & Farriols, 2007). Depression, suicidal ideation, social avoidance, posttraumatic sensations, substance use, and problems at the time of forming and maintaining interpersonal relationships are all part of the emotional dysfunction mentioned above (Birchwood, 2003). When using DBT, the goal is to treat the emotional dysfunction by using the skills learned. To this purpose, we asked Ana to fill specially formatted diary cards to track relevant emotions and behaviors:

1. It is well known that emotional problems contribute to the development of delusional ideas and the maintenance of hallucinations (Freeman & Garety, 2003). In Ana's case, identifying her emotions and learning how to observe them helped to reduce the anguish that accompanies these experiences.
2. We also dealt with the so-called postpsychotic PTSD, which relates to the avoidance, hyperexcitability, and distress caused by the psychotic experience (Shaw et al., 2002).

In Ana's case, these were the skills that were tackled during therapy. We came up with a model based on the emotion regulation script that helped us to deal with her auditory hallucinations. We followed the following script:

Triggering event: In her case, we mean the effect of the auditory hallucinations of the patient, which she situated inside her head.

Interpretating the event: In Ana's case, we mean the way in which she gave a status of absolute truth to her hallucinations and to the thoughts that the insulting nature of the voices came from people who wanted to harm her.

Vulnerability factors: This item refers to past traumatic events in Ana's history (i.e., physical and sexual abuse) to which we need to add Ana's insomnia and her tendency to drink excessive quantities of caffeine.

Experimenting and expressing emotions: At times, Ana could experience a sensation of paralysis of all her body; she could not move; some other times, Ana would clench her fists and would punch the wall or self-lacerate.

Labeling the emotions: Ana would display two emotions frequently, fear and rage.

Another skill that became especially relevant in Ana's recovery was her tendency to "check the facts." We suggested a "survey method" consisting of asking friends or trusted people about their opinion of what was happening to her at the time or if her interpretation of the events was a valid one. This strategy allowed her to gain a new perspective of the facts.

Another skill we centered on was the "take the opposite action" skill, which was particularly useful since her emotions did not coincide with the facts. This skill was crucial when managing her fear. We also insisted on the need for her to take care of her physical health and her sleeping habits. Finally, we emphasized the need to increase pleasant emotions and to develop her own values. She started to exercise physically, which she had done since she was a little girl. She also started a cooking course in the context of Gaining a Meaningful Employment program.

24.1.11 *Personal Effectiveness Skills*

One of the main challenges in the process of recovery of patients who suffer from psychosis is, in the words of Anthony (1993), "living a satisfactory life, with hope and contributing to life even with the limitations caused by the illness." Some of the recovery goals are the connection with others, building up optimism and hope, a positive self-identity, finding a meaning in life, and empowerment in the management of your own life (Leamy et al., 2011). In the case of DBT, the skills would help for each of the listed items as principles of recovery. The said skills can be summarized as follows:

1. The attendees must learn to become skilled achieving what they want and need from others.
2. They need to build new relationships and finish those that are destructive.
3. They need to walk a midway in the path of relationships. They need to achieve a balance between acceptance and change.

Patients also need to identify their support systems, including family, friends, peers, mentors, online communities, spiritual and/or religious communities, and health care workers who are part of a stable social environment.

We also worked with patients in widening their social network; if the disorder starts during adolescence or when they are in their 20 s, it is possible that they feel unable to make friends. This is the time when we develop our identity, when we explore our interests, and when we learn to build relationships. If psychosis emerged at this time, it is likely that it took priority over everything else and became an obstacle to building relationships. As a result, the skills to make friends are poor or inappropriate. Making friends can be difficult if you have isolated from the rest of the world. A way of making friends is through sharing common interests, such as hobbies, values, or shared activities. There is always the possibility of finding resources in the community (associations, groups, activities, etc.).

In Ana's case, she was able to break with toxic relationships and to be capable to become more assertive and firmer when defending what she loved and liked in a relationship and avoiding relationship based on dependence.

24.1.12 *Evolution*

After completing the skills group, Anna clearly improved in all the problematic areas. At the time of preparing this chapter, she was dating a young man whom she had met when taking the cooking course; she had not been admitted to hospital for a while and had not self-lacerated. She had also accepted her auditory hallucinations and had improved emotionally too.

24.2 Conclusions

Schizophrenia and psychosis in general are still subjects that generate a great deal of controversy in mental health (Luhrmann & Marrow, 2016). When listening to persons who suffer from mental illness, it is possible to discern those behaviors are modeled when these persons must confront situations that are extremely disturbing and negative, such as traumatic events, abuse, and poverty (Boyle & Johnstone, 2020). Psychosis and schizophrenia amplify the traumatic experiences we have mentioned and, as we have suggested, the division between personality and psychosis appears more imaginary than real.

In the field of psychosis/schizophrenia, using the skills of DBT can be very helpful in the process of recovery, keeping in mind the necessity to keep a transdiagnostic mind, which reflects clinical reality instead of the categorical criteria and the hard core biological perspectives used so far, which have deep and serious limitations.

Disclaimer Clinical cases presented in this chapter do not include real names or personal information of real persons.

References

Anthony, W. A. (1993). Recovery from mental illness: The guiding vision of the mental health service system in the 1990s. *Psychosocial Rehabilitation Journal, 16*(4), 11–23. https://doi.org/10.1037/h0095655

Bentall, R. (2006). Madness explained: Why we must reject the Kraepelinian paradigm and replace it with a 'complaint-orientated' approach to understanding mental illness. *Medical Hypotheses, 66*(2), 220–233. https://doi.org/10.1016/j.mehy.2005.09.026

Birchwood, M. (2003). Pathways to emotional dysfunction in first-episode psychosis. *British Journal of Psychiatry, 182*(5), 373–375. https://doi.org/10.1192/bjp.182.5.373

Bleuler, E. (1993). *Demencia precoz. El Grupo de las Esquizofrenias*. Hormé.

Boggiano, J. P., & Gagliesi, P. (2018). *Terapia Dialéctico Conductual: Introducción al tratamiento de consultantes con desregulación emocional*. Tres Olas.

Boyle, M., & Johnstone, L. (2020). *A straight talking introduction to the power threat meaning framework: An alternative to psychiatric diagnosis* (The straight talking introductions series) (English edition). PCCS Books.

Chmura Kraemer, H., Periyakoil, V. S., & Noda, A. (2002). Kappa coefficients in medical research. *Statistics in Medicine, 21*(14), 2109–2129. https://doi.org/10.1002/sim.1180

Fienstein, A. R. (1970). The pretherapeutic classification of comorbidity in chronic disease. *Journal of Chronic Disease, 23*, 455–468.

Freeman, D., & Garety, P. A. (2003). Connecting neurosis and psychosis: The direct influence of emotion on delusions and hallucinations. *Behaviour Research and Therapy, 41*(8), 923–947. https://doi.org/10.1016/s0005-7967(02)00104-3

Gross, J. J. (1998). The emerging field of emotion regulation: An integrative review. *Review of General Psychology, 2*(3), 271–299. https://doi.org/10.1037/1089-2680.2.3.271

Hansson, L., Eklund, M., & Bengtsson-Tops, A. (2001). The relationship of personality dimensions as measured by the temperament and character inventory and quality of life in individuals with schizophrenia or schizoaffective disorder living in the community. *Quality of Life Research, 10*, 133–139.

Hervás, G., Cebolla, A., & Soler, J. (2016). Intervenciones psicológicas basadas en mindfulness y sus beneficios: estado actual de la cuestión. *Clínica y Salud, 27*(3), 115–124. https://doi.org/10.1016/j.clysa.2016.09.002

Jansen, J. E., Gleeson, J., Bendall, S., Rice, S., & Alvarez-Jimenez, M. (2020). Acceptance- and mindfulness-based interventions for persons with psychosis: A systematic review and meta-analysis. *Schizophrenia Research, 215*, 25–37. https://doi.org/10.1016/j.schres.2019.11.016

Kabat-Zinn, J. (2004). *Vivir con plenitud las crisis: Cómo utilizar la sabiduría del cuerpo y de la mente para enfrentarnos al estrés, el dolor y la enfermedad* (Tra ed.). Nirvana Libros, S.A. de C.V.

Kretschmer, E., & Sagarra, J. S. (1959). *Delirio sensitivo paranoide* (3rd ed.).

Leamy, M., Bird, V., Boutillier, C. L., Williams, J., & Slade, M. (2011). Conceptual framework for personal recovery in mental health: Systematic review and narrative synthesis. *British Journal of Psychiatry, 199*(6), 445–452. https://doi.org/10.1192/bjp.bp.110.083733

Lecomte, T., Spidel, A., Leclerc, C., Macewan, G., Greaves, C., & Bentall, R. (2008). Predictors and profiles of treatment non-adherence and engagement in services problems in early psychosis. *Schizophrenia Research, 102*(1–3), 295–302. https://doi.org/10.1016/j.schres.2008.01.024

Linehan, M. (1993). *Cognitive-behavioral treatment of borderline personality disorder*. The Guilford Press.

Linehan, M. (1994). Acceptance and change: The central dialectic in psychotherapy. In S. C. Hayes, N. S. Jacobson, V. M. Follete, & M. J. Dougher (Eds.), *Acceptance and mindfulness. Expanding the cognitive-behavioral tradition* (pp. 243–260). Guilford Publications.

Luhrmann, T. M., & Marrow, J. (2016). *Our Most troubling madness, 11: Case studies in schizophrenia across cultures* (Illustrated ed.). University of California Press.

Mansueto, G., Palmieri, S., & Faravelli, C. (2018). Parental style and Cloninger's model in psychosis. *Psychiatry Research, 269*, 221–228. https://doi.org/10.1016/j.psychres.2018.08.066
Morrison, A. P., Frame, L., & Larkin, W. (2003). Relationships between trauma and psychosis: A review and integration. *British Journal of Clinical Psychology, 42*(4), 331–353. https://doi.org/10.1348/014466503322528892
Mullen, M., & Turkington, D. (2021). *The dialectical behavior therapy skills workbook for psychosis: Manage your emotions, reduce symptoms & get back to your life*. New Harbinger Publications.
Palma Sevillano, C., & Farriols Hernando, N. (2007). Las emociones en la intervención del primer episodio psicótico. *Aloma, 20*, 307–327.
Pérez-Álvarez, M., García-Montes, J. M., Perona-Garcelán, S., & Vallina-Fernández, O. (2008). Changing relationship with voices: New therapeutic perspectives for treating hallucinations. *Clinical Psychology & Psychotherapy, 15*(2), 75–85. https://doi.org/10.1002/cpp.563
Read, J., Bentall, R., Mosher, L., Read, J., & Dillon, J. (2013). *Models of madness: Psychological, social and biological approaches to psychosis* (The International Society for Psychological and Social Approaches to psychosis book series) (English edition) (2nd ed.). Routledge.
Sadock, B., & Sadock, V. A. (2018). *Kaplan y Sadock. Manual de psiquiatría clínica* (4th ed.). LWW.
Safran, J., & Segal, Z. V. (1996). *Interpersonal process in cognitive therapy*. Ars Aequi Libri.
Schneider, K. (1997). *Psicopatología clínica*. Tricastela.
Shapiro, S. L., Carlson, L. E., Astin, J. A., & Freedman, B. (2006). Mechanisms of mindfulness. *Journal of Clinical Psychology, 62*(3), 373–386.
Shaw, K., McFarlane, A. C., Bookless, C., & Air, T. (2002). The aetiology of postpsychotic posttraumatic stress disorder following a psychotic episode. *Journal of Traumatic Stress, 15*(1), 39–47. https://doi.org/10.1023/a:1014331211311
Widiger, T. A., & Smith, G. T. (2008). Personality and psychopathology. In O. P. John, R. Robin, & L. A. Pervin (Eds.), *Handbook of personality: Theory and research* (3rd ed., pp. 743–769).

Chapter 25
Mindfulness and Compassion as a Path to Recovery and Personal Discovery: A First-Episode Schizophrenia Case Study

Gerardo Rivera, Reiner Fuentes-Ferrada, Edwin Krogh, and Álvaro I. Langer

25.1 Introduction

Interventions based on acceptance and mindfulness, also known as third-generation cognitive-behavioural therapies (Hayes & Hofmann, 2017), have gradually been shown to have a positive impact on the well-being of people with psychosis (Khoury et al., 2013; Li et al., 2021; Louise et al., 2018). A number of protocols have been used in mindfulness-based interventions for psychosis (MBIp); however, researchers have tended to follow the guidelines proposed in the seminal study by Paul Chadwick and colleagues (Chadwick et al., 2005). In contrast, compassion-based therapies have developed more slowly in this field, but they have been shown to be

G. Rivera
Instituto de Neurociencias Clínicas, Facultad de Medicina, Universidad Austral de Chile, Valdivia, Chile

Instituto de Estudios Psicológicos, Facultad de Medicina, Universidad Austral de Chile, Valdivia, Chile

Servicio Nacional de Salud, Región de los Ríos, Chile

R. Fuentes-Ferrada
Instituto de Estudios Psicológicos, Facultad de Medicina, Universidad Austral de Chile, Valdivia, Chile

Centro de Salud Universitario, Universidad Austral de Chile, Valdivia, Chile

Núcleo Milenio para Mejorar la Salud Mental de Adolescentes y Jóvenes (Imhay), Valdivia, Chile
e-mail: reiner.fuentes@uach.cl

E. Krogh
Instituto de Neurociencias Clínicas, Facultad de Medicina, Universidad Austral de Chile, Valdivia, Chile
e-mail: edwin.krogh@uach.cl

J. A. Díaz-Garrido et al. (eds.), *Psychological Interventions for Psychosis*,
https://doi.org/10.1007/978-3-031-27003-1_25

feasible and safe for this population, especially compassion-focused therapy (CFT) (Braehler et al., 2013). CFT integrates multiple fields of research, including developmental psychology, attachment theory, Buddhist psychology, cognitive-behavioural therapy, and depth psychology, focusing on compassion to facilitate changes in the way people feel and relate to their experiences (Gilbert, 2010, 2017).

In this promising context, it is necessary to continue generating scientific evidence obtained through randomized-controlled trials (RCT) and clinical practice (Chadwick, 2014) in order to ensure the implementation of these therapies in usual clinical work, identifying the most suitable one according to the patient's profile, both in high-risk mental states and in first-episode schizophrenia (Langer et al., 2016). However, the maintenance of positive outcomes in the long term and the continuity of mindfulness practices in the transition from research to clinical contexts remain practically unexplored. Also, researchers have paid little attention to the movement of MBIs to compassion training and to how these approaches can complement one another. In this chapter, we seek to address these issues by presenting the case of a young woman with first-episode schizophrenia who took part in an RCT and then continued receiving clinical treatment, at which point CFT was implemented after an increase in the severity of her psychotic symptomatology. To meet these goals, we describe the case and the course of the therapy; furthermore, we present the results of quantitative and qualitative evaluations that complement our analysis of the clinical case.

25.1.1 Case Description

P. is a 25-year-old woman who was diagnosed with schizophrenia in October 2016. The patient describes an uneventful childhood and adolescence. She reports that her family has no history of mental illness. She highlights a period of bullying in her early adolescence and her parents' divorce when she was 13 years old. During that period, she reports being "very shy and anxious around other people". However, she managed to cultivate stable social relationships. Since then, and until the onset of her disease, she painted as a hobby.

Á. I. Langer (✉)
Instituto de Neurociencias Clínicas, Facultad de Medicina, Universidad Austral de Chile, Valdivia, Chile

Instituto de Estudios Psicológicos, Facultad de Medicina, Universidad Austral de Chile, Valdivia, Chile

Instituto Milenio para la Investigación en Depresión y Personalidad (MIDAP), Santiago, Chile

Facultad de Psicología y Humanidades, Universidad San Sebastián, Valdivia, Chile
e-mail: alvaro.langer@gmail.com

At age 19, while pursuing technical studies, roughly over a 6-month period, she began to exhibit symptoms such as feeling watched and having ideas of reference linked to her past bullying experiences, grounded in the notion that unknown people were aware of her situation, together with depersonalization symptoms such as not feeling herself in her body, all of which caused her to withdraw from social activities.

Afterwards, she began exhibiting involuntary movements of her upper limbs and head, associated with psychomotor slowdown and stereotypies which consisted in moving her neck to one side along with both arms, together with the delirious idea that people were laughing at her for wetting herself in public and auditory hallucinations of multiple people telling her about these embarrassing events. These symptoms co-occurred with formal thinking blocks and symptoms of anguish.

The patient's symptomatology became increasingly problematic in her daily functioning and resulted in an intense fear of leaving her home because of the people mocking and criticizing her. In October 2016, her family took her to the psychiatric urgency ward of her city's hospital, where she was diagnosed with first-episode schizophrenia according to DSM-IV-TR criteria.

Her clinicians initiated a psychopharmacological treatment with 1 mg risperidone, with her dosage being increased to 3 mg until she was referred to a specialized centre. They prescribed paroxetine in the subsequent weeks to deal with her anxious symptomatology. The narcoleptic treatment was especially useful in controlling positive symptoms; however, it was fairly ineffective with respect to the patient's negative symptomatology, which included apathy, psychomotor slowdown, and a lack of initiative, while also failing to tackle the persistence of stereotypies, anxiety, and social inhibition. The patient's negative symptomatology increased when a neuroleptic therapy was adopted one month after diagnosis (see Table 25.1).

Afterwards, P. was placed in day hospitalization. This regime was maintained for 5 months, until March 2017. During this period, occupational therapy, psychoeducation, and pharmacological adjustment interventions were conducted. Table 25.1 summarizes the pharmacological interventions implemented since the initial diagnosis.

25.2 Course of the Therapy

The course of the therapy can be divided into four stages: Phase A (only mindfulness-based interventions, from December 2017 to September 2018), phase B (compassion-based therapy, from October 2018 to February 2020), phase C (formal incorporation of both approaches since March 2020 during the pandemic), and phase D (follow-up every three months since 2021 to date). A general description of these phases is presented below.

As part of a research project aimed at evaluating the effectiveness of mindfulness-based interventions (MBIs) for psychosis, P. was given the chance to participate in an 8-session program based on mindfulness training. The intervention was conducted between December 2017 and February 2018 (A.1). Over the following

Table 25.1 P.'s pharmacological treatment

Medication	Maximum daily dose	Duration	Reasons/comments
Antipsychotics			
Risperidone	3 mg	1 month, 2016	Suspended due to low efficacy and increase in negative symptoms
Olanzapine	30 mg	15 months. From November 2016 to March 2018	Replaced risperidone due to low efficacy and increase in negative symptoms
Olanzapine	20 mg	4 months, 2018	Dose was reduced due to metabolic effects, weight gain, and hepatic effects
Olanzapine	15 mg	November 2016 to date	
Antidepressant			
Paroxetine	20 mg	23 months. From November 2016 to October 2018; at this point, dose was reduced to 10 mg due to clinical improvement	Reduced
Paroxetine	10 mg	November 2018 to date	Progressively reduced due to clinical improvement after start of CFT

Table 25.2 Phases of the mindfulness- and compassion-based interventions

Interventions by phase	Duration
Phase A.1, Group MBI	2 months, December 2017–February 2018
Phase A.2, Individual MBI	6 months, April–September 2018
Phase A.3, In-person group MBI	2 months, August–September 2018
Phase B, CFT	October 2018–February 2020
Phase C, MBI and online compassion intervention	March 2020–March 2021 (telemedicine format)
Phase D, MBI and individual compassion intervention	Follow-up every 3 months in person and online as of December 2021

months, she continued to receive individual mindfulness-based treatment with her psychiatrist (A.2), complemented with group exercises in another mindfulness-based program (A.3). Once her baseline pathology re-entered an acute phase, she received individual compassion-based training (B) through CFT (compassion-focused therapy). Afterwards, weekly follow-ups were performed, complemented with group mindfulness-based interventions and compassion practices delivered online from March 2020 to March 2021 due to the COVID-19 pandemic (C). From March 2021 to date, individual interventions combining MBI and compassion (D) have been conducted trimonthly. Table 25.2 summarizes the interventions based on mindfulness and CFT implemented and their duration.

25.2.1 Phase A of Treatment: Introduction to Mindfulness

During the first stage of the mindfulness-based treatment (*Phase A.1*), the patient took part in group sessions. Here, she was trained in breathing and body exploration exercises aimed at familiarizing patients with mindfulness practices and encouraging observation and acceptance.

Afterwards, the patients practised returning to the present, paying attention to their breathing and body, complemented with stretching and mindful walking exercises. Then, they watched an introduction to compassion: a video entitled "compassion for voices" (Charlie Heriot-Maitland, King's College London). In order to help the participants to find ways of reducing the degree of identification with what they are thinking and encouraging them to see thoughts as thoughts, a number of metaphors were used, including "the river with leaves that simply float away" or "the clouds in the sky". This methodology made it possible to identify signs of relapse and establish an action plan. Also, a collage was produced to represent signs and symptoms that one is not feeling well, based on which coping strategies were developed. Finally, relational exercises in pairs were conducted for the participants to analyse what they had learned.

With respect to the patient's pharmacological treatment, olanzapine was reduced from 30 to 20 mg due to metabolic and hepatic alterations found. Metabolic alterations were corrected as a result of this change and no clinical repercussions were observed when reducing psychoactive drugs, except for residual symptomatology. This included motor symptoms, consisting in occasional stereotypies and negative symptomatology, especially social inhibition, which according to P.'s perception had improved during the group workshop.

During this stage (*Phases A.2, A.3*), the patient continued to attend check-ups with a specialist and received individual MBI training, mainly based on breathing and body awareness practices. In addition, she participated in another program of her own accord because she wanted to continue working with other people, which made her feel "relaxed and not judged".

25.2.2 Phase B: The Patient's Psychotic Symptomatology Re-enters an Acute Phase; She Receives Compassion Training

During 2018 (*Phases A.2, A.3*), the patient continued to implement MBI practices in her daily home life, which she mainly used to "relax, concentrate, and be able to pay more attention to things".

During her clinical follow-up, the patient's psychoactive drug dosage remained unchanged, however, her condition re-entered an acute phase in September 2018. This situation was characterized by thinking blocks, increased fear of other people, symptoms of psychotic anguish, and the reappearance of stereotypic movements of the upper limbs and neck, along with the delirious idea of wetting herself and "being judged" by other people, who would become aware of her disease due to this. These stereotypic movements and the delirious fear of wetting herself were associated with strong feelings of embarrassment and self-criticism, together with frustration due to being unable to attain the well-being that she had expected by using the mindfulness-based interventions that she had learned some weeks earlier.

In addition, although lab tests showed that the patient was still suffering from metabolic and hepatic side effects, the decision was made not to fully halt her pharmacological therapy because of the acute state of her clinical condition. Her pharmacological treatment was permanently supervised.

At this treatment stage (*Phase B*), and due to the patient's acute psychotic symptomatology and psychotic anguish, together with high levels of embarrassment and self-criticism, which pharmacological therapy and mindfulness practices had been unable to address, the patient and her clinicians decided to complement their approach with compassion-focused therapy (CFT) instead of the usual mindfulness practices. This new approach, which is presented below, was more helpful in dealing with the patient's acute and subacute stages.

25.2.3 Compassion-Focused Therapy (CFT)

In this specific case, the patient took part in exercises and imagery of compassionate mind training. The exercises sought to elicit feelings that would stimulate a mental state consisting in the ability to generate and sustain compassionate mind images in order to change her mental and emotional states through images that activate her calm and affiliation system. In turn, this system should reduce the activity of the threat system, which, in this patient, consisted in intense anguish associated with the recurrent idea of wetting herself in front of others and her deep embarrassment due to her stereotypic movements and feeling ill again.

The compassion-focused therapeutic approach initially consisted in reminding P. of the mindfulness process, that is, telling her that her mind wanders and that her thoughts are just thoughts and not facts, as are her emotions and movements, which are part of experience. The clinicians explained to her that her mental wandering would persist throughout the practice process and that it was important for her to notice when her mind started to wander, as she would need to return–kindly and gently–to her breathing; however, from this point onwards, she was instructed to do her breathing exercises more slowly and deeply than usual (calm breathing), which made it possible to reduce her anxious symptomatology and increase her feeling of confidence. Over the following sessions, the use of imagery techniques continued, introducing a colour to represent compassion (the "compassionate colour" technique) and generate a feeling of calm and peace that even led to a reduction in her stereotypic movements. The safe place and the compassionate ideal imageries were employed next, with the patient imagining a person she knew and who represented compassion for her due to his/her possession of the essential qualities of compassion, such as wisdom, inner strength, and kindness. Then, the compassionate self-practice was conducted, in which the patient imagined herself as exhibiting the qualities of compassion. The latter practices significantly reduced the patient's anguish symptomatology by opening up space for the characteristic symptoms of her disease without judging them. This led to a reduction in her motor symptomatology through an approach based on a compassionate attitude. In brief, the patient learned to accept her symptomatology and became increasingly capable of preventing and relieving her suffering without judging herself.

25.2.4 Phase C: Clinical Follow-Up with MBI and Compassion During the Pandemic

P. continued to attend regular individual sessions complemented with relational exercises with her mother, using audio recording of techniques that she had already learned. In addition, she attended weekly group sessions as part of her follow-up which consisted in mindfulness and compassion exercises. This situation continued unchanged until February 2020, when in-person sessions were halted due to the COVID-19 pandemic.

However, given the impossibility of holding in-person follow-up sessions, P. joined some of her mental training peers and attended the online program entitled "Mindfulness and compassion in the time of COVID-19" (Phase C). P. took part in weekly sessions, during which she continued to perform mindfulness practices. This program was expanded, being implemented regionally, nationally, and internationally.

In this program, P. continued to engage in practices that she had first learned in 2017:

> Thanks to this online program, I've been able to practice more than before. When COVID-19 reached Chile and my workshops and activities were all suspended, I thought I had no choice but to resign myself and wait for things to return to normal one day, but I got this opportunity to do the online workshop and practice with a computer screen. I really enjoyed the idea of being closer to my peers and reconnecting with them.

During her clinical process in 2020 (*Phase C*), individual online and in-person sessions were conducted in parallel every 3 months. Over a 3-year period, P. received the same pharmacological treatment dosage–the minimum effective doses for her–which benefited her by reducing the classic adverse effects of neuroleptics (weight gain, metabolic effects, extrapyramidal symptoms) and generating a positive impact on her self-esteem. As her positive schizophrenia symptoms disappeared, she became more accepting of her mental disease and more willing to prevent and relieve her motor symptoms whenever they occurred (occasionally), without avoiding the experience but instead being present to deal with them. She remained clinically stable, with no new outbreaks, and exhibited improvements in motivation and functionality. In this context, she developed an interest in going to university at age 24. She enrolled in a visual arts program and simultaneously joined a drawing course.

25.2.5 Phase D: Recovery, Social and Functional Integration

When she entered university (March 2021), she continued attending individual follow-up sessions every 3 months (*Phase D*) but stopped taking part in the online community program that had been set up during the pandemic due to scheduling clashes with her studies. However, she continued to engage in formal contemplative practices every day from Monday to Friday, specifically mindful breathing practices associated with visualization exercises learned in CFT, which she performed while listening to audio recordings personalized by her psychiatrist. These recordings were useful to her in 2021 given her inability to participate in the weekly online meetings that she used to attend.

P. acknowledges that, upon entering university, she experienced intense anxiety symptoms in times of high academic stress. In the most difficult period, she exhibited residual positive symptoms of schizophrenia, mainly motor symptoms, with stereotypies and mental blocks associated with intense anguish that she had struggled with in the past. In these cases, she tended to employ generative practices that she had learned in her individual sessions and then practised relationally with other people. Through CFT, by imagining and visualizing a compassionate ideal or colour, or a being that represented compassion for her, she generated experiences of warmth, safety, and calm, encouraging self-compassion in hard times. In this context, she said: *"I don't mind if I feel another crisis coming, if it comes, I accept it, and I know I have a tool inside me that I can access when I'm in a crisis"*. This was beneficial to P. when interacting with other people, as she did not stigmatize herself due to her mental disease and *"freed herself from the embarrassment"* of having this chronic disease.

The patient has found it easier to imagine and visualize a compassionate figure when she is in a crisis, which enables her to adopt an open attitude and feel safe when a crisis emerges thanks to her mindful state and self-knowledge. She is now aware that her mind is more creative and artistic and knows that generative exercises are more useful in those times. She has discovered that breathing helps her to concentrate at the beginning; then, she is able to calm down and manages to reach the visualization that she has practised and which inhabits her mind.

Feeling more fulfilled and integrated into society, she has managed to make progress in the first year of her program, free from the stigmatization and the self-belief that having a severe mental disease would prevent her from going to university.

Her current symptomatology is only residual. She no longer has delirious ideas and her anxious symptomatology has been reduced, with only occasional motor stereotypies remaining. Given the reduction in her panic symptomatology and her positive and negative symptomatology, along with her feelings of well-being and integration into her social role regarding her peers, students, and teachers, and visualizing her future as an artist, she developed the motivation to study art therapy and integrate her knowledge of mindfulness and compassion to become "a bridge to help others" who are affected by severe mental health pathologies.

25.3 Clinical Follow-Up Results

25.3.1 Quantitative Evaluations

To evaluate the patient, in addition to the clinical evaluation, 6 questionnaires were administered before and after the intervention over a 4-year follow-up period, with evaluations at 3, 9, 12, and 44 months. The following areas were evaluated: general symptomatology (DASS-21), worry (PSWQ-11), affect (PANAS), self-esteem (Rosenberg Scale), well-being (Ryff Scales), and mindfulness (FFMQ). Mean scores are presented in Table 25.3.

To establish whether any statistically significant variations existed between the evaluations, we calculated the Reliable Change Index (RCI) (Jacobson et al., 1984). The RCI determines the smallest change in a self-report measure score that can be considered statistically reliable. This criterion has been used to determine clinically significant changes in mental health research (Ferguson et al., 2002). The RCI formula presented by Jacobson and Truax (1991) is the following: $RCI = (xX - xY)/$

Table 25.3 Mean scores of the scales used to evaluate the effect of MBI and CFT

		MBIp			CFT and MBIp		
Measures	Dimension	Pre	Post	3 months	9 months	12 months	44 months
Mindfulness	Observing	27	28	29	27	31	37
	Describing	33	36	30	30	33	39
	Acting with awareness	24	27	24	25	33	31
	Nonjudging	37	34	26	34	40	34
	Nonreactivity	27	27	33	22	26	30
	Total score	147	152	142	138	163	171
Psychological well-being	Autonomy	20	19	19	19	20	26
	Environmental mastery	25	25	23	25	23	25
	Personal growth	20	20	20	19	20	11
	Positive relations with others	25	25	22	25	25	21
	Purpose in life	25	25	22	24	25	25
	Self-acceptance	20	19	19	19	20	21
	Total score	135	133	125	131	133	129
Affects	Positive affects	33	32	34	33	32	28
	Negative affects	22	21	19	19	11	11
Self-esteem	Self-esteem	38	39	38	39	39	38
Worry	Worry	14	22	16	12	11	14
Depression, anxiety, stress	Depression	1	1	0	1	0	0
	Anxiety	3	2	1	2	2	1
	Stress	3	1	0	2	1	1
	Total score	7	4	1	5	3	2

σ_{diff}, where $\sigma_{diff} = \sqrt{2}(1 - rxy)$. Thus, the RCI is calculated using the difference between the averages of the single case before the intervention (xX) and after the intervention (xY), with this difference being divided by the standard error of the difference (σ_{diff}). Statistical significance is demonstrated if the RCI is equal to or higher than 1.96, being equivalent to a 95% confidence interval (Iverson, 2017).

Mindfulness After the mindfulness-based intervention, the total FFMQ score increased by 4 points and then decreased at 3-month follow-up; however, after the CFT and MBI were completed, it was observed that they had a significant effect on the increase in all the facets of mindfulness. Specifically, the RCI analysis shows that the change between the pre and post scores of the MBIs was significant (RCI = 11.02), as well as at 9- and 44-month follow-up (RCI = 19.83) (see Fig. 25.1).

Psychological Well-being exhibits relatively stable scores across all its dimensions (see Table 25.3). A significant increase can be observed between 9 and 12 months, the period during which CFT and MBI were applied (RCI = 2.11). However, at 44-month follow-up, a statistically significant decrease in the total score (RCI = –6.35) can be observed relative to the pre-intervention score (see Fig. 25.2)

Positive and Negative Affect The positive affects subscale exhibits rather stable results, with a slight decrease at 44 months. The negative affects subscale shows a constant, statistically significant decrease, with the largest effect being found between 9 and 44 months during the compassion-based therapy intervention and MBI (RCI = –31.83) (see Fig. 25.3)

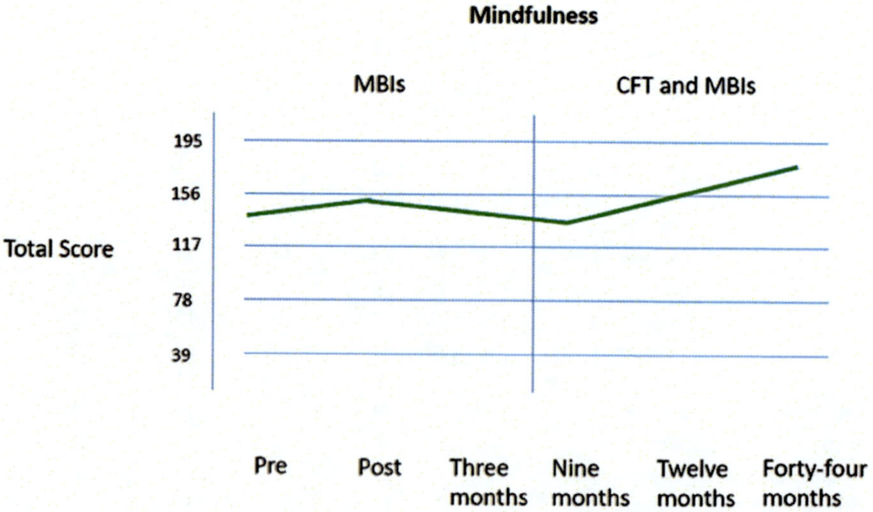

Fig. 25.1 Total scores for the five facets of the mindfulness questionnaire at the six moments of evaluation

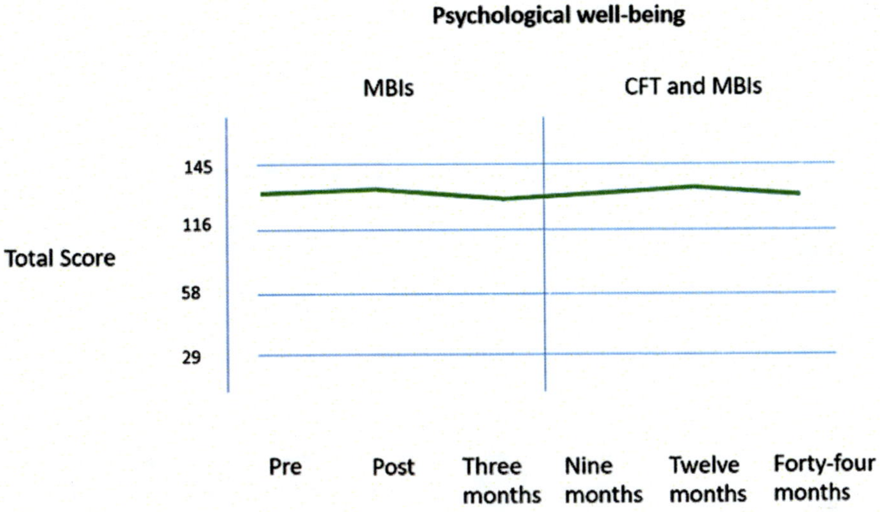

Fig. 25.2 Total scores for the Ryff Scales of psychological well-being at the six moments of evaluation

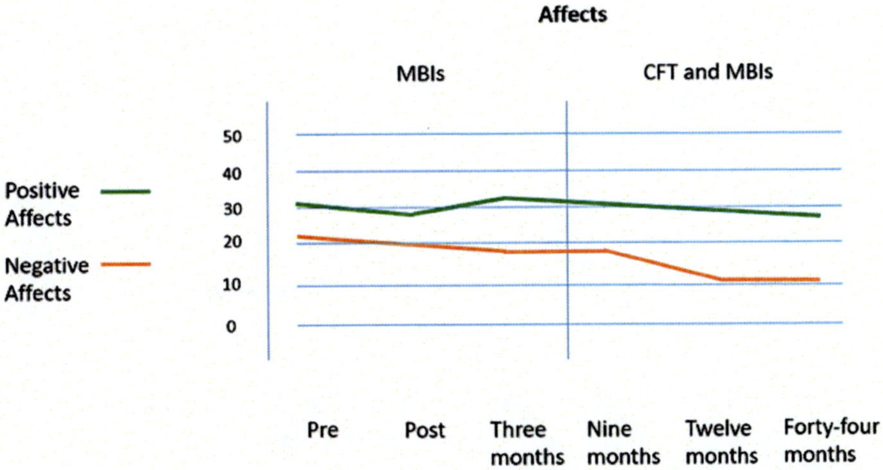

Fig. 25.3 Total scores for positive and negative affects at the six moments of evaluation

Self-Esteem The scores remain stable with single-point variations between evaluations. Only the pre–post MBI increase is slightly significant (RCI = 2.24) (see Fig. 25.4)

Worry Worry scores exhibit a significant increase between the pre- and post-measurements of the first stage of MBI (RCI = 14.15). However, a significant

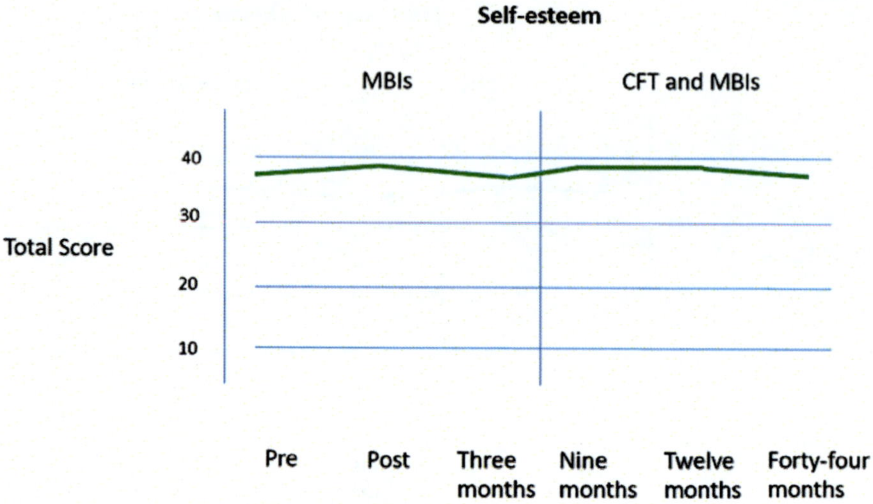

Fig. 25.4 Total scores for Rosenberg Scale at the six moments of evaluation

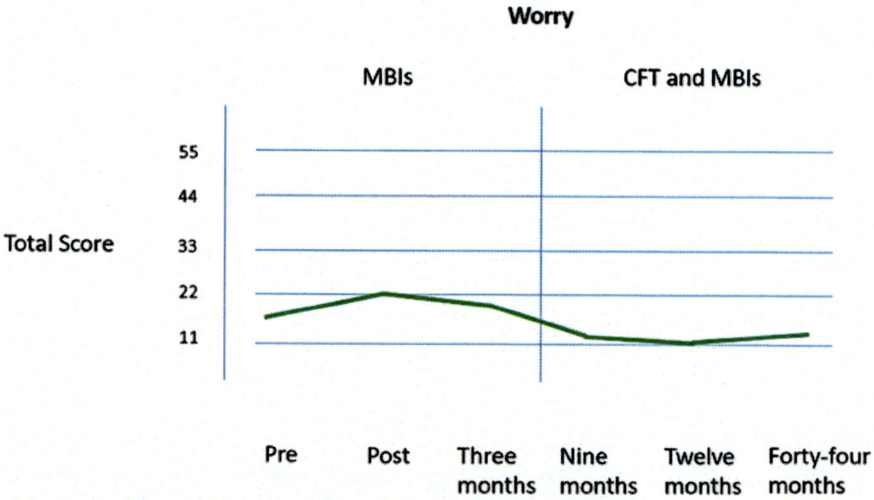

Fig. 25.5 Scores for the Worry Scale at the six moments of evaluation

decrease can be observed between the last MBI follow-up score and the post-measurement of the CFT and MBI (RCI = –19.46) (see Fig. 25.5)

Depression, Anxiety, and Stress A constant, significant decrease in total scores can be observed at pre–post and at 3-month follow-up for the MBI (RCI = –22.09). Likewise, a statistically significant decrease can be observed between the 9- and the 44-month evaluations (RCI = –11.04) (see Fig. 25.6)

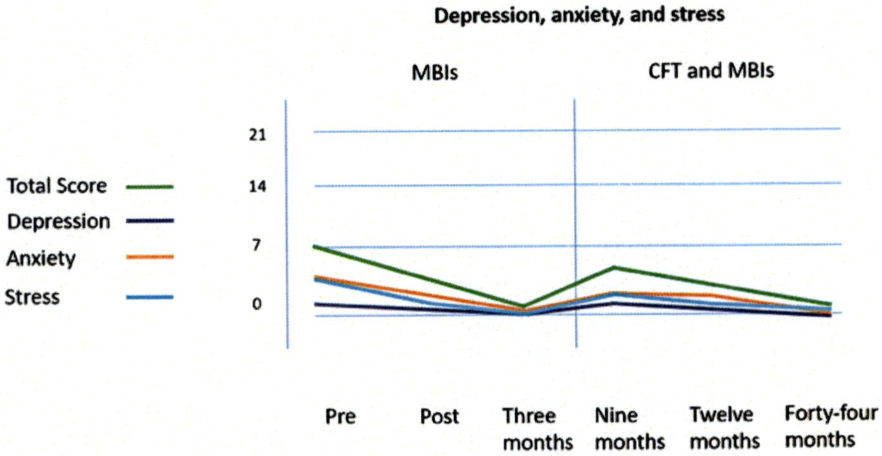

Fig. 25.6 Depression, anxiety, and stress scores at the six moments of evaluation

25.3.2 *Qualitative Evaluations*

This section covers the differences and similarities between mindfulness and compassion practices based on a semistructured interview with P. conducted 12 months after the completion of the first mindfulness training intervention. Specifically, we explored 9 dimensions of both interventions, regarding which P. mentions benefits, difficulties, bodily aspects, and impact on social relationships, among other elements. With respect to compassion, P. highlights her increased ability to recognize and self-regulate her emotions, which enabled her to experience things without judging herself as emotions passed by; in addition, she noticed an improvement in her self-esteem mediated by compassion, which manifested itself through greater affective openness to others and resignified her interpersonal relationships and thus her relationship with herself. She interprets the latter as a "personal tool that can help her find her own path to recovery". The vignette includes verbatim phrases used by the patient when referring to the dimensions studied (see Table 25.4).

25.4 Discussion

In this clinical case, we explored the experiences of a young patient who was dealing with fist-episode schizophrenia. She took part in an RCT (Langer et al., 2017); later on, at her clinical centre, her mindfulness practice was reinforced through individual and group interventions (during Phases A, B, C, and D of her treatment). Regarding the results obtained, the questionnaires administered (pre-, post-, and three-month follow-up measures) do not reflect the importance that P. attaches to mindfulness practice (apart from a slight increase in some dimensions of the FFMQ

Table 25.4 Differences and similarities between MBI and CFT practices in P.'s experience

Dimension	Mindfulness	Compassion
Concept	"It's a practice that is within me, which allows me to concentrate and recognize my breathing and my body"	"It's a tool that allows me to feel love and compassion towards others and also towards myself, through imagination"
Benefits	Indirect self-esteem benefits: "being more relaxed around other people… makes me feel better"	Direct self-esteem benefits. "I use compassion and feel love for myself when I use it with others"
	Attention and concentration improvements; for instance, when she reads, writes, and draws	
Difficulties	"It takes more effort at the beginning". High levels of self-criticism when she fails to attain her objective	"It takes less effort", fewer self-critical feelings. "Compassion practice is more natural"
Most frequent practices	Body scan and breathing-focused mindfulness	Being compassionate/self-compassion
Feelings/ corporality	Emotions connected to a specific area. With respect to breathing, she "feels it on her back"	"General emotion throughout my body, with a feeling that breathing is softer and more pleasant"
Interpersonal and social relationships	"It's an exercise I do with myself, which relaxes me and helps me nearly every time I'm surrounded by other people"	"It's a more fluent exercise that allows me to approach myself and others more kindly. This allows me to interact with people better"
	"I can practise this in a group"	"I can practice on my own and with others"
Emotionality/ affectivity	"I feel peace and calm due to the relaxation that it produces in me"	"I feel love, compassion, and kindness towards others and then towards myself"
Conclusions	"Mindfulness has always been inside me, I can do it on my own, I just need to stop regularly, using my 5 senses"	"These practices have been hugely helpful, because of the love and compassion I feel towards others, that way I can feel compassion for myself and then accept myself". "It's the best tool I've discovered"

and a decrease in general symptomatology). The patient's first-person experience highlights impacts and benefits to her attention, concentration, and memory, which improved her reading capabilities: she noticed that, after conducting mindfulness practices, it was easier for her to remember and integrate what she read. In addition, P. used brief mindfulness exercises as a method for controlling stress and anxiety, noting that *"when I'm surrounded by other people, I use body scan to reduce my anxiety"*. These benefits have also been observed in other qualitative studies (Abba et al., 2008; Dennick et al., 2013), especially in patients with first-episode schizophrenia who have received mindfulness training (Ashcroft et al., 2012). These results confirm the benefits and the feasibility of using mindfulness in a variety of sociocultural contexts and in the clinical treatment of patients with psychosis (Potes et al., 2018).

Throughout P.'s treatment, her symptoms entered another acute phase (phase B) and a subacute phase (phase D). The mindfulness-based tools that the patient was trained to use, together with pharmacological support, were insufficient for coping with these phases. Thus, by incorporating CFT, P. began to manage and accept her abnormal movements and her ideas associated with them. The patient's gradual compassion training led to a decrease in worry and negative affect, which had an impact on the evaluations of the subacute and stabilization phases at 9 and 12 months, respectively. In the stabilization phase, improvements were also observed in the FFMQ dimensions nonjudging, observing, and–mainly–acting with awareness. Therefore, it can be hypothesized that CFT helped the patient to embody the essential qualities of compassion, which include love, wisdom, inner strength, and goodness (Gilbert, 2010, 2017; Neff & Germer, 2013). This allowed P. to see herself more positively and with no prejudices. To exemplify this point, P. says: *"I used to look outside for healing, for a solution to the problem, various therapies, but I realized the problem wasn't outside of me, I realized the disease doesn't define me, but use mindfulness to know myself as I cope with this disease."*

Consider P.'s therapeutic process as a whole, mindfulness training appears to have laid the groundwork for her to benefit from compassion training. Western-style mindfulness and compassion training comprises three dimensions: (1) focused attention, (2) open monitoring, and (3) the cultivation of loving goodness and compassion. However, MBIs prioritize the first two dimensions, whereas the third is the main target of compassion-focused therapies (Salzberg, 2011). Researchers agree that the training of focused attention and open monitoring creates a mental state that encourages the development of compassionate attitudes (Gilbert, 2017). Compassion and self-compassion training can be difficult for meditation novices. Compassion training requires a higher state of intentionality that allows the person who meditates not to resist suffering and opening himself/herself to it (Gilbert, 2017). This intentionality can be achieved by through the practice of mindfulness as such, which P. possibly managed to attain thanks to prior MBIs. It has been observed that mindfulness-based training increases self-compassionate attitudes by 19%, whereas compassion-based therapies increase said attitudes by 43% (Neff & Germer, 2013). In the same vein, Brito and colleagues (Brito-Pons et al., 2018) evaluated whether MBIs were as effective in encouraging compassionate attitudes as compassion-based interventions. Their study compared the ability of MBSR and compassion cultivation training (CCT) to foster compassion, concluding that the latter therapeutic strategy more successfully manages to cultivate self-compassion. Thus, based on the available literature, it can be asserted that even though some common elements can be strengthened through mindfulness and compassion training, these approaches boost specific dimensions of compassion and self-compassion.

Embarrassment was an especially intense symptomatic element in P.'s case; therefore, the benefits of CFT that she observed may indicate that embarrassment is a clinical dimension that can be tackled much more effectively using this therapeutic approach than mindfulness as such (Kirby, 2017). Another interesting aspect of P.'s case was the impact of compassion training on her motor disorder. These abnormal movements are a symptomatic group present in some cases of schizophrenia (Ayehu et al., 2014; Whitty et al., 2009). However, no cases have been reported to date in which mindfulness or compassion training have been able to modify this symptomatic dimension. This observation encourages us to pay closer attention to the possible therapeutic effects of mindfulness training on specific symptoms of schizophrenia. However, it is worth noting that there was nearly no concordance between the self-report questionnaires administered and the patient's experience in domains such as psychological well-being and self-esteem, which were even lower at the last measurement, when P. was starting to attend university and had to deal with more academic stress while interacting with others online. In this context, we can hypothesize that, during this stage (D), P. became more aware of what was happening to her and even managed to identify more clearly her disease-related symptoms and her anxious symptoms that react to her environment. Based on her prior MBI and compassion training (stages B and C), she learned to shift her focus away from what was happening to her, not identifying with her symptoms and responding more efficiently and compassionately to her unpleasant experiences secondary to stress.

It is worth mentioning that we did not use questionnaires developed specifically for this population, nor did we use scales specifically made for psychotic symptomatology or compassion, which could have made it possible to evaluate the patient more accurately. Yet, we consider that it is highly relevant to determine, considering each patient's specific symptoms and the course of his/her disease, when it would be adequate to employ interventions focused on mindfulness or compassion. Although it is not possible to differentiate the additive effect of MBIs on CFT, we can hypothesize that the development of compassion enabled the patient to increase her ability to accept others without judging them or herself, thus resignifying her own attempts to help as compassionate acts and reducing criticism when she "failed" to achieve the desired effect of mindfulness exercises. Regarding her experience with contemplative practices and her increasing familiarity with them, she says: *"In the past, before going out of the house, I often thought, 'I have to think about this or do this other thing to avoid having a crisis'… I was running away from my crises, instead, to accept a crisis is to say 'okay, let it happen' (…) nowadays I let it happen, I have no expectations because I don't know when the crisis can come, so I try to say to myself 'if it happens, that's okay because I can still enjoy the present'"*.

In this context, it would be interesting to study the relationship between mindfulness, compassion, and social cognition in schizophrenia, since authors are nowadays working on cognitive remediation in this field (Rose et al., 2015). Beyond P.'s particular situation, it is interesting to highlight the role of social cognition (SC) and its relationship with practices based on mindfulness and compassion. SC consists in the "psychological processes required to perceive, encode, store, retrieve, and regulate social information" (Mediavilla et al., 2019). Based on this definition of SC, authors have suggested that there exists a relationship of continuity between SC, meditative practices, and psychopathology, ranging from healthy people to others with psychosis or bipolar disease. More specifically, healthy people who meditate are found near the pole with better SC-related skills and those who do not meditate and suffer from severe psychopathology are located near the opposite pole (Gallagher & Varga, 2015). Likewise, there is evidence that SC deterioration is directly related to the negative and depressive symptoms associated with schizophrenia and that MBIs can help to reduce these symptoms; therefore, MBIs can be hypothesized to be effective in improving SC in people with chronic psychosis (Louise et al., 2018). Recent findings in chronic patients show that mindfulness-based interventions aimed at improving SC do not only strengthen this skill, but also help to increase self-care skills, as illustrated by P.'s case (Mediavilla et al., 2021). In this regard, P.'s case can lay the groundwork for more specific studies on the relationship between meditation, compassion, psychosis, and SC, with first-episode psychosis offering rich opportunities for further research development. P. states: *"I'd like to do meditation, I study art to become an art therapist for other people", "Maybe I could help other people to get better, people who have gone through the same things I did, I could help them feel what I feel".*

The present clinical case illustrates how some elements that had not been explored in the mindfulness and compassion literature can be applied to first-episode psychosis (Li et al., 2021), revealing the clinical richness of a patient who manages to continue his/her training in mindfulness and compassion skills after the completion of a study. This was achieved because the treating psychiatrist had received training in said interventions, which enabled him to modify the standard treatment. Furthermore, during the COVID-19 pandemic, the treating psychiatrist generated an online community intervention to continue delivering care through mindfulness and compassion practices, which are essential for strengthening a sense of affiliation and shared humanity among multiple people, both with and without diagnosed mental diseases. P. expresses this in her own words:

> Thanks to the practices of each session, I've learned to connect with what keeps me alive, which is breathing. I've also learned to connect with perseverance, and I see that now I'm more patient and compassionate with myself and others. I've gained more self-esteem, confidence, and tranquillity. I've noticed some changes in my mental disease that make me feel proud and encourage me to keep meditating, so I always try to recommend practices of this type to all those who need them. This is a sort of virtual meeting that brings us together around the emotion of the heart. It teaches us and guides us in our daily lives. I remember one time a partner at the healthcare centre workshop said all this would become huge one day, and now what she said has come true. We're a big community of love and compassion that, in my opinion, has grown and will continue to grow because it is good for us, it heals us and frees us.

Another relevant aspect to consider is that the patient's clinical follow-up lasted nearly 4 years. This period made it possible to get a broad view of the clinical course of the patient's disease, including her second acute phase and her entry to university in 2021. Therefore, all the strategies used played a key role in helping P. to develop a personal base of confidence and empowerment, allowing her to integrate her disease as one of many aspects of her life without depriving her from a meaningful life.

25.5 Conclusion

It can be noted that both mindfulness and compassion (in their various formats) are used as of this writing by P. according to her needs and requirements in a way that is harmoniously integrated into her life. In this context, the patient concludes that one of the main lessons of this whole process is that *"the power of healing is within me and comes from within myself... that's the best tool I've discovered, and it's been helpful"*. This quote reinforces and illustrates the view that a comprehensive and timely care-based approach to schizophrenia is essential for achieving recovery and allowing patients to find themselves.

Acknowledgements The authors wish to thank P. for her generous decision to share her experience during the treatment process. This study was partly funded by FONDECYT No. 11150846, ANID–Programa Iniciativa Científica Milenio [Millennium Scientific Initiative]–NCS2021_081e ICS13_005.

Ethical Statement This study was conducted in accordance with the Declaration of Helsinki. We obtained the patient's informed consent in writing before publication. The patient grants her permission for her information to be published in this case report.

References

Abba, N., Chadwick, P., & Stevenson, C. (2008). Responding mindfully to distressing psychosis: A grounded theory analysis. *Psychotherapy Research, 18*(1), 77–87. https://doi.org/10.1080/10503300701367992

Ashcroft, K., Barrow, F., Lee, R., & MacKinnon, K. (2012). Mindfulness groups for early psychosis: A qualitative study. *Psychology and Psychotherapy: Theory, Research and Practice, 85*(3), 327–334. https://doi.org/10.1111/j.2044-8341.2011.02031.x

Ayehu, M., Shibre, T., Milkias, B., & Fekadu, A. (2014). Movement disorders in neuroleptic-naïve patients with schizophrenia spectrum disorders. *BMC Psychiatry, 14*(1), 1–7. https://doi.org/10.1186/s12888-014-0280-

Braehler, C., Gumley, A., Harper, J., Wallace, S., Norrie, J., & Gilbert, P. (2013). Exploring change processes in compassion focused therapy in psychosis: Results of a feasibility randomized controlled trial. *British Journal of Clinical Psychology, 52*(2), 199–214. https://doi.org/10.1111/bjc.12009

Brito-Pons, G., Campos, D., & Cebolla, A. (2018). Implicit or explicit compassion? Effects of compassion cultivation training and comparison with mindfulness-based stress reduction. *Mindfulness, 9*(5), 1494–1508.

Chadwick, P. (2014). Mindfulness for psychosis. *The British Journal of Psychiatry, 204*(5), 333–334.

Chadwick, P., Taylor, K., & Abba, N. (2005). Mindfulness groups for people with psychosis. *Behavioural and Cognitive Psychotherapy, 33*(3), 351–359.

Dennick, L., Fox, A., & Walter-Brice, A. (2013). Mindfulness groups for people experiencing distressing psychosis: An interpretative phenomenological analysis. *Mental Health Review Journal.* https://doi.org/10.1108/13619321311310096

Ferguson, R., Robinson, A., & Splaine, M. (2002). Use of the reliable change index to evaluate clinical significance in SF-36 outcomes. *Quality of Life Research, 11*(6), 509–516.

Gallagher, S., & Varga, S. (2015). Social cognition and psychopathology: A critical overview. *World Psychiatry, 14*(1), 5–14. https://doi.org/10.1002/wps.20173

Gilbert, P. (2010). *Compassion focused therapy: Distinctive features. The CBT distinctive features series*. Routledge.

Gilbert, P. (Ed.). (2017). *Compassion: Concepts, research and applications*. Taylor & Francis.

Hayes, S., & Hofmann, S. (2017). The third wave of cognitive behavioral therapy and the rise of process-based care. *World Psychiatry, 16*(3), 245.

Iverson, G. (2017). Reliable change index. *Encyclopedia of Clinical Neuropsychology*, 1–4. https://doi.org/10.1007/978-3-319-56782-2_1242-2

Jacobson, N., & Truax, P. (1991). Clinical significance: A statistical approach to defining meaningful change in psychotherapy-research. *Journal of Consulting and Clinical Psychology, 59*, 12–19.

Jacobson, N., Follette, W., & Revenstorf, D. (1984). Psychotherapy outcome research: Methods for reporting variability and evaluating clinical significance. *Behaviour Therapy, 15*, 336–352.

Khoury, B., Lecomte, T., Gaudiano, B., & Paquin, K. (2013). Mindfulness interventions for psychosis: A meta-analysis. *Schizophrenia Research, 150*(1), 176–184. https://doi.org/10.1016/j.schres.2013.07.055

Kirby, J. N. (2017). Compassion interventions: The programmes, the evidence, and implications for research and practice. *Psychology and Psychotherapy: Theory, Research and Practice, 90*(3), 432–455. https://doi.org/10.1111/papt.12104

Langer, Á., Van Carmona-Torres, J., Gordon, W., & Shonin, E. (2016). *Mindfulness for the treatment of psychosis: State of the art and future developments. Mindfulness and Buddhist-derived approaches in mental health and addiction* (pp. 211–223). Springer.

Langer, Á., Schmidt, C., Mayol, R., Díaz, M., Lecaros, J., Krogh, E., et al. (2017). The effect of a mindfulness-based intervention in cognitive functions and psychological well-being applied as an early intervention in schizophrenia and high-risk mental state in a Chilean sample: Study protocol for a randomized controlled trial. *Trials, 18*(1), 1–9. https://doi.org/10.1186/s13063-017-1967-7

Li, Y., Coster, S., Norman, I., Chien, W. T., Qin, J. L., Tse, M., & Bressington, D. (2021). Feasibility, acceptability, and preliminary effectiveness of mindfulness-based interventions for people with recent-onset psychosis: A systematic review. *Early Intervention in Psychiatry, 15*(1), 3–15. https://doi.org/10.1111/eip.12929

Louise, S., Fitzpatrick, M., Strauss, C., Rossell, S. L., & Thomas, N. (2018). Mindfulness-and acceptance-based interventions for psychosis: Our current understanding and a meta-analysis. *Schizophrenia Research, 192*, 57–63. https://doi.org/10.1016/j.schres.2017.05.023

Mediavilla, R., Muñoz-Sanjose, A., Rodriguez-Vega, B., Bayon, C., Lahera, G., & Palao, A. (2019). Mindfulness-based social cognition training (SocialMind) for people with psychosis: A feasibility trial. *Frontiers in Psychiatry, 10*, 299.

Mediavilla, R., Munoz-Sanjose, A., Rodriguez-Vega, B., Lahera, G., Palao, A., Bayon, C., et al. (2021). People with psychosis improve affective social cognition and self-care after a mindfulness-based social cognition training program (SocialMIND). *Psychiatric Rehabilitation Journal*.

Neff, K. D., & Germer, C. K. (2013). A pilot study and randomized controlled trial of the mindful self-compassion program. *Journal of Clinical Psychology, 69*(1), 28–44.

Potes, A., Souza, G., Nikolitch, K., Penheiro, R., Moussa, Y., Jarvis, E., et al. (2018). Mindfulness in severe and persistent mental illness: A systematic review. *International Journal of Psychiatry in Clinical Practice, 22*(4), 253–261. https://doi.org/10.1080/13651501.2018.1433857

Rose, A., Vinogradov, S., Fisher, M., Green, M. F., Ventura, J., Hooker, C., et al. (2015). Randomized controlled trial of computer-based treatment of social cognition in schizophrenia: The TRuSST trial protocol. *BMC Psychiatry, 15*(1), 1–16. https://doi.org/10.1186/s12888-015-0510-1

Salzberg, S. (2011). *Real happiness: The power of meditation*. Workman.

Whitty, P. F., Owoeye, O., & Waddington, J. L. (2009). Neurological signs and involuntary movements in schizophrenia: Intrinsic to and informative on systems pathobiology. *Schizophrenia Bulletin, 35*(2), 415–424. https://doi.org/10.1093/schbul/sbn126

Chapter 26
Compassion-Focussed Therapy for Voices and Unusual Experiences

Andrew Fleming and Charlie Heriot-Maitland

26.1 Overview

In this case study, we show how compassion-focussed approaches helped a young woman – Ffion (a pseudonym to respect confidentiality) who was troubled by several voices and other unusual experiences.

Compassion-focussed therapy (CFT) is an integrative therapeutic approach grounded in an evolutionary psychological model. CFT can be a particularly helpful model of therapy for people distressed by their unusual experiences. Rather than viewing challenging emotional and psychological experiences as something to be got rid of, CFT invites us to develop a compassionate and understanding relationship with challenging inner experiences.

Even in the midst of her deepest distress, Ffion's wisdom was guiding us to focus on the importance of listening to and validating emotions. Compassion-based interventions enabled Ffion to reconnect to her body wisdom through movement and dance. Ultimately it was this compassion-based movement work and the freedom she rediscovered through dance that enabled Ffion to overcome a significant emotional block and move forward on her road to recovery.

A. Fleming (✉)
Bangor University, Bangor, Wales, UK
e-mail: ndf21tjc@bangor.ac.uk

C. Heriot-Maitland
Balanced Minds, Edinburgh, Scotland, UK

J. A. Díaz-Garrido et al. (eds.), *Psychological Interventions for Psychosis*,
https://doi.org/10.1007/978-3-031-27003-1_26

26.2 Why CFT for Psychosis?

In the UK, the NICE Guidelines for treatment of schizophrenia and psychosis recommend cognitive behaviour therapy for psychosis (CBTp) as the psychological treatment of choice (National Institute for Health and Care Excellence, 2014/CG178 Section 1.3.7). However, a recent meta-analysis for CBTp (McGlanaghy et al., 2021) shows that there remains room for improvement in the effectiveness of the therapy.

Birchwood and Trower (2006) advocate focussing CBTp towards addressing the emotions underlying psychotic experiences rather than simply directing interventions towards the elimination of psychotic "symptoms". Gumley et al. (2010) suggest that compassionate mind approaches may be a helpful addition to established CBTp practice as well as helping inform how practitioners develop therapeutic relationships and influencing how services are delivered. They particularly highlight the role of CFT in preventing future psychotic relapse. It may be that fear of future relapse and hospitalisation, coupled with feelings of guilt, shame and embarrassment about letting down loved ones or others in the support system, can become a trigger for threat-based emotions that in turn contribute to further relapses.

People's relationship with voices can have a significant impact on levels of shame and self-criticism as well (Mayhew, 2015). CFT is an evolution-informed approach to therapy that draws on influences from CBT and other psychotherapeutic approaches to address the psychological problems experienced by people with high levels of shame and self-attacking (Gilbert, 2010).

Helping people to develop their compassionate capacities may be an alternative route to recovery for people with distressing voices and beliefs, and there is an ever-increasing body of work describing how CFT for psychosis can be helpful (Heriot-Maitland & Russel, 2018; Heriot-Maitland & Levey, 2021; Kennedy & Ellerby, 2016; Mayhew, 2015; Wright et al., 2014). A recent review of compassion-based approaches for psychosis (Mavituna et al., 2022) has concluded that they may hold promise of effective clinical benefit; however, further research is needed.

CFT is similar to other process-orientated therapies in that it focusses less on the content of people's unusual experiences and more on understanding the emotional function of their experiences. It explores the relationship that people have to their unusual experiences and helps people to see that they are separate from those experiences and their lives do not have to be dictated by their diagnosis or symptoms (Martins et al., 2017).

As this book describes, there are several different process-orientated approaches to therapy with psychosis, including acceptance and commitment therapy, mindfulness, dialectical behaviour therapy, metacognitive training and compassionate mind training and CFT (Martins et al., 2017). As is evident in the other case studies described in this book, there are many areas of overlap in these approaches. However, one thing that all of these approaches have in common is a hopeful message about recovery.

There is an important movement and paradigm shift that is emerging out of all of the process-orientated approaches to CBTp. These approaches have grown out of the shared experience and wisdom of both people experiencing psychosis and clinicians alike. Increasingly we are hearing the important voices of people with lived experience of psychosis in the literature (Kennedy & Ellerby, 2016; Ellerby, 2013, 2014, 2017; Heriot-Maitland & Levey, 2021; Parker et al., 2021).

26.3 Listening to and Learning from Our Shared Human Story

CFT proposes that our minds do what they do because they have been shaped by evolutionary influences over millions of years (Gilbert, 2015). Once born into the world, the developing human mind sets out on a lifetime of responding to stimuli and learning. The mind is "hard wired" to do the best it can to adapt to the challenges of our physical and social environments. Unfortunately some of the strategies that our minds use to cope with threats and challenges can have problematic unintended consequences.

Holding this perspective allows space for very different conversations about extreme states of mind and distressing unusual experiences. Hearing voices, having visions and other modalities of hallucination is a common human experience. As we know from literature, religious texts and other cultural traditions, people have heard voices and had visions for millennia. Such experiences are not always indicative of illness. Indeed, in historical record, we hear of figures like Julian of Norwich and Joan of Arc who were revered and respected in their lifetime and continue to be sources of inspiration to spiritual and political life to this day. In shamanic cultures, unusual perceptual experiences are valued as potentially rich sources of spiritual information and growth to be shared with the community.

Normalising the diverse range of human experiences is an important de-shaming strategy used throughout the literature on psychological interventions for psychosis. The psychoeducation that underpins all CFT work provides a sound evolutionary scientific explanation for using this strategy. It is important to stress that the normalising of unusual perceptual disturbances is not done with the intention of belittling or romanticising distressing states of mind. Rather it is a reminder that distressing and disturbing states of mind are on a continuum with normal human thinking and could even be a source of learning and growth for an individual and their community when the experiences are viewed through the lens of compassion (Razzaque, 2014).

Human minds evolved to seek meaning and make connections. We cannot stop ourselves trying to make sense of things that may seem unexplainable. It is part of our humanity. We love getting together to tell and share tales of mystery and adventure. For centuries and across hugely different cultures, the telling and passing on of myths have helped us to process and come to terms with dealing with power, pain, suffering and loss.

We also have minds that evolved to make shortcuts in thinking. Being able to jump to conclusions quickly is a highly adaptive strategy for keeping safe when in danger. We all descended from early humans that needed "better safe than sorry" thinking styles in order to stay alive. This particular cognitive bias will come on line more frequently when we are under greater stress. Intuitively this makes a lot of sense; when we are facing danger, it is highly adaptive to have a mind and body that can quickly direct all our mental and physical energy into mobilising all of our threat protection resources. Evidence has shown that prolonged periods without sleep can lead to feelings of paranoia and episodes of auditory hallucinations (Waters et al., 2018).

The mind can even be a bit tricky in less stressful situations. For instance, have you ever had the experience of mistakenly hearing your name being called out in noisy social environments, or experienced deja vu, or seen something fleeting in the corner of your eye that disappeared once you turned towards it or perhaps you were thinking about family or a friend and then moments later got a phone call or text from them? How did you make sense of these experiences?

Tricky minds hey!? This is what it is to be human. CFT puts a lot of effort into getting more familiar with the workings of our "tricky minds," and most importantly, it helps us to develop a compassionate relationship towards the "tricky mind" that gets expressed in ourselves, in others and in the broader community when a whole bunch of tricky minds get together.

Most forms of psychotherapy aim to help people understand and make sense of their personal life story. CFT extends this by stressing the importance of bringing compassionate understanding to not just our own story but the shared human story of how we all find ourselves in the flow of life on this planet.

So in that same spirit of valuing the telling and sharing of a story to shed light on things that may at first seem mysterious, we will introduce you to Ffion the protagonist of this case study.

26.4 Ffion's Story

At the time of her referral to Early Intervention in Psychosis services, Ffion was a 19-year-old woman living with her family. She is bilingual and her first language is Welsh. Her education had been disrupted by her difficulties. She has a love of music, making collages, reading and dancing.

Ffion found social situations a real challenge. She learned to suppress her emotions and be socially submissive and avoidant at a young age. Ffion is highly sensitive to emotions expressed by others around her, especially anger. Within her family, Ffion developed a peace-making role and felt obliged to ensure others in the family were happy.

26.5 Ffion's Voices

Ffion hears several voices. They speak to her in a mixture of both Welsh and English. When they are being critical of her, they mostly speak in English, which may reflect the unwelcome dominance of the English language and culture in the area where she lives (Hadden et al., 2019). One female voice has always been in her life. When she was younger, it used to instruct her on how to fit in with her peers. Increasingly this voice became very bossy towards her. As is often the case with other young voice hearers, new voices developed during adolescence and when there was increased social pressure and significant life events happening for her. Her voices changed over time and now some were telling her to kill herself. Ffion had made several high-risk suicide attempts and was lucky to be alive. Sometimes Ffion felt her voices expressed views similar to how she thought about herself. When we first met, Ffion did not think the voices were at all helpful and she wanted to get rid of them.

26.6 Other Interventions

Ffion had transitioned to adult mental health services from CAMHS. Whilst under CAMHS, she had been offered CBT, EMDR and treatment for an eating disorder. During her first hospital admission, she received a diagnosis of schizophrenia. Her poor response to medication led to Ffion being prescribed Clozaril, which is recommended for psychosis when two other anti-psychotics have been found ineffective (NICE CG178 [1.5.7.2], 2014).

During subsequent stays in hospital, pharmacological treatment was steadily increased, with little impact on her presenting symptoms, but with a marked increase in side effects from medication, such as weight gain and drowsiness. Initially this made any therapy very difficult. It was hard for Ffion to concentrate and she could rarely recall our work in between therapy sessions. An important initial intervention was to advocate for medication to be reduced as it was adversely impacting on our therapy with little impact on her overall mental health.

26.7 The Therapist's Story (First Author AF)

My personal experience of extreme states of mind and unusual experiences also began at an early age. My mother spent many years in psychiatric institutions and had several episodes of psychosis; the early trauma she experienced that arguably was the root cause of her mental suffering was overlooked and tragically never even heard by a treatment system that viewed her mostly through the lens of having a severe biological mental illness.

I have a professional background in mental health nursing and work as a psychological therapist within an Early Intervention Service in Wales. For most of my career, I have focussed on working alongside people who live with the experience of psychosis. In my early career, this was with people who were street homeless. Most had lived with psychosis for many years in extremes of poverty and with very little support for their overall well-being, let alone their mental health. Witnessing first-hand the limits of what medication had to offer people dealing with such extreme challenging difficulties led me to seek alternative ways of helping people and undertaking training in psychosocial interventions for psychosis.

Seeing all of these different expressions of human suffering, in both my personal life and professional life and having a desire to try to make sense of it all drew me to the compassionate mind work of Paul Gilbert (2009) and CFT.

26.8 Validating the Concerns of Voices

Right from the start of our work together, I was open with Ffion that my role was not to get rid of her voices. I wanted her voices to hear that message too. It is never a great place to start working with voices, or anybody that we work with for that matter, if they feel threatened in anyway. It helps to explain this explicitly to voice hearers and their voices. Meeting new people for the first time, working out if someone can be trusted and being open to the possibility of change are all understandable sources of threat. It makes a lot of sense to be wary of or sceptical about the intentions of apparently well-meaning therapists.

Trust needs to be earned; it should never be taken for granted. A common experience when therapists start to work with voice hearers is for a voice to advise their hearer, "Don't trust them!" "Don't listen to them – they don't know what they are talking about!" "They are only saying this because they are paid to, they don't really care about you." Voices that give expression to such doubts are demonstrating a great deal of wisdom. When we first met, Ffion's voices had some very dismissive views about me!

It is important to acknowledge and validate the concern expressed by voices and even to express gratitude for their opinion and for their understandable desire to protect the voice hearer from being hurt again.

26.9 The Flow of Therapy

There are three interrelated phases to the flow of CFT: (1) evolutionary psychoeducation, (2) training the compassionate mind and (3) putting the compassionate mind into action.

Ffion presented with many complex underlying difficulties and there were significant blocks and resistances to her engaging in the therapeutic work with many false starts along the way. We detail here a selection of the CFT practices that helped

Ffion negotiate her blocks and resistances. CFT stresses the importance of committing to practice and values repetition. Some practices when first introduced to Ffion appeared to make no impact on her at all, and yet towards the end of therapy they would become essential tools for her personal compassionate mind kitbag. The compassionate mind kitbag is a personalised range of objects and activities that can help us to bring our compassionate minds on line quickly (Lucre & Clapton, 2021).

26.10 Introducing Compassion and the Core Principles of CFT

Before developing the compassionate mind, it is important to explore an individual's understanding of compassion. People's early experiences and their pre-conceptions about compassion need to be attended to. Some people have a view of compassion as something that is soft and fluffy and possibly even a sign of weakness. For others, compassion may have become associated as a precursor to something bad happening to them. There are some people who sadly have never experienced any form of compassion and it may seem a very alien concept for them.

Ffion's view of compassion was that she did not deserve to be receiving it and she thought that compassion was something to appease others with.

So what exactly do we mean by compassion?

26.11 The CFT Definition of Compassion

Paul Gilbert (2009) based his definition of compassion on the teachings of the Dalai Lama.

In CFT, compassion is described as having:

A sensitivity towards the nature and causes of suffering that arise in ourselves and others and as a response to that sensitivity having the desire, commitment and motivation to alleviate and prevent suffering in ourselves, others and the human community.

Compassion is for everyone, not just for the few. It is essential for those that are in need of healing and it is equally essential for those that are in the business of healing.

In order to be compassionate, we need to develop intentions and motivation to be helpful and not harmful, in how we think, act and behave towards ourselves and others. This is a key message to embody and communicate in all of our therapeutic interactions.

Compassion can flow:

- From the self to another.
- From another to the self.
- From self to self.

We can have strengths and blocks within all three of the flows of compassion. Training up our compassionate minds involves undertaking and repeating practices that exercise all three of the flows, building all the time on our strengths, capacities and past experiences of being in the flows of compassion.

26.12 Hardwired to Be Compassionate?

In our practice of CFT, we want to help people discover compassionate resources and wisdom that are already within them. The ability to be compassionate may actually be at the heart of what it is to be human. There is archaeological evidence that over a million and half years ago, very early humans were caring for weaker members of their social groups for extended periods of time (Spikins, 2017). Spikins argues that the ability to be emotionally committed to and enter into collaborative relationships with others may have been what gave humans an evolutionary advantage leading to further brain developments that set us on the pathway to present-day human social functioning. Spikins (2017) notes that the archaeological evidence for pro-social behaviours appears much earlier and is more widespread than evidence of violent social behaviours in early humans.

Stellar and Keltner (2017) summarise several studies that provide evidence of an evolved network of integrated pro-social biological processes incorporating the autonomic (parasympathetic nervous system), neural (activation in the periaqueductal gray) and hormonal (oxytocin) systems that counters arguments that humans evolved only to be selfish.

They suggest that the psychophysiology of humans indicates the importance of how compassionate abilities enabled us to downregulate biological threat-based responses in order to be able to bond with infants, form nurturing relationships and to be able to tolerate proximity to others for sustained social relationships, in order to live in co-operative social communities. They extend the ideas of Steven Porges' (2003, 2007) Poly Vagal Theory, that it was the evolutionary emergence of the myelinated section of the vagus nerve (the tenth cranial nerve) arising in the nucleus ambiguus in the brain which enabled the biological basis for compassionate qualities to arise: specifically the ability to tune into the needs of other members of the social group and then to set up the physiology to be able to take care of another (Stellar & Keltner, 2017). Every time we take a breath in, vagus nerve activity is tuned down; when we breathe out, the activity of the vagus nerve increases and slows heart rate down. It is argued that this calming effect on heart rate helped to facilitate affiliation and bonding in our evolutionary history. Focussing on the slowing effect of the out-breath is a key part of the ground work for developing a soothing breathing rhythm that helps to prepare for all CFT practices.

Stellar and Keltner (2017) also outline how the neural connections of the vagus nerve acting on face muscles, voice tone and the perception of human voices are all needed for effective social communication especially for feeling genuine safe connection to another. A smiling face can affect how we function (Niedenthal, 2007).

Even when we simply recall or bring to mind a smiling face and a warm voice tone, this can have a soothing impact on our physiology. Perhaps you could take a moment to explore this for yourself now? All of these important pro-social qualities of human biology are utilised in training up the compassionate mind.

26.13 Presenting CFT Psychoeducation

All of us find ourselves in the "flow of life," not choosing the time, place, families and genes we are born with. We are shaped by our formative experiences also not of our choosing. Nature has gifted us with highly evolved "new brain" capacities of creativity, imagination and rumination. Our "new brains" with highly evolved social mentalities, focussed on social rank, status, dominance and submission, are constantly receiving and sending a myriad of complex social signals, utilising all of the physiological systems outlined above. These interact with and activate "old brain" emotional systems that are focussed on protecting us from danger (threat protection system), the acquisition of resources and finding a mate (drive system) and systems that help us to feel content connected and safe (soothing system) (Gilbert, 2009).

As part of our therapy, Ffion was given a tailor-made CFT work book that we developed together. The work book and her own journaling of therapy provided a resource that we added to as new CFT exercises were introduced and practised.

The following is an extract from her work book summarising CFT psychoeducation:

1. **The Flow of Life**
   Like all living beings, we are part of the flow of life in the universe. We did not choose to be born with a human mind, and we did not choose the family that we are born into or the country, culture or language that we are born into.
2. **Tricky Human Brain**
   Our brains evolved over millions of years. Our brains work in ways that were helpful thousands of years ago when there were many more dangers to deal with. So, now our brains have a natural tendency to look for and focus on threats all the time. Our minds can get caught up in loops between our old brain systems (e.g., emotions and motives) and our new brain systems (e.g., thinking and ruminating).
   We (and you!!!) did not design our brains to work this way – so it doesn't make sense and is certainly not helpful when we blame ourselves for when our brain is struggling with difficult emotions.
3. **The Three-Emotion Regulation Systems**
   A simple way to understand our "old brain – emotional system" is to group it into three-coloured circles (see Fig. 26.1).
   Red: threat protection system – helps to keep us safe from danger.
   Blue: drive system – helps to motivate us and get us to move towards our goals in life.

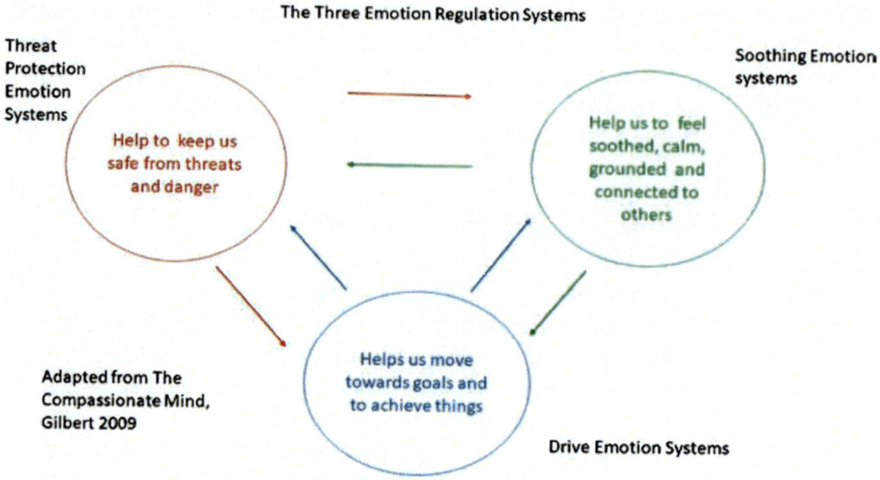

Fig. 26.1 The three-emotion regulation systems

Green: soothing/connection system – helps us to feel calm and to feel safe around other people.
The "new brain" is the part of our brain that gives us language, culture and creativity. It also helps us to think about things, imagine things, worry and ruminate about things. (This is the extra tricky bit of our tricky brains!!!)

4. **We Are Shaped**
All of us are shaped by the families and societies that we are born into, just as our parents, grandparents and great, great, great grandparents were.
If you were born into a drug gang family living in central London, instead of the family you were born into would the same version of you still exist today?

5. **Not Our Fault – Wisdom**
Because of all these points, it is not our fault that our minds get caught up in unhelpful loops of worry and negative thinking. It is how our minds have been shaped by nature (genes) over millions of years. In fact it can be more helpful to think of our minds as actually being nature's mind expressed in and through us – pretty cool.
This is an important step towards developing wisdom about the nature of being human and can help us to respond more compassionately to ourselves and to each other, once we realise that we are all in this together.
As we did not design or choose our tricky minds, it does not make sense when we give ourselves a hard time when we notice worry thoughts or negative thoughts arising in our minds.

6. **What We Can Do About It**
So although it is not our fault that we are born with minds like this, we do have responsibility for understanding our tricky minds with wisdom, compassion and acceptance.

Think of it like learning to ride a bike! We didn't design or make the bike but we have to learn to be able to ride it in a safe and responsible way.
Oh and here's an extra bit of tricky mind wisdom to get your head around – it is not even our fault when we notice that our minds have a natural tendency to blame and shame us for nature's mind being expressed in us. The evolving human mind worked out that it can be easier to live with a thought that something is our fault (even when it clearly isn't) in order for us to have a feeling of control about things. Our evolved human mind tends to feel better about itself when it feels in control of things, even if that means we have ended up blaming ourselves. Super tricky minds!

26.14 CFT Formulation

Formulation is informed and rooted in this CFT psychoeducation. It can be as simple as inviting people to draw out circles to represent their three emotional systems (Gilbert, 2009).

When we take time to draw out our own three circles we create a reflective distance from where we can observe our emotional experiences without judgment. The act of stepping back and developing a non-judgemental observing perspective is a useful compassionate skill in itself.

Drawing out the circles or using some other creative medium to represent the three emotional systems provides a focus for exploring the relationships between all of the three emotional systems and how each system in turn impacts on the others.

Regularly drawing out the circles throughout the course of therapy not only helps to reinforce CFT psychoeducation, but it can also demonstrate that the systems do not represent a fixed state but are always in a dynamic interaction.

As this can be a particularly useful exercise to do, some CFT therapists recommend having a white board handy with coloured maker pens so that circles can be easily drawn and rubbed out when needed. Drawing out the three circles can provide a useful visual tool for explaining the rationale for compassionate mind skills that aim to shape up the healing capacities of the soothing system.

At the start of therapy Ffion's initial three-circle formulation was dominated by a threat system that she drew out as a very large red circle – The space it occupied on the paper sent a stark message that there was little space for anything else in her life. I invited her to divide up her red threat protection circle into the different emotions of fear, anger and shame. Fear and shame were the dominant emotions, and there was very little space for anger. Later in the course of therapy we discovered that what had appeared initially to be a threat protection system with very little anger in it was not quite how it first seemed (see Fig. 26.2).

We discovered that the large segment of shame and self-disgust was linked to repressed feelings of anger. Some strongly felt emotions can serve a function of protecting the mind from other emotions that may be perceived as destructive, harmful or frightening. Ffion was very sensitive to anger being expressed by others

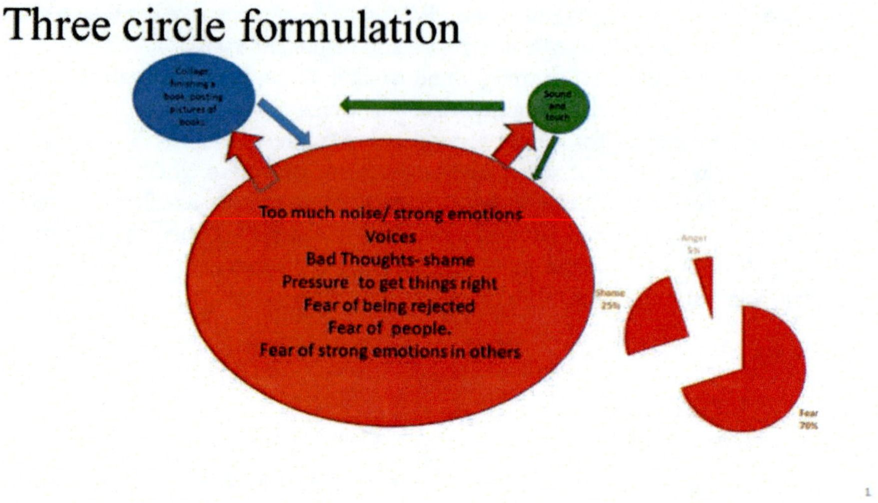

Fig. 26.2 Three-circle formulation

and this in turn had led her to become fearful of her own anger. Ffion's mind worked hard to "micro manage" anger in herself and wherever possible in others. In stark contrast the circles that she drew to represent her drive and soothing systems were very small.

Over the course of therapy we worked on practices that would help her grow both her drive and soothing emotional systems to help downregulate her very well-developed threat protection system.

26.15 The CFT Threat-Focussed Formulation

A threat-focussed formulation is another opportunity to reintroduce and reinforce the key de-shaming psychoeducation message that human minds are doing the best they can to cope with sources of threat that arise from the external environment that we grow up and live our lives in and from internal sources of threat that arise from what the mind thinks of itself and how the mind relates to itself (see Fig. 26.3).

Ffion felt different from her peers and family members for as long as she can remember. She had no explanatory model for this difference that made sense to her until, during her admission to hospital, she was diagnosed with ASD. It took her a long time to process and accept this new way of understanding herself.

In order to cope with her difference Ffion developed her own set of strict rules for life in order to appease others and to minimise the chance of anger being expressed around her. This had the unintended consequence of invalidating her own emotional needs leading to a firmly held belief that others were dangerous, anger was bad and

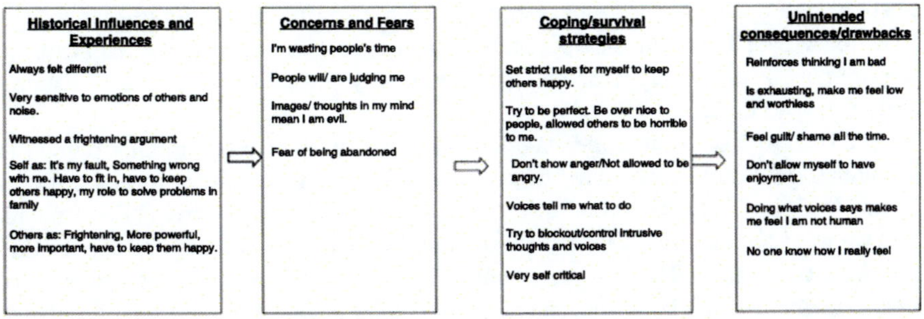

Fig. 26.3 Ffion's threat-focussed formulation

she was worthless. This reinforced her firmly held belief that she did not deserve compassion and that people would be better off if she were no longer alive.

Her voice hearing was initially perceived as a source of help and company to a very frightened isolated young mind, but in time became a further source of internal threat as voices barked instructions to her in a desperate bid to make sure that she did not mess up, make mistakes or upset others.

Heriot Maitland and Levey (2021) propose that some voices that arise in the mind following early traumatic events can be formulated as a rapid way for the mind to switch on essential threat protection responses of submission, withdrawal and scan for danger. As we have discovered already the automatic "better safe than sorry" reactions of the mind provide an "act now and don't ask questions later" response with the sole purpose of keeping us safe. The evolved pathways in the mind that drive these automatic responses come online so quickly, utilising old brain capacities that functionally have no time or capability for considering the impact and unintended consequences of using the strategy. Ffion had found some of her early life experiences overwhelming and traumatising.

Ffion had spent a life time of putting others' needs first and it had almost become habitual for her to not attend to or listen to her own needs. This had been an essential coping strategy to help her manage social interactions both at home and at school.

26.16 Learning to Listen Again

As we began to practice compassionate mind training by using simple attention focus and mindfulness exercises, Ffion realised something profound. She was starting to learn to listen and observe herself without critical judgement, even if her voices continued to express criticism. It dawned on her that she had been lacking this all her life – she needed to learn to listen and validate her needs, and more importantly she needed others to really hear her.

Unfortunately some of the traditional treatment approaches to psychosis can reinforce a potentially unhelpful message. Sometimes when people are in acute hospital settings there can be a systemic pressure and rush to fix and resolve things. If we only ever focus on the "symptoms" and problems, we can lose sight of the importance of connecting with our shared humanity and we can sometimes systemically forget to listen.

The rush to "fix" is an understandable reaction. When we see another human in emotional pain and distress, we want to put things right, we want to make things better. And surely this is a good thing? But perhaps our rush to "treat" Ffion meant that we were not making space to actually listen to her? The expressions of her mind that were being formulated as symptoms to be got rid of were sitting on top of emotional needs that had been longing to be heard for a long time. Unless we helped create the environment for Ffion to learn to listen and validate the emotions that sat underneath the "symptoms," we would be caught up in an unhelpful dynamic of trying to shut down important sources of potentially helpful information.

It is interesting to note that it wasn't until a brave psychiatrist made the decision to reduce and stop Clozaril treatment, which had made little to no difference to her voices, that Ffion was really able to notice benefits from her compassionate mind training.

26.17 Compassionate Mind Training

Compassionate mind training flows from the psychoeducation and formulation and is introduced to help support the unintended consequences of how a mind had to deal with the pain of difficult early attachments and traumatic events. The overall aim is to help someone develop and internalise a more understanding and compassionate response to the various expressions of their hurting mind.

The CFT therapist has an important role of embodying and modelling compassionate responses to human pain and suffering based on their personal compassionate mind practices. The quality of the therapeutic relationship and the quality of our presence in the therapy space play an important part in compassionate mind training. However, we must be cautious not to inadvertently portray compassion as some super human ability to live in an idealised state of tranquillity and balance. Compassion is about recognising, facing up to, turning towards and entering the muck and messiness of life. At times it needs fierce and determined qualities to overcome the challenges of life. Indeed the image of the lotus flower that is often used to represent the wisdom of compassion is a useful image to explore, because this beautiful serene looking flower can only grow out and through the reality of the mud and dirt that it is rooted within. So when we undertake compassionate mind training, we want to communicate a message that it is ok to be fallible and make mistakes. Our imperfections and flaws are to be welcomed and celebrated with warmth and humour as a potential source of learning and growth for our developing compassionate minds.

26.18 Introducing Playfulness and Curiosity

Lucre (2021) stresses the importance of bringing a lightness and playfulness to the healing work undertaken in her CFT groups by embodying and modelling these principles. Some of the things that the human mind can throw back at us is not pretty at all, and facing this with an openness and warmth is essential lest we get overwhelmed by our emotions. As we saw from Ffion's formulation she had coped with the pressures of growing up by making a great effort to please her teachers and parents alike. She worked extra hard to be as unnoticeable as possible by trying to be perfect in everything that she did. And as she came to learn this strategy had painful unintended consequences for her. An important focus of therapy would involve encouraging Ffion to expose herself to making mistakes and letting go of the protective role of perfection – so bringing playfulness and curiosity to our therapy would be an important stylistic approach to embody.

As we saw earlier when Ffion drew out her three circles, we identified that both her drive and soothing emotional systems needed some compassion-focussed attention; we turn now to how we helped Ffion develop her soothing system in order to downregulate the expressions of threat protection in her emotional systems. It was later towards the end of her course of therapy that we found a way to use her drive system to help overcome blocks to giving expression to tricky emotions.

26.19 Activating the Soothing System

There are two elements to our emotional soothing system: (1) Sensory soothing which can be accessed by any aspect of our perception systems and (2) the feeling of safe non-striving contentment that comes with emotional connection to another. This feeling of safe connection can not only be gained by being in the presence of someone that we have a secure connection with, it can also be derived from a feeling of safe connection to a place, object or animal. Like most of the workings of the mind, there is an overlap between the sensory soothing and the felt safe connection elements. Furthermore we can use our "new brain" capacities of memory, imagery and imagination to stimulate and bring on line our soothing system. What we bring to mind through memory or via the creative domains of our "new brain" systems will be felt in our body. CFT utilises this built-in wisdom of our body to help us downregulate our threat protection system, and we will look at the power and usefulness of imagery in a little more detail later.

Ffion was particularly sensitive to sensory stimulation. This had been a mixed blessing for her throughout her life. Some noises and smells were very aversive for her. For example, she could hear to the point of almost feeling it the electricity in her home electric circuitry. It was very hard to be around some electrical appliances. Growing up with this sensitivity in both the home and school environment was very triggering for her threat protection system.

On the other hand touching soft things was a very powerful way for Ffion to feel soothed. CFT uses guided discovery to help people tap into the wisdom of their body and their lived experience. There is no one-size-fits-all approach to how to do this. Right at the start of our work together we explored this aspect of her sense of touch. I encouraged Ffion to notice and observe what happened in her body when she touched and stroked soft objects. At the start of every session we practiced together holding and exploring with our fingers or brushing on our faces a small piece of felt. This simple tactile practice is how we started all our initial sessions, and alongside attending to posture and slowing down of the breath, it became a practice that we used to cue in that we are about to step into the compassionate mind and body.

26.20 Preparing the Mind by Preparing the Body

All CFT practices stress the importance of preparing the body to help prepare the mind for compassion. Several studies of biofeedback have demonstrated how posture and stance can impact on how we feel and perform. Wilson and Peper (2004) report how it is easier to recall positive thoughts when adopting an upright posture. Peper and Lin (2012) reported decreases and increases in subjective reports of energy levels simply by changing posture. The findings of these and other studies on embodied cognition theory (Niedenthal et al., 2005; Niedenthal, 2007) reflect already known spiritual wisdom that posture affects how we feel. Many forms of meditation, prayer and yoga begin by purposefully adopting an upright and wakeful open posture.

Similarly in compassionate mind exercises and therapy practices an upright open stable sitting posture is adopted with feet placed flat on the floor roughly shoulder width apart and the back either supported to be in an upright position or held that way by the body. The head is held in an upright position with eyes facing forward and gently closed or focussed on the middle distance. Shoulders and the chest area are gently encouraged to open up, with the hands resting in an open fashion on the lap.

When introducing this practice in the therapy setting, a useful form of guided discovery can be to explore together how the body feels and what it communicates to the mind when a slumped posture is adopted. We observe the breath when sitting slumped forward in a closed up posture and compare this with how our body feels when we breathe with an open upright posture and of course with a warm smile on our face!

For some, even these initial steps can prove challenging and they may report feeling exposed. We can use this discovery as an opportunity to discuss and explore their current body wisdom, explaining this is how their body has learnt to feel safe, and gently encouraging them to dip their toes into just one part of open body posture practice.

Having taking time to settle into an open stable posture a soothing breathing rhythm is adopted. There are different ways of introducing and cuing in a soothing breathing rhythm. It is thought that a breath rate of approximately five breaths per minute is the optimum rate to move towards; however, everybody is different and for some this suggested rate will be far too slow a breathing rate to achieve so it is more helpful to let people discover the breathing rate that is most helpful for them by listening to their own body wisdom rather than imposing a specific pattern and rate of soothing breathing rhythm. When first learning to use a soothing breathing rhythm to calm the body it can help to slowly say "body slowing down" and again, "mind slowing down" on the out-breath.

26.21 Using Wilderness and Nature to Tone Up the Soothing System

At this very moment, the Earth is above you, below you, all around you, and even inside you. The Earth is everywhere....Everything outside us and everything inside us comes from the Earth. We often forget that the planet we are living on has given us all the elements that make up our bodies. The water in our flesh, our bones, and all the microscopic cells inside our bodies come from the Earth and are part of the Earth. The Earth is not just the environment we live in. We are the Earth and we are always carrying her within us. (Thich Nhat Hanh, 2013)

CFT is a relational therapeutic model that draws from evolutionary psychology as well as practices and wisdom from Buddhist spiritual traditions. As evolved creatures in the flow of life on earth, our biology, psychology, language and culture have been shaped by our relationship to our natural environment over millions of years of adaptation and change. Tapping into this wisdom can bring an added richness to our therapeutic work especially when we are using guided discovery to explore and tone up the soothing system.

It is perhaps understandable that when we connect mindfully, purposefully and with helpful intention with our natural environment we will find that our bodies and minds will respond accordingly. It is as if we are getting in touch with a deep wisdom that has been imprinted in our genes and continues to be somehow held in our bodies. Much of how we live our lives today can disconnect us from the natural world, but our ancestors lived in ways that depended on having a safe connection to and intimate knowledge of the environment and natural resources. We can use compassionate mind training to help us restore a more balanced relationship with our natural environment.

Just as certain images and sounds from nature can be viscerally frightening for us – think for a moment about how it would feel walking alone through a dense woodland in the dead of night and hearing the sound of a branch cracking or a sudden rustle of leaves?

Other sounds and images from nature can have a profoundly soothing and calming effect on human biology – Think for a moment now of the sound of slowly flowing water, or the rhythmical lapping of the sea on a beach, or the feel and sound of a gentle summer breeze, the feel and scent of warm sunlight on skin, or the sight of dappled sunlight shining through a woodland glade. Have you ever experienced being caught in a moment of awe when seeing the sun rise or set or catching a glimpse of a large full moon rising low on the horizon as if for the first time?

Of course we all respond differently to these archetypal stimuli from the natural world and CFT is wise to the knowledge of how our tricky minds can easily build connections between traumatic events and their location. For this reason it is very important that when using guided discovery to explore using the natural environment to help recovery that we check out first that certain sounds and sights will not be triggering of memories of past painful events.

Ffion and myself are fortunate to live and work in a part of the world close to a mountainous national park and several areas of outstanding natural beauty. With such a rich resource on our doorstep it would have been negligent not to use the natural environment in our therapeutic work. When Ffion was an inpatient on a busy, noisy acute unit, I would use whatever opportunity I could find to facilitate our compassionate mind training sessions in an outdoor setting of her choosing.

We conducted mindfulness and compassionate attention practices under trees, by the sea shore and in the mountains. In this way, we were able to explore what sounds, sights and physical sensations were the most helpful for Ffion to bring her sensory soothing system on line in the most effective way.

Our initial work outdoors not only helped with our engagement at a time when Ffion was feeling very disconnected, but it helped her to discover that she already had within her capabilities and qualities that she could draw on to help her when she needed. Ffion was discovering that there were things she could easily do that would enable her body to slow down her automatic threat responses. She was drawing on her own inner wisdom.

26.22 Putting the Compassionate Mind to Work

Once Ffion began to get comfortable and more confident about activating her soothing system we used this grounding to help Ffion develop her compassionate self-identity. We did this through the use of compassion-based imagery, chair work, voice dialogues and action-based embodiment practices.

The CFT Multi selves exercise (Irons & Beaumont, 2017; Kolts et al., 2018) was introduced to illustrate that we are a multiplicity of emotional selves with different needs and motivations that are in a dynamic relationship with each other. Compassionate mind training helps us to develop a compassionate self to hold and guide the various needs of our other selves such as anxious self, angry self, sad self, etc. We can think of the compassionate self as being like a skilful captain of a ship sailing through stormy waters, all of the different selves are essential crew members and each have an important role to play. Some crew members are more dominant than others and the compassionate captain of the ship needs to draw on the strengths of each crew member not just the dominant ones. To provide a wonderfully visual idea of multi selves we watched a short clip from the Disney Pixar animated movie "Inside Out" (Docter & Del Carmen, 2015) and we frequently viewed and reflected on the compassion for voices animation (Heriot-Maitland & Anderson, 2015) to help guide our work.

CFT pays special attention to the self-critic. Ffion's self-critic and some of her voices held similar views about her and this had impacted Ffion's initial view of what compassion was. She had learnt to be submissive in social interactions in order to "fit in" and keep people happy around her. Ffion had a similar submissive relationship towards her self-critic and her voices.

Heriot Maitland and Levey (2021) suggest that compassionately attending to and working with the underlying needs and function of the self-critic can be useful preparatory work before undertaking voice dialogue work with critical voices.

26.23 Fears, Blocks and Resistances (FBR)

When we had started to explore the CFT definition of compassion, Ffion's voices told her that she did not deserve compassion because she was a bad person.

Fears, blocks and resistances (FBR) to compassion are very common once when we start to explore and experience care-giving and care-receiving social mentalities (Gilbert, 2010). And the belief that we do not deserve compassion is a significant block to work around. In CFT when a FBR shows up, this is a clue that there is something very important in a person's life story to attend and listen to. Similar to the self-critic, FBR will also be serving an important function that needs to be understood. There is a good chance that there is a painful emotional back story that is being protected by the FBR.

Earlier in our work Ffion had revealed how the compassionate skill of listening without critical judgement was important to her; indeed there was a sense of sadness that this was something that she had lacked in her life experiences. Ffion also had a strong view about social justice. She believed that people should not be unfairly judged, but at the same time she never challenged the harsh judgements about herself that she received from her voices. Ffion had an all-or-nothing thinking style that was reflected in the views and attitudes of her voices. The belief that she did not deserve to receive compassion was accepted as a fact by her voices and there was no point challenging this.

However, rules and following rules was very important to Ffion. Rather than getting into an unhelpful debate with her about deserving compassion we looked at an important set of internationally agreed rules that even governments are expected to abide by. Following an idea presented in a training session delivered by Mary Welford (2019) we reviewed the statements in the Universal Declaration of Human Rights (1948). The declaration made it clear that the right to be treated with dignity and respect is a fundamental human right that applies to all human beings no matter what they have done in life. As this was set down in internationally agreed rules Ffion accepted this as fact and she didn't think her voices had more authority than the United Nations! Even if it were true that Ffion was fundamentally bad she still had a right to receive compassion.

So although we still needed to attend to the story and needs that sat behind her block to compassion at least we had found a way for Ffion to give herself permission to explore her compassion mind training further and we did this through imagery and embodiment practices.

26.24 The Important Role of Imagery-Based Work in CFT

Imagery is used in a range of therapeutic approaches. Humans have related to images for thousands of years. We love to communicate images through the telling and sharing of stories and this in itself can take a therapeutic form (Gersie, 1997). Core archetypal images emerge across thousands of years and thousands of miles of vastly different human cultures (Gilbert, 2017). CFT draws on this wisdom of millennia of human culture by tapping into the power that soothing compassionate images can have on human psychology and physiology.

A key part of compassionate mind psychoeducation involves exploring the impact that imagery can have on activating and triggering the limbic system of the brain, and the impact this can have on other physiological systems in the body (Gilbert & Irons, 2005; Gilbert, 2009, 2010). If we imagine tasty food or food that has gone off and looks disgusting, our body can respond to the created image in our mind in the same way as if we were actually faced with these foods. Mentally recalling and focussing on a time when we were bullied or threatened can activate our threat response system as if we are threatened in the present moment. In CFT, time is spent drawing out and exploring examples like this to illustrate what can happen in our minds and bodies when the mind becomes self-critical. This helps to set the scene for the rationale of mindfully using supportive compassionate images to help self soothe and regulate emotional systems that are responding to threat (Gilbert & Irons, 2005; Gilbert, 2010). Stimulation of the soothing system through the use of imagery is central to compassionate mind training. As well as a tool to activate the soothing system, CFT image work is used to help to create an inner safe haven and secure base from which suffering and the causes of suffering can be approached rather than avoided. Practices such as recalling a memory of when you gave or received care, imagining being welcomed and greeted by a dear friend, who delights to see you and be in your company, imagining a welcoming compassionate safe place, focussing on a compassionate colour and creating an imagined ideal compassionate other are all used to help strengthen the compassionate self.

26.25 Using Imagery to Put Ffion's Compassionate Self to Work

Ffion was a keen reader of a series of fantasy novels, and when we were exploring how to help her develop her compassionate self, we used characters and settings from the novel that helped her to relate to the different qualities of the compassionate self that she needed. We would always begin by attending to posture, friendly facial expression, using sensory soothing cues, and soothing rhythm breathing. Once we felt settled and prepared to begin, I would lead Ffion through imagining the different courtiers in her compassionate court. Each had a different compassionate quality, such as wisdom, understanding, courage, strength, warmth, freedom from judgement, that she could turn to for help and encouragement. We rehearsed this several times together, and Ffion was given an audio and video recording of the exercise, and in time, she learnt to step into the court whenever she needed to get the guidance of her compassionate self. Through this exercise, her imagined compassionate courtiers helped her to feel that she was not alone when she was struggling, and they gave voice to much-needed supportive messages.

26.26 Embodiment Practices

A common reaction to undertaking compassionate mind training is that some people do not think it is possible for them to be able to express the different qualities of compassion. This reaction is very understandable if sadly you have had a limited experience of receiving compassion. In CFT, we validate this perspective and explain that one of the wonders of our new brain capacities is that when we visualise something in our mind we can feel it in our body. And when we act in compassionate ways, we will feel this in our bodies too. Just like an athlete training for a competition or a musician learning to play an instrument, we need to practice how to be compassionate and repeat these patterns over and over again to help shape up supportive compassionate mind and body states. It is a bit like a method actor; they have to study what it would be like and imagine how they would feel, talk and hold their bodies as they step into the role they are portraying, whether it is an action hero or a villain or a passionate lover. CFT uses similar techniques to help people embody and practice being compassionate, using posture, voice tone and facial expressions. Initially, Ffion found doing this sort of work very challenging, especially in the presence of an older male therapist.

As a way to overcome her understandable resistance to doing this work we conducted a session where instead of Ffion being the actor she was invited to be the director of the action. We used a willing psychology trainee to act out the role of a strong and powerful compassionate courtier based on a character from one of the novels.

Ffion directed her compassionate actor to hold his body in a particular way – helpfully her ideal compassionate other had powerful wings that could enfold, support and carry. Ffion instructed her actor to hold a confident strong open upper body posture as if he had these wings. Using messages from earlier sessions we guided him to give voice to some of her compassionate messages. Messages that Ffion wanted to hear but had found hard to accept could be offered to her. It was fascinating to see the physical change, in posture, facial expression and voice tone in her actor as she gave him directions. More significantly as she did this, her own posture began to mirror what she was directing in her actor. I noticed small signs of quiet, strong, supportive confidence appearing in the facial expression of Ffion as she directed the exercise. We had negotiated a way around a small block to training the compassionate mind, and Ffion was starting to get the feel of compassionate qualities in her body.

Later we would use this same ideal compassionate character to be a strong companion standing alongside her younger self as we revisited a significant trauma memory.

26.27 Addressing Anger Part One

In the initial three-circle formulation work, we identified that Ffion's threat protection system was mostly made up of fear and shame. The more detailed threat-focussed formulation identified how some of this was related to a fear of anger being expressed in others and by her. We needed to use the skills she had developed in her compassionate mind training to support Ffion to engage in working with anger. We approached this by first undertaking exposure work to seeing and tolerating anger expressed in others. In the spirit of playfulness outlined earlier we began this work by watching short animated cartoon expressions of anger. Even this apparently gentle approach took a great deal of courage for her to engage with and could only be done once she had undertaken the compassionate mind grounding work to prepare herself for the exercise. Gradually over time she learnt to build resilience to her learnt natural reactions to seeing anger expressed in others and found anger expressed in others easier to tolerate. However, giving herself permission to express anger was a much tougher ask.

26.28 Revisiting Blocks

When dealing with blocks and resistances to tricky emotions we can take a similar approach to dealing with blocks to compassion. We bring compassionate wisdom and curiosity to understand why the block needed to be there. We discovered that Ffion's sensory sensitivity, neuro-diversity and early traumatic events all played a part in the life story of the block to expressing anger.

We used brief chair work to facilitate a role-taking exercise to curiously have a dialogue with her block to anger (Lucre, 2021). First, Ffion was invited to sit in a chair and imagine being her block. I took the role of a curious interviewer and enquired how long the block had been in her life, wondered what it was like taking on this job for her and what the block feared would happen if she were no longer there for Ffion. The block revealed that it did not want her to get into trouble and face rejection as a consequence of expressed anger. After helping Ffion de-role from playing her block, we explored how she might validate the understandable fear of rejection and the pain that the block was giving voice to. Then Ffion was invited to step into her compassionate self as she switched into a chair that we nominated to represent her compassionate self. Speaking from her compassionate self she told her block.

"I know that you are worried that I might spiral out of control and hurt someone if I express my feelings."

"I hear you have concerns about me and I am grateful that you want me to be safe, but I am going to be ok with this." "It's alright I will be ok now."

Although through this work and other practices and dialogues Ffion could understand cognitively what she needed to do, actually allowing herself to express anger remained very tricky.

As we discovered through the dialogue work her block to expressing anger openly had been in her life a very long time and it was not quite ready to give up its important protective role.

Ffion needed to be able to give expression to anger rather than letting voices be the only parts of her that sounded angry. Perhaps if we could help Ffion to express her anger in a way that was acceptable to her, her voices might not need to sound so angry themselves?

26.29 A Quiet Clue from Ffion's Past

Growing up Ffion learnt to cope with her difficulties by being very controlled and submissive in social situations. This led to her being withdrawn and restricted in emotional expression and interactions. It took a long time for Ffion to learn to let go of this strategy, and ultimately it was listening to her body wisdom that opened the door to more freedom of expression.

During one of her early inpatient stays, Ffion was feeling overwhelmed, helpless and hopeless. In our session she presented in an emotionally flat and blunted way. Sitting with her in purposeful and present silence I could feel the weight of her despair and suffering.

Curious to know more about the other parts of Ffion's life, the parts that didn't get much opportunity to be expressed, I wondered if Ffion had ever experienced a sense of freedom and lightness of being. After more silence and in barely a whisper Ffion replied "Dancing." As she spoke that word, for the briefest of moments there was a lightness about her facial expression that I had not seen before. The micro muscles in her face and around her eyes were sending me a social signal that there was something very important to pay attention to here. But as quickly as that beautiful expression appeared it was closed down again by her protective strategies.

That one word and flash of emotional expression that had escaped her protective defences had a powerful impact. I felt a surge of emotion: a mixture of joy and deep sadness, it was as if a window had opened for a moment to reveal a view showing a possible way ahead. Those feelings that I experienced then were like a compass pointing the direction to follow. There would indeed be sadness to address in our work ahead but ultimately it would be Ffion rediscovering the importance of dance in her life that would help to set her free and would also help her to find a way to give expression to anger.

At this point in our compassion-focussed journey, Ffion found it impossible to let down her protective guard. It was too early in our work to even try to tackle this as Ffion lacked enough internal signals of safeness to draw upon and both voices and self-critical parts were telling her that she did not deserve any positive experiences. But it was something very important that we needed to return to.

26.30 Addressing Anger Part Two – The Window Opens

Paradoxically it was to be another acute admission to hospital during the Covid pandemic that gave us an opportunity to work on the unfinished business of helping Ffion free herself from some of her protective social inhibitions and give expression to anger.

For several months the rhythm of our work had been interrupted by health authority social distancing policies as a result of the Covid pandemic. Ffion was starting to struggle with increased voice hearing and suicidal urges. One of the causes of her distress and despair was related to her difficulties in expressing anger. Sadly Ffion was admitted to hospital again but the admission enabled us to meet in person once again.

We started to meet twice a week in a spacious area away from the ward environment. Ffion welcomed the opportunity to practice the posture, breathing and sensory grounding work that was our cue for stepping into the compassionate mind. We revisited familiar practices and started to extend them. Ffion was now more confident about acting into the part of her compassionate other. Recalling our earlier session and the briefest flash of longing to dance that I had seen upon her face, I took this opportunity to introduce her to some of the movement-based practices from Rufus May and Elisabeth Svanholmer's work (https://openmindedonline.com/). We discovered that standing up and stomping our feet was very helpful for releasing frustration at being on the ward again (we both shared this frustration and the sense of release that the practice gave us!). We added shouting to the stomping. Her anger was starting to find an outlet. Ffion tried out the yoga boxing practice she had watched in one of Rufus's videos (https://rufusmay.com/). She was not too keen on this practice, but she found more release for her anger by using a pillow borrowed from the ward as a punch bag that I held up for her.

In every session we used the stomping practice, and then we started to do this in time to music that Ffion played on her phone. Gradually over a few sessions we explored different types of movement. With up-beat music playing we engaged in an exercise where we would take it in turns to make a movement that the other had to repeat before adding a new one of their own. Before we knew it and without naming it as such we had made up a dance routine.

Out of respect to the parts of her that still held some social awkwardness we would in time finish our movement-based practices with Ffion choosing a music track of her choice, then standing with our backs to each other in a different corner of the room we would have a free dance session.

These movement- and dance-based sessions finally opened the window for Ffion to safely express anger that had been waiting to be heard for a long time. Reflecting back it was these sessions that were the real turning point for Ffion. However, we were only able to reach this point by carefully building up her compassionate mind and sensitively validating and working alongside the parts of her that were fearful of letting go of their protective function.

Dance was to become an integral part of her compassionate kitbag and daily practice.

At the same time as rediscovering dance Ffion was learning to value and celebrate what it was to be neuro-diverse. She researched more about her condition and tried different forms of sensory stimulation and reduction. Noise-cancelling headphones proved to be revolutionary for her. Her own research and discoveries gave her a new sense of identity and freedom. As Ffion grew in self-confidence her relationship with voices began to change. She started to view them as aspects of her own thinking and not something that she needed to ignore or get rid of.

As we drew our compassion-based work to a close and were reflecting and summarising on her therapy journey, Ffion realised that her voice hearing had become much more problematic when she supressed the parts of her that gave expression to her neuro-diversity and in particular when she stopped herself from dancing. It was now that she had found a way to give herself permission to enjoy dancing again coupled with accepting that being neuro-diverse was a strength to be celebrated that she was able to move forward with her life.

Ffion wrote this summary for her medical notes so that her version of her story could be heard alongside the medical version.

"My understanding of my mental health problems is that as a result of being undiagnosed autistic, I developed severe depression at a very young age. This presented itself as voices that I could hear. As I went through childhood, every time a big change would happen I would develop more voices. These voices had a protective form, although they didn't do this very effectively. They tried to make sure that I fit in and wouldn't be rejected, they did this by being very negative and critical towards me. This constant dialogue caused me to develop anxiety and an eating disorder. These, again, were caused by my suppressed autism. My mental health deteriorated very quickly at the age of 18, and I was admitted to hospital for the first time at 19. For the next 3 years I was in and out of hospital and was on many medications, one was clozapine. This was prescribed as the diagnosis at the time was schizophrenia, but this medication didn't help and made things worse, and I don't identify with that diagnosis. I had a lot of negative side effects from this medication. In my last hospital admission, the doctors took more time to review me and realised (as well as myself and family members) that autism is what was causing all the other problems. From that admission I have been accepting my diagnosis and I am coping well with all my mental health problems."

26.31 Conclusion

CFT for psychosis offers a potentially liberating and acceptable treatment paradigm. When our interventions, whether it be psychological or pharmacological, focus solely on symptom reduction there is a danger that we inadvertently overlook some very important sources of information and wisdom that hurting and distressed minds need us to hear. As Eleanor Longden (2013) so beautifully describes in her TED talk, even our most critical voices and parts can be expressing long overlooked or disowned emotional needs, holding echoes of past trauma, loss and rejection. If we learn to let go of the security of the dominant biomedical view of psychosis as something to be treated, silenced or ignored, we can open a window on the wisdom and messages hidden in the emotional needs that lie beneath unusual experiences. As we saw with Ffion, it was through listening, dialoguing and relating compassionately with voices and emotional blocks that Ffion found her way forward to recovery.

At the heart of CFT is an understanding and wisdom that suffering is an intrinsic part of the human condition. It is understandable for all humans to want to avoid this reality, but it is through the development and training of our compassionate minds that we can learn to relate to our hurt and suffering in a more helpful way.

Being truly compassionate is a challenge for us all as individuals and for society. It draws us to approach the dark mud of the mind wherever we may find it with warmth, strength and courage (Gilbert & Choden, 2013). Doing so unlocks an amazing potential for much-needed transformational change of whole social and economic systems and perhaps nowhere needs this more than our mental health systems. As Paul Gilbert says in his collection of essays "Living like Crazy":

As some of the contemplative sciences have shown for thousands of years, and science is beginning to reveal, compassion is one of the most important courageous and healing motivations that nature ever came up with. Not to cultivate it and use it for the benefit of us all would be to continue living like crazy. (Gilbert, 2017, Second Edition p. 536).

Disclaimer Clinical cases presented in this chapter do not include real names or personal information of real persons.

References

Assembly, U. G. (1948). Universal declaration of human rights. *UN General Assembly, 302*(2).

Birchwood, M., & Trower, P. (2006). The future of cognitive-behavioural therapy for psychosis: Not a quasi-neuroleptic. *The British Journal of Psychiatry, 188*(2), 107–108. https://doi.org/10.1192/bjp.bp.105.014985

Cupitt, C. (Ed.). (2018). *CBT for psychosis: Process-orientated therapies and the third wave*. Routledge.

Docter, P., & Del Carmen, R. (Director). (2015). *Inside Out* [Film]. Pixar Animation Studios.

Ellerby, M. (2013). Schizophrenia, Maslow's hierarchy, and compassion-focused therapy. *Schizophrenia Bulletin, 42*(3), 531–533. https://doi.org/10.1093/schbul/sbt119

Ellerby, M. (2014). How compassion may help me. *Psychosis, 6*(3), 266–270. https://doi.org/10.1080/17522439.2013.81633

Ellerby, M. (2017). Resisting voices through finding our own compassionate voice. *Schizophrenia Bulletin, 43*(2), 230–232. https://doi.org/10.1093/schbul/sbu035

Gersie, A. (1997). *Reflections on therapeutic storymaking: The use of stories in groups*. Jessica Kingsley Publishers.

Gilbert, P. (2009). *The compassionate mind*. Robinson.

Gilbert, P. (2010). *Compassion focused therapy: Distinctive features*. Routledge.

Gilbert, P. (2015). An evolutionary approach to emotion in mental health with a focus on affiliative emotions. *Emotion Review, 7*(3), 230–237. https://doi.org/10.1177/1754073915576552

Gilbert, P. (2017). *Living like crazy*. Annwyn House.

Gilbert, P., & Choden. (2013). *Mindful compassion: Using the power of mindfulness and compassion to transform our lives*. Hachette UK.

Gilbert, P., & Irons, C. (2005). Focused therapies and compassionate mind training for shame and self-attacking. In *Compassion* (pp. 263–325) Routledge.

Gumley, A., Braehler, C., Laithwaite, H., MacBeth, A., & Gilbert, P. (2010). A compassion focused model of recovery after psychosis. *International Journal of Cognitive Therapy, 3*(2), 186–201. https://doi.org/10.1521/ijct.2010.3.2.186

Hadden, L. M., Alderson-Day, B., Jackson, M., Fernyhough, C., & Bentall, R. P. (2019). The auditory-verbal hallucinations of Welsh–English bilingual people. *Psychology and Psychotherapy: Theory, Research and Practice*. https://doi.org/10.1111/papt.12234

Hanh, T. N. (2013). *Love letter to the earth*. Parallax Press.

Heriot-Maitland, C., & Anderson, K. (2015). *Compassion for voices: A tale of courage and hope* [online]. Available at: https://www.youtube.com/watch?v=VRqI4lxuXAw

Heriot-Maitland, C., & Levey, V. (2021). A case report of compassion-focused therapy for distressing voice-hearing experiences. *Journal of Clinical Psychology, 77*(8), 1821–1835. https://doi.org/10.1002/jclp.23211

Heriot-Maitland, C., & Russell, G. (2018). Compassion-focused therapy for relating to voices. In *CBT for psychosis: Process-orientated therapies and the third wave* (pp. 114–130). Routledge.

Irons, C., & Beaumont, E. (2017). The compassionate mind workbook: A step-by-step guide to developing your compassionate self. .

Kennedy, A., & Ellerby, M. (2016). A compassion-focused approach to working with someone diagnosed with schizophrenia. *Journal of Clinical Psychology, 72*(2), 123–131. https://doi.org/10.1002/jclp.22251

Kolts, R. L., Bell, T., Bennett-Levy, J., & Irons, C. (2018). *Experiencing compassion-focused therapy from the inside out: A self-practice/self-reflection workbook for therapists*. Guilford Publications.

Longden, E.(2013). *The voices in my head* [Video]. TED conferences. https://www.ted.com/talks/eleanor_longden_the_voices_in_my_head

Lucre, K. (2021). *Role taking in CFT – Online webinar*. Compassionate Mind Foundation.

Lucre, K., & Clapton, N. (2021). The compassionate kitbag: A creative and integrative approach to compassion-focused therapy. *Psychology and Psychotherapy: Theory, Research and Practice, 94*, 497–516. https://doi.org/10.1111/papt.12291

Martins, M. J. R. V., Castilho, P., Carvalho, C. B., Pereira, A. T., Santos, V., Gumley, A., & de Macedo, A. F. (2017). Contextual cognitive-behavioral therapies across the psychosis continuum. *European Psychologist*. https://doi.org/10.1027/1016-9040/a000283

Mavituna, S., Hahn, E., Hahne, I., Bergmann, N., Pijnenborg, M., Ta, T. M. T., et al. (2022). Compassion-based approaches: A systematic review of their effectiveness and acceptability in schizophrenia spectrum disorders. *Current Psychology*, 1–15. https://doi.org/10.1007/s12144-022-02908-3

Mayhew, S. L. (2015). Compassion focused therapy for people experiencing psychosis. In *Innovations in psychosocial interventions for psychosis* (pp. 111–130). Routledge.

McGlanaghy, E., Turner, D., Davis, G. A., Sharpe, H., Dougall, N., Morris, P., et al. (2021). A network meta-analysis of psychological interventions for schizophrenia and psychosis: Impact on symptoms. *Schizophrenia Research, 228*, 447–459. https://doi.org/10.1016/j.schres.2020.12.036

National Institute for Health and Care Excellence. (2014). *Psychosis and Schizophrenia in adults: Treatment and management* (NICE clinical guidelines (CG178)). National Institute for Health and Care Excellence. https://www.nice.org.uk/guidance/cg178

Niedenthal, P. M. (2007). Embodying emotion. *Science, 316*(5827), 1002–1005. https://doi.org/10.1126/science.1136930

Niedenthal, P. M., Barsalou, L. W., Winkielman, P., Krauth-Gruber, S., & Ric, F. (2005). Embodiment in attitudes, social perception, and emotion. *Personality and Social Psychology Review, 9*(3), 184–211. https://doi.org/10.1207/2Fs15327957pspr0903_1

Parker, I., Schnackenberg, J., & Hopfenbeck, M. (2021). *The practical handbook of hearing voices – Therapeutic and creative approaches*. PCCS Books.

Peper, E., & Lin, I. M. (2012). Increase or decrease depression: How body postures influence your energy level. *Biofeedback, 40*(3), 125–130. https://doi.org/10.5298/1081-5937-40.3.01

Porges, S. W. (2003). The polyvagal theory: Phylogenetic contributions to social behavior. *Physiology & Behavior, 79*(3), 503–513. https://doi.org/10.1016/S0031-9384(03)00156-2

Porges, S. W. (2007). The polyvagal perspective. *Biological Psychology, 74*(2), 116–143. https://doi.org/10.1016/j.biopsycho.2013.02.013

Razzaque, R. (2014). *Breaking down is waking up: The connection between psychological distress and spiritual awakening*. Watkins Media Limited.

Spikins, P. (2017). Prehistoric origins: The compassion of far distant strangers. In *Compassion* (pp. 28–42). Routledge.

Stellar, J. E., & Keltner, D. (2017). Compassion in the autonomic nervous system: The role of the vagus nerve. In *Compassion* (pp. 120–134). Routledge.

Waters, F., Chiu, V., Atkinson, A., & Blom, J. D. (2018). Severe sleep deprivation causes hallucinations and a gradual progression toward psychosis with increasing time awake. *Frontiers in Psychiatry, 9*, 303. https://doi.org/10.3389/fpsyt.2018.00303

Welford, M. (2019). *Why wait for adulthood CFT for young people*. Workshop for PG Diploma, CFT Birmingham University.

Wilson, V. E., & Peper, E. (2004). The effects of upright and slumped postures on the recall of positive and negative thoughts. *Applied Psychophysiology and Biofeedback, 29*(3), 189–195. https://doi.org/10.1023/b:apbi.0000039057.32963.34

Wright, N. P., Turkington, D., Kelly, O. P., Davies, D., Jacobs, A. M., & Hopton, J. (2014). *Treating psychosis: A clinician's guide to integrating acceptance and commitment therapy, compassion-focused therapy, and mindfulness approaches within the cognitive behavioral therapy tradition*. New Harbinger Publications.

Chapter 27
Clinical Case: Compassion-Focused Therapy

Maria João Martins and Marta Alonso Maynar

27.1 Introduction

According to Gilbert et al. (2000), there are a few underlying factors in which psychotherapy is rooted in and evolved from: the process of natural selection, what humans evolved to do (e.g., motivations and social roles), and which physiological mechanisms are behind those actions and motivations (Gilbert et al., 2000). One might also add the nature of human suffering as one of the essential understandings from which psychotherapy should be conceptualized.

The human brain is a product of evolution, has been shaped following the Darwinian "selection for function" (Panksepp, 2004), and has been conceptualized as having a "tricky" nature. The major trade-off of human brains is the combination and interaction of "old brain" emotions and motivations (shared with other animals) and "new brain" abilities, such as complex thinking, theory of the mind, symbolic representation, observing, sense of self, and self-identity (Gilbert, 2014b). The capacity to pay attention to, reflect on, and interpret mental states (e.g., sensations, thoughts, feelings, and emotions) of the self and others can stimulate threat emotions and maintain these physiological systems in a state of activation in the body, even when the (perceived) threat is no longer present (Gilbert, 2014b).

Compassion-focused therapy (CFT) takes an evolutionary functional view to emotions in which three evolved functions of emotions emerge, namely, to alert for threat and activate defensive strategies; to inform on availability of resources/rewards activating seeking engagement strategies; and to inform on safeness and

M. J. Martins (✉)
University of Coimbra Medical Services, Coimbra, Portugal
e-mail: m.joao.martins@sas.uc.pt

M. A. Maynar
Center for Mindful Self Compassion, San Diego, CA, USA
e-mail: marta@centerformsc.org

J. A. Díaz-Garrido et al. (eds.), *Psychological Interventions for Psychosis*,
https://doi.org/10.1007/978-3-031-27003-1_27

allow for non-action in the form of contentment and openness (Gilbert, 2014b). These functions are described and conceptualized in the three affect regulation systems' model (Gilbert, 2005).

The three affect regulation systems' model (Gilbert, 2005) derives from research in the area of neurophysiology and neuroscience of emotion. It suggests the existence of three different but interactive emotion regulation systems (one underpinning negative affect and two positive affect related), sensitive and responsive to different types of stimuli (Depue & Morrone-Strupinsky, 2005). The threat defense system refers to focusing attention, detecting, and appropriate responding to different types of threats. In the presence of a potential threat, this system quickly, automatically, and unconsciously activates a series of emotional (anger, anxiety, disgust, shame), behavioral (fight, flight, immobilization, submission), cognitive, and physiological responses. The system may also remain active after the threat disappears with the focus remaining on the consequence of that threat (damage or loss) (Gilbert, 2014a). The drive system is a system of positive affect oriented towards the quest for resources geared towards survival and well-being. Bound predominantly in reaching and getting, and linked to the dopaminergic system, the emotions elicited by this system are usually experienced as exciting and activating (e.g., vitality, excitement, enthusiasm, and energy). This system is also often linked to competitive motives, dominance and social status (Gilbert, 2014b). Finally, the soothing system is usually characterized as a more specialized positive affect system linked to endorphin and oxytocin systems that can downregulate threat activation (Depue & Morrone-Strupinsky, 2005). Especially linked to the caring mentality and particularly linked to attachment and connection to others, the soothing system gives rise to positive emotions, such as connectedness, warmth, contentment, happiness, and well-being.

Gumley and collaborators have further explored the three-system model and applied it to a formulation of recovery in people with psychosis (Gumley et al., 2010).

Considering the three systems model, in psychosis, there would be an imbalance in the affect regulation systems, with threat activation arising from several internal and external sources creating an overly stimulated threat system (hypersensitivity to threat). This overactivation of the threat system would be combined with few sources of soothing and safeness resulting from an underdeveloped soothing system unable to counter the easy and fast activation of the threat system. This imbalance between the frequency and intensity of activation of the different systems would have its origins in evolved mechanisms (derived from the consequences of humans having a "new brain" that allows us to anticipate negative consequences, ruminate on past events, and self-criticizing, thus maintaining vicious circles of threat-based responses – Gilbert, 2010), combined with aversive early experiences (Gilbert, 2005), as well as genetic predisposition (Gilbert, 2004). This threat-based functioning rooted on aversive interpersonal environment and experiences is fuelled by the presence of several internal and external perceived sources of threat (Gumley et al., 2010). In fact, it has been argued that problems in affect regulation systems might cause subsequent maturation of frontal cortical processing systems with, for instance, people oriented to threat – instead of safeness – processing in early life having difficulties in feeling safe in the social world (Gilbert, 2004). These emotional experiences and external world perceptions often co-occur with cognitive/perceptual changes (e.g., subclinical psychotic symptoms) that constitute themselves as internal threats potentially leading to relapse. Fear of relapse has been described as an internal threat prevalent in people with psychosis. The associated external threat of psychiatric interventions is also important (Gumley et al., 2010, 2015).

Compassionate responding emerges as an emotional recovery-oriented alternative to threat-based responses to external and internal threats. Learning to switch from a threat-based social mentality oriented by threat-based processing to a caring mentality characterized by sensitivity, sympathy, distress tolerance, empathy, nonjudgement, acceptance, and warmth may be key in psychotherapy for people with psychosis (Gumley et al., 2010).

Understanding of the origins and organization of the threat and safeness processing has been argued as important in intervening with people with psychosis (Gilbert, 2004). In fact, authors have recommended that along with reducing the sense of threat there is also the need to stimulate and learn to activate the soothing–safeness system (Gumley et al., 2010).

A Brief Overview of CFT and CMT Research in Psychosis
Compassion-focused approaches and CMT have been used to promote recovery in psychosis with promising results. Improvement has been found regarding social comparison, shame, self-esteem (Laithwaite et al., 2009), self-criticism, fears of compassion, compassion, clinical improvement (Braehler et al., 2013a, b; Martins et al., 2018), and distress associated with psychotic experiences (Hickey et al., 2021). Processes studies have found that increases in compassion were significantly associated with reductions in depressive symptoms and perceived social marginalization (Braehler et al., 2013a, b). The compassionate self-acceptance process, which implies both acceptance and change in relationship with the self, was considered essential to recovery, growth, and empowered action (Waite et al., 2015).

27.2 Case Description[1]

27.2.1 Sociodemographic Data and Referral

Miguel is a 22-year-old, male, medical student, living with his parents and sister (Ana, 15, student).

[1] The clinical case presented in this chapter is a combination of several real patients and therapeutic processes.

Miguel comes to the first psychology appointment referred by his assistant psychiatrist after a 1-month hospital stay – "patient with a first episode of psychosis about a month ago. Persecuting delusional ideation present, with partial insight, and auditory-verbal hallucinatory activity. Medicated with Paliperidone 100mg IM monthly and Clonazepam 2mg per day at night".

27.2.2 *Mental State Examination*

Miguel comes to the first psychology appointment with his parents, although asks to be alone in the appointment. He was cooperative throughout the session, although with some difficulty in maintaining eye contact, and articulated himself clearly, answered questions spontaneously, although at a slow rate and speed. Miguel was alert and orientated to time and place, and did not exhibit any formal thought disorders. He was able to answer questions and recall his past, although sometimes was not sure about symptoms that occurred during the psychotic episode. Presented signs of mild anxiety throughout the session. When questioned about his health condition, Miguel spontaneously reported having had a "psychotic break" and "needing help to manage [his] symptoms and preventing relapse."

27.2.3 *Disease Evolution and Current Symptoms*

Miguel has always felt mildly anxious in social contexts and when he started higher education the symptoms worsened. He suffered from performance anxiety throughout the first years of his medical degree ("always extremely anxious during evaluations", missing oral exams) although his functioning was mostly maintained, and never sought professional help. One month ago, during the exam period, Miguel reports starting to become more aware of other people's thoughts and feelings about him. This progressed to paranoia and then persecutory delusions "I was constantly thinking people wanted to harm me, even kill me if they could, and I didn't understand why," "a conspiracy," and self-referential delusions "always watching me, talking about me." With the high levels of anxiety, Miguel struggled with everyday activities including self-care and leaving home for classes/other tasks. Sleep disturbances emerged, with a period of severe insomnia ("For three days I wasn't able to sleep") leading to the first occurrence of hallucinations. Hallucinations were always auditive-verbal – voices – and invariable caused high levels of distress. Miguel describes his voice as "a male, with a powerful, profound and frightening tone of voice," "always saying difficult things, calling me names, trying to discourage me to do the things I want/need to do." When questioned if he knows the owner of the voice, Miguel states, "I don't know him but he seemed to know me very well, that was frightening," "still his voice always seemed familiar."

Currently, Miguel has insight related to his positive symptoms. As a medical student, he refers to them as delusions and hallucinations. At the first appointment, Miguel identified some paranoid thoughts when in stressful social situations ("they are after me," "don't want me to succeed," "will harm me and my family"). These thoughts are anxiety provoking and the acknowledgment as only thoughts only occur after the situation has ended. He still occasionally hears voices ("only one or two words now," "one or two times per month," "difficult words, usually about me, such as dumb, stupid, failure," "always the same male voice") which still is a significant cause of suffering.

Following his hospitalization, Miguel reports the appearance of negative symptoms, such as anticipatory anhedonia ("it seems that I don't have the motivation to go out and do things I used to like, but if my friends 'force' me I usually go and have some fun"), lack of energy and "feeling kind of numb, it seems like sometimes I'm not able to feel things normally" (blunted affect was observable during the assessment stage).

Regarding social and academic areas, Miguel also reported feeling significantly anxious in most social and performance situations (not always associated with paranoia but thoughts of inadequacy and inferiority). Troubles in concentration were also reported.

27.2.4 *Instruments Used[2] for Assessment*

Clinical interview for psychotic disorders (CIPD, Martins et al., 2015, 2019)[3]

Semi-structured clinical interview for the assessment of psychotic disorders. In addition to evaluating psychotic symptoms in a diagnostic perspective, the CIPD also assesses their psychosocial correlates, namely, the relationship one establishes with their symptoms, the interference in one's life caused by the symptoms, the sense of empowerment, and hope.

Miguel had a schizophreniform disorder diagnosis according to the DSM5 (APA, 2013). CIPD scores showed that positive symptoms had a moderate interference in everyday life, while negative symptoms' interference was high (particularly in social and academic areas). Empowerment regarding both positive and negative symptoms was perceived as low.

[2]Assessment tools were used throughout the sessions in order to assess difficulties and monitor progress and also as a way of eliciting important content to be discussed with Miguel.

[3]Available from the first author.

27.2.5 Clinical Goals and Therapeutic Plan

At the end of the first session, after brief psychoeducation regarding the therapeutic relationship (roles of both Miguel and the therapist) and therapeutic process (as a collaborative one), Miguel was asked to reflect on his therapeutic goals during the time between sessions. In the following session, Miguel's ideas were discussed and the therapeutic team (Miguel and therapist) established the following clinical goals:

- Build self-confidence.
- Manage negative symptoms.
- Manage anxiety symptoms.
- Manage paranoia in social and academic settings.

The proposed therapeutic plan included three parts: individual therapy (Part 1) and group therapy (Part 2), both based on compassion-focused therapy, and relapse prevention (Part 3). Miguel would start with one-to-one therapy and then he would be included in a therapeutic group for people living with psychosis (COMPASS – COMPassionate Approach for Schizophrenia and Schizoaffective disorder[4]). Although experiencing some reluctance regarding group therapy, Miguel accepted that being in a group (after some competencies had been built and trained) would be an important experience both to acquire (and practice) new competencies and strategies for giving/receiving compassion, and connecting with people with similar experiences. He also expected that individual therapy would "prepare [him] to not dread the group so much."

Miguel continued with psychopharmacological treatment throughout the therapy sessions and close articulation was assured between the therapist and his assistant psychiatrist.

27.3 Part 1: Individual Psychotherapy[5]

27.3.1 Phase 1: Establishing the Therapeutic Relationship and Psychoeducation

Notes to Therapists

Mindfulness in the context of the therapeutic relationship is recommended as it has been defined as a way of paying attention with empathy, presence, and ability to listen in depth (Hick & Bien, 2008) and seems to increase the quality

[4] In this chapter, only the individual therapeutic process will be described, although we provide a brief description of COMPASS contents and process.

[5] Since different patients may present different needs and paces in the therapeutic process, therapy in this chapter will be described through phases, which may have different lengths. Examples of specific session content, practices, and clinical feedback will be provided.

perception of the relationship (Wexler, 2006) and even improve the results of the therapeutic process (Grepmair et al., 2007). It is intended that therapists facilitate a helping relationship, which is based on principles, such as being present moment by moment, presenting a non-judgmental understanding, and loving attitude of acceptance with the constant perspective that the suffering that patients experience is part of a common humanity. Therefore, it is also important that therapists maintain a moment-by-moment awareness of their inner private experience (emotions, thoughts, sensations) as well as an accepting attitude, without reacting to them (Gilbert & Leahy, 2007). This awareness will also allow a deeper understanding of people's difficulties. The therapist also has an important role in modelling compassionate behaviors and attitudes towards themselves and in the interaction with the patient. It is important to embody the compassionate qualities (Gilbert, 2014b), and therefore, the therapeutic relationship may function as the first source of compassionate relationships activating the patient's soothing system.

As a way of introducing the therapeutic plan, Miguel watched in session the video "Compassion for Voices: a tale of courage and hope"[6] (King's Cultural Community, 2015, February 23). Previously established goals for therapy were revisited from the perspective of compassion-focused therapy as presented in the video: managing symptoms through a different relationship with them, the self, and others, and the compassionate self as a secure base from which he can engage with difficult thoughts and feelings.

Following the explanation present in the video, the three-system model was explored. Miguel was asked to draw his three systems as they usually are in the past month: the bigger the circle drawn, the higher the intensity of emotions/thoughts, and the easiest and frequent activation of the system. Discussion regarding the specific cognitive, emotional, physiological, and behavioral outputs of each system more frequent in Miguel followed. Miguel's three systems' drawing with information of the discussion is shown in Fig. 27.1.

The concept of "tricky brains" was then introduced. It was important for Miguel to realize that the activation of the threat system "by default" was not his fault, but the consequence of an old brain–new brain loop-inducing interaction. Miguel identified some of his loops and they were recorded for future sessions (see Table 27.1).

With the "not our fault" premise established, therapy focused on providing Miguel with a more individualized account of how his specific difficulties emerged, developed, and were being maintained. An idiosyncratic formulation of Miguel's difficulties was built together using guided discovery (see Fig. 27.2).

[6] Available from https://www.youtube.com/watch?v=VRqI4lxuXAw

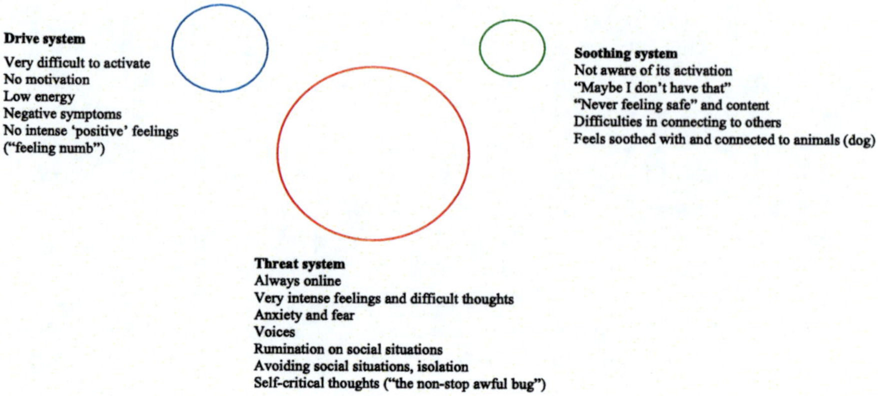

Fig. 27.1 Miguel's drawing of the three systems – annotated during the discussion with the therapist

Table 27.1 Miguel's loops

Old brain motive	New brain ability	How does the loop look like?	Consequences/ defensive behaviors (old brain)
Status	Rumination Worry Theory of mind self-criticism	Ruminating after social situations on perceived mistakes. Worrying about what others might think, worry about future situations	Anxiety, frustration Impulse to avoid future social situations
Harm avoidance	Anticipating Planning Self-monitoring	Planning ahead social situations, going over everything that might go wrong. Self-focused attention during social interactions monitoring and judging every anxiety symptom	Increased anxiety Freeze response Submissive behaviors
Social connection Harm avoidance	Self-criticism Rumination	Self-critical thoughts about being a failure, different, having a disease Ruminating on the meaning of the voice	Fear of relapse Excessively engaging with the voice

27.3.1.1 Instruments Used

Other as Shamer Scale (OAS, Goss et al., 1994).

The OAS aims to explore expectations of how others see or judge the self (external shame).

Miguel presented high levels of external shame with the most significant statements being "I think other people look down at me," "People see me as unimportant compared to others," and "Other people see me as defective as a person." Miguel reports feeling this way before the first episode of psychosis but states that these feelings intensified after his hospitalization "people now know I'm different, weak and that I have a disease."

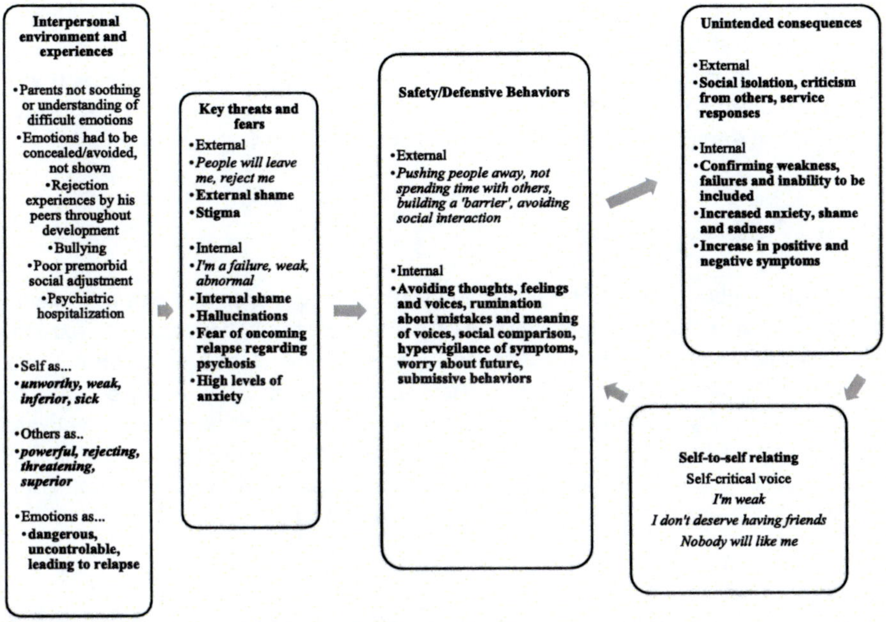

Fig. 27.2 Idiosyncratic formulation of Miguel's difficulties

Forms of Self-Criticism and Reassurance Scale (FSCRS, Gilbert et al., 2004).

The FSCRS measures self-criticism and self-reassurance through statements regarding how people respond to perceived failure and setbacks. It measures two types of self-criticism (hated self and inadequate self) and self-reassurance.

Miguel scored high in the self-criticism scales, particularly in the inadequate self, as expected. There is a clear view of the self as not good enough and inadequate, and this is often met with criticism, rumination on failures and shortcomings, and difficult emotions (disappointment, sadness, and frustration). Miguel does not report the want or need to hurt himself and the hated self is less present. These levels of self-criticism are combined with severe difficulties in self-reassurance. Miguel referred that when in situations of perceived failure, he has difficulties in still feeling that he deserves love and acceptance, forgiving himself, and being able to remind himself of positive qualities he has. In these situations, he finds it very difficult to deal with these thoughts and feelings with gentle and genuine care and support for himself.

His answers to the scales were used to discuss the activation of the threat system both in social interactions/relationships and in the relationship with the self. Miguel identified, with help from the therapist, thoughts and emotions arising from the activation of the threat systems and some threat-based patterns were discussed: anxiety, fear, and shame associated with social relationships (others as powerful, superior, and threatening; self as inadequate, inferior, and weak) leading to flight-freeze responses. On the other hand, thoughts and emotions towards the self were discussed and self-criticism was identified as a strategy (highly frequent) Miguel uses to deal with this negative view of the self and the emotions arising (shame, fear, sadness). Self-reassurance was briefly introduced as an alternative strategy and Miguel showed some resistance to it ("I don't know how to do that," "what if I do that and bad things happen?" "I have to be strong and stop feeling this way").

27.3.1.2 Clinical Feedback

At the end of phase 1, Miguel was able to identify the activation of the three systems (with the threat system being the most easily activated) throughout his daily routine. He was more aware of his threat-based loops and understood their origins (both regarding the evolutionary perspective and the role of his early experiences). He could also identify the situations in which he would like his drive system to activate (e.g., situations in which he lacks motivation/energy) and interactions with others/self in which he would like to be able to soothe and reassure himself, thus activating the soothing system.

27.3.2 *Phase 2: Associating Psychotic Symptoms and the Threat and Drive Systems. Introducing Mindfulness and Grounding*

Positive psychotic symptoms, delusions and hallucinations, were conceptualized as an output of an overly active threat system. Such as, when activated, the threat system "sends" us particular emotions (such as fear, anger, or disgust) and behavioral tendencies (fight-flight-freeze responses), it also shapes our way of thinking (negative cognitions about the self, others, future) that in an extreme state can cause delusions to occur (e.g., persecutory delusions), as well as our perception, which is the case of hallucinations (extreme alterations in perception). Although these outputs can feel very intense, it was explored with Miguel that he has a choice (similarly to when threat-based emotions or thoughts occur): being carried away by emotions (either by overidentifying or overinvolvement with them), or being able to observe them, with understanding and kindness and without reacting or confusing them with the self.

Miguel attributed the cause of his negative symptoms to side effects of medication. The difference between primary and secondary negative symptoms was explained and Miguel and the therapist concluded that the majority of Miguel's negative symptoms were primary.[7] This conceptualization helped Miguel better understand his negative symptoms, decrease resistance regarding antipsychotic

[7] Primary negative symptoms are part of the disease process itself, that is, are not secondary to other factors (e.g., depression, drug-induced effects) (Carpenter et al., 1988)

medication, and gain a sense of empowerment to deal with them (as with other symptoms, reducing the passive resignation which he usually meets side effects of medication). Negative symptoms were conceptualized as a reflection of the under-activation of the drive system. Drive system outputs were revisited and symptoms such as anhedonia, lack of energy and motivation, and blunted affect were clearly identified as a sign of a blocked drive system. Intervention was then proposed to also focus on practices (e.g., compassion, loving-kindness meditations) that would boost positive emotions which would in turn a) enhance personal resources to deal with negative symptoms improving motivation, and anticipatory pleasure, and b) foster psychological recovery through feelings of hope, environmental mastery, self-acceptance and feeling of purpose in life (Johnson et al., 2009).

Notes to Therapists

Mindfulness and compassion have been described as co-creating one another (Tirch, 2010). Neff and Dahm (2015) argue that mindfulness and (self)compassion are able to mutually enhance one another since mindfulness provides the basis for the compassionate response to be free of avoidance tendencies (e.g., being kind to avoid pain) and compassion provides the secure base in order to mindfully experience difficult internal experiences.

Specifically, regarding compassion-focused therapy, mindfulness and compassion complement one another although the primordial focus is on developing compassionate relationships with self and others through compassionate mind training.

Mindfulness has been described as a way of accessing the soothing–safeness system helping people shift from a "doing mode" to a "being mode." In the two psychologies or mindsets of compassion, attention sensitivity as the ability to search for and be attentive to suffering is described as an important engagement attribute (Gilbert, 2014b). The rationale for applying mindfulness to psychosis, developed by Paul Chadwick and collaborators, states that a mindful response (characterized by an accepting, non-judgmental and "letting go" attitude) to a distressing psychotic experience potentiates a cycle of clear awareness (instead of being lost in reaction) (Chadwick et al., 2005), potentiating recovery.

All practices suggested to Miguel were adapted in order to meet the recommendations and adaptations of mindfulness practices for people with psychosis, namely, regarding the duration of practice (<15 min), type of meditations (mostly based on mindfulness of breath), fewer "silence" periods, more specific and frequent instructions, among others (Chadwick et al., 2005; Shonin et al., 2014).

Mindfulness was suggested as a way of accessing the soothing–safeness system helping people focus and ground their attention in a non-judgmental way and engage in an accepting way with difficult internal experiences that might arise in informal and formal compassion-based practices. It was also discussed that mindfulness would help Miguel step out and observe the loops of the mind (old brain–new brain: rumination, worry, self-criticism) and prepare for the development of the compassionate mind (reminding the video on CFT from the first phase).

In the first few sessions of this phase, Miguel practiced mindfulness of the breath (5–10 min) and grounding practices (focusing on soles of feet – 3–5 min). The idea of focusing on the present moment (while our minds tend to wander between past and future) was particularly interesting to Miguel ("I'm almost never in the present and I didn't even notice"). When the ability to ground and take a step back to being able to engage with difficult experiences, a brief version of soothing rhythm breathing was introduced (10 min). Miguel struggled to find a rhythm that felt calm and soothing at first but with practice and instructions more focused on letting the breathing be and observing the slowing of the body (not necessarily slowing the breathing down which increased anxiety) and the mind, Miguel became more comfortable. Counting was not considered helpful, but focusing on a longer out-breath helped Miguel gain a sense of grounding and tranquillity.

Miguel was suggested to keep practicing mindfulness, breathing rhythms, and grounding as a way of slowing down, returning to the present, and not being carried away by emotions in challenging situations in which difficult thoughts, feelings, or experiences (voices) emerge.

27.3.2.1 Clinical Feedback

After some practice, grounding exercises were particularly pleasant to Miguel. Although Miguel understood that the goal was not relaxation per se, mindfulness helped him feel more stabilized, grounded, and safe. He reported feeling "calmer, more relaxed, and in control." He struggles with regular formal practice and, although formal practices kept being encouraged, Miguel and the therapist developed a list of informal practices that he was confident he could implement in daily life (only practices rated, in a 0–5 scale, as a 3 or higher, with 3 meaning "moderately confident I can implement this," were accepted into the list), for example, using the 5 senses for a few minutes when outside, feeling feet on the floor while in waiting lines, taking a brief moment to observe breathing and/or find a soothing rhythm breathing, and stretching slowly and mindfully.

27.3.3 Phase 3: Being Aware of and Managing Fears of Compassion

Notes to Therapists

Considering the developmental pathways commonly experienced by people with psychosis, it is understandable that people with psychosis often struggle with countering the activation of the threat system through the engagement with the affiliative one. Even in the presence of soothing-affiliative clues and adequate responses to suffering (e.g., giving and receiving compassion to/from self/others), people with psychosis might activate threat-related responses, which can result in the avoidance of compassionate behaviors (Gilbert, 2009; Gilbert et al., 2011), and possibly limit the efficacy of psychological interventions. Fears and blocks to compassion may be related to conditioning processes (wherein early memories of seeking comfort and closeness become associated with negative outcomes), reactivation of early memories of emotional distress coded in the affiliation system, and lack of key competencies necessary for compassion, like mentalizing or emotion processing skills (Gilbert et al., 2012; Liotti & Gilbert, 2011). Other reasons might involve negative beliefs or misconceptions about compassion and external blocks within the individual's environment, such as stigmatization towards compassionate behaviors (Gilbert, 2019).

As a way of eliciting some misconceptions about compassion, Miguel was asked what compassion means to him. Miguel associated compassion with religion and acts of "kindness, doing good and the 'turning the other cheek' thing."

Miguel filled in the Fears of compassion scales (see "Instruments used") and his responses were discussed with the therapist and served as a baseline starting point for the work on fears of compassion. Information on fears of compassion was presented and discussed in dialogue format. Fears of compassion were explained as an activation of the threat system when in contact with compassion that can happen due to several aspects. The ones that Miguel identified with were not being encouraged to expose suffering as a child, and society passing the message that "big boys don't cry." Difficulties in activating the soothing system were also explored and Miguel recognized that he had "few opportunities to be/feel soothed" because emotions had to be concealed and avoided, also his "parents did not believe in comforting us, they always wanted us to be strong and independent and solve our own problems." He pointed out his bullying experiences as reinforcing these ideas and patterns (avoiding appearing vulnerable, needing to be alert and prepared all the time). These experiences were then linked to his drawing of the three systems (see Fig. 27.2) and the activation of the threat system with subtle signs of danger (even if the danger is a "positive" emotion) was normalized considering the experiences discussed. Fear of "positive" emotions was briefly introduced at this stage to reinforce the understanding of fears of compassion (positive emotions as unfamiliar, not able to maintain, giving expectations, thus causing the threat system to activate).

The definition of compassion by Paul Gilbert – "a sensitivity to suffering in self and others, with a commitment to try to alleviate and prevent it" – was presented and each of its components was explored: sensitivity to and engaging with suffering (first psychology of compassion) and alleviate suffering (second psychology). His responses from the fears of compassion scales were discussed in the light of this definition and qualities of courage, strength, dedication, and wisdom were introduced.

Practice was stressed as an aspect facilitating compassion and therapy was reminded as a safe place to be able to develop, practice, and explore compassionate competencies. Moreover, as homework, Miguel was encouraged to expose himself to compassion throughout the time between sessions. The rationale for exposure was presented and the intention "to develop the soothing system and let my threat system know it can rest a bit" was set. The exposure was graded starting with being aware and observing any acts of kindness and compassion in everyday life (e.g., between other people, with animals, acts benefiting the community, etc.), paying attention to the emotions and thoughts that arise at the moment. Being aware of thoughts and emotions when being compassionate to others or receiving compassion from others was then suggested and remained as an ongoing homework throughout the intervention.

27.3.3.1 Instruments Used

Fears of Compassion Scales (FCS; Gilbert et al., 2011).

The aim of the FCS is to measure the three types of fears of compassion: for others, from others, and self-compassion.

Miguel scored high in all three scales, showing intense activation of the threat defense system when in contact with all three flows of compassion. Some of the most significant aspects of Miguel's responses were related to beliefs of not deserving compassion (e.g., "I feel that I don't deserve to be kind and forgiving to myself"), being uncomfortable with emotional proximity from others (e.g., "Feelings of kindness from others are somehow frightening") and misconceptions of what compassion is (e.g., "Being compassionate towards people who have done bad things is letting them off the hook").

27.3.3.2 Clinical Feedback

At the end of this phase, Miguel reported feeling less uncomfortable in trying to be more compassionate towards others and the self. He described compassion as "a way of being able to take care of myself and others even when we mess up. It seems like a difficult thing to do, and uncomfortable, so I do believe it takes courage to try this." Misconceptions about compassion seemed no longer endorsed (e.g., "I was confusing compassion with pity, but I understand now that compassion means doing something about it and not just saying 'oh well, that's too bad' and walking away"). Activation of the threat system during the following sessions' exercises was normalized, and Miguel was motivated to pursue the therapeutic plan. This issue was also approached and discussed throughout the rest of the intervention in a normalizing, non-judgmental way (the therapist often shared her own fears of compassion), and Miguel was asked to be aware and share, if willing, when such fears arise (in order to be able to train to receive compassion and understanding both from the therapist and himself).

27.3.4 Phase 4: Developing the Compassionate Mind and CMT

Notes to Therapists
People with psychosis often struggle with several internal (e.g., symptoms, shame) and external sources of threat (e.g., stigma). Moreover, there is usually a lack of abilities to (self)sooth and experience positive affect (e.g., safeness). Thus, authors recommend that along with reducing the sense of threat there is also a need to learn positive affect regulation strategies (Gumley et al., 2010). CMT focuses in developing a compassionate mind (Compassionate Mind Training) that promotes affiliation and self-soothing, and stimulates compassionate qualities (e.g., distress tolerance, empathy, non-judgement) and skills (e.g., compassionate thinking, behaving).

In order to prepare for the development of the compassionate self, the first sessions of the CMT were devoted to exploring the three qualities of compassion: wisdom (tricky brains that can learn new ways of dealing with difficulties), strength (courage to engage with and tolerate distress), and caring commitment (motive of caring for, others, and the self).

One session was dedicated to exploring how might be the body posture of the compassionate self. The therapist introduced this training as if Miguel was an actor and was exploring a new role. At first, Miguel and the therapist tried several body postures associating them with the three systems (in a playful way). Some scenarios were read and Miguel and the therapist enacted the congruent body posture (e.g., winning the lottery, petting a small dog, listening to favorite music, giving a speech). After that, Miguel and the therapist experimented with body postures associated with emotions – how sadness/anger/anxiety/excitement/relaxation feel in our bodies? Finally, Miguel explored embodying the three qualities of compassion: first standing and then walking. Compassionate smile exercise was introduced in order to stimulate a compassionate facial expression. Miguel also imagined how his tone of voice would sound like. From this body posture, Miguel practiced the "Imagining the Compassionate Self" exercise.[8]

As therapy evolved, Miguel practiced bringing the Compassionate self and the compassion qualities to everyday struggles. Since they caused major distress, Miguel tried to respond in a compassionate way to voices through the question: How would the Compassionate Miguel respond? Miguel and the therapist agreed that the first step was grounding, focusing in the present moment, and being aware of the voice, the distress emerging, but also his surroundings (other sounds what he can see, touch, and smell). Compassionate touch was also promoted as a further level of grounding, a compassionate way of grounding in difficult situations. Then, Miguel stated that "compassionate Miguel would listen to the voice but then move on," "perhaps saying that's ok, you are trying to protect me but that's not reality" and "I think I'm not able to be friends with the voice, neither I want that to happen because it has harmed me in so many ways, but I think I can develop compassion for it, I understand that it's my fear of others trying to keep me away from people, protected," "there are other ways to feel safe while connecting to others and doing what matters to me." The three qualities of compassion in Compassionate Miguel's response were discussed and are summarized in Table 27.2.

The compassionate self was also the basis to work on self-critical loops identified in phase 1. When a loop was identified in session, Miguel and the therapist agreed that the therapist would ask Miguel to pause, identify the loop, and do a brief grounding practice. He would then, try to embody his compassionate self and see what would emerge regarding the situation and the loop itself. Some ideas regarding the self-criticism loop were: "here's the self-critical bug again," "it's not new, you can deal with it," "it just wants you to do good and be all right, but you can do it in a different way." A strategy that helped Miguel deal with self-criticism was his compassionate post-its (based on compassionate letter writing instructions).

The concept of compassionate interactions was then introduced. The flows of giving compassion to others and receiving compassion from others were explored and fears in those fears of compassion were reminded from phase 3. First, considering the session on fears of compassion that revealed that the giving flow might be easier to begin, Miguel practiced directing compassion to others starting with compassion for his dog and then moving to familiar people (starting with his sister). He struggled moderately with imagery therefore pictures were used to begin with these exercises, he was then able to imagine the picture and then the animal/person.

When approaching the idea of receiving compassion from others, Miguel experienced increased anxiety and sadness. He stated "I feel kind of empty, sad that I can't remember someone being compassionate towards me." Considering the graded exposure to compassion and compassionate practices that oriented the entire intervention, and in order for the practice to feel less threatening, Miguel started to work on creating his ideal compassionate other discussing its characteristics with the therapist (appearance, posture and voice tone, facial expression, ways of relating to

[8] All the scripts used on this phase can be found in Gilbert (2010).

Table 27.2 Miguel's compassion qualities

Compassion qualities	Description	Verbalization
Wisdom	Knowledge that voices are not his fault nor a reflection of reality. Understanding that they are rooted on fear and the ultimate function they are serving is a protective one	"That's ok, you are trying to protect me but that's not reality" "I understand that it's my fear of others trying to keep me away from people, protected"
Strength	Courage to keep doing what's important when the voices are present (neither avoiding them or being overinvolved with them).	"Compassionate Miguel would listen to the voice but then move on"
Caring commitment	Developing compassion for a part of Miguel (the voice) Taking care of himself while dealing with difficulties and pursuing a valued path	"I think I can develop compassion for it" "There are other ways to feel safe while connecting to others and doing what matters to me"

Miguel). After this exercise, using guided discovery, his ideal compassionate other was described in the following way: "An old lady, as I imagine my grandmother would be from the photos I have of her. She would be small and all dressed in black, grey hair and kind, brown eyes. She would speak softly but I could hear her voice clearly, she would sound confident and calm," "she would not touch me, she would know better! But she would stay close and I think, with time, her presence would be comforting." Miguel was not sure how he would relate to his compassionate other but felt comfortable to train receiving compassion from this ideal compassionate other. As was done with exposing to fears of compassion, Miguel was reminded to keep observing acts of kindness and compassion between other people and from other people towards him.

27.3.4.1 Instruments Used

Compassionate Engagement and Action Scales (CEAS, Gilbert et al., 2017).

The CEAS invites people to record how they respond when confronted by their own suffering, the suffering of others, or they experience compassion from others. The first part measures engagement with suffering (first psychology) and the second part of each scale assesses the ability to pay attention to, learn about, and act on what is helpful (second psychology).

Miguel revealed difficulties in both psychologies of compassion and those difficulties were more severe regarding self-compassion compared with the other flows (giving compassion to others was the one with better scores). Regarding engagement with distress, motivation to engage was generally present, as well as being aware and sensitive to suffering; however, distress tolerance with empathic insight had very low levels (e.g., "I avoid thinking about my distress and try to distract myself and put it out of my mind." was scored as "Always"). Regarding ways of actively and compassionately coping with distressing emotions, thoughts, and situations (from self or other people), Miguel struggles to find out what are the compassionate and helpful actions that might alleviate suffering. Regarding the perception of receiving compassion from others, Miguel feels that other people do not engage in helpful or supportive actions.

27.3.4.2 Clinical Feedback

Although all flows of compassion were practiced in this phase, more attention was given to self-compassion since it was the flow Miguel struggled the most (and that had the most interference in his well-being) and the others would have the opportunity to be trained in a group setting.

Although Miguel has seen some evolution regarding the flows of compassion involving others, due to his social anxiety those flows were still quite difficult to address. In the next phase, social anxiety was specifically targeted in one-to-one therapy format, and to further develop his abilities to give to and receive compassion from others, Miguel then started a CFT-based group therapy (see Part 2: Group intervention).

27.3.5 Phase 5: Working with Associated Symptoms (Social Anxiety)

Notes to Therapists

Social anxiety is a prevalent comorbidity among people with psychosis, although its origin is not well understood. Social anxiety disorder rates of 25% were found in people with the first episode of psychosis and rates of above 11% reported severe difficulties in social situations (Michail & Birchwood, 2013). Moreover, when comparing people with social anxiety disorder and psychosis and social anxiety disorder only, comparable levels of social anxiety, autonomic symptoms, and avoidance were found, and social anxiety in people with psychosis was not associated with positive psychotic symptoms (Michail & Birchwood, 2013).

Social anxiety was conceptualized as an exacerbated activation in the threat system when in social situations: both interaction related and performance related. A list of situations Miguel fears was made and negative automatic thoughts arising in these situations were explored. Situations included oral presentations, exams, eating/walking alone, being in a group (more than 3 people). Miguel worked on identifying the activation of his threat system focusing on three types of outputs: emotional (anxiety, fear, frustration with himself), cognitive ("I will embarrass myself," "I don't know what to say," "People will think I'm weird"), including self-critical thoughts ("I'm a failure," "Nobody likes me," "I'm different"), and behavioral (avoiding, hiding). Loops identified in phase 1 were revisited and Miguel trained to be aware of them while they were happening. A protective function was identified: "keeping me from getting hurt," "my mind doesn't want others to disappoint me." Fears of affiliative emotions were also explored (e.g., fear of proximity with others) and normalized as a part of the activation of the threat system.

Miguel relied on the three qualities of his compassionate self (strength, wisdom, and caring commitment to alleviate his suffering) and described his compassionate self in social situations: "Compassionate Miguel would know (and remember!) that social anxiety is normal, all humans that value others feel a certain degree of (social) anxiety. I know that my experiences (including psychosis) have shaped my threat alarm to go off with very small clues of rejection. Compassionate Miguel is strong enough to be anxious and deal with anxiety in social situations. He can be grounded and take care of himself while doing something difficult."

Miguel also had a set of rigid rules about a successful social interaction, for instance, "always being spontaneous," "being a good company for others," and "avoiding conflict at all costs." When reflecting on the question "How would the compassionate Miguel feel about these rules?" Miguel found out that these were very rigid and perfectionism-based rules that he would not be able to maintain in the long run. He also identified that they were fear-based protective strategies that were promoting avoidance and/or increasing the likelihood of unsuccessful interactions (e.g., not talking with the fear of not being spontaneous).

A series of graded exposure exercises were then practiced, embodying his compassionate self. Additional helpful strategies for Miguel while doing exposure included grounding (focusing on 5 senses in the social interaction/context), compassionate touch (hand in heart), and remembering the intention of wanting to further connect with others. Miguel was also encouraged to bring a curious attitude to social situations and to repeat some brief compassionate phrases ("I'm doing something really important," "It's ok to be anxious, I am safe," "I've done this before").

27.3.5.1 Clinical Feedback

Miguel chose to start the exposure exercises with the performance situations that caused anxiety ("These have more consequences for me right now"). However, some social interaction situations were arising and discussion in the session focused on how he could generalize strategies used in performance situations. Although anxiety levels reduced only slightly, with the continuity of exposure Miguel felt more confident to deal with his increases in anxiety in social contexts (increased sense of empowerment). Avoidance behaviors significantly reduced (particularly those felt as automatic, increasing awareness regarding avoidance patterns).

27.4 Part 2: Group Intervention

27.4.1 How COMPASS Was Introduced

COMPASS was introduced as a way of further developing and training Miguel's compassionate mind. Being in a group has the advantage of being able to practice giving compassion to others in the group, receiving compassion from others, and practicing self-compassion in a secure social context. Miguel had been working on his social anxiety and paranoia in social contexts; therefore, the group was also presented as an experiment he could try in order to observe how his threat system reacts and how his compassionate mind might "jump in" to help.

27.4.2 Brief Description of COMPASS

COMPASS is a manualized (Martins et al., 2020) group-format intervention. It was primarily based on the compassion-focused therapy rationale as it was adapted for psychosis (Gumley et al., 2010), in general, and in the group intervention protocol from Braehler et al. (2013b) and patients' and clinicians' feedback from previous clinical studies, in particular. Being more affiliative than contemplative in nature COMPASS combines intrapersonal practices (e.g., mindfulness and (self)compassion meditations) with interpersonal ones (e.g., training receiving, giving, and observing compassion). It comprises 12 weekly sessions (approximately 3 months), and evolves through three phases: "Building Trust and Group as a Safe Place" (Sessions 1–4); "Compassionate Mind Training" (Sessions 5–10); and "Revisiting Recovery and Compassionately Planning Ahead" (Sessions 11 and 12). Preliminary results showed improvement both in objective and subjective recovery aspects: positive and negative symptoms and social functioning on one hand, and fears of self-compassion and self-criticism on the other (Martins et al., 2018).[9]

27.4.3 Individual Support During COMPASS

As defined for the COMPASS intervention (each participant has the possibility to have 2 individual sessions throughout the intervention), Miguel had two individual sessions in which he was able to express some difficulties he was having.

The difficulties addressed were regarding giving and receiving compassion from others. In the first individual session, Miguel reported feeling ashamed and embarrassed when interacting with others. The activation of the threat system in social interactions was normalized and explored. Misinterpretations of compassion were

[9] Further results from the clinical trial are available from the first author.

still emerging, such as "if I need compassion it means I'm weak, unable to deal with my own stuff," and therefore, fears of compassion were again addressed. It was practiced in session giving and receiving compassion from the therapist while being mindful of thoughts that might encompass these misinterpretations. In the second individual session, Miguel and the therapist reflected on how would the compassionate mind respond to these situations. Compassionate phrases were generated while embodying his compassionate self, and Miguel wrote them in order to remember how he can respond to distressing situations in the group, and in life. Miguel's compassionate phrases at this stage, to use in social situations and particularly in the group, were "Its normal to be anxious and this is a safe place," "You are able to do this, you've been in these sessions before," and "You are not alone, probably other people in the group are feeling the same way."

Like all participants, Miguel also had direct contact with the therapeutic team (if needed) and received a weekly compassionate message.

27.5 Part 3: Relapse Prevention and Looking Forward

Notes to Therapists

Research has shown that the competencies developed and trained in compassion-focused therapy are key to relapse prevention. Shame and self-attacking further stimulate an overly active threat system, creating a vicious circle (Longe et al., 2010) that, combined with the unintended consequences of threat-based safety strategies (e.g., social withdrawal, limiting awareness to distressing internal experience), can potentiate relapse and further impairment (Gumley et al., 2010). Decreases in shame and self-criticism are thus essential in recovery and relapse prevention (Gumley et al., 2010), as well as regulating feelings of self-blame, usually associated with relapse (Gumley et al., 2006). An intervention focused on the activation of the safeness system (Gumley et al., 2010) is of utmost importance for relapse prevention since this system is essential for stress regulation and promotion of social bonding and affiliative behaviors (Gumley et al., 2014). Compassionate self-acceptance would, therefore, foster the maintenance cycle of well-being and recovery leading to feelings of empowerment, hope, and agency regarding psychosis, culminating in post-traumatic growth (Waite et al., 2015). On the other hand, "acting with awareness" has important benefits for developing skills to identify and respond to early warning signs of relapse (e.g., Birchwood et al., 2000).

Miguel maintained monthly sessions with the therapist to enhance his practicing of mindfulness and compassion. Sessions are dedicated to applying the compassionate self's wisdom, strength, and caring commitment to everyday situations, difficulties, and decisions.

Relapse prevention was also addressed. Residual symptoms and idiosyncratic warning signs were discussed (lacking sleep, increases in paranoia, social isolation), as well as more specific cues to psychological suffering: self-criticism increasing in everyday life and higher involvement in strategies to avoid difficult thoughts and feelings (e.g., shame). As a way of promoting empowerment and hope, Miguel watched Eleanor Longden's Ted Talk regarding her experience with psychosis[10] (TED, 2013, February) and several key aspects were discussed with the therapist, namely, important aspects facilitating recovery, resources and social support network, and relationship with symptoms (function of symptoms, e.g., voices).

Based on the discussion of the Ted Talk, Miguel and the therapist discussed what can be meant by recovery. Differences and complementarity between objective (reduction in symptoms – psychotic and associated symptoms, meeting developmental milestones and goals, and being effective in different social roles) and subjective (self-determination, empowerment, hopefulness, sense of purpose, self-confidence) recovery was also discussed. Recovery was then conceptualized as an ongoing active process with both aspects of recovery seen as independent (though sometimes related). Examples were elicited from different periods in Miguel's life where objective and subjective recovery aspects were not necessarily related (e.g., symptom stabilization in hospital but no hope, self-determination, or sense of empowerment; living with lower levels of medication, higher levels of anxiety but making meaningful choices, and getting out of comfort zone – higher sense of empowerment and self-determination). Compassionate responding to oneself, others and situations was reminded as a sign of subjective recovery, since it may be the basis of living a personally meaningful life as integral member of a community.

27.6 Conclusion

Compassionate acceptance has been argued to be a context in which people experiencing mental distress may develop their unique way of accepting, coping and living with their difficulties (Spandler & Stickley, 2011). The basic motivation for any therapeutic team is a compassionate motivation rooted in the caring social mentality and, specifically, from a compassion-based perspective, is to be able to identify and recognize the signs of suffering of the other and to implement effective actions to alleviate it (Gilbert, 2014b; Gilbert & Irons, 2005).

Therefore, the helping relationship should be based on principles, such as being present moment by moment, presenting a non-judgmental understanding, and loving attitude of acceptance with the constant perspective that the suffering that participants experience is part of a common human experience. Therapeutic contexts should constitute themselves as safe and affiliative environments, rooted in an

[10] The voices in my head: TED Talk by Elanor Longden, available from https://www.ted.com/talks/eleanor_longden_the_voices_in_my_head?language=pt

affiliative-cooperative mentality, that facilitate courage and exploration (safe/secure base) on one hand, and discourage high expressed emotion and shaming experiences on the other. Mutual helping has also been stressed as key in feelings of belonging and recovery, since the combination of receiving care and caring for others helps people form affiliative relationships and regulate emotions (Veale et al., 2015). This is particularly important for improving health care for people with psychosis since evidence has shown psychiatric treatment and hospitalization in this context to be a potentially distressing and traumatic experience (Paksarian et al., 2014).

Compassion-focused therapy for psychosis, as an empirically validated intervention, particularly developed for people with high levels of shame and self-criticism, has the potential to help people who struggle with an overly active threat system giving them the competencies to self-regulate and self-soothe. Additionally, people with psychosis, as illustrated in Miguel's case, often have few sources of safeness both internal and external, rooted in insecure attachment styles and maintained through (avoidance-based) defensive strategies with major unintended consequences. Miguel's therapeutic process illustrates how compassion-based psychotherapeutic intervention can help people with psychosis develop a more balanced, wise, strong, and care-focused mind state (as opposed to a threat-focused mind), which constitutes as a secure base from which they can thrive and live meaningful lives, while taking care of themselves in moments of suffering.

In summary, it is important that compassionate health care contexts include components, such as acceptance, understanding of suffering and psychosis as intelligible within individual experience and history, and a common humanity-based perspective. Compassion would be therefore a quality needed as a basis of all new innovations, policies, and practices (Spandler & Stickley, 2011). This particular therapeutic focus, in which acceptance, common humanity, equanimity, and mindful presence are important vectors and compassion is the key motivation, has the potential to be more ethically responsible in terms of the general goal for mental health care interventions (de Zulueta, 2015).

References

American Psychiatric Association. (2013). *Diagnostic and statistical manual of mental disorders* (5th ed.). American Psychiatric Association.

Birchwood, M., Spencer, E., & McGovern, D. (2000). Schizophrenia: Early warning signs. *Advances in Psychiatric Treatment, 6*, 93–101. https://doi.org/10.1192/apt.6.2.93

Braehler, C., Gumley, A., Harper, J., Wallace, S., Norrie, J., & Gilbert, P. (2013a). Exploring change processes in compassion focused therapy in psychosis: Results of a feasibility randomized controlled trial. *British Journal of Clinical Psychology, 52*(2), 199–214. https://doi.org/10.1111/bjc.12009

Braehler, C., Harper, J., & Gilbert, P. (2013b). Compassion focused group therapy for recovery after psychosis. In C. Steel (Ed.), *Cognitive behaviour therapy for schizophrenia: Evidence based interventions and future directions* (1st ed., pp. 235–265). Wiley-Blackwell. https://doi.org/10.13140/2.1.3956.2886

Carpenter, W. T., Heinrichs, D. W., & Wagman, A. M. I. (1988). Deficit and non-deficit forms of schizophrenia: The concept. *American Journal of Psychiatry, 145*, 578–583.

Chadwick, P., Taylor, K. N., & Abba, N. (2005). Mindfulness groups for people with psychosis. *Behavioural and Cognitive Psychotherapy, 33*(3), 351–359. https://doi.org/10.1017/S1352465805002158

de Zulueta, P. C. (2015). Suffering, compassion and "doing good medical ethics". *Journal of Medical Ethics, 41*(1), 87–90. https://doi.org/10.1136/medethics-2014-102355

Depue, R. A., & Morrone-Strupinsky, J. V. (2005). A neurobehavioural model of affiliative bonding: Implications for conceptualizing a human trait of affiliation. *The Behavioural and Brain Sciences, 28*(3), 313–395. https://doi.org/10.1017/S0140525X05000063

Gilbert, P. (2004). Threat, safeness, and schizophrenia: Hidden issues in an evolutionary story. *Behavioural and Brain Sciences, 27*(6), 858–859. https://doi.org/10.1017/S0140525X04260198

Gilbert, P. (2005). Compassion and cruelty. In P. Gilbert (Ed.), *Compassion: Conceptualizations, research and use in psychotherapy* (pp. 9–74). Routledge.

Gilbert, P. (2009). Introducing compassion-focused therapy. *Advances in Psychiatric Treatment, 15*(3), 199–208. https://doi.org/10.1192/apt.bp.107.005264

Gilbert, P. (2010). *Compassion focused therapy: Distinctive features*. Routledge/Taylor & Francis Group.

Gilbert, P. (2014a). Compassion-focused therapy: Preface and introduction for special section. *British Journal of Clinical Psychology, 53*(1), 1–5. https://doi.org/10.1111/bjc.12045

Gilbert, P. (2014b). The origins and nature of compassion focused therapy. *British Journal of Clinical Psychology, 53*(1), 6–41. https://doi.org/10.1111/bjc.12043

Gilbert, P. (2019). Explorations into the nature and function of compassion. *Current Opinion in Psychology, 28*, 108–114. https://doi.org/10.1016/j.copsyc.2018.12.002

Gilbert, P., & Irons, C. (2005). Focused therapies and compassionate mind training for shame and self-attacking. In P. Gilbert (Ed.), *Compassion: Conceptualisations, research and use in psychotherapy* (pp. 263–325). Routledge.

Gilbert, P., & Leahy, R. L. (Eds.). (2007). *The therapeutic relationship in the cognitive behavioral psychotherapies*. Routledge/Taylor & Francis Group.

Gilbert, P., Bailey, K., & McGuire, M. T. (2000). Evolutionary psychotherapy: Principles and outline. In P. Gilbert & K. G. Biley (Eds.), *Genes on the couch: Explorations in evolutionary psychotherapy* (pp. 3–27). Brunner-Routledge.

Gilbert, P., Clarke, M., Hempel, S., Miles, J. N. V., & Irons, C. (2004). Criticizing and reassuring oneself: An exploration of forms, styles and reasons in female students. *British Journal of Clinical Psychology, 43*, 31–50. https://doi.org/10.1348/014466504772812959

Gilbert, P., McEwan, K., Matos, M., & Rivis, A. (2011). Fears of compassion: Development of three self-report measures. *Psychology and Psychotherapy: Theory, Research and Practice, 84*, 239–255. https://doi.org/10.1348/147608310X526511

Gilbert, P., McEwan, K., Gibbons, L., Chotai, S., Duarte, J., & Matos, M. (2012). Fears of compassion and happiness in relation to alexithymia, mindfulness, and self-criticism. *Psychology and Psychotherapy: Theory, Research and Practice, 85*, 374–390. https://doi.org/10.1111/j.2044-8341.2011.02046.x

Gilbert, P., Catarino, F., Duarte, C., Matos, M., Kolts, R., Stubbs, J., Ceresatto, L., Duarte, J., Pinto-Gouveia, J., & Basran, J. (2017). The development of compassionate engagement and action scales for self and others. *Journal of Compassionate Health Care, 4*(4). https://doi.org/10.1186/s40639-017-0033-3

Goss, K., Gilbert, P., & Allan, S. (1994). An exploration of shame measures—I: The Other as Shamer scale. *Personality and Individual Differences, 17*(5), 713–717. https://doi.org/10.1016/0191-8869(94)90149-X

Grepmair, L., Mitterlehner, F., Loew, T., Bachler, E., Rother, W., & Nickel, M. (2007). Promoting mindfulness in psychotherapists in training influences the treatment results of their patients: A randomized, double-blind, controlled study. *Psychotherapy and Psychosomatics, 76*(6), 332–338. https://doi.org/10.1159/000107560

Gumley, A., Karatzias, A., Power, K., Reilly, J., McNay, L., & O'Grady, M. (2006). Early intervention for relapse in schizophrenia: Impact of cognitive behavioural therapy on negative beliefs about psychosis and self-esteem. *British Journal of Clinical Psychology, 45*, 247–260. https://doi.org/10.1348/014466505X49925

Gumley, A., Braehler, C., Laithwaite, H., MacBeth, A., & Gilbert, P. (2010). A compassion focused model of recovery after psychosis. *International Journal of Cognitive Therapy, 3*(2), 186–201. https://doi.org/10.1521/ijct.2010.3.2.186

Gumley, A. I., Taylor, H. E., Schwannauer, M., & MacBeth, A. (2014). A systematic review of attachment and psychosis: Measurement, construct validity and outcomes. *Acta Psychiatrica Scandinavica, 129*(4), 257–74. https://doi.org/10.1111/acps.12172. Epub 2013 Jul 3. PMID: 23834647.

Gumley, A., Macbeth, A., Reilly, J. D., O'Grady, M., White, R. G., McLeod, H., Schwannauer, M., & Power, K. G. (2015). Fear of recurrence: Results of a randomized trial of relapse detection in schizophrenia. *British Journal of Clinical Psychology, 54*(1), 49–62. https://doi.org/10.1111/bjc.12060

Hick, S. F., & Bien, T. (2008). *Mindfulness and the therapeutic relationship*. The Gilford Press.

Hickey, T., Nelson, B., Enticott, J., & Meadows, G. (2021). The MAC-P program: A pilot study of a mindfulness and compassion program for youth with psychotic experiences. *Early Intervention in Psychiatry, 15*(5), 1326–1334. https://doi.org/10.1111/eip.13085

Johnson, D., Penn, D., Fredrickson, B. L., Meyer, P. S., Kring, A. M., & Brantley, M. (2009). Loving-kindness meditation to enhance recovery from negative symptoms of schizophrenia. *Journal of Clinical Psychology, 65*(5), 499–509. https://doi.org/10.1002/jclp.20591

King's Cultural Community. (2015, February 23). *Compassion for Voices: a tale of courage and hope* [Video]. YouTube. https://www.youtube.com/watch?v=VRqI4lxuXAw

Laithwaite, H., O'Hanlon, M., Collins, P., Doyle, P., Abraham, L., Porter, S., & Gumley, A. (2009). Recovery After Psychosis (RAP): A compassion focused programme for individuals residing in high security settings. *Behavioural and Cognitive Psychotherapy, 37*(5), 511–526. https://doi.org/10.1017/S1352465809990233

Liotti, G., & Gilbert, P. (2011). Mentalizing, motivation and social mentalities: Theoretical consideration and implications for psychotherapy. *Psychology and Psychotherapy: Theory, Research and Practice, 84*, 9–25. https://doi.org/10.1348/147608310X520094

Longe, O., Maratos, F. A., Gilbert, P., Evans, G., Volker, F., Rockliff, H., & Rippon, G. (2010). Having a word with yourself: Neural correlates of self-criticism and self-reassurance. *NeuroImage, 49*(2), 1849–1856. https://doi.org/10.1016/j.neuroimage.2009.09.019

Martins, M. J., Barreto Carvalho, C., Castilho, P., Pereira, A. T., & Macedo, A. (2015). The "Clinical Interview for Psychotic Disorders" (CIPD): Development and expert evaluation. *International Journal of Clinical Neurosciences and Mental Health, 2*(7). https://doi.org/10.21035/ijcnmh.2015.2.7

Martins, M. J., Barreto Carvalho, C., Macedo, A., Pereira, A. T., Braehler, C., Gumley, A., & Castilho, P. (2018). Recovery through affiliation: A compassionate approach to schizophrenia and schizoaffective disorder (COMPASS). *Journal of Contextual Behavioral Science, 9*, 97–102. https://doi.org/10.1016/j.jcbs.2018.07.009

Martins, M. J., Palmeira, L., Xavier, A., Castilho, P., Macedo, A., Pereira, A. T., Pinto, A. M., Carreiras, D., & Barreto-Carvalho, C. (2019). The Clinical Interview for Psychotic Disorders (CIPD): Preliminary results on interrater agreement, reliability and qualitative feedback. *Psychiatry Research, 272*, 723–729. https://doi.org/10.1016/j.psychres.2018.12.176

Martins, M. J., Castilho, P., Barreto Carvalho, C., Macedo, A., Braehler, C., & Pereira, A. T. (2020). *Compaixão e Recuperação na Psicose: Manual clínico de implementação do programa COMPASS*. Pactor.

Michail, M., & Birchwood, M. (2013). Social anxiety disorder and shame cognitions in psychosis. *Psychological Medicine, 43*(1), 133–142. https://doi.org/10.1017/S0033291712001146

Neff, K. D., & Dahm, K. (2015). Self-compassion: What it is, what it does, and how it relates to mindfulness. In B. D. Ostafin, M. D. Robinson, & B. P. Meier (Eds.), *Handbook of mind-*

fulness and self-regulation (pp. 121–137). Springer Science & Business Media. https://doi.org/10.1007/978-1-4939-2263-5

Paksarian, D., Mojtabai, R., Kotov, R., Cullen, B., Nugent, K. L., & Bromet, E. J. (2014). Perceived trauma during hospitalization and treatment participation among individuals with psychotic disorders. *Psychiatric Services, 65*(2), 266–269. https://doi.org/10.1176/appi.ps.201200556

Panksepp, J. (2004). *Affective neuroscience: The foundations of human and animal emotions*. Oxford University Press.

Shonin, E., Van Gordon, W., & Griffiths, M. D. (2014). Do mindfulness-based therapies have a role in the treatment of psychosis? *Australian & New Zealand Journal of Psychiatry, 48*(2), 124–127. https://doi.org/10.1177/0004867413512688

Spandler, H., & Stickley, T. (2011). No hope without compassion: The importance of compassion in recovery-focused mental health services. *Journal of Mental Health, 20*(6), 555–566. https://doi.org/10.3109/09638237.2011.583949

TED. (2013, February). *Eleanor Longden: The voices in my head* [Video]. TED. https://www.ted.com/talks/eleanor_longden_the_voices_in_my_head?language=pt#t-839921

Tirch, D. D. (2010). Mindfulness as a context for the cultivation of compassion. *International Journal of Cognitive Therapy, 3*(2), 113–123. https://doi.org/10.1521/ijct.2010.3.2.113

Veale, D., Gilbert, P., Wheatley, J., & Naismith, I. (2015). A new therapeutic community: Development of a compassion-focussed and contextual behavioural environment. *Clinical Psychology and Psychotherapy, 22*(4), 285–303. https://doi.org/10.1002/cpp.1897

Waite, F., Knight, M. T. D., & Lee, D. (2015). Self-compassion and self-criticism in recovery in psychosis: An interpretative phenomenological analysis study. *Journal of Clinical Psychology, 71*(12), 1201–1217. https://doi.org/10.1002/jclp.22211

Wexler, J. (2006). The relationship between therapist mindfulness and the therapeutic alliance. *Dissertation Abstracts International: Section B: The Sciences and Engineering, 67*(5-B), 2848.

Chapter 28
The Wall of Disconnection

Olga Runciman

I wish to start my chapter rather philosophically by doing a brief meander into the philosophy of mind and matter where I ask the question, "What is consciousness" and if we can't answer *what is consciousness* then I would in the same breath like to ask, how then, can we explain sanity and madness?

There is an accepted consensus that mental distress and actual physical disorders affecting the brain are fundamentally different. Alzheimer's disease, multiple sclerosis, Parkinsonism, strokes, and brain tumors are all examples of physical disorders affecting the brain and people affected by these illnesses tend to go to a neurologist and not a psychiatrist. Distress of a non-physical origin such as great sadness, or hearing things that others cannot, generally involves going to a psychiatrist. Thus, one can be tempted to say neurologists deal with physical ailments of the patient's brains and psychiatrists deal with people's minds and their ability to be aware, to feel, plan, think, and to make choices, in other words the uniqueness of being a conscious being. However, this brings in the awkward question, what is consciousness? And how does psychiatry cope with such a concept?

There exist many ideas, theories, and ways of looking at consciousness, and if we were to relate them to the enigma of insanity, we can ask *can they be separated?* For, just as in the studies of consciousness where we seem to inevitably hit the proverbial brick wall –*what is consciousness really*? – so too, do we hit the same brick wall when we ask ourselves – *what is madness really*? Or indeed what is normality? I want, therefore, to look at both phenomena in relation to each other since in my everyday work within the mental health system I find so many attempts at explanations and yet when it comes to the "hard question" – *does madness exist* – we are in the same boat as the "hard problem" (Blakeslee, 1996) present when we attempt to explain consciousness. The "hard problem" is a term coined by David Chalmers,

O. Runciman (✉)
Psycovery, Frederiksberg, Denmark
e-mail: psykolog@psycovery.com

J. A. Díaz-Garrido et al. (eds.), *Psychological Interventions for Psychosis*,
https://doi.org/10.1007/978-3-031-27003-1_28

professor of philosophy and director of the center for consciousness at the University of Arizona. He phrases the hard problem as this: What is the nature of subjective experience? Why do we have vividly felt experiences of the world? Thus far, nothing in physics or chemistry or biology can explain these subjective feelings, Chalmers says. "What really happens when you see the deep red of a sunset or hear the haunting sound of a distant oboe, feel the agony of intense pain, the sparkle of happiness or meditative quality of a moment lost in thought?" he asks. "It is these phenomena, often called qualia, that pose the deep mystery of consciousness."

Consciousness is one of the last frontiers of science, but what is consciousness? If someone was to ask you to define love, you might answer, "If you have to ask that, then you have not been in love." We can say the same when trying to define consciousness. And in the same way when one is trying to describe consciousness and conscious mental states, many of us will be mixing subjective and objective conceptions of these states together. We are not separating the feelings, which are subjective from the objective physicality of the experience, the *-what is it like to have this experience, such as seeing red or biting into a juicy apple-* from what is happening on an objective biological level in our eyes, brain and taste buds, though we can separate the two should we wish to do so. It is this dualism that prompted the philosopher Thomas Nagel to ask his famous question, "*What is it like to be a bat?*" (Nagel, 1974). Looking at how it might be like to be a bat from our point of view, we might describe that as living mostly in the dark, hanging upside down a lot of the time and hearing a tremendous amount of screeching. However, it is unlikely bats experience life like that. For them echolocation is natural, and they view the world through echo probably like we view the world through vision, in both cases we are aware of physical objects in our world, not sound waves in the bats' case or light waves in our case. Hence, in Nagel's paper "What is it like to be a bat," he explores the private experience of consciousness and concludes that no matter how much we know about a bat's brain and body we will never know what it is *like* to be a bat.

Taking this a step further one can say the same thing about one person in relation to another. I will, for example, never know what it is like to be my closest friend, and we will have things in common, such as language, an ability to describe experiences, and be able to agree that we are both looking at the color red, but what it actually *feels* like to *be* my friend, looking and experiencing the world through *her* eyes when she is looking at *her* experience of red is something I will never know. These private qualities are unique to the individual.

I suggest therefore that it is reasonable to say that – if viewing the world from Nagel's viewpoint of phenomenal consciousness – no one is able to know what it is *like* for another person's experience of sanity or madness. If I experience green as red, is the problem a question of language or do I really see red as green or do I experience something completely different involving other colors or sensations? Perhaps I see the true colors and it is the rest of the world that is wrong or maybe I see red as green but have learned to say red for green and then nobody would be any the wiser as to me being different. I would be deemed normal (sane) even though what I experienced was not normal (insane) if it was objectively measurable. In terms of looking at this through the lens of consciousness we will accept that we have hit upon one of the *hard problems*. However, when we look at the experience of sanity and madness in psychiatry, the lens changes and psychiatry becomes blind to the hard problems which are also present here and this blindness often has tremendous consequences for the patient. For though the psychiatrist does not know and will *never* know what that other person is *actually* experiencing, the psychiatrist will nevertheless be able to impose his own subjective opinion upon the other and define the others' experience as if it were a measurable biological fact.

In other words what is being introduced here is the concept that no amount of scientific description will ever convey the subjectivity of the conscious experience, and therefore, the next big challenge is to explain how the phenomenal experience of consciousness fits into the objective world and our knowledge of the brain.

Here it is worth looking at the *hard problem* (Chalmers, 1995), highlighting the explanatory problem of how the brain gives rise to subjective experiences. This contrasts with the *easy problems* of consciousness which include the ability to react to stimuli, integrate information, attention, and the difference between being awake and asleep. One can say that this discussion on *hard* and *easy* problems is a modern-day version of the traditional mind body problem which has intrigued humankind for hundreds of years. Interestingly, in traditional psychiatry the *hard* problem (i.e., *the felt/phenomenological aspects of experience*) often appears to be forgotten or ignored with the major focus being directed toward the *easy* problems resulting in an almost complete disregard to the subjectivity of the experience. Thus, the main thrust of focus in psychiatry is on the perceived brain defects, resulting in talk of chemical imbalances, defective genes, and "broken" brains, and begs the question, why psychiatry? Why not just neurology? If all we want to do is focus on the easy problems, then in theory psychiatry should not exist as a separate specialty from neurology and yet it does. Perhaps this is because psychiatry is so highly adept at ignoring the obvious discrepancy between focusing on assumed brain defects (easy problems) and claiming they are addressing the subjective/phenomenological experiences (hard problems) that they can justify their existence as a science?

Chalmers is one of the few modern-day dualists and he argues for science to expand its horizons and include phenomenological consciousness as a basic feature in nature. *"The argument is complex, but the basic idea is simple: the physical structure of the world—the exact distribution of particles, fields, and forces in spacetime—is logically consistent with the absence of consciousness, so the presence of consciousness is a further fact about our world"* (Chalmers & Searle, 2022).

Descartes thought of mind and matter as two separate substances which never mixed, *substance dualism*, each having their own properties, whereas Chalmers less extreme version of dualism, *property dualism*, sees the mind as not split off from the body and existing as two separate entities. He is quite happy to allow the possibility of just one unified substance in humans but proposes this substance has two distinct properties.

Another angle to this dualism is G. Leibniz's approach (Leibniz, 1714) via knowledge where he describes a machine which can think, feel, and perceive and then he enlarges it (we could use a modern-day analogy of an enlarged computer or brain). What would you see? Parts that are moving, pushing, and pulling or substances swirling around but there would be nothing that could explain feelings or perceptions. The modern version of Leibniz's knowledge argumentation is Frank Jackson's science fiction story of Mary (Jackson, 1986) living in a black and white world but who has access to all available knowledge also that on color. One day she walks out of her door and sees a red rose and for the first time sees color. If you believe this would be a completely new experience for her, then it follows that once again there is a difference between conscious properties and the physical properties.

If we were to look at sanity and madness with this form of dualistic viewpoint, then it stands to reason that something has gone wrong on the subjectivity level rather than biological level, as most people experiencing mental distress describe their plight subjectively. This would contradict modern-day treatments which attempt to repair the physical brain with drugs, electroshock, etc. In theory, treatment should fail because it is not the physical brain but the conscious properties that are distressed, something we still do not know what is, yet here in this context we know it is separate from the physical.

Modern-day eliminative materialists (Ramsey, 2022), in other words, those who view the subjective experience of consciousness *as purely biological*, see the problems we have with understanding consciousness today, as changing the more we find out about the brain. Basically, the assumption is we just need more knowledge or as psychiatry is often seen, as having its roots firmly planted in the period of enlightenment. This is highlighted in psychiatry's constant search for the genes of madness, which they claim is just around the corner, and when they find them, they will finally have their explanation. Behaviorism, also a form of eliminative materialism, was an attempt to explain behaviors as occurring through stimuli devoid of consciousness. Yet even here when looking at consciousness biologically, it is clear that we *still* know too little about the brain and like consciousness, "sanity and madness" are needed, in this context, to be discovered biologically. Therefore, the assumption that we "know" how to fix the broken brain by chemical means is extremely naïve even though traditional modern-day psychiatry's major focus is to be found here within the confines of eliminative materialists.

In conclusion to my original question, can consciousness, sanity, and madness be separated, I would posit no saying *that the concepts of sanity and madness cannot be separated from consciousness and therefore share the same explanatory problems as does the enigma of consciousness.* The difference between the two specialties is as follows: one, those who study consciousness acknowledge that the answer is still waiting to be found, whereas psychiatry boldly claims it has found the answer to sanity and madness; secondly, the debate on consciousness does not have such a direct effect as does the debate on sanity and madness on a large group of people whose lives are directly affected by the outcome of the solution. A solution which means the dice has fallen on the side of eliminative materialism and with it the idea that we "know" what is wrong with the broken brain and how to "fix it" resulting in treatments directly affecting the brain and body. This is so, even though sanity, madness and the concept of normality are still as mysterious as consciousness is.

They called me mad, and I called them mad, and damn them, they outvoted me. – Nathaniel Lee on being consigned to a mental institution.

28.1 Maria

Maria was a woman from Brazil who had moved to Denmark many years ago when she had married a Dane. She was musical and had for many years been a concert pianist. When I met her in my group for people who hear voices or have other unusual experiences, she had been in psychiatry quite a number of years and spoke of demons taking her music from her and that she could fly like an angel. The staff defined her as severely schizophrenic and that to cure her of her plight she need daily medication and ECT when she began to talk about the demons taking her music from her as that was indicative of a potential depressive period starting. It quickly became clear to all of us in the group that the demons she spoke of represented the staff whom she was terrified of as they would force her to undergo ECT, a treatment she attributed to having caused her to not remembering how to play the piano like before. However, it was the description of flying like an angel which she said she literally did that had been one of the reasons the staff said she was mentally ill. She would even insist she was flying when the staff saw she was clearly not. She told us of times when she had literally flown up in the air throughout her life fascinating the group. However, it was when she for the first time "flew" in our group and through the interest and curiosity of those present that it became clear Maria was using a completely different terminology to describe happiness. Maria was describing "red as green" and by viewing her use of words as biological markers she was deemed insane by psychiatry and treated for brain defects through drugs and ECT. Perhaps had there been an interest in cultural differences and a curiosity to explore why Maria described "red as green" Maria's plight might have been very different.

28.2 The Hearing Voices Network

Having been a psychiatric nurse working many years in the psychiatric system as well as being a voice hearer and experiencing the psychiatric system in my own body and mind I can attest to the consequences of being viewed as a being devoid of a contextualized and meaningful life story. This is why the Hearing Voices Movement (HVM) is so important. It arose to address the lack of meaning making in madness providing safe spaces for those typically deemed schizophrenic to talk about their voices and their lives connecting the two to create meaning and find ways to heal, something psychiatry has consistently been unable to provide for the majority of those it labels schizophrenic.

The Hearing Voices Network (HVN) which has existed for more than 30 years was inspired by the innovative research by Professor Marius Romme and Dr. Sandra Escher, who because of their research advocated a radical new approach and a profound shift in perspective on the symptoms traditionally associated with schizophrenia: hearing voices. These symptoms have traditionally been viewed as symptomatic of a biological disease with a genetic etiology; however, they established that the voices were meaningful and make sense when viewed in conjunction with the traumatic life events that provoked them (Romme & Escher, 2006). They and others show that at least 75% (Read et al., 2005; Johnstone, 2011; Hammersley et al., 2008; Moskowitz & Corstens, 2008) who hear voices have had some traumatic experience connected to their voices.

HVN is an influential grassroots movement which openly critiques traditional psychiatry's relational roles of "passive, recipient patient" and "dominant, expert clinician" and has instead created spaces where people across many disciplines can work together to gain a better understanding about those who hear voices, see visions, and feel tactile sensations and other sensory experiences. The HVN has created a strong self-help tradition where people can meet in a safe place and share experiences, "*without the threat of censorship, loss of liberty or forced medication, a common feature of disclosure in traditional psychiatric settings*" (Rapley et al., 2011). Likewise, they have developed, researched, and published their own methodologies, techniques, and narratives as separate from psychiatry to help those who have problems with their voices, visions, etc. One such book, *Living with Voices*, (2010), comprising 50 anthologies from voice hearers from many different countries who have learned to live with their voices by accepting them, has highlighted several key themes:

- Voices are a survival strategy pointing at past and present problems often using the language of metaphors representing emotions split off from self and telling tales of often dreadful events while attacking yet protecting the person's identity.
- Trauma is a dominating theme ranging from sexual abuse, emotional neglect, physical abuse, and bullying, and it becomes clear that these events play a profound role in the development of alternative beliefs/experiences.
- Recovery is not about getting rid of the voices but about understanding their message(s) and changing the relationship so that the voices may become helpful and cease to be so damaging.
- Interestingly, another theme that came out of the 50 anthologies was that recovery had only become possible outside of psychiatry.

Thus, with the HVM, madness is placed in a context where it can become accessible as understandable which challenges those who view these experiences as irrational, or as symptoms of an underlying biological phenomenon. Therefore, depending on which perspective one approaches symptoms typically ascribed to schizophrenia, different realities can appear or disappear. For though psychiatry can identify focus objects in schizophrenia, its inability to convincingly link them to schizophrenia means that they must continually address these inconsistencies, resulting in their interrelations becoming opaque, contested, ideological, etc.

Hearing voices is also filled with controversy engendering powerful emotions yet the realities regarding voices are created for the most part by the dominant practices surrounding those who hear voices and rarely by those who hear them. Therefore, as a voicehearer myself and as someone who has both worked in the psychiatric system entrenched in the dominant biological narrative as well as having experienced the consequences of this dominant narrative in my body I wish to create a bridge between the two understandings. By creating a possible bridge, I hope to focus on the silenced voices and bring that non-dominant perspective into the forefront and allow those of you who only have access to the dominant narrative a glimpse into what lies on the other side. A side where life stories play a profound role in why people suffer and that by not listening and insisting that one's own truth is the right one, we make people suffer even more.

28.3 Trauma

The evidence linking trauma and psychosis is overwhelming, with poverty, sexual and physical abuse, bullying, neglect, death of mother/primary caregiver, living in foster care/adopted, etc., playing a profound role.

It is important to note though that trauma is not a prerequisite to hearing voices though it is very common (Luhrmann et al., 2019). There are many people who hear voices and are not distressed by them likewise many cultures who value those who can hear and communicate with the religious deities of their culture. Research shows some evidence that those who have not had trauma are not so distressed by their voices, tend to have more positive voices, and do not hear them as often (Bless et al., 2018). Many people who seek the voice of their God or their spiritual guides can actively cultivate hearing voices (Luhrmann, 2016).

It is only fairly recently, that meta-analyses looking at the relationship between trauma and psychosis started. The first one in 2012 (Varese et al., 2012) looked at six specific childhood traumas, sexual abuse, physical abuse, emotional abuse, neglect, bullying, and parental death from 41 robust studies of which 18 also compared non-psychotic controls with psychotic patients. The odds ratio they found was parental death 1.7, bullying 2.4, sexual abuse 2.4, neglect 2.9, physical abuse 2.9, and emotional abuse 3.4 (Read, 2022).

This has also been shown to be dose related. That is, the more trauma in childhood the more likely to develop psychosis. For example, if you have experienced one kind of trauma you are 1.7 times more likely to develop psychosis than people who have not experienced trauma. If you have had three types of traumas, then you are 18 times more likely to develop psychosis and if you have had five types of trauma you are 193 times more likely to develop psychosis (Shevlin et al., 2007).

Unfortunately, the impact of trauma and the link between trauma and psychosis are mostly ignored in psychiatry. If the trauma is known, then it is typically not recognized as playing an important role. The dominant narrative is that you are dealing with an illness that needs to be treated with medication with limited access to other help such as therapy.

Let me take you by the hand so that we may cross the bridge and you can meet the counter narrative, that of the typical voice hearer. I will do this by introducing some of the ideas of postpsychiatry as I believe that the HVN is an excellent example of a postpsychiatric enterprise and share with you the approach or philosophy I use when I work with people who hear voices including redacted stories to elucidate and inspire you.

28.4 Postpsychiatry and HVM

The philosophy of postpsychiatry resonates with me and slots into ideology of the HVM. Postpsychiatry, like the HVM, is linked to postmodernism and does *not* seek to find solutions within psychiatry. Instead, both advocate we should be moving beyond psychiatry, encouraging an acceptance that not all human problems can be grasped in a modernist technological manner and having "the *imagination* to think what a post-technological or a postpsychiatry would look like" (Bracken, 2012).

Patrick Bracken and Philip Thomas are the main actors in postpsychiatry, viewing psychiatry arising as a modern enterprise based on the enlightenment period or the age of reason as it is also known.

Although they support the criticisms voiced by critical psychiatry they specifically advocate for the deprofessionalism and demedicalization of psychiatry and by placing mental distress firmly in a social context, advocate that diagnoses is a matter of negotiation between client and the psychiatrist.

In particular they view academic psychiatry as being guided "*by a profound ideological commitment to what is known as reductionism*" (Bracken & Thomas, 2009). In other words they see psychiatry as trying to explain subjective reality through the use of non-meaningful entities such as neurotransmitters and genes. This reductionistic approach is guided by the concept that it is only experts who hold privileged positions of power who can define the others experience.

They, like the HVM, also question the paradigm of recovery which in psychiatry is often viewed from a perspective of a reduction or lessening of intensity of symptoms. Instead they promote supporting that it is the person herself who defines her recovery. For example in the HVM getting rid of the voices is not seen as a goal such as psychiatry aims for. Rather it could be an acceptance of the voices as being a part of the person's daily life or any other myriad of ways someone can choose to live or not with their voices.

Postpsychiatry has commonalities with antipsychiatry; however, Bracken & Thomas want to avoid the polarization that was created by the antagonism that existed between psychiatry and anti-psychiatry (Double, 2002). In other words they are hoping for dialogue, something antipsychiatry expressed little interest in, or more likely saw as unimportant in that they, like psychiatry, believed that there was a correct way to frame madness. Postpsychiatry and the HVM do not believe there is a correct way to frame madness instead, they view madness as opening up spaces where other perspectives can assume a valid role. Significantly postpsychiatry argues for the voices of survivors and (ex)users of psychiatry to assume center stage. Bracken & Thomas therefore advocate a joining of professional expertise with that of the laypersons experience and give such a prominent role to service users that according to some critics of postpsychiatry "*psychiatrists appear mainly sidelined*" (Kecmanovic, 2009). So though anti/critical/postpsychiatry share elements with each other the advocacy of a true joining of those who use and have used services is extremely important to postpsychiatry. This is born out in practice within the HVM in that it actively encourages both voice hearers and others be they professionals or laypeople to join the movement if it resonates with them. Thus, all over the world most HVNs are composed of voicehearers and non-voicehearers.

28.5 Postpsychiatry and Postmodernism

Postpsychiatry draws on the critique of the modern mind by in particular Michel Foucault, Martin Heidegger, and Ludwig Wittgenstein working toward a hermeneutics of distress. Bracken and Thomas's focus is on power and moving beyond a Cartesian explanation of phenomenology (as defined by Karl Jaspers inspired by Renee Descartes and Edmund Husserl, an explanation which continues to infuse modern-day psychiatry. Bracken and Thomas are concerned with the way psychiatry sees people and the problems they have as expressed in psychiatry's Cartesian approach and the power of "the gaze" as described by Foucault. This approach allows psychiatry to disempower by separating the body from the context of human experiences and the potentiality of meaning making. This is because Jaspers' approach concerns itself with identifying psychiatric symptoms by separating the *form* of the symptom from the *content* opening up for the power of the gaze. He saw the *forms* of psychopathology as being universal and occurring inside the individual, whereas the *content* was socially and culturally mediated context and of secondary value, something that is evident in psychiatry's medical model of madness.

Heidegger therefore plays a significant role introducing the concept of meaning as a non-scientific issue through his two main areas of inquiry, the ontological and the ontic. To use Bracken and Thomas's metaphor, Jaspers' view of human psychology is like an avocado, the pip is where universal processes occur which are context independent and Jaspers' scientific psychopathology comes about through trying to grasp *the nature* of the pip. Therefore, to gain access to the pip so as to expose the pip to a true scientific gaze, the flesh around the pip must be removed, which here represents the world of context and meaning and where the individual's psychology, or one can also say consciousness, resides. A hermeneutic phenomenology as represented by Heidegger is likened to an onion with no central core, just layers representing there is no human psychology without context.

Wittgenstein introduces the concept of the mind and language and the fact that according to him there is a one-to-one relationship between the person and the world they are relating to through words, i.e., he regards language as a social and human phenomenon. This he says can be thought of as rules in the terms of games, where the rules are flexible to account for changing times and different cultures but that language is about its place in human activities and lived life. He addresses the issue that what we feel/our inner world is different from the agreed upon rules for engaging with the outside world, for though we agree upon and describe such things as a feeling of happiness it will remain uniquely our own experience and we will never know if the happiness we feel is the same as the next person's. This has, says Bracken and Thomas, tremendous consequences for psychiatry, for when psychiatry imposes a positivistic reductionism of lived life with stories of trauma and loss, e.g., rating scales such as the Hamilton scale which attempts to measure sadness even though sadness is an unmeasurable entity, psychiatry *acts* as if it was a measurable entity. However, because the mind, our inner worlds, is unmeasurable and inseparably linked to context, emotions, values, and beliefs exist as if they were physical entities, yet remain outside the realm of physicality. What Wittgenstein does is show that we cannot discuss our inner knowledge of the mind in a Cartesian manner for what we say about our inner mind is intimately connected to our outside world of cultural social and historical contexts and makes us according to Bracken and Thomas "*above all else embodied social and cultural beings*" (Bracken & Thomas, 2009).

Accordingly, postpsychiatry has, by questioning the validity of the biomedical model and the reductionism of modern psychiatry and engaging fully with the user movements, created three major goals.

1. The importance of contexts, in other words, political, social, and cultural contexts should be center stage in understanding mental distress. A context centered approach allows for non-cartesian models of mind as exemplified by Wittgenstein and Heidegger with an emphasis on the term hermeneutic which here means priority is given to meaning and interpretation.
2. Ethical rather than technological orientation, meaning a move away from the belief that science guides clinical practice in psychiatry to acknowledging that psychiatry is primarily concerned with beliefs, moods, and behaviors and that values and assumptions regarding these issues are what underpins psychiatric classifications. If this is ignored, dangers arise as can be seen by the problematic encounters with those diagnosed schizophrenic or people suffering distress from other cultural backgrounds.
3. Rethinking the politics of coercion. Many who use psychiatric services question the medical model of psychiatry and are outraged that this forms the basis for force. Postpsychiatry wishes to relinquish the right to detain and/or force treat the mentally distressed and advocate a principle of reciprocity meaning any legislation allowing force has to have safeguards such as advance directives and advocacy.

28.6 Olga

I recall the day I was told I was suffering from a dire lifelong illness. I sat across from the psychiatrist who very sincerely and with great sorrow studied me from across his large desk. "Olga," he says, "You have a very severe illness." "Oh," I say "and what is that?" "You have schizophrenia, or to be more specific you have paranoid schizophrenia." I looked back at him, panic surging through me because I knew what that meant as I had seen it happen so many times to innumerable other patients from at that time the perspective of a psychiatric nurse. Now it was happening to me. "No I don't," I said, "You are completely wrong." With that recognizable look of dismissal I have seen on many a professional's face when contradicted along with the glancing at the clock, he said, "The very fact that you deny that you are ill, proves that you are ill as you are expressing what we call 'lack of illness insight.' You must learn to both accept your illness and that your life will never be the same." And thus I entered into, or perhaps more fittingly crossed the bridge into from my perspective, the Kafkan world of psychiatry. For you see at no point were any tests of a biological nature ever taken for this biological disease that I was perceived to be suffering from. Nor were any biological tests ever taken to see if the many drugs I took over the next 10 years were correcting the alleged neurotransmitter imbalances of my defective brain from this inherited disease called schizophrenia. All it was, was words. Very powerful words. Words that the second they were uttered completely changed my life and left me as a chronic incurable schizophrenic on the highest disability pension as I was assumed to be totally incapable of ever contributing to society again. The chemical treatment rendering me to a shuffling shadow of myself and the vast array of side effects as further symptoms of my schizophrenia. It was a world I had never seen before because, being a psychiatric nurse, I had been taught to define the descriptions and behavior that people shared, as part of an illness, an illness that we as the experts knew more about than our patients. Crossing that bridge albeit involuntarily has been the single most profound game-changing experience I have ever had. It has profoundly altered me and resulted in among other things the development of my philosophy/approach which I have called "The Wall of Disconnection" first introduced 2016 Gothenburg (Runciman, 2016) *and described here in this chapter. This includes both the thinking behind it and in action.*

28.7 What Is This Thing We Call Psychosis?

Paris Williams "Rethinking Madness" (Williams, 2012) describes existential crises as a key cause, and I very much agree. But since existential crises are universal, how is it that some react so strongly that they become psychotic, and others do not? This can be illustrated by looking at two common existential dilemmas.

We all need an ongoing balance between being independent, free, and self-determining in relation to the need for love, dependence, and acceptance. The balance between the two poles is the art of creating sustainable relationships with other people, a dilemma that everyone can recognize.

The other more airy, intangible existential dilemma, is the need to have a stable sense of self in relation to the universe, understood from the outside of the great philosophical questions about the meaning of life, death, and existence itself.

In order not to be overwhelmed by this, it is essential to develop mental constructs in which to create meaning, truths, and a framework of understanding to navigate daily life. This helps build a sense of predictability/solidity, where the world is experienced as stable and safe, and a stable sense of self can be developed. The flip side is that you can create an illusion that the world and your sense of self are more stable and secure than they really are. In the event of a crisis/trauma, one's mental constructs can become so shaken that they become very unstable. For some this can be a life-changing experience, but for others it can open the door to the overwhelming anxiety of discovering that one's worldview, which was stable and reliable, is no longer. In the often desperate process of regaining their footing, many experience the psychic phenomena of disconnection with their everyday and the world around them, in other words becoming what is referred to as psychotic.

Psychiatry chooses to divide psychotic crises into separate illnesses and then treat them as if they were separate bio/genetic diseases. But psychosis is something anyone can experience. The outcome, whether you recover or not, is in turn very different, depending on the help you get.

From my personal experience and the scientific research, I find it more meaningful and fruitful to look at "madness" and "normality" from the outside and see how much the common reality matches one's inner reality. In my daily work I use the words I use in relation to myself, distinguishing between the "*private world*" versus the "*common world.*" The *common world* is the one we are all part of, where we are connected to each other culturally, emotionally, and feel we belong in a meaningful way. It is also the place where we can usually agree there exists a *joint reality* that we are present in together. The joint reality is to be understood as the space where there is shared consensus about the reality that is taking place. At the same time, it is also about the degree to which one is emotionally affected, and how stable/unstable one is when one's experiences are significantly different from the rest of the world.

In short, reality, along with emotion and stability, together determine whether one is considered "mad" or not. At one end, one is "normal" when one's "private world" is in line with the "common world," i.e., when there is consensus between inner and outer reality, between the person and her culture. However, what is "normal" in one culture may be considered "mad" in another.

One can experience discrepancy between one's "private world" and the "common" without this being an obstacle. Personally, I hear "voices" no one else in the "common world" can hear; they are real to me. Yet I thrive. Others may have strange beliefs, or ways of seeing the world that seem outlandish, yet they thrive. Conversely, enough people believe in God, that Jesus walked on water and Mary was a virgin, that these are recognized as "normal" beliefs.

Then one can experience discrepancies between private and shared reality, where one is emotionally affected, yet not unstable. Many will experience being diagnosed here but, again, the evidence shows that one can recover with the right support. For example when I worked in psychiatry as a psychiatric nurse, I heard voices and I knew that that meant I was seriously ill with an incurable disease as that is what I had been taught. I had to hide that discrepancy and was emotionally affected as fear became a daily companion – fear of being mad and fear of being discovered as mad. Yet I was stable and continued to work and to the outside world to all intents and purposes normal.

Finally, we have the condition where, along with the inconsistencies of reality, one is emotionally affected and unstable. In this situation the person is no longer able to separate the private from the common world the private world spills over into the common world alerting those around them that something is wrong. In this state, one is most often considered to be highly psychotic. Again, research shows that many recover despite psychiatry's pessimism. I am one of them.

Problems, therefore, are not about inconsistencies between the inner, "private world" and the outer, "common world," but rather about the ability to cope with and relate to the "private world." Help is about reducing the anxiety that is most often present and help to find meaning and understanding from the reality that one is now experiencing in the "private world" and not having to agree with the majority in the "common world".

28.8 The Private World

Normally when people are well functioning and able to deal with their lives and the challenges of the everyday they do so because they are connected, connected to the world around them, with meaningful relationships and networks. They have purpose and direction and can place themselves and understand the world around them in a contextualized and meaningful manner. Indeed, I would posit that one is able to deal with very challenging situations if one is connected. However, what happens when people start to have difficulties connecting? They start to disconnect? The *private world* is the world which only exists for the individual. We all have a private world, and we cannot share these unique qualities of our private world in the sense it is completely subjective as described so well by Nagel in his paper, "What is it like to be a bat?" Therefore, I will, for example, never know what it is *like* for my client to hear the voices in her head nor she mine. We all interpret our experiences in the common world through the lens of our private world and share these interpretations with others using language and behavior to communicate and connect to others about our experiences creating a shared reality. Therefore, in the private world the person is mind-wise alone with their unique subjective experiences. However, if they are able to communicate and connect in an emotional and meaningful way with others, we will be on the whole deemed "normal." This means many live their lives connecting and communicating their experiences that if analyzed through the lens of psychiatry could be deemed delusional. Also, if enough people share and able to connect a common belief that would normally render an individual alone with that belief as mad, they are protected by it being a group belief. For example, in the USA, 12 million people believe that the country is run by genetically modified lizard–human hybrid race called the "Babylonian Brotherhood" (Parramore, 2021) and there is a lot of overlap between the lizard–people theory and QAnon. The QAnon movement alleges that there exists a "deep-state cabal" of human traffickers and pedophiles many are well-known figures, who apart from molesting children kill their victims, extracting a life-extending chemical called adrenochrome (Roose, 2021). Again, if this was presented in isolation, in other words nobody else shared this interpretation of the common world, it would likely lead to being admitted into the psychiatric hospital. So when I talk of the private world of people who come to me for help I am referring to a world that is usually causing the person great distress, that they are alone with and often they have become so separated from the common world that the private world dominates (see Fig. 28.1). They have in a sense switched the worlds around. For though their body exists in the common world, they live in the private world some completely others more subtly. They are interpreting the private world using cues from the common world and trying to share these interpretations within the private world using language and behavior to communicate and connect to others about what is happening. However, the problem is they are no longer able to connect to the common world in a meaningful way for others. This means that they are now seen as not normal, that they have "gone mad," and more often than not they are now in psychiatry and deemed ill with a brain disease called schizophrenia.

A typical trajectory is that the person has usually experienced traumatic things in their childhood that they have been alone with. Often, they have started to drift into their private world which is viewed from the outside, as the person beginning to change. If they are at school, their grades may start to fall, or they start to miss out on school, drug use and truancy can start to occur or they become introverted avoiding others and isolating themselves. Gradually the behavior becomes more and more noticeable and people around them will begin to react. At some point, psychiatry can become involved though usually if there is contact with their nearest and dearest, various avenues will have been tried before they reach out to psychiatry.

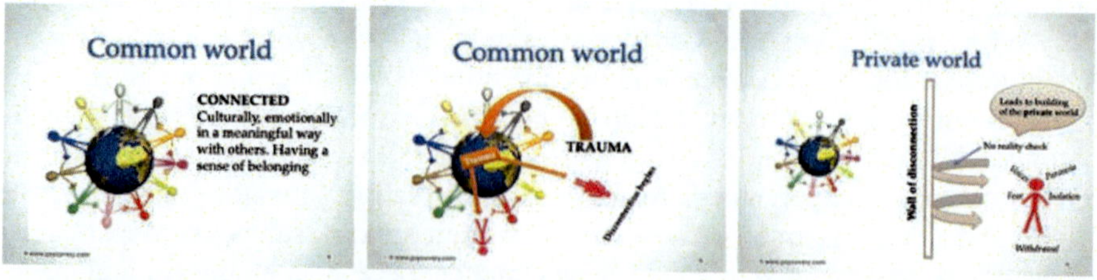

Fig. 28.1 The process of disconnection from the common world. From Olga Runciman's PowerPoint illustrating "The wall of disconnection"

Another trajectory I meet is where someone has been in psychiatry many years often living in a residential home and I have been asked to help the person. In such cases it is no longer just the private world that is the source of distress or problems but institutionalization along with the consequences of long-term drugs that play a profound role. Sometimes that means a return to normal life outside of the institution proves to be no longer possible but does not mean that things cannot change.

28.9 Amalia

Amalia had been institutionalized for many years no one could remember how long but before she had come to the residential home she had been living in a locked ward for a couple of years. When she came to the home the hospital staff wrote in her papers, she was a through and through schizophrenic. I came regularly to this residential home and on this occasion, I had been invited to do some teaching which was open to both staff and residents and Amalia would sit at the back talking to, it turned out, her private world family. Amalia was on a community treatment order which meant she was force medicated every month. She was overweight and had a large beard due to the hormonal disturbances believed to have been caused by the many psychiatric drugs she had been and was on. She would spend her everyday talking to those who inhabited her private world rarely responding to those who worked or lived in the home. On this occasion something had resonated with within her and she came to me when I was finished teaching and said she wanted to explain her world. Very surprised I immediately said yes. We fetched a large piece of paper, drawing a line down the middle, and she said her private world was to be placed higher on the paper than the common world indicating that her private world was more important than the common world. She then began to describe her world while I wrote things down according to her instructions.

In her ***private world*** *she was married to Thomas, and Thomas was able to go into the common world as the only one who could. If all the aunts, uncles and cousins were counted, then her family was 173 members. She had a wedding ring on her ring finger, and time was fluid in that she could be a grandmother in the morning, giving birth to her first child in the afternoon and be dealing with teenagers in the evening. She was a real estate agent, which suddenly made sense for why she would wait in the morning to gather all the newspapers and cut out property announcements. Something that nobody had understood and caused frustration as people were annoyed over the damaged newspapers. She was also a sports journalist on the side, which also made sense as to why she would always turn the communal TV back to the sports channels. In her private world people believed her when she talked about her life and she had meaning and purpose.*

In the ***communal world*** *she said no one believed her, especially that she had family or work, she felt people mocked her and laughed at her. No one could see her wedding ring as the skin had grown over it. She was, she told me, attacked and force injected by something that made her feel confused for a couple of days and she* *worried she was unable to be a proper mother during that period. When she was in the communal world, it was Thomas who would fetch her when she needed by the family in the private world. Suddenly it became clear why she would, when it was nearing the time for her forced injection, become extremely anxious and agitated, talk of constant danger to the children and that it was important that they be taken to safety and calling to Thomas to hide the children from danger.*

I remember sitting there when she was finished, stunned, and very moved, and I said to her I can see why you spend most of your time in your private world. The common world has so little to offer you. Sensing how present she was in this moment of shared reality, I suggested that we could perhaps meet in the common world for tea, and she agreed to that. For the next year I would visit, and she surprised us all as she would set a beautiful tea table for my visit and we would talk about the past. She would talk about holidays she had been on, countries she had visited, and old movies she had seen. Whenever we came too close to something that was difficult, she would get a certain expression of "disappearance," look to the right and say "Thomas is calling me." In that way I knew we should change the conversation or that our meeting over tea was over. Meeting over tea was where Amalia would truly be present in the communal world as long as we kept to the safe topics. Meeting for tea also changed the relationships she had with the staff who began to engage with her very differently. She has since passed away, but I often think of her and the remarkable ability of the human mind to survive circumstances that are so unbearable that moving into the private world is the only possible way to live.

28.10 Disconnection

I like to describe the wall of disconnection as being like a glass wall, it is invisible yet there. Once the person is behind it, they are more engaged with what is unfolding in their private world than the common world, the voices, the visions, and the powerful emotions where often fear is very much present. Indeed, research has shown us that a primary difference between people who hear voices and are in psychiatry versus those who hear voices but are not in psychiatry is that the person in psychiatry is afraid of their voices and feels that the voices are more powerful than them (Romme & Escher, 2009).

The common world is now there to corroborate what is going on in the private world. For example, someone can believe that car number plates are codes to unlock the secrets to saving the world. I would be able to see the car number plates too but I would be viewing them through the culturally accepted ideas of registration. However, for that person the numbers have taken on a special significance that are no longer subjected to the same reality checks and balances that occur between people when one is emotionally connected in a meaningful and purposeful way to one's every day in the common world. Instead meaning-making constructions can be based on private logic, private interpretations, voices, signs, and visions that are to be found primarily in the private world. But behind it all is a message, an important message, a message with its roots in the past, triggered by the present and waiting to be understood.

Having been on both sides of the psychiatric system and knowing what it is like to move between the common and the private worlds, I see myself today as a bridge builder (see Fig. 28.2). A bridge builder between the service users subjected to the power of the system and the psychiatric system which has the power. A bridge builder creating a bridge between the two worlds, the private and the common world. In this process the purpose is never to eliminate the private world of people only that they can find ways to navigate the two and ideally function well in both. Many, myself included, continue to hear voices; the difference is I can clearly separate them and my private world from the common world. My private world is not spilling out into the common world creating disturbances and distorting my way of being.

We can all become bridge builders each in or own way for it is about meeting the person where she is and creating a relationship that can act as a guiding light to help the person find their way back to their society where they can be reconnected with what is meaningful emotionally and culturally and finding purpose in the common world.

There are many ways to being a bridge builder, and being trauma informed is of course very helpful. Being able to offer within the psychiatric system various therapeutic approaches which do not look to removing the voices but rather help with finding coping strategies that help reduce the stress and increase functioning such as CBT for psychosis can be helpful. Open Dialogue in Western Lapland is an example of a psychiatric system that has the best results in the world when it comes to supporting people suffering from psychotic breaks. Their approach is network based, dialogical and the distress is viewed as that something has happened in the life of that person and not an illness-based approach. Hearing voices groups encourage exploration through focusing on listening to the voices and encouraging the creation of meaning-making, changing the relationships with voices and connecting with others in a safe environment (Dillon & Hornstein, 2013). Indeed Open Dialogue and the HVM have much in common (Runciman & Twamely, 2021).

To give an example of bridge building I will tell the story of Magnus.

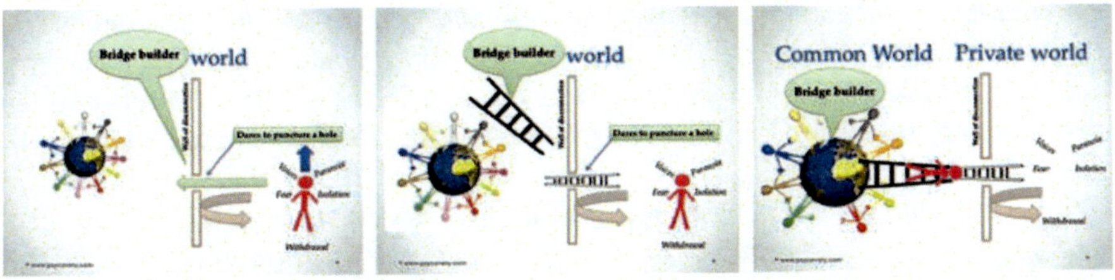

Fig. 28.2 Building bridges between the private and the common world. From Olga Runciman's PowerPoint illustrating "The wall of disconnection"

28.11 Magnus

Magnus was around 30 when I met him the first time. I met him at the psychiatric residential home where he lived where I had just started as a consultant as there was a wish to learn more about alternative ways of understanding "schizophrenia." Those residents who wanted could meet me along with workers of their choice with the idea that both residents and staff could come to understand each other better. The first time I met him had been because his key worker had suggested it and when I asked him what might he like to talk about he said there was no point, nobody had ever understood nor did they believe him.

His key worker had suggested meeting with me as they were at a loss and didn't know how to approach the situation as Magnus insisted that the original Magnus was dead and he was a copy and was 5 years old. The psychiatrist told the staff that he was severely mentally ill and had gradually increased his medication over time which had made Magnus reluctant to meet with the psychiatrist at all and resulting in him withdrawing more and more from the other residents and the staff. Magnus was forced to live at the home as he was on a forensic treatment order because he had attempted to murder a man in his remote fishing village many years ago. The staff were cautious as is so often the case when people are viewed as ill with a mental disease and violence is seen as being a symptom of said disease. This feeds into systemic and societal stigma which is particularly prevalent when people are viewed as different because they are suffering a biological illness and feeds into the concept of meaningless violence as a symptom.

I said I would be very interested to listen to his story and try and understand if he wanted to give me that chance. I remember him studying me for a while before saying it is very complicated to which I replied I will do my best to understand and hoped he would have patience with me. He agreed to give me a chance to understand his story. I suggested that perhaps we could start with a bit about who he was, his life story, as that would help me better understand his life as a copy. He agreed.

As is often the case when someone starts telling their story for the first time to others it is disjointed and fragmented but with time the person can unite the fragments creating a whole. Magnus told us he was a copy and the original was dead and that there were other copies of him he believed there were maybe 5 or 6 in all but he had most contact with 3 of them. The original Magnus had died 12 years ago. Since then various copies had appeared and he was the youngest of the copies. He had contact with the copies who were to be found in town and he knew they were also in his village. I suggested that perhaps the copies could help tell his story as they were all older than him and so it was through the copies that he was able to piece his story together. Each had a birth date for when they appeared, and it turned out that it was not just random birth dates, they were in actual fact connected to highly significant events. For example, one copy replaced the original Magnus who died on the day he had attacked the village teacher with a knife, severely injuring him. This copy went to court and was unjustly accused of attempting to kill this teacher and was deemed criminally insane. Magnus had never been outside of his village and when he was taken out of the local prison where he had been during the investigation and court case and taken far away from his village to the locked forensic hospital, a new copy appeared to keep the first copy company. It turned out he was desperately lonely, and the second copy could comfort the first copy, who had been unjustly accused and now punished by being banished from the only place he knew, his village. They were together for the first 6 or so years while he was in the hospital, and then Magnus was transferred to the residential home as he was deemed safe enough to leave the forensic hospital and move to where I met him or as he was at that time the 5-year-old copy. The 5-year-old copy's birth date was when Magnus was moved to the home and was the one I met. The two older copies were now living in the city, and he saw them regularly in the supermarket or on the streets.

It took a while for Magnus to refer to the three copies still in the village whose ages turned out to represent important events. Two were children and one was an angry teenager. The youngest child copy was 6 years old, and the older child was around 12. The teenager copy around 16. They carried the stories of his childhood and the sexual abuse he had been subjected to. When he was 6, the teacher he had stabbed as an 18-year-old had started to abuse him. The teacher was well liked in the village and played an important role as a popular figure in local politics. He would give gifts to Magnus while threatening bad things would happen to his family if he said anything. His family were proud of the teacher's interest in their son and so it became his secret. When he was around 12 or 13 and beginning to come into puberty, the teacher lost interest in him. Magnus discovered that there was a new little boy that had replaced him. He was relieved but at the same time wracked with guilt that now another little boy was exposed to the same thing he had been. He recognized the same patterns and saw a repeat unfolding. When he was 16 or 17 he overheard some of the villagers talking about the teacher insinuating that he was a sexual abuser yet at the same time saying he couldn't be because he was such a nice person and popular. It was then he realized that perhaps it was not such a secret and he began to feel that everyone knew what the teacher had done to him. One day he came home and his father was sitting with the teacher chatting and Magnus became enraged. He accused the teacher of molesting him and his father furious at Magnus for falsely accusing the teacher of such filth threw Magnus out of the house. It was then that Magnus began to drink and smoke dope and increasingly felt the whole village was somehow in collusion with the teacher ultimately resulting in him drinking heavily one night and then stabbing the teacher.

It became clear the copies originated from the sense of repetition that he saw unfold with the other boy and the intense guilt he felt for not stopping it while at the same time feeling the enormous relief that the teacher no longer abused him anymore. The sense of betrayal when his father chose to stand by the teacher cemented the sense that the village was in cahoots with teacher choosing to turn a blind eye because of his prominent role in the village along with the fact he too let a "copy" another small boy replace him and not stop it. The enormous emotional toil of conflicting emotions was just too overwhelming. When he woke up in the police cell and was accused of attempted murder he became a copy and Magnus the original from the village who was guilty of attempted murder and carried within him overwhelming emotions, died.

The bridge building involved how to invite Magnus who now was more connected to his private world interacting with his copies, than the common world back into to the common world. To do that it was important to together create a shared reality, but also to see if it was possible to make the common world inviting enough so that he would be motivated to reconnect.

It took time but very importantly when the staff heard his story for the first time in a different context, it made complete sense to them. Suddenly their viewpoint of this man changed. Previously he had been seen as a man who, despite never having shown any signs of violence in the home, never drank or smoked dope, continued to instill fear in the staff. This was because they knew he had attempted to kill, according to the notes, an innocent man and that he had done so because he was mentally ill. They now found it understandable that he had attacked the teacher, not that that was OK they said, but it was relatable. That he was a copy and talked to his other copies made much more sense to them. This changed their relationship with him and they began to engage with him for who he was rather than someone whom they could not understand and saw as "mad" and whom they had feared. By talking openly about what had happened his reality which had previously been denied began to become a shared one. The staff supported him in beginning to reduce his medication, arguing his case to the psychiatrist. It was also decided to look at his treatment order and they supported him in ending it which they were successful in, 3 years later.

During those years we worked with his trauma, in particular, the guilt and shame. Two of his sisters lived in the city and they, Magnus would say, only "saw" the copies. But by involving them and talking about what had happened they helped Magnus revive the Original by accepting him and what he had done as well as what had happened to him as a child. Thus, over time he stopped being a copy and began to become the Original. Initially the Original was just the guilty one, the one that had papers defining him as a criminal. Yet by becoming the Original one he was accepting that he had attacked the teacher something he had disconnected from by becoming a copy and denying he had anything to do with.

The copies, though, continued to exist and they were multifaceted in their personalities. They were the bright student, the sporty football player, the fun joker, the kind brother, and the loving son, all disconnected from the revived Original. We talked about how the copies who possessed the things he valued could perhaps be reintegrated with the Original to create a Magnus of today. Magnus said initially that they never could be a whole but when we began to work with his hopes and dreams it became clear he had a burning wish to come back to the village and most importantly he dreamt of being welcomed by his father.

His father had not had any contact with him in all the years he was in psychiatry. Magnus would say his father was in contact with the copies but not the Original and that his father would never see the Original. It became clear that this was an important relationship and if that could be reestablished perhaps it could help with reintegrating the copies. Once again his two sisters came to play another extremely important role by facilitating a bridge back to his/their father.

Magnus's father had been filled with shame when his son had been accused of attempted murder and guilt that it was his son who had done that to the teacher so he had vowed to never speak to Magnus again. The teacher recovered but at some point the rumors began about his interest in small boys and he ceased to be a popular figure. One day he just moved. In many ways Magnus was right, the village always suspected but turned a blind eye because of who the teacher was. His father could not bear the thought that perhaps his son had not lied when he had accused the teacher that afternoon in front of him and his guilt, anger, and sorrow kept him from connecting with Magnus during all those ensuing years. Magnus' sisters helped create a bridge so that father and son could reconnect and healing to occur. It was a big day for all when Magnus' dream that his father would say welcome home came to fruition. It was first then when his father could see the Original in other words accept him fully that the copies began to fill less and less as they reintegrated into the Original to become whole. Another source that helped his healing was the local nurse who created a group for adult children of abuse and there he found others who had also been abused by the same teacher. However, he never found the other little boy who became the source for his copies.

Today Magnus is working in the fishing industry.

28.12 Conclusion

We can all become bridge builders and help those who are lost behind a wall of disconnection to reconnect. When we let go of the concept that extreme distress and psychosis is a biological phenomenon and instead listen to and meet the person where they are then we can become helpful.

There is enormous metamorphic potential in psychosis. In order to become a butterfly, the caterpillar must go through a process of complete dissolution and then reconstruct itself as the beautiful butterfly that it is destined to be. Similarly, when a person experiences such a huge crisis that their worldview no longer works and ordinary strategies are not enough, the psyche, as a last resort, can enter a state where the self is fragmented and one's meaning structure disintegrates. As the recovery literature so clearly shows, the possibility of reintegrating and coming through the process as a stronger person is greater, provided the person receives the right support. For many, the process can end with an experience of feeling better than ever before.

Unfortunately, academic psychiatry with its biomedical approach is an obstacle for many. This is something that can be seen in the numbers who become marginalized and passive recipients of government support as described in Robert Whitaker's "Anatomy of an Epidemic." People are very vulnerable when they are in crisis and more often than not the encounter with psychiatry happens when one is in a disintegrated and fragmented state where the self is at risk. Therefore, for the many who enter into psychiatry, the imposed diagnosis, such as schizophrenia, becomes their new identity and meaning structure. One becomes "schizophrenic" with all the implications of the diagnosis, rather than the butterfly one was meant to be.

I hope this chapter can inspire you to reconsider the implications of a biological approach to crises of the mind and the phenomenon of hearing voices, seeing visions, and other unusual experiences. I also hope this chapter can encourage interest in becoming a "bridge builder," walking alongside the one in crisis in dialogue, working together to decipher the symbolism of the voices, visions, and other unusual experiences.

As someone who used to work in psychiatry believing what I had been taught that people were ill and the way to fix them was through the mechanical means of psychiatric drugs or ECT, I am today in awe of the human mind, its amazing ability to heal, and the myriad of ways of surviving the most awful situations. So many have invited me to connect with them when they were lost behind their walls of disconnection and to share their journeys as they find their way back to the common world. Journeys that I am eternally grateful for as each and every one who has invited me to join them has taught me so much and expanded my horizons. We all suffer, but when we are met with ears that will listen, hands that reach out, and a willingness to be met even though it is in our darkest of places, we have a far greater chance of surviving even the most terrible of circumstances.

Therefore,

Let us join together and create the butterflies people were meant to be, and not schizophrenics.

Disclaimer All stories are compilations and not referring to one specific person apart from my own "Olga."

References

Blakeslee, S. (1996). The conscious mind is still baffling to experts of all stripes. *New York Times*. https://www.nytimes.com/1996/04/16/science/the-conscious-mind-is-still-baffling-to-experts-of-all-stripes.html. Accessed 29 Sept 2022.

Bless, J., Larøi, F., Laloyaux, J., et al. (2018). T2. Do adverse life events at first onset of auditory verbal hallucinations influence subsequent voice-characteristics? Results from an epidemiological study. *Schizophrenia Bulletin, 44*, S113. https://doi.org/10.1093/schbul/sby016.278

Bracken, P. (2012). *Postpsychiatry – Reaching beyond the technological paradigm in mental health.* https://slidetodoc.com/postpsychiatry-reaching-beyond-the-technological-paradigm-in-mental/. Accessed 2 Oct 2022.

Bracken, P., & Thomas, T. (2009). *Postpsychiatry: Mental health in a postmodern world.* Oxford University Press.

Chalmers, D. (1995). Facing up to the problem of consciousness. *Journal of Consciousness Studies, 2*, 200–219.

Chalmers, D., & Searle, J. (2022). 'Consciousness and the philosophers': An exchange. *The New York review of books*. https://www.nybooks.com/articles/1997/05/15/consciousness-and-the-philosophers-an-exchange/. Accessed 29 Sept 2022.

Dillon, J., & Hornstein, G. (2013). Hearing voices peer support groups: A powerful alternative for people in distress. *Psychosis, 5*, 286–295. https://doi.org/10.1080/17522439.2013.843020

Double, D. (2002). The limits of psychiatry. *BMJ: British Medical Journal, 324*, 900–904. https://doi.org/10.1136/bmj.324.7342.900

Hammersley, P., Read, J., Woodall, S., & Dillon, J. (2008). Childhood trauma and psychosis: The genie is out of the bottle. *Journal of Psychological Trauma, 6*(2–3), 7–20. https://doi.org/10.1300/J513v06n02_02

Jackson, F. (1986). What Mary didn't know. *Journal of Philosophy, 83*, 291–295.

Johnstone, L. (2011). Can Traumatic Events Traumatize People? Trauma, Madness and 'Psychosis'. In: Rapley, M., Moncrieff, J., Dillon, J. (eds) De-Medicalizing Misery. Palgrave Macmillan, London. https://doi.org/10.1057/9780230342507_8

Kecmanovic, D. (2009). Postpsychiatry: How to throw out the baby with the bath water. *Schweizer Archiv für Neurologie und Psychiatrie, 160*, 27–33. https://doi.org/10.4414/sanp.2009.02032

Leibniz, G. W. (1714). *The monadology*. https://www.plato-philosophy.org/wp-content/uploads/2016/07/The-Monadology-1714-by-Gottfried-Wilhelm-LEIBNIZ-1646-1716.pdf. Accessed 29 Sept 2022.

Luhrmann, T. (2016). Diversity within the psychotic continuum. *Schizophrenia Bulletin, 43*, 27–31. https://doi.org/10.1093/schbul/sbw137

Luhrmann, T., Alderson-Day, B., Bell, V., et al. (2019). Beyond trauma: A multiple pathways approach to auditory hallucinations in clinical and nonclinical populations. *Schizophrenia Bulletin, 45*, S24–S31. https://doi.org/10.1093/schbul/sby110

Moskowitz, A., & Corstens, D. (2008). Auditory Hallucinations: Psychotic Symptom or Dissociative Experience?. *Journal of Psychological Trauma, 6*:2–3, 35–63. https://doi.org/10.1300/J513v06n02_04

Nagel, T. (1974). What is it like to be a bat? *The Philosophical Review, 83*, 435. https://doi.org/10.2307/2183914

Parramore, L. S. (2021). Like QAnon's Capitol rioters, the Nashville bomber's lizard people theory is deadly serious Bonkers? Sure. Harmless? Definitely not. *NBC News*. https://www.nbcnews.com/think/opinion/qanon-s-capitol-rioters-nashville-bomber-s-lizard-people-theory-ncna1253819. Accessed 2 Oct 2022.

Ramsey, W. (2022). Eliminative materialism. In *The Stanford encyclopedia of philosophy* (Spring 2022 Edition).

Rapley, P., Moncrieff, D., & Dillon, M. (2011). *De-medicalizing misery* (pp. 141–158). Palgrave Macmillan.

Read, J. (2022). Traumas, adversities, and psychosis: investigating practical implications. *Psychiatric Times*. https://www.psychiatrictimes.com/view/traumas-adversities-and-psychosis-investigating-practical-implications. Accessed 2 Oct 2022.

Read, J., van Os, J., Morrison, A. P., & Ross, C. A. (2005). Childhood trauma, psychosis and schizophrenia: A literature review with theoretical and clinical implications. *Acta Psychiatrica Scandinavica, 112*, 330–350.

Romme, M., & Escher, S. (2006). *Accepting voices*. MIND Publications.

Romme, M., & Escher, S. (2009). *Living with voices*. PCCS Books.

Roose, K. (2021). What is QAnon, the viral pro-Trump conspiracy theory? *New York Times*. https://www.nytimes.com/article/what-is-qanon.html. Accessed 2 Oct 2022.

Runciman, O. (2016, October 15). *Psych-drugs risks and alternatives 1 – Olga Runciman*. Youtube.com. https://www.youtube.com/watch?v=-2HwfOf0dR4. Accessed 2 Oct 2022.

Runciman, O., & Twamely, I. (2021). An invitation to dialogue: What we can all learn from open dialogue and hearing voices networks. In M. Hopfenbeck, I. Parker, & J. Schnackenberg (Eds.), *The practical handbook of hearing voices: Therapeutic and creative approaches*. PCCS Books.

Shevlin, M., Houston, J., Dorahy, M., & Adamson, G. (2007). Cumulative traumas and psychosis: An analysis of the national comorbidity survey and the British Psychiatric Morbidity Survey. *Schizophrenia Bulletin, 34*, 193–199. https://doi.org/10.1093/schbul/sbm069

Varese, F., Smeets, F., Drukker, M., et al. (2012). Childhood adversities increase the risk of psychosis: A meta-analysis of patient-control, prospective- and cross-sectional cohort studies. *Schizophrenia Bulletin, 38*, 661–671. https://doi.org/10.1093/schbul/sbs050

Williams, P. (2012). *Rethinking madness*. Rethinkingmadness.com. http://rethinkingmadness.com/wp-content/uploads/2021/12/Rethinking_Madness_completeBook.pdf. Accessed 2 Oct 2022.

Chapter 29
Learning to Relate Differently to Hearing Voices

Rufus May and Kerry Middleton

29.1 Introduction

Learning to relate differently to hearing voices is a challenge for all of us not just people who hear voices. In this chapter we will look at approaches that have come out of the hearing voices movement and share stories of how people have made use of these developments.

R. May (✉)
Greater Manchester Mental Health Trust, Bolton, UK
e-mail: rufus.may@gmmh.nhs.uk

K. Middleton
Southern Health, Southampton, UK
e-mail: kerry.middleton4@nhs.net

J. A. Díaz-Garrido et al. (eds.), *Psychological Interventions for Psychosis*,
https://doi.org/10.1007/978-3-031-27003-1_29

29.1.1 What Attracted Us to Trying to Better Approach and Understand Hearing Voices?

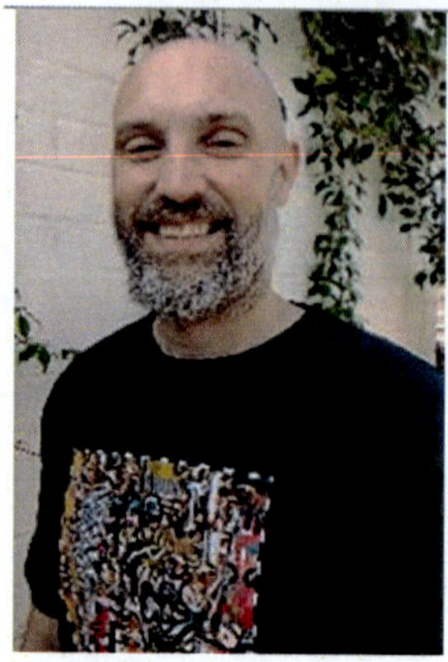 RUFUS	I don't hear voices but my partner does and has done so ever since she can remember. We do not see her experiences as pathology rather as a different way to experience human consciousness. I first came across the hearing voice network in 1999. I had recently qualified as a clinical psychologist. I was looking for a space to integrate my role as a clinical psychologist with experiences as a young person of psychosis and of psychiatric treatment (which I was quite critical of). At the age of 18 I had had strong beliefs others deemed as psychotic and experiences of an altered sense of reality. In 1999 I gave a talk about my experiences: how I had found the diagnosis of Schizophrenia unhelpful and what seemed to help my recovery. I went on to reflect on how these influenced my practice as a psychologist. The conference was organised by members of the English Hearing Voices network. Because I was interested in developing psychological approaches for people given psychotic diagnoses, I became increasingly interested in how to help people who hear voices. I remember going to a workshop facilitated by Marius Romme (one of the founders of the hearing voices movement) in 2001. He asked participants why they were afraid to work with the voice hearing experience. I reflected that as a therapist I felt very de-skilled to help someone who hears voices because I did not have the experience of voice hearing. I felt like a blind person trying to teach a sighted person how to drive. It is through working closely with hearing voices peer support groups since 2001 as a facilitator and co-facilitator I have become confident in talking with people about their experiences and exploring ways for them to improve their relationship with their voices.

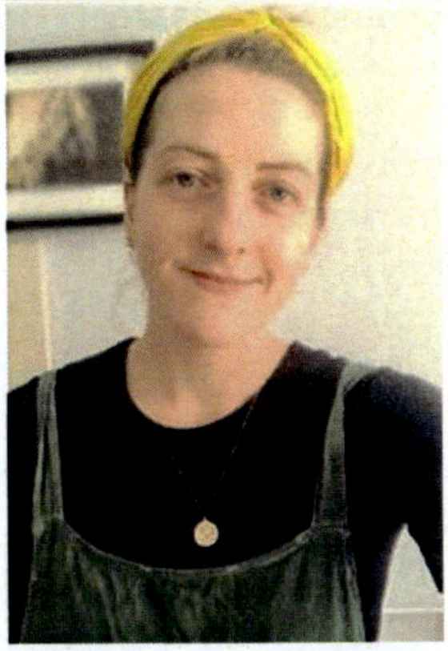

KERRY

I have been interested in therapeutic approaches for voice hearing for some time, having completed a Masters in 'Early intervention in Psychosis' (EIP) at King's College London and worked in an EIP service in London before training as a Clinical Psychologist. I have also grown up as a young carer with family members who hear voices, but was always dissatisfied with the care they had received in services; both in terms of the limited availability of talking therapies which considered the experience of voice hearing and professionals inviting conversation around it more generally.

This led me to discovering the work of the Hearing Voices Movement and wanting to both share these ideas with relatives and find opportunities to bring them into my work as an assistant and trainee psychologist. I qualified as a Clinical Psychologist from Salomons Institute for Applied Psychology in 2021 and completed my DClinPsy thesis alongside Rufus May and Anne Cooke (Clinical Psychologist. Principal Lecturer and Clinical Director, Salomons Institute for Applied Psychology). The thesis is divided into two parts: a scoping review of dialogical approaches for people who hear distressing voices and a qualitative study of people's experiences of the 'Talking with Voices' approach.

29.2 Background

29.2.1 'Voice Hearing as an Understandable Experience': Founding and Growth of the Hearing Voices Movement

The hearing voices movement began in the late 1980s when voice hearers and non-voice hearers (therapists, family members and academics) began to come together and gather research on voice hearing experiences and organise learning events and self-help/peer support groups. What quickly emerged was that understanding the social context within which hearing voices developed was crucial to making the experience more understandable and less frightening. What also came apparent was that an accepting approach to voice hearing made the experience easier to talk about and relate to.

Marius Romme, a Dutch psychiatrist, and Sandra Escher, his co-researcher, were at the forefront of this movement. A key tool that they developed originally as a research questionnaire, and later as an intervention itself, was the Maastricht interview. This interview asked about the characteristics of each voice the person heard and relevant social contexts. For example, what was happening in the person's life prior to each voice's appearance and how difficult life experiences might be linked to themes the voices focused on (Corstens, 2021).

The hearing voices movement was inspired by research into voice hearers who felt comfortable with their voice hearing experiences. These voice hearers had people around them who respected their experiences and frameworks of understanding the experience. They used less distraction strategies and were confident to be assertive and negotiate with their voices. They had a coherent narrative that gave meaning to their voices and that other people around them respected. In contrast voice hearers who struggled with their voices reported being much more isolated with their voices, they tended to rely more on distraction techniques. Furthermore, they could not dialogue with or negotiate constructively with their voices. They had low self-confidence and did not have a narrative that gave meaning to their experiences other than the fairly limited idea that their voices were caused by mental illness.

29.2.2 *The Power of the Relationship*

An important finding of Romme and Escher's original research was the power relationship between the person and the voice (see Table 29.1). The people living well with their voices had a more equal relationship with their voices, like one has with a friend or a respectful colleague; they felt they had choices in this relationship and could assert their needs with the voices. They also felt able to set boundaries when they needed to with the voices they heard. The voice hearers who struggled with their voices had a more unequal relationship with their voices such as the relationship between a child/submissive person and a domineering parent or bully. They did not feel they had choices or could assert or negotiate their needs with the voices.

Another interesting finding was that many of the voice hearers who were living well with their voices had alternative frameworks to a rational world view, for example, spiritual and paranormal understandings and narratives about their voices. Romme and Escher concluded from this that it was important to respect a range of explanatory frameworks if we were to genuinely support voice hearers to become more empowered in their relationships with their voices.

Table 29.1 Differences between people who coped and didn't cope with their voices

People who could cope with voices	People who could not cope with voices
Experienced themselves as stronger	Experienced themselves as weaker
Experienced more positive voices	Experienced more negative voices
Experienced less imperative voices	Experienced more imperative voices
Set more limits to the voices	Did not dare set limits to them
Listened selectively to the voices	Tried to escape from the voices by using more distraction techniques
Communicated more often about their voices	

Romme (1998)

29.2.3 *Accepting and Living with Voices*

The first book Marius Romme and Sandra Escher wrote about their research was called Accepting Voices (1991). In it they proposed that rather than see voices as pathology that needed to be eliminated, voices should be accepted and learned to live with. They were not denying that voice hearing could be an extremely challenging and distressing experience. Rather they suggested the pathology or difficulty lay in the relationship with the voices rather than the voices themselves.

The hearing voices movement grew internationally through conferences and networking events and the development of networks of hearing voices self-help/peer support groups. The belief that if voice hearers could be given the right support and resources they could grow in confidence and change the relationship with their voices. Testimonies emerged supporting this proposition. What also became clear was that social attitudes that were negative and fearful towards voices were a barrier and that these needed to be challenged. The image of Joan of Arc on the cover of Romme and Escher's book Accepting Voices pointed to a time when people (not just voice hearers but the wider community) could be inspired by voices rather than terrified of them. Joan of Arc was a farm girl who guided by voices she saw as saints, became a mascot for the French army, helping them win many battles against the English. In contrast in modern society hearing voices is a taboo experience that is both often associated with moral depravity and mental illness.

The hearing voices movement as it grew in confidence made the argument that hearing voices was just another way to experience consciousness and should not be in itself seen as pathological. At the 2011 hearing voices conference in Italy a Kenyan participant stated: 'When the community panics about voices the voices panic'. An accepting approach to voices is as much about changing community attitudes to voice hearing as supporting individual change.

29.3 Approaches to Hearing Voices to Create Support and Understanding

We would like to present three approaches to hearing voices that aim to help create more social support and understanding in relation to the experience and assist someone to improve the relationship with the voices they hear so they can get on with their lives:

1. Hearing voices peer support groups,
2. Formulating voice hearing guided by the principles of the Maastricht interview, and
3. Talking with voices.

In the second part of this chapter, we will explore how two people have found these approaches based on their contribution to a qualitative research project conducted by the authors of this chapter, Rufus and Kerry.

29.3.1 *Hearing Voices Peer Support Groups*

Hearing voices groups done well create an emancipatory environment where people who hear voices can find greater self-confidence and self-acceptance. In the context of this accepting supportive context voice hearers can become more creative in how they navigate their lives living with voices.

Hearing voices groups are confidential spaces for people who hear voices to come together and share experiences, ideas and strategies that can be helpful to the process of living with voices. I (Rufus) have been involved in a Hearing Voices group in Bradford, Yorkshire since 2003. With recent lockdown policies there has been a growth of online hearing voices groups to enable people to still meet when face to face meetings are not possible.

29.3.1.1 The Values of Hearing Voices Groups

The values of a group are important. For example, the Bradford hearing voices group holds the values that each person has expertise and wisdom about their experiences and the world and that different ways of seeing and understanding experiences and the world are respected.

Value 1: Every Person Has Wisdom and Expertise About Their Experience

The first value that each person has wisdom and expertise about their experience and the world offers a challenge to expert lead approaches. The elevating of subjective knowledge and wisdom is an important and unique feature of the hearing voices approach. This is in contrast with a medical perspective that the subjective perspective is only of value if it is 'insightful' in that it agrees with the dominant viewpoint.

The group is democratically organised in that all decisions about the group, where it meets, how often, who can attend, what the ground rules are, etc., are decided by the group. People who may have been treated in a paternalistic way because they are viewed as 'mentally ill' are in contrast encouraged to take responsibility for decision-making and the running of the group. The group is affiliated to the English Hearing Voices Network and has assisted other groups to be set up in the region.

When we help launch new hearing voices groups, our group will do a presentation. As part of this, group members want to take 10 min each to share experiences of how they live with their voices and how attending a group has been helpful. These testimonies to an audience can be deeply inspiring to both voice hearers and their supporters.

Jack for a number of years believed his voices were his family members talking to him. His family denied this but he was certain that they were lying. It was only once he had been to a hearing voices conference and saw people giving talks about how they lived with their voices he changed his mind. He explained that prior to this conference he had thought that if he believed he heard voices he would just be 'a schizophrenic'. But seeing role models made him realise that one could hear voices and be cool.

Many people in explaining how they find the group empowering highlight the value of realising that they are not alone and that their experience of voice hearing shares much in common with other group member's experiences. By speaking up about their experiences of voice hearing, a new respect for voice hearing is being constructed. This is an example of how hearing voices groups fit a community development approach to voice hearing where the emphasis is on education, networking and confidence building. What we have found in hearing voices groups is that if family members are not supportive of an accepting approach towards voices, the person struggles to change their relationship with their voices. As a consequence, the Bradford group has decided that family members are welcome to attend the group. Family members/partners/friends have then reported how coming to the group has helped them better understand and empathise with the voice hearer. Groups are spaces where different ways to cope with voices are shared including relevant online resources (e.g. www.understandingvoices.com, www.voicecollective.co.uk, www.openmindedonline.com).

Value 2: Respect Different Versions of Reality

The second value that the hearing voices group aims to respect different versions of reality also contrasts with medical approaches to hearing voices which tend to privilege frameworks such as diagnosis and an ensuing language that poses as being objective. Biological psychological, social and spiritual frameworks are all respected. Whilst members will have their preferred frameworks and may seek to influence how others see things we also try to respect different viewpoints and warn against trying to privilege one way of seeing things. I (Rufus), for example, have a bias towards more psychological and dissociative models of voice hearing (for example, see Longden et al., 2012b) but recognise that if I talk about this in a fundamentalist way (that these are the best ways to understand all voice hearing experiences) I will be being oppressive. Thus, hearing voices groups can be seen as open-minded spaces as opposed to an environment where it is assumed there is one best way to see the world. It is likely that this acceptance of plural realities is going to be less alienating for individuals attending. As one hearing voices group member, Felix, a local musician, recently told me (Rufus) 'I hate seeing psychiatrists, they always just tell me I am delusional'. My sense is in the group this member feels valued as an equal citizen with qualities that are valued by others rather than someone who is reduced to clinical descriptions.

29.3.2 Using the Maastricht Approach

The Maastricht approach is to understand the person's voice hearing experience in the context of their life history. This can be done by using the structured questionnaire: The Maastricht interview or a slightly more informal approach that will be outlined later. The Maastricht interview focuses on the following areas (adapted from Corstens, 2021):

1. The nature of the experience, including how the voice communicates with the person.
2. The characteristics of the voices (e.g. how old the voices sound, their gender, how they communicate, associated imagery).
3. Life history up to the onset of the voices and the circumstances at first onset of each voice.
4. What triggers the voices.
5. What the voices say.
6. How a person explains the origin of the voices.
7. What impact the voices have on a person's daily life.
8. The relationship the person has with their voices, from the perspective of the person and their voices.
9. How the person copes with the voices when they are challenging.
10. Questions relating to the person's childhood (emotional neglect, attachment issues, bullying, sexual abuse and so forth).
11. The person's medical history.
12. The person's social network.

Once the interview has been worked through by the voice hearer either by themselves or with a supporter a narrative is written up, which Romme and Escher called the 'construct', to give a meaningful account of the person's voice hearing experience in the context of their social and emotional experiences. This narrative or construct aims to answer two related questions:

1. Who or what do the voices represent? (Do they resemble people you have known or certain attitudes that have affected you?).
2. What underlying social and emotional problems could the voices be related to? (Corstens, 2021).

From answering these two questions we may want to focus on a third question: What might need to change in how you relate to your voices, yourself and people in your life and what resources might support this?

The process of giving meaning to the voices and their relationship with the voice hearer can be done more informally than using the Maastricht Interview for people who are put off by a large questionnaire. In such circumstances I (Rufus) ask voice hearers the following questions.

- How many voices do you hear?
- Do the voices have names?

- For each voice – What gender does it sound like? How old does it sound? What kind of things does it say? When is it more active, does anything seem to trigger the voice?
- How do you feel about yourself in relation to what the voices say?
- When in your life did each voice come along? – What was happening at that time in your life?
- What are important relationships in your life and how could these be related to the voices you hear?
- Have you had significant challenges in your life? (e.g. bereavement, bullying, abuse, displacement, neglect). How do you respond to your voices? (e.g. ignoring, selective listening, negotiating, setting boundaries, reasoning, listening).

Both the Maastricht interview and this more informal questioning allow the voice hearer and their supporter(s) to map out the voice hearing experience in the context of their life and relationship history (Longden et al., 2012a, Shnackenberg et al., 2021).

Jenny, who was 47 years old, heard a voice who called himself the General. She had heard him since she was 11 years old. The voice had always been domineering, telling Jenny she was worthless and urging her to keep quiet and be obedient to him and others and at times self-harm. Jenny had been sexually abused by an uncle from the age of 8 to 14 and had kept this secret until she told a counsellor in her mid-thirties. The age that Mary started hearing her voice (11) was significant as that was when she realised sex with a relative was not normal and began to feel great shame about what had happened and was happening. In some ways the voice related in a similar way to how her uncle had related to her but Jenny felt there were differences too in that the voice could sometimes be quite philosophical. When we looked together at the purpose of the voice, we concluded it probably came along to help her keep quiet about the abuse and suppress her upset feelings. She had had a valid fear that disclosing (about the abuse) would destroy the family; the voice thus protected her from this scenario.

Jenny and her therapist concluded that the challenge for her was to now learn to be compassionate to herself and to learn to set boundaries with her voice and people around her. Over time Jenny learned to see herself in a more compassionate way. She also learned assertiveness skills to let people know what she was feeling and needing. Through dialoguing with the voice she explained to the voice whilst she understood why he had dominated her in the past, she now wanted that relationship to change. Gradually through such negotiations Jenny became less afraid of the General and the voice became more of a companion renaming himself Mr. G.

29.3.3 Talking with Voices

29.3.3.1 Setting Boundaries

As the early hearing voices research has demonstrated (Romme, 1998), many voice hearers who struggle with their voices fear setting boundaries with their voices. Therefore, it is important for voice hearers to improve their confidence and assertiveness skills so they can apply them with their voices.

Assertiveness role plays are recommended to help voice hearers rehearse how they might say no to a voice that is demanding they do a certain action (e.g. self-harm or stay at home or keep quiet, etc.). A number of therapies have been developed that focus on teaching voice hearers assertiveness skills (e.g. Relational therapy, Hayward et al., 2017, and Avatar therapy, Ward et al., 2020). However, we would see assertiveness as just one strand of helping someone change the relationship with their voices rather than the central focus of an approach.

One strategy many people find helpful is to write down the demanding things a voice might say to the person. Once this list is created the voice hearer and supporter can together generate constructive and assertive responses the voice hearer is comfortable stating. Then together they practise in a role play responding to those commands or derogatory comments with assertive and self-affirming statements. These exchanges are repeated many times to help the person get comfortable with a more assertive and self-affirming way of relating. Below are some examples of role plays a supporter might have with a hearer:

Example 1

A supporter role plays a voice saying 'Cut yourself' to the person and the person practises saying assertive and affirming statements like 'Thank you for telling me I am in distress I will find other ways to manage these feelings'.

Example 2

A supporter role plays a voice saying 'Kill yourself' and the person practises responding: 'I have thought long and hard about this and I have decided I want to live' Or simply 'I want to live' (it can help if the person has done some work on this, for example, generating a list of 10 reasons why they want to live).

Example 3

A supporter role plays a voice saying derogatory statements like 'You are worthless'. The person practises self-affirming responses, like 'I respect myself'.

Example 4

A supporter role plays a voice which blaming and frequently, saying things like 'It's all your fault' and the person can practise replying: 'I am compassionate to myself and know I am doing my best'. Or simply 'I am doing my best'.

Being cruel to the voice and trying to bully it in return is not encouraged. However, some people do find swearing can help them be self-protective and assertive (e.g. show me some f**king respect!). This response style therefore needs to be done somewhere where they will not cause offence to others or where the people around them understand the rationale for this approach. I (Rufus) have used boxing pad work or physical wrestling whilst the person is saying affirming statements and I'm saying things the voice might say. This physical approach seems to help someone access their sense of authority. It can also be confidence building for voice hearers to swap roles and say the things their voices say and the supporter plays them responding assertively. This can make the content of what the voices say less frightening, help the person understand the strategy and emotions which the voice is using and help the voice hearer be less afraid of the voice.

29.3.3.2 Using Voice Dialogue with Voices

As was mentioned earlier, Sandra Escher and Marius Romme noticed in their original research that voice hearers who lived well with their voices often had a more dialogical relationship with their voices. So that rather than being talked at or about as if they were not there, they were able to have two-way conversations with their voices and make choices in that relationship. An important strategy for people in the hearing voices movement was to find approaches that could assist voice hearers to change how they relate to their voices.

Origins of the Approach: Voice Dialogue

Voice Dialogue is a self-development approach that was developed by two Jungian psychologists, Sidra and Hal Stone, that has been adapted to work with voice hearers (Lafferty & Allison, 2021). The adapted version has been variously called Talking with voices and Voice Dialogue with voices.

A central premise of Voice Dialogue is that rather than having one personality we all have many subpersonalities or selves. We have strong or primary selves that we have relied on to represent our needs to the world (such as pleaser, the competitive and caring selves) and disowned selves that we have denied and suppressed. The aim is to be more conscious of how different parts of us or selves influence our behaviour so we might make more conscious choices rather than be controlled by one or a group of selves.

Sidra and Hal Stone originally used the approach to better understand dynamics happening in their marriage/relationship with each other. After mapping out parts they observed in themselves and each other, they took it in turns to interview each other' different selves shifting chairs to help them get in tune with the different characters they were exploring. They called the process of interviewing selves facilitating and the person who did this they called the facilitator.

A key attitude in Voice Dialogue is being non-judgemental towards different selves. Acceptance therefore is important and curiosity in trying to understand the meaningful aims and values of the self in question. When a facilitator interviews a self they are encouraged to explore the intentions and motivations of the self rather than trying to change it in some way. It is recognised that change through dialogue may well happen, but this is not something the facilitator should strive to initiate or achieve.

The aim is not get all selves to agree but rather to live with the tension of differing perspectives and for the person to learn to make decisions that take these diverse viewpoints into account (Stone & Stone, 2011).

Adapting Voice Dialogue with Voices

Voice Dialogue with voices is also called 'Talking with Voices' to avoid confusion with Voice Dialogue for parts work. Talking with Voices is a technique that allows a supporter to enter a dialogue with a voice hearer and their voice (Corstens et al., 2012; Longden et al., 2021a, b). In the late nineties people from the hearing voices movement, such as Marius Romme and Dirk Corstens, became more curious how the principles and techniques used in Voice Dialogue could be used to help voice hearers. The approach appeared very compatible with the ethos of the hearing voices movement. For example, the emphasis on acceptance and non-judgemental attitudes and the concept of facilitator which was used in both hearing voices groups and in Voice Dialogue practice. In Voice Dialogue, mapping out of selves is encouraged and this has many commonalities with the formulating mapping out process described earlier used in the Maastricht approach. Below, we outline how Voice Dialogue might typically be carried out with the use of chairs:

Conducting Talking with Voices using chairs

Preparation Work

Firstly, the person wanting to explore their voices will have already done some mapping out work using Maastricht interview style questions. From this they are encouraged to choose a voice they would like to better understand through dialoguing with it.

Prior to talking with the voices it is recommended both facilitator and voice hearer become centred and grounded. This might include some brief physical exercise, mindfulness and or breathing exercises. If the person who hears voices is anxious about the process time can be spent looking at writings and media that describe the philosophy and practice of talking with voices/Voice Dialogue (e.g. Engaging with Voices videos at openmindedonline.com, the animation Compassion for Voices on YouTube, Corstens, May & Longden's online Talking with Voices article).

It is important for the facilitator to have a positive attitude towards both the voice hearer and the voice who is being dialogued with. So we need to be compassionate to how the voice hearer feels and also mindful of the feelings of the voice. Many voices will expect facilitators to be wanting to get rid of them. So countering this with a clear message that the aim of the work is to help the person improve their relationship with their voice not get rid of them is important.

In preparation for the dialogue, the facilitator can ask the voice hearer if there are any questions or subjects that they would like the facilitator to explore with the voice.

When Not to Talk with a Voice

We only go ahead with a dialoguing session if the voice is agreeable to being conversed with. If the voice chooses not to want to try the process, we respect that.

We could then do some more work on introducing the person to an accepting approach to voices with the hope the voice would pick up on this non-aggressive approach. Or we can ask if there are any other voices who would like to try the dialoguing process.

Facilitation of a Voice

Classically we ask the person to sit in a different chair to relate what the voice is saying. However, if the person feels more comfortable not moving this is respected. We also collectively need to make a decision whether to use direct or indirect questioning. Direct questioning is where the facilitator asks a question directly to the voice and the person says verbatim what the voice is saying. For example, 'How long have you been in Michael's life?' Michael then repeats what he hears his voice saying: 'I came along when he was fifteen'. Indirect questioning is where the facilitator asks the person to ask their voice the question, e.g. 'Can you ask your voice how long he has been in your life? And the person then responds indirectly, e.g. 'He is saying he first came along when I was fifteen'. Some people prefer the greater level of control they feel using the indirect approach, others find it easier and less tiring to use the direct approach.

Dissociation

Sometimes when people act as a spokesperson for their voice, they can dissociate and lose awareness of what is happening. It is important to discuss this possibility with the person and how they would like such a scenario to be managed. This to some degree happens in general Voice Dialogue and is one of the reasons for using chairs and always returning to the original chair to debrief after a dialogue with a voice has taken place. It is important for the facilitator to write down everything that is said by the voice and when the person comes back to their original chair, they are then informed of everything has been expressed. Some people are comfortable with losing awareness and being debriefed afterwards. For others this does not feel a safe enough process. I (Rufus) tend to check in regularly with the person about whether they are still aware and present during the dialoguing process. If there is evidence, they are not (and the person has made it clear they are uncomfortable with this) I will bring them back to their original chair and encourage them to become re-oriented to their surroundings.

Creative Approaches to Dialoguing

We can be creative with the process of trying to establish a dialogue between a facilitator and the voice of the person who is hearing it. If speaking out loud what the voices are saying is too anxiety provoking, we can conduct the session using writing. The facilitator can write questions to the voice and the person hearing the voice can write back what the voice is saying. Some people prefer doing dialoguing whilst going for a walk in a quiet area with their supporter. Some people have found it useful to make finger puppets of their voices or decorate spoons to assist the dialoguing process (May & Svanholmer, 2021).

Questions to Ask the Voices in a Dialogue Session

It is important to start the conversation in a warm and welcoming fashion and to finish the conversation thanking the voice. By relating to a voice in a respectful way that is honouring of their presence in the person's life we are modelling a way of interacting that the person and their voice can learn from. Sometimes I (Rufus) might ask the voice if it wants to know more about me and my values before it engages in a conversation with me. The facilitator asking that voice questions about its relationship to the person its needs and aims.

Examples of questions:

Hello how are you?	How long have you been in ….'s life?
What do you see as your job?	What made you come along and start speaking to …. at that time?
What are you trying to achieve for …….?	What do you like about ……?
Do you have any advice for ……..?	Do you have any advice for……?
What would ….'s life be like if you were not there?	Is there anything …. could do to help you feel more relaxed?

The facilitator is encouraged to pay attention to physiological, emotional and verbal information during the dialoguing process. If the facilitator senses the conversations becoming too tense it can be useful to check out with person if they want to continue the dialogue.

Debriefing

When the interview is completed, the person returns to their original chair and reflects with the facilitator on what has been learned. As in general Voice Dialogue this 'Talking with voices' debrief is a crucial process where the person gets an opportunity to reflect on and process any new information that has been gleaned from the dialogue. For example, often voices that are domineering and critical when interviewed in a curious and respectful way will disclose that they are trying to protect the person from danger. When a voice hearer learns that it can help them re-orient themselves to a more accepting attitude towards the voice, the process can also help the person who hears voices develop some ideas about the purpose of the voice and continue to build their understanding of this, which in turn can make the experience less intimidating.

The aim of facilitating a dialogue with a voice is also that the person gets confidence to start to relate to their voice differently themselves. Some members of the hearing voices group I volunteer with have chosen to have one or two dialoguing with voices sessions with myself. I then encourage them to carry on dialoguing with their voices and feeding back to the group how the process is going. There is a danger that if the person is not encouraged to dialogue with their voice themselves, they can become reliant on an external person to talk with their voices and dependent upon them for insights about the motivations of the voices they hear.

Table 29.2 Feelings and needs list

Feelings when needs are met

Happy	Amused	Excited	Interested
Encouraged	Confident	Playful	Moved
Relieved	Curious	Compassionate	Trusting
Secure	Relaxed	Joyful	Adventurous
Amazed	Alert	Inspired	Energised
Grateful	Friendly	Hopeful	Alive
			Peaceful

Feelings when needs are not met

Needs

Safety	Peace	Empathy/love	Creativity/play	Autonomy	Contribution	Community
Protection from harm	Acceptance	Consideration	Joy	Power	Meaning	Support
Emotional Safety	Awareness	Understanding	Fun	Integrity	Purpose	Belonging
Predictability	Balance	Presence	Spontaneity	Honesty	Learning	Trust
Confidence	Simplicity	Respect	Openness	Choice	Participation	Mutuality
Relaxation	Harmony	To be seen and heard	Humour	Continuity	Competence	Co-operation
Trust	Recreation	Acknowledgement	Passion	Authenticity		Inclusion
Honesty	Space	Communication	Movement	Creativity		Shared values and understandings
Transparency	Appreciation	Clarity	Exercise	Meaning		
	Responsibility	Love		Self-worth		
	Contribution	Sexual expression				
	Emotional safety	Intimacy				

Over the last 10 years the Bradford group has become more and more interested in more friendly approaches to voices. We have often found that compromising with different voices' needs and desires has led to the voices being less controlling in their relationship with the voice hearer. For example, if voices are supported to listen to music or other media (e.g. films, cartoons, reading) at times during the week, they often become more amenable and friendly towards the voice hearer (May & Svanholmer, 2021).

However, if these efforts are only done half-heartedly and the person secretly harbours a wish to get rid of their voices, the voices will pick up on this and be less cooperative. It can be invaluable for the person who hears voices to reassess their intentions and commit to living more harmoniously with the voices. Some people have found this or an adapted version of this affirmation helpful to recite daily to help them convey to their voices a more accepting and collaborative attitude:

> We are in this together. I will try to respect you and in return I would like you to try to respect me. I don't want to get rid of you, I want us to find ways to live together with mutual respect. I know when you are threatening to me you are feeling frightened, and I want to find ways to help you feel safer. I want to live a life that I choose but I also want to spend time each day listening to you and trying to find things to do that we both enjoy. I will try to keep you informed about my plans each day so that you feel more confident and aware of what is happening.

I (Rufus) with my partner Elisabeth have developed a self-help guide for voice hearers looking at how to talk with their voices (May & Svanholmer, 2019a, b). This aims to assist voice hearers with ideas of how to creatively dialogue with their voices.

Using Non-violent Communication with Voices

Non-violent communication (Rosenberg, 2015) is an approach to communication and awareness that enables people to give themselves empathy and better understand judgmental communication. We have found it a useful strategy to support the process of talking with voices (May & Svanholmer, 2021). A 'feelings and needs inventory' is a simple tool voice hearers can use to both understand their own and the voices' feelings and needs (see Table 29.2, for example). Voices people struggle with tend to use quite judgmental language. We can use the inventory to give the voice a chance to say what it feels and needs and thereby communicate less aggressively. We can show the voice a list of feelings and needs and ask it to choose words that describe how it is feeling and what it is needing. This is a simple way for voice hearers to regularly check in with their voices or explore the deeper feelings and needs (that may lie beneath the surface communication) with them. Using the inventory regularly can help teach voices new ways to communicate that might be more constructive for both the person and their voice(s).

29.4 Voice Dialogue with Voices: Voice Hearer Perspectives

This section provides first-hand accounts of Voice Dialogue with voices by Angela* and Dan*.

29.4.1 Angela

29.4.1.1 A Bit About Me and Voices

Voices became a part of my life in 2012 following a traumatic incident. The following morning, I got up and I had this ringing in my ears. It subsided for a couple of weeks and then a couple of months later it came again. It developed into whispering and eventually voices.

When this first happened, I didn't know what was going on. I was scared 24/7 as the voices were frightening and often critical of what I did or said. I came to believe things like I had a chip in my head and the police were talking to me. So, for example, if I then went outside and saw a police car, I was convinced that they were following me.

When I first started hearing the voices, I used to write a lot of what they said down to try and understand what they were saying. I thought that getting them out of my head onto paper would help but it didn't. Otherwise, I would try to ignore them, but this didn't work either. In fact, it made them worse. So I would just live in fear and you know what it's like when you're living in fear. You struggle to see how things could be better. It was really hard to see beyond that.

Around 12 months after the incident, I remember just getting up one morning and saying to my daughter that I think I needed to go to the doctor because I wasn't coping. My doctor then referred me to a psychiatrist who I saw regularly for the next few months.

29.4.1.2 What Led You to Voice Dialoguing?

I first found out about the idea of talking with voices via a hearing voices network (HVN) group. It took me 6 months to pluck up the courage to go because my voices didn't like the idea at first. When I did go along, I remember somebody in this group mentioned that they had names for their voices because it helps them communicate with them. Initially, I wasn't sure how I felt about this, but I just listened to people's stories. I admired their ability to talk about these things openly. They just seemed to cope better with the voices than I did at the time.

The group members said it would be a really good idea to name my voices so that they become like people, rather than just viewing them as something I needed to ignore or try to get rid of. The group members introduced me to different ways to talk with my voices by speaking about what they had found helpful. After these conversations, I then thought I would give it a try.

My confidence grew overtime as I talked with my voices. It took a few years until I felt comfortable talking with my voices and listening to them. The opportunity then arose to start more structured dialoguing sessions with a facilitator. I decided to give this a try, but I did this once I had become comfortable with talking with them myself first.

29.4.1.3 First Impressions

I have to be honest and say that talking with voices in general didn't appeal to me at first. I remember feeling quite embarrassed about even naming my voices in the beginning. I just hoped that they would stop.

On the same day the group members recommended I named my voices, I went home and asked one of my voices whether they liked the name 'Kojak'. I found a time when it was quiet and sat down with a cup of tea and just said 'how do you like the name "Kojak?"'. He said, 'I love it, I really like it' and that was the first positive conversation I had with him. After this experience, and because I then knew that it could be easier to talk with him, I would sit and talk to him all the time after that. Not that this always made my voices quieter. They were just easier to talk with. Talking with my voices connects me to them and they feel like they're being listened to.

29.4.1.4 Trying Out Dialogue Sessions with a Facilitator

Although I had already had a lot of experience of talking with my voices prior to trying out facilitated dialoguing, there are a few changes I think that having some structured sessions with a facilitator helped with.

I would say that this process helped me understand the motives of my voices. I spent time trying to make sense of why my voices could still be quite critical of me, tell me to harm myself, or say things like I would be better off dead. My facilitator worked with me and my voices to try and understand the reasons behind why they had often been so critical. It was from this dialogue that I came to learn that they were often trying to protect me. Telling me things like I was better off dead, for example, was coming from a voice who had witnessed trauma themselves and was a wish for me to be away from trouble in the world.

It helped me think more about my voices having needs which I could ask about and cater for. I will now put some time aside in the day for my voices to ask me about these things. I might then do things such as putting on a particular TV programme, listening to music or cooking something which they like.

29.4.1.5 Was There Anything You Found Challenging or Unhelpful About Facilitated Voice Dialoguing?

Yeah, it's very tiring. It tires you out. Because you're having to really concentrate on what the voices are saying. Having to try and balance their needs with my own can also be hard as we can't always agree!

29.4.2 Dan

29.4.2.1 A Bit About Me and Voices

I first started hearing voices about 20 years ago when I was in my early twenties. They were pretty infrequent and unintrusive then, and although I worried about it, I just managed to put it out of my mind and get on with my life. It wasn't until 20 years later when things got a lot worse that I was then forced to take notice of it. At this time in my life, I was living abroad and had just been through a difficult break up. I noticed immediately that there seemed to be more voices and what was also strange is that they seemed to be speaking from different perspectives. It was bewildering and frightening at the time. I had no idea what was happening to me, but I knew I needed to do something about it.

29.4.2.2 What Led You to Voice Dialoguing?

I started by doing some research online about voice hearing to try to figure out what the hell was going on with me. It was then that I came across Marius Romme's work and bought a book titled 'Living with Voices: 50 stories of recovery' which Romme had co-authored. From here I got the idea that hearing voices is a complex reaction to something, usually trauma. I wanted to understand my voices more and I would do various things like setting time aside to listen to my voices and note down what they said to try and make sense of it. That was the informal beginning if you like.

I tried to get help from psychiatric services, but my experience of these services was that they were no help at all. Over a few years, I had seen a number of psychiatrists who diagnosed me with different things, everything from depression to schizophrenia. In these instances, I never seemed to receive anything helpful in terms of understanding. It often felt that I was put on one trial of antipsychotic or antidepressant after another. Any meaningful help seemed hard to find and this made me feel angry and in despair at times.

So, I ultimately turned away from services and tried to search for help elsewhere. It was from here that I found out about a hearing voices group, and I was also very fortunate to have a friend who I confided in. Both the group and my friend introduced me to Voice Dialogue ideas. It was my friend who helped me get started with talking with my voices. Well, she actually talked to one of my voices before I did. I knew this friend and trusted her completely. I think it was quite a rare thing to find somebody who knew what to say and how to say it. This was largely possible due to the fact that she had read some very good professional literature on trauma, dissociation, voice hearing and Voice Dialogue with voices. So, her interaction with my voice was informed by that. I then tried out sessions with another person trained in Voice Dialogue with voices around 2 years later.

29.4.2.3 First Impressions

I didn't realise that what I was experiencing was of a kind that I could establish a dialogical relationship with my voices. Initially, it was one way. I would just sit down; they would say things to me and I listened. When I started to establish a dialogue with them, I found this fairly astonishing.

29.4.2.4 Trying Out Dialogue Sessions with a Facilitator

There were parts of me that I didn't even know about until I started doing the dialoguing. I was completely cut off from them and the dialoguing helped me to get in contact with that. Before, I was aware of these intrusive type experiences, but I couldn't make sense of them. It is hard to describe it was an intrusive feeling if you like. It's perhaps easier to describe it metaphorically. It was like a torrent of water pushing on a dam and threatening to break through, and these feelings were really debilitating. Through dialoguing, I found out that the voices were related to this force. That these experiences were to do with dissociative parts of me. Dialoguing with my voices brought this to my conscious awareness.

Once I began to be aware of these things, dialoguing helped me find ways to meaningfully engage with my voices, which led to some profound changes for me. To give an example, my main voice at the start of dialoguing was a voice who represented an abusive adult figure. The voice would say not very nice things to me and it was very critical and blaming of everything I did. At first, I didn't really know how to engage with that voice. All I'd really been doing up until that point was writing some stuff down, but mainly trying to ignore it and distract myself. When my friend started to dialogue with this voice, it became clear that this voice, which I viewed to be a part of me, turned out to be a defensive part that was defending a younger part inside by imitating somebody who had hurt me in childhood. What we found was that the more my friend expressed an understanding for the part which was doing a defensive job and the more I developed a proper relationship with it, the more this part slowly dropped its mask of the perpetrator and became more ordinarily protective. Later in the dialogue, this then seemed to allow another part of me to emerge which was a voice of a very young child. So later dialogue work became about supporting the persecutory part to be protective in a way that allowed me to develop a relationship with this child part. It was really quite profound. So, I essentially went from experiencing something quite threatening and persecutory, to gaining a good mother part of me and a child who I could nurture and support to grow up.

29.4.2.5 Was There Anything You Found Challenging or Unhelpful About Facilitated Voice Dialoguing?

I would certainly say that dialoguing with voices can be very intense and so you need to have a stable base before considering starting it. In other words, you can't do it if you're in survival mode. My recovery has very much been two steps forward and one step back and there were certainly moments where I wasn't in a good place to be able to engage with my voices in a meaningful way. During these times, I just had to focus on getting myself stable in a very basic sense, for example, getting some sort of income, having a place to live and trying to build in some social structure in my life. I spent a couple of years just doing that. I think this probably then enabled me to get more out of the dialoguing when I did feel ready to do it too.

29.4.3 Reflections on Angela and Dan's Stories of Learning to Relate Differently to Voices

The interviews with Angela and Dan demonstrate how individual each persons route is when they are able to change their relationship with their voices. At the time of writing they themselves are helping other voice hearers as hearing voices group facilitators. We hope that Angela and Dan's account of changing the relationship with their voices bring alive how important it is we co-create a listening community for the voice hearer and their voices. Peer support features strongly for both Angela and Dan had a friend and a therapist facilitate dialogue with his voices at different times and Angela had two sessions from the facilitator of the hearing voices group she was attending and carried on the dialoguing herself with support from the hearing voices group. This demonstrates the importance not only of individual therapy work but also how as therapists we can be strong allies to hearing voices groups, voice hearers' families, and friends to really grow the 'accepting voices' approach.

29.5 Conclusion

In this chapter we have outlined some key components of the hearing voices approach that started in Holland in the 1980s and since now has networks in many countries around the world. The key elements we have focused on are hearing voices groups, the Maastricht approach and the use of Voice Dialogue with voices. Hearing voices groups when set up democratically help to build supportive environments for people who hear voices and help them to gain confidence in their ability to navigate their experiences in the social world. The Maastricht approach, whether administered formally or informally, supports people to understand their voices in the context of their social and cultural lives. Voice Dialogue with voices enables supporters to assist voice hearers to better understand and negotiate with the voices they hear. We think these three approaches help creatively support voice hearers to become empowered in their relationship with their voices. Not to have power over their voices and to dominate them into submission but rather to learn to live with them, to listen selectively and be able to set boundaries and dialogue with them. Both Angela and Dan's stories show how accepting friendships and support networks helped them. And once there was more stability in their lives, dialoguing with a facilitator and by themselves, helped them change the relationship with their voices in a meaningful way. If both therapists and the community can be educated in these approaches, we can respond with curiosity and a desire to understand them in the context of the person's social and relational history.

References

Corstens, D. (2021). The Maastricht Approach: social and personal perspectives on hearing voices. In I. Parker, J. Schnackenberg, & M. Hopfenbeck (Eds.), *The practical handbook of hearing voices: Therapeutic and creative approaches* (pp. 13–23). PCCS books.

Corstens, D., May, R., & Longden, E. (2012). Talking with voices. In M. Romme & S. Escher (Eds.), *Psychosis as a personal crisis: An experience based approach* (pp. 166–178). Routledge.

Hayward, M., Jones, A., Bogen-Johnston, L., Thomas, N., & Strauss, C. (2017). Relating therapy for distressing auditory hallucinations: A pilot randomized controlled trial. *Schizophrenia Research, 183*, 137–142. https://doi.org/10.1016/j.schres.2016.11.019

Lafferty, R., & Allison, R. (2021). Voice Dialogue. In I. Parker, J. Schnackenberg, & M. Hopfenbeck (Eds.), *The practical handbook of hearing voices: Therapeutic and creative approaches* (pp. 194–202). PCCS Books.

Longden, E., Corstens, D., Escher, S., & Romme, M. (2012a). Voice hearing in a biographical context: A model for formulating the relationship between voices and life history. *Psychosis, 4*(3), 224–234. https://doi.org/10.1080/17522439.2011.596566

Longden, E., Corstens, D., Morrison, A. P., Larkin, A., Murphy, E., Holden, N., et al. (2021a). A treatment protocol to guide the delivery of dialogical engagement with auditory hallucinations: Experience from the talking with voices pilot trial. *Psychology and Psychotherapy: Theory, Research and Practice*. https://doi.org/10.1111/papt.12331

Longden, E., Corstens, D., Pyle, M., Emsley, R., Peters, S., Chauhan, N., et al. (2021b). Engaging dialogically with auditory hallucinations: Design, rationale and baseline sample characteristics of the talking with voices pilot trial. *Psychosis, 1–12*. https://doi.org/10.1080/17522439.2021.1884740

Longden, E., Madill, A., & Waterman, M. G. (2012b). Dissociation, trauma, and the role of lived experience: Toward a new conceptualization of voice hearing. *Psychological Bulletin, 138*(1), 28. https://doi.org/10.1037/a0025995

May, R., & Svanholmer, E. (2019a). Retrieved from Guía de autoayuda para hablar con las voces. Ideas para personas que oyen voces y quieren dialogar con ellas; de Rufus May y Elisabeth Svanholmer https://primeravocal.org/guia-de-autoayuda-para-hablar-con-las-voces-ideas-para-personas-que-oyen-voces-y-quieren-dialogar-con-ellas-de-rufus-may-y-elisabeth-svanholmer (Spanish version).

May, R., & Svanholmer, E. (2019b). Retrieved from https://openmindedonline.files.wordpress.com/2019/09/self-help-guide-to-talking-with-voices-r.-may-and-e.-svanholmer-sep-2019.pdf

May, R., & Svanholmer, E. (2021). Creative ways to engage with voices. In I. Parker, J. Schnackenberg, & M. Hopfenbeck (Eds.), *The practical handbook of hearing voices: Therapeutic and creative approaches* (pp. 194–202). PCCS Books.

Romme, M. (1998). *Understanding voices: Coping with auditory hallucinations and confusing realities*. Handsell Press.

Rosenberg, M. (2015). *Nonviolent communication: A language of life*. Puddledancer Press.

Shnackenberg, J. K., Lusco, O., & Debesay, S. (2021). Experience focussed Counselling (Making sense of voices). In I. Parker, J. Schnackenberg, & M. Hopfenbeck (Eds.), *The practical handbook of hearing voices: Therapeutic and creative approaches* (pp. 180–193). PCCS Books.

Stone, H., & Stone, S. (2011). *Embracing ourselves: The voice dialogue manual*. New World Library.

Ward, T., Rus-Calafell, M., Ramadhan, Z., Soumelidou, O., Fornels-Ambrojo, M., Garet, P., & Craig, T. K. (2020). AVATAR therapy for distressing voices: A comprehensive account of therapeutic targets. *Schizophrenia Bulletin, 46*, 1038–1044. https://doi.org/10.1093/schbul/sbaa061

Further Reading and Resources

Compassion for Voices film. https://www.youtube.com/watch?v=VRqI4lxuXAw&t=1s

Engaging with Voices film series. https://openmindedonline.com/portfolio/engaging-with-voices-videos/

Talking with voices online paper. https://rufusmay.com/2011/01/26/talking-with-voices/ [object HTMLSpanElement]

Chapter 30
Psychological Intervention with Relatives of Patients with Psychotic Disorders

Gloria Roldán-Maldonado, Gloria María Bonilla-Roldán, and Rosalia Guardia-García

'I never thought that at my age I could learn and change so much. Just thank you for this unique space.' (Family)

Since 1989, psychotherapy groups have been conducted with patients diagnosed with Psychosis, first in the Community Health Team and, subsequently, in the Mental Health Day Hospital of the Virgen de las Nieves University Hospital, Granada, Spain. They are integrative interventions oriented to the needs of the person in his or her context.

A *permanent psychotherapeutic group space* was created. The methodology integrates competency training models (social skills, problem solving, emotional regulation, coping strategies, etc.) with acceptance and commitment therapy (ACT) and Mindfulness (compassion and self-compassion). The aim is to achieve the recovery or the acquisition of cognitive and behavioural repertoires that allow them to act in the direction of their personal values, following their existential goals, as well as to break with behavioural paralysis (experiential avoidance). Working with metaphors, experiential exercises, creative despair, distancing and deliteralization, together with training in skills aimed at achieving valuable existential goals, proved to be a very powerful psychotherapeutic tool. Disorders of thought and perception (delusions, hallucinations, etc.) ceased to be an insurmountable obstacle and became companions on the journey.

At the same time, there was a growing need to work with the family. Relatives and patients made the demand explicit and verbalized, in the groups, how important

G. Roldán-Maldonado (✉)
Hospital Universitario Virgen de las Nieves, Servicio Andaluz de Salud (SAS), Granada, Spain

G. M. Bonilla-Roldán
Málaga, Spain

R. Guardia-García
Granada, Spain

J. A. Díaz-Garrido et al. (eds.), *Psychological Interventions for Psychosis*,
https://doi.org/10.1007/978-3-031-27003-1_30

it would be for their families to have experiences of this type. This gave rise to the research '*Evaluación e Intervención Psicológica sobre los problemas emocionales de los familiares de pacientes con Trastornos Mentales Graves*' ('*Evaluation and Psychological Intervention on the emotional problems of relatives of patients with Severe Mental Disorders*'), *a* project funded by the Consejería de Salud de la Junta de Andalucía SAS111215. The results obtained in the different studies are presented in this chapter. The needs of the families were detected and the effectiveness of the intervention programme was demonstrated. It has been created a permanent space for group psychotherapeutic intervention with relatives.

30.1 Introduction

Psychotic disorders are considered Severe Mental Disorders (SMDs) and are considered to be clinical problems that are persistent throughout life, or that, being transitory or episodic, cause a significant degree of disability and dependence that affect the individual, his or her family and social environment.

It is common to observe in patients attending the Mental Health Day Hospital (HSDM) that, when they have been diagnosed very young and have followed only treatments aimed at symptom management for years, they settle into experiential avoidance and isolation predominates and they only relate with health institutions. As they experience improvement and get out of the disease model, they become aware of their deficits and difficulties for interpersonal relationships and claim, themselves, to be provided with tools to be able to join the different social spaces involved in resuming their lives (Roldán et al., 2017). For this reason, the HSDM maintains a permanent training group in Daily Life Skills (Social Skills, Identification, Emotional Regulation and Expression, Contextual Therapies): ACT and Mindfulness).

The role that families play in providing support is undeniable. Preliminary results of an international survey, conducted by EUFAMI (European Federation of Associations of Families of People with Mental Illness, 2014), point to the fact that 72% of caregivers of people with psychotic disorders are primarily or solely responsible for caring for them, with the consequent emotional and physical burden that this entails. In addition, the international scientific community states that between 2.5% and 3% of the adult population presents an SMD (Porcar et al., 2015) and, specifically in Spain, in one out of every four families, there is at least one person with some mental disorder, revealing that the numbers seem to be increasing. According to Desviat (2000), the provision of health care in Spain by informal caregivers (family) accounts for 88% of total care.

Therefore, it is inevitable that psychotic disorders do not only affect those who suffer from them but also those who are responsible for their long-term care (Guardia, 2010). This responsibility often falls on the closest relatives, whether parents, spouses or siblings, generally women. To assume the role of caregiver, the relative has to reorganize his or her life according to the new needs of the patient and, in some cases, set their personal needs or desires aside.

Naturally, taking care of a person with a psychotic disorder is not a simple task as it involves time, effort, economic investment and emotional wear (Tartaglini et al., 2011). For caregivers, this can have repercussions on subjective well-being, interpersonal relationships, leisure time, routine, work and other activities. In most extreme cases, these concerns could lead to a sense of overload (Hidalgo, 2013). The scientific literature affirms that family caregivers present high levels of "psychological distress", that is, they experience a wide variety of overwhelming feelings and emotions (apathy, grief, anger, anguish, sorrow, hopelessness and guilt) (Magaña et al., 2007), as well as mood disorders (mostly depressive and anxiety) (Steele et al., 2010). For example, it has been found that caregivers of patients with bipolar disorder and schizophrenia suffer mostly from depressive and anxiety disorders (Rascón et al., 2010).

Likewise, Wittmann and Keshavan (2007) propose that it's common to observe a grieving process after the diagnosis of psychosis, which is a fundamental experience that both the patient and the family have to cope with. This grieving is complex because the 'lost' person has not disappeared; he or she has rather changed and with that all the expectations which were placed on him or her. Loss has been described by some authors as non-finite, psychic, ambiguous and intangible, but real and painful (López de Arróyabe & Calvete, 2005). Research suggests that these symptoms of loss and grief include intrusive thoughts and emotions, avoidance, preoccupation with their relatives' mental illness and difficulties accepting their circumstances (Godress et al., 2005). Escalante and Gavlovski (2011) agree that, over time, a notion of permanent suffering seems to be constructed, as it becomes chronic over time and arise from perceiving the relative as a person who has a mental illness that will not disappear quickly. This pain is related to the feeling of guilt.

In addition, relatives often present health problems, social isolation, economic problems, social problems (stigma or social rejection, Stengler-Wenzke et al., 2004), a decrease in their performance in other vital areas (work or study), a significant loss of socio-labour opportunities, a lack of interest in leisure and, in general, in everything that once attracted them. Unfortunately, these conditions, in the form of a vicious circle, bring in return other types of aversive consequences, such as loss of employment, decrease in income, abandonment of social life or a professional or personal project (getting married, having one's own family), thus increasing vulnerability to psychological problems (Scheirs, 2007). Thomen (2020) confirms this affirmation and states in his research that when there is a relative with psychotic disorder, they present a less favourable family functioning.

Taking into account the gender perspective, mothers, more than fathers, report a greater number of problems and needs related to a higher level of stress and the burden of their children's mental illness (Wancata et al., 2008), and this makes them a group that requires significant therapeutic support to cope with the situation.

Up to date, most of the programmes conducted with relatives of patients with psychotic disorders are focused on positively influencing evolution. Most of these types of interventions or programmes are psychoeducational in nature and the most effective have been those that have included cognitive behavioural strategies, such as assertiveness training, problem solving and communication (Girón et al., 2010; Gutiérrez-Maldonado & Caqueo-Urízar, 2007; Society of Clinical Psychology, APA, 2010). This represents an important advance in the care and assistance that can be provided to relatives and, according to Vallina and Lemos (2003), has been shown to have a positive influence on the patient's clinical variables (e.g. reduction of clinical symptoms, relapses and hospitalizations).

From our perspective, it is necessary to create spaces for direct attention to the needs of relatives, since our experience shows that they present emotional disorders that require psychotherapeutic interventions. Among the most important issues to be considered within the intervention proposals are alterations in mood; the appearance of emotions such as guilt and shame; and the management of uncertainty, anxiety, stress levels and coping strategies in general. It is also worth mentioning the components that support the patient's recovery and improve the family's level of control over the disease situation (Babacan, 2008), which is why it is necessary to work on disease education, communication training and problem solving training. Likewise, it is important to accommodate the most appropriate management of problems related to living with a relative with a SMD, including high emotion expressed (emotional over-involvement); criticism and hostility; social problems (e.g. stigma, isolation); occupational problems (e.g. sick leave, job loss, etc.); economic problems; distribution of household chores and management of their leisure time.

In this line, one of the main challenges we face in the care of HDSM users is the assistance with the psychological needs of relatives of patients with SMD. Although psychoeducational programmes are being offered nowadays, they are not enough to cover their own emotional problems.

As we have demonstrated in our clinical experience, it is common to find problems of anxiety, depression or stress among relatives of patients who are being treated there. They report serious problems in their relationships, do not know how to deal with them and present communication problems, which generates a tense family environment. It is common, after receiving their relative's diagnosis, that they abandon important areas of their lives and focus on caregiving. Most of them settle in a great experiential avoidance and remain stuck to pain, to the past and to the anguish-laden anticipation of the future by predicting negative evolutions and considering that their lives are broken with any possibility of recovery. They stop living in the present and the feelings of guilt make them abandon spaces for fun, culture, leisure and relationships with friends and other relatives, which are significantly reduced. This means that, on many occasions, they deal alone with their pain, and distance themselves from their partners, which facilitates the appearance of emotional disorders (Roldán et al., 2015).

Therefore, the aim of offering the patients' relatives a psychological intervention programme with cognitive-behavioural and third generation therapies (ACT and Mindfulness) is to achieve the recovery or acquisition of cognitive and behavioural repertoires that allow them to act in the direction of their personal values, following their existential goals and breaking with behavioural paralysis (experiential avoidance), thus increasing their psychological flexibility.

To this effect, and confirming the previous statement, in the pioneering study we conducted (Roldán et al., 2015) we detected the presence of emotional and health problems in relatives and we demonstrated the effectiveness of a group intervention programme, based on acceptance and communication training in order to reduce them. On the other hand, Bonilla (2018) in his study evaluates the presence of depression, anxiety, stress and grief in 32 relatives, as well as the level of interference of the diagnosis in their lives and the level of experiencing ambiguous and difficult emotions. The results of this study confirm that relatives present emotional disorders and grief reactions after the diagnosis. There is a fusion between beliefs and fears about what it is considered to be a 'serious chronic' mental illness and the behaviours become coherent with thoughts and emotions, installing the experiential avoidance 'stop doing what goes in the direction of my life project…, it is not possible because of the disease'. As the important and valuable areas of life are abandoned, distress, discomfort, avoidance, suffering and pain increase. This is reinforced by the prevailing power, institutions and society, established knowledge and context.

The family is a victim of these beliefs, unaware of other models and acts without being aware of it, reinforcing the experiential avoidance that ends up becoming a rigid, destructive pattern. In this way, they become isolated and the relationships become strained and emotions of helplessness and hopelessness increase. In most of the cases depressive sadness and anger reveal, a great discouragement similar to a dysfunctional chronic pathological grief.

After observing so much pain, *a radical paradigm shift in the care of people diagnosed with psychosis and their families is urgently needed.*

30.2 Research and Needs Detected in Relatives of Patients with Psychotic Disorders

The theoretical-scientific review presented above empirically justifies the importance of developing and implementing programmes to meet the needs of relatives of patients with psychotic disorders, given the positive impact it has during the course of the disease. However, scientific research and clinical practice have revealed important psychological needs in these relatives, which further support the obligation to be considered the target of attention within the psychotherapeutic process.

30.2.1 Sociodemographic and Clinical Profile of Patients with Severe Mental Disorders

The sociodemographic and clinical profile of 116 caregivers of 80 patients with a Severe Mental Disorder (SMD) treated at the Mental Health Units of the Hospital Universitario Virgen de las Nieves (Granada, Spain) was studied.

The diagnosis distribution of Severe Mental Disorder (SMD) (according to ICD-10) was: 53.75% with schizophrenia, schizotypal disorder and delusional disorders, 18.75% with personality disorders, 16.25% with bipolar disorder and 11.25% still unspecified. Patients were between 19 and 79 years old (M = 54.96; SD = 12.67) 54.96; SD = 12.67), most of them were old (55.2% between 51 and 65 years old and 17.2% were 66 years old or older). Women predominated (69.8%), married/partnered (70.7%), completed their compulsory education degree (68.1%) and had an employment (39.7%) or were housewives (26.7%). Caregiving work was distributed mainly between only the mother (27.5%), both parents (25%), the partner (20%) and both parents and a sibling (8.8%). As for the number of caregivers, 56.3% of the time there was only one caregiver. 45.7% have not received any therapeutic help related to the relative's SMD, some of whom have attended psychoeducation (23.3%) and support groups (14.7%). 52.6% have symptoms of depression, 51.7% have symptoms of anxiety and 47.4% have an average level of health.

These data lead to think about the *vulnerability of caregivers,* due to the scarcity of relatives who perform this work, to the fact *that* it is performed by older adults (most of the time, mothers), who are currently *psychologically and physically affected and who have received very little help related to their role as caregivers.*

30.2.2 Coping Strategies and Self-Rated Health in Caregivers of Patients with Severe Mental Disorder

The aim of this chapter is to examine the relationship between coping strategies and perceived health by 118 caregivers of people with SMD. Of all those evaluated, 70.3% were women and the average age was of 55.1 years (SD = 12.6). The patients (n = 82) had a psychotic disorder (64.6%), personality disorder (33.0%), bipolar disorder (1.2%) or a SMD not yet specified (11.1%) and were being treated at the Mental Health Units of the Virgen de las Nieves University Hospital of Granada (Spain).

It was detected that the most commonly used coping strategies were desiderative thinking, social isolation and problem solving and the least used were cognitive restructuring, self-criticism and emotional expression.

By analysing the relationships with the health dimensions evaluated with the SF-36 Spanish questionnaire, it was observed that those who had *less social isolation* played a *better physical role, emotional role* and reported *less body pain*; those who used more problem solving strategies had a better physical role and greater vitality; those who used more cognitive restructuring strategies had a lower perception of body pain, greater vitality and better emotional roles and those who turned less to self-criticism had greater vitality and better emotional roles, being all these relationships significant ($p \leq 0.05$).

It could be concluded that the use of *strategies oriented to solve problematic/difficult situations have the best positive impact on the different aspects of health.*

30.2.3 Assertiveness, Coping and Psychological Distress of Caregivers of People with Severe Mental Illness

The aim of this work was exploring whether the coping strategies and assertiveness of the family caregiver were related to their psychological distress (anxiety, depression, stress). A total of 118 family caregivers participated.

It was detected that there was a *significant relationship between not being assertive with anxiety* (84.2% have anxiety in contrast to the 15.8% who do not have it). The same occurs with *depression* (78.9% of non-assertive people have depression in contrast to 21.1% of assertive people). With regard to the perceived state of health, it was detected that the relationship with the physical role, body pain and vitality was significant, the assessment of the non-assertive ones being worse.

The relationship with social functioning was significant, the non-assertive ones presenting worse functioning compared to the assertive ones. Assertiveness was significantly related to mental health. The non-assertive ones (89.5%) have worse mental health compared to 10.5% of the assertive ones.

30.2.4 Family Caregivers of Patients with Severe Mental Disorder: Sociodemographic Characteristics, Health Perception and Coping Strategies

The aim of this study was to understand the *sociodemographic characteristics*, health status perception and coping strategies of family caregivers of patients with severe mental disorder. Total 101 relatives of 70 patients with severe mental disorders participated.

Most part of family caregivers live with the patients (90.2%) and are *women* (70.6%). The average age of the participants was 54 years and the kinship was distributed as follows: mother 47.1%, father 18.6%, partner 15.7% and sibling 12.7%. On the perceived state of health in the last month: 77.6% had some *emotional problem* (mental health), 70% *felt tired* (vitality), 68.3% believed that *their health was not good* (general health) and 51% experienced some *physical pain* that interfered with their usual work/activity (physical pain).

30.2.5 Assertiveness and the Health of Family Caregivers of Patients with Severe Mental Disorder

The aim of this study was to evaluate the assertiveness of family caregivers of patients with psychotic disorders and the relationship between assertiveness and physical and psychological health.

A total of 140 caregivers (139 relatives and one friend) of 94 patients with a diagnosis of psychotic disorder, personality disorder or bipolar disorder who were being treated at the Mental Health Units of the Virgen de las Nieves University Hospital of Granada (Spain) participated.

Regarding the relationship between assertiveness and anxiety, depression and perceived stress, it is observed that assertiveness is significantly related to these three psychological aspects. Those relatives who *are assertive do not have clinical problems of anxiety, depression or perceived stress*, compared to non-assertive relatives.

Taking into account the relationship between assertiveness and the perceived health of relatives, those relatives who are assertive have a better assessment of physical role, vitality, mental health, social functioning, general health, bodily pain social functioning, as well as global health status, compared to relatives who are not assertive.

It is confirmed that *lack of assertiveness correlates with anxious-depressive problems*, with greater *perceived stress and more health problems*, and is a risk factor for developing and maintaining it. Therefore, it highlights the importance of using an assertive training with relatives of psychosis patients.

30.2.6 Psychological Assessment and Intervention on the Emotional Problems of Relatives with SMD Patients

The daily practice at the HSDM showed the researchers that relatives of patients with SMD frequently presented emotional disorders that required psychotherapeutic interventions. In this line, they conducted a study in which 118 caregivers were evaluated and subsequently offered a weekly group space of psychotherapeutic intervention.

This led to a research project funded by the Andalusian Health Service (SAS 111215 SAS 2011).

The aims were to (1) detect the emotional problems of relatives of patients with SMD and (2) evaluate the efficacy of a psychological intervention programme for these problems.

In this study, it was detected that 64.7% suffered from *depression* (27.1% mild, 18.8% moderate and 18.8% severe). *Anxiety* was present in 52.2% of the patients (22.9% mild, 18.8% moderate and 10.4% severe). Additionally, a high correlation was found between psychological problems.

The programme based on competency training, *ACT and Mindfulness, proved to be effective* since, after its application, the levels of depression, anxiety and stress decreased significantly.

This study proved to be effective in significantly reducing clinical variables and improving assertive behaviour, physical health, problem-oriented adaptive coping strategies, reducing isolation and experiential avoidance.

30.2.7 Grief and Emotional Disturbances in Relatives of Patients with Severe Mental Disorder

The presence of emotional problems (depression, anxiety, stress and grief) in relatives of patients with SMD, and other protective variables (resilience and post-traumatic growth) and the relationship between them were studied in 32 subjects. Secondly, the differences between men and women were analysed and the presence of relationships between the difficult emotions experienced and the level of interference in the diagnosis of the relative's life and emotional problems (depression, anxiety, stress and bereavement) was verified. In addition to that, a qualitative analysis of the interviews conducted with relatives was carried out in order to learn more about the emotions experienced after the diagnosis, the changes that have occurred in their lives and the experience of loss.

After analysing the results, it was found that 56.38% of the relatives presented *significant depressive symptoms*, distributed according to sex: 53.9% of men and 63.3% of women. This is aggravated by the fact that 21.1% of women present severe depression and another 21.1% moderate depression. The same occurs with *anxiety* in which 53.14% of the relatives present anxious symptoms (53.9% men, 57.6% women). In the *perceived stress* in the last month, it was detected that there is a high level, for 84.2% of women medium (68.4%) and high (15.8%). In men, 69.2% presented medium stress. As for the *caregiver grief*, according to the data obtained, its value is high in 100 % of men and 94.7 % of women. In the feelings and emotions of grief after diagnosis, 69.2% of men presented a high level compared to 78.9% of women. Scores remain high at present, they have dropped a bit for men (61.5%) and remain the same for women.

On the other hand, the *age* correlates positively with anxiety and depression levels. The older they get, the higher the levels and the other way round, the older they get the less possibility of post-traumatic growth.

Levels of *depression correlate positively with levels of anxiety, perceived stress, caregiver grief and grief at the moment of diagnosis and the present and negatively with resilience and post-traumatic growth.* At the same time, post-traumatic growth and resilience correlate positively and, as expected, negatively with clinical and grief variables. Therefore, the more resilience and post-traumatic growth, the less pathological emotional reactions and, in turn, these are more frequent in young people. In this sense, the same occurs with *interference in vital areas*, the more the interference (family, leisure, self-care, friendship, etc.) the higher the levels of depression, anxiety, sustained grief and stress, and of course, there is an inverse relationship with resilience.

In terms of emotions, *sadness, fear, pain, anxiety, helplessness and anger* stand out as those experienced most intensely after the diagnosis of the relative, and in lesser proportion resentment, injustice, resentment and shame. Resilience correlates significantly negatively with pain, resentment, anxiety, fear and helplessness. However, the significant positive correlation with rage, resentment, injustice and anger is curious. It seems that certain levels of anger are good for fighting and coping and not the experiential avoidance that is often linked to sadness, fear or hopelessness.

The qualitative analysis of the data obtained through the semi-structured interviews goes in the same direction as the previous ones and confirms *emotional reactions of grief*. The relatives highlighted emotions of sadness and grief upon learning of the diagnosis of their relative with severe mental disorder. They also noted difficulty and disbelief and feeling very frightened about the future and the development of the disease. Some also felt *guilt, rage and anger*. In addition, after the diagnosis, their lives changed significantly, with a decrease of *time constraints* (due to the care of the relative) and *social and leisure activities*. Likewise, they expressed loss of illusion, peace of mind and freedom. Also, a subgroup pointed out how the family nucleus worsened, with a greater number of arguments and increased tension in family relationships.

Regarding the conceptualization of the relative's illness as a grieving process, there was great variability. Most expressed *intense emotional pain and similarity to the loss of a loved* one. In several cases, it is considered even worse than the death of a relative because the person is not really gone.

30.3 Evaluation

The instruments described in Table 30.1 were used to evaluate and obtain relevant data on the presence of emotional alterations (anxiety, depression, stress, grief), health status as well as protective variables (resilience, post-traumatic growth), assertiveness, coping strategies and acceptance, in relatives of patients diagnosed with psychotic disorders. This has made it possible to contrast pre-, post- and follow-up measures to assess the effects of the intervention programmes.

30.4 Intervention Plan

Once the needs detected in the different research studies with relatives of patients with psychotic disorders were analysed, we found that they matched those observed in routine clinical practice in our HSDM. These were also expressed by patients when they attended psychotherapeutic groups, in which they stated that their relatives needed to participate in psychotherapeutic experiences of this kind.

Table 30.1 Evaluation instruments

Semi-structured interview	An interview is prepared containing questions about the time of the relative's diagnosis, feelings about it, worries, abandonment of activities they used to do, feelings of loss and changes in expectations and projects. A Likert-type scale is included in which the scores range from 1 to 5 for relatives to indicate the level of interference in the different vital areas that the relative's diagnosis had had and the level to which they had experienced a series of difficult and ambiguous emotions as a result of the diagnosis.
Beck Depression Inventory II (Beck Depression Inventory II, BDI-II; Beck et al., 1996).	It measures the magnitude of depression by means of 21 items with four response alternatives that are ordered according to severity. The person should choose the option that best describes his or her situation during the last 2 weeks.
Beck Anxiety Inventory (BAI; Beck et al., 1988).	Through 21 items it measures the degree to which anxiety-related physical symptoms are experienced during the last week.
Perceived Stress Scale (PSS; Cohen et al., 1983).	Evaluates the level of stress perceived during the last month. It has 14 items with five Likert-type response options (0 = never; 4 = very often). Higher scores indicate a higher level of perceived stress.
Connor-Davidson Resilience Scale (Connor-Davidson Resilience Scale, CD- RISC; Connor & Davidson, 2003).	A 25-item self-administered questionnaire that evaluates, on a Likert-type frequency scale, from 0 'do not agree at all' to 4 'strongly agree', how the participant has felt in the last month. The maximum score is 100. Higher scores reflect greater resilience.
Post-traumatic *Growth* Inventory (PTGI; Spanish validation, Weiss & Berger, 2006).	21 items assessing the 9 positive changes that people may experience after experiencing a traumatic or adverse event on a scale from 0 ('I did not experience this change at all/no change') to 5 ('I experienced this change to a great extent'). It includes 5 scales that indicate different dimensions of growth: Relationships with others; new possibilities; personal strengths; spiritual changes and appreciation of life. High scores on this questionnaire indicate a higher degree of perceived post-traumatic growth.
Caregiver Grief Scale (The Caregiver Grief Scale, CGS; Meichsner et al., 2016).	Spanish adaptation of this scale. Since the test was not available in our language, the authors were contacted to indicate that an adaptation to Spanish would be made. A translation–retranslation process was carried out with the participation of linguistic experts. The scale consists of four dimensions: Emotional pain, relational loss, absolute loss and acceptance of loss with a Likert-type score from 1 (strongly disagree) to 5 (strongly agree).
The *Texas* Revised Inventory of Grief (ITRD; Faschingbauer et al., 1987) has been adapted to Spanish and validated by García-García et al. (2005).	Questionnaire of 21 items with 5 response categories (Likert type) from 'completely true' (1 point) to 'completely false' (5 points). It is divided into two parts: Part I explores the behaviour and feelings of the bereaved in the immediate aftermath of the death; part II explores the current feelings of the bereaved in relation to the deceased.

(continued)

Table 30.1 (continued)

Assertion Inventory (AI; Gambrill & Richey, 1975)	Formed by 40 items in which the person has to evaluate the level of discomfort/anxiety experienced in the proposed situations and the probability of using the assertive behaviour described in these situations. In both cases a five-point Likert response format is used. A score equal to or higher than 105 indicates problems in performing the behaviour (lack of assertiveness).
Health questionnaire (SF-36; Vilagut et al., 2005).	It allows to know the assessment of positive and negative states of health by the person. It has 35 items with Likert-type response format distributed in eight subscales: Physical functioning, physical role, bodily pain, general health, vitality, social functioning, emotional role and mental health and the item assessing the change in general health status from the previous year. Scores vary according to the subscale and, in general, higher scores indicate a better assessment of the aspect of health to which it refers.
Coping Strategies *Inventory* (CSI; Spanish adaptation of Cano et al., 2007).	It consists of eight subscales that correspond to coping strategies for stressful situations: Problem solving, self-criticism, emotional expression, desiderative thinking, social support, cognitive restructuring, problem avoidance, social withdrawal. It contains 40 items that are scored on a five-point Likert scale to indicate the degree of use of that strategy in the stressful situation described by the person (from 0 = 'not at all' to 4 = 'completely').
Acceptance and Action Questionnaire. (Action Questionnaire -II, AAQ-II; Bond, Hayes, Baer, Carpenter, Orcutt, Waltz and Zettle; Spanish adaptation by Barraca, 2004).	It is an instrument that allows measuring both experiential avoidance and psychological flexibility, depending on the orientation of its ten items. Responses to the items are made on a seven-point Likert-type scale, ranging from 1 (never true) to 7 (always true). Low scores reflect psychological flexibility, while high scores represent an experiential avoidance cognitive style.
Ad hoc survey	Survey about the treatment programme and the effects observed in their lives from their participation in it. This survey consists of five questions. Three of them collect the participants' evaluation of the programme (on a Likert scale from 0 = 'not at all' to 10 = 'very much') and two open-ended questions on the aspects learned in the sessions that they have put into practice and the concrete actions carried out according to their personal values.

For these reasons, it was essential to develop a psychological intervention programme by creating a permanent psychotherapeutic care space open to relatives in need. It is carried out in groups integrating third generation therapies (ACT and Mindfulness) and training in competencies and communication.

The intervention is based on the Albee Competency Model (1985) reformulated by Costa and López (2006), according to which when access to resources and opportunities to maximize competencies, coping capacity and support systems is facilitated, sources of stress are controlled and the incidence of problems is reduced. According to the model, we all have some probability of having a health problem depending on the needs or critical situations we go through, for example, stress. In this sense, the increase in personal, social and economic resources would reduce the incidence of problems. It is integrated into Functional Contextualism, highlighting the third generation therapies, ACT and Mindfulness–compassion.

The objective is not the reduction of discomfort nor the cure of the symptoms, but learning competencies and skills to manage and cope with the situations that influence the vulnerability of the person to present different emotional and relational problems.

'Patients' are contemplated as people capable of learning and applying competencies. The therapeutic relationship provides an interpersonal environment for learning attitudes and behaviours that the person can apply to solve present and future problems, in a context where acceptance (understood as the human capacity to experience being aware of the here and now, of sensations, thoughts, feelings, emotions, memories, images, events, etc., i.e. private events), together with the commitment to carry out actions in accordance with personal values and linked to the necessary change strategies to increase psychological flexibility, is a constant throughout the therapeutic process (ACT and Mindfulness).

The therapist through the clinical processes, the Socratic method for guided discovery of group interactions, promote that people can see themselves in their functioning, contact and can be fully aware of their reactions, and choose whether to let their thoughts and/or emotions appear in their consciousness or choose to notice them, accept them and focus their attention on changing their behaviour in the direction of what is valuable. Acceptance and psychological flexibility are promoted. To do so, you will need to:

- *Discriminate* their operants and the consequences they entail in the short, medium and long term.
- *Identify* contextual cues, private events, rules, self-instructions and the consequences of such behaviours.
- *Differentiate* your public or private reactions (the self-contents, thoughts, memories, images, sensations, rules…) the self-contained vs. the self-context, putting them in perspective 'I think', 'I feel' but 'I am not a thought', 'I am much more than what I feel and think'. This is done with defusion techniques.
- *Establish* what is important, the *values* and from there, choosing your behaviour without making it consistent with your private events. Defusion skills training. We cannot change what we feel and think, but we can change our behaviour.
- *Choose* the course of *action* to follow. Everything approached in the context of values in a sense for them.

For each experience they live between sessions, the following is raised: what happened, description of the situation, context, what did you feel, what did you think, what did you do, what happened next, how did it affect you, was that what you wanted to achieve, what did you want, how could you achieve what you wanted, what were the obstacles, the barriers, what kind of person do you want to be, did your behaviour bring you closer to your values or did it push you away?

The principles of Learning Psychology are moulded, reinforced, modelled and put into action for the acquisition of behavioural repertoires that facilitate different behavioural patterns that lead to the desired direction and the consequences are different and do not increase discomfort.

The group context provides a space that enriches the exchange of roles, the contributions from peers and the reconstruction of the live experience, facilitating the acquisition of therapeutic objectives and enhancing the motivation for change. The sessions are very rich in terms of experiences in which self-discovery and behavioural rehearsals are tremendously useful for self-knowledge and change. In this game of interactions, the learning of skills is included when necessary in a dynamic, dialectic way, adapting to the group process.

The fact that it is arranged in sessions is for didactic purposes, but it does not have to be that way. In each group, they may occur differently, but the clinical components, methodology and *philosophy* guiding the group process are the same based on Functional Contextualism, relational frame theory and radical behaviourism. It is this philosophy that surrounds and directs the entire psychotherapeutic process and guides the training in emotional regulation and communication skills.

The discovery that what we do is the result of our biographical history and the socio-cultural-historical context in which we live, increases suffering and constitutes part of the problem, produces great pain (creative despair), awakens very strong feelings and emotions of guilt, rage and shame and triggers destructive self-criticism. Helping to develop loving kindness, a sense of shared humanity and Mindfulness, self-compassion and compassion with the relative, enhances emotional health and the strengths in order to face life's diversities. Recognizing the pain, the suffering, being able to observe it, accept it and develop a different relationship with it generates unconditional love and alleviates that pain by covering affective needs in ourselves and others. Developing compassionate empathy in relatives, towards oneself and others.

In all sessions, Mindfulness and compassion exercises are performed during the last 15 min from the established and approved programmes within the Contextual Third Generation Therapies, which enjoy empirical evidence that have demonstrated their beneficial effects in various fields (Germer, 2011; Simón & Alonso, 2013; Gilbert, 2015; Kabat-Zinn, 2016; Neff & Germer, 2020).

The psychological intervention consists of approximately 16–24 sessions per week, with a duration of two and a half hours per week. The aims are as follows:

(a) To learn cognitive and behavioural strategies that allow them to live more fully, to resume their existential project and to act in the direction of their personal values, breaking with behavioural paralysis (experiential avoidance).
(b) To reduce clinical anxiety-depressive symptoms and the level of perceived stress, as well as to improve perceived health status, assertiveness and the use of adaptive coping strategies.
(c) To promote their resources and potential.
(d) To achieve psychological flexibility and increase adaptability.

(e) To facilitate the elaboration of grief (loss of illusions, expectations and projects deposited in the relative). To discover the function of the behaviour and its relationship to the context. To establish the relationship between thought, emotion, behaviour and consequence.
(f) To learn to express opinions, feelings, desires and defend one's own rights while respecting those of others. To acquire communication and interpersonal skills.
(g) To identify, recognize and express emotions. To manage anxiety and hostility.
(h) To learn to accept, manage and distance yourself from negative emotions and thoughts so as not to get trapped by them. To break the avoidant pattern of negative emotions and negative thoughts.
(i) To learn to live in the present moment with Mindfulness.
(j) To reduce useless suffering.
(k) To clarify values and act towards them.
(l) To differentiate the self-context from the self-content, between the evaluating mind and the observing mind.
(m) To learn to distance themselves (defusion) from private events (emotions and thoughts) that constitute traps to keep moving in the direction of what is important in their lives.
(n) To develop compassion and self-compassion skills.

In short, the aim is to break the cognitive and emotional fusion, clarify values, live in the present moment, accept discomfort and commit to maintain actions in the direction of those values. Recover their existential project with meaning.

In this protocol of psychotherapeutic intervention, integrative, oriented to the needs of each person, psychoeducation, unlike what happens in other treatment models, is not aimed at explaining what concerns the disorders and their evolution (symptoms, aetiology, treatment, etc.). The aim is that, through a Socratic dialogue, the identification, knowledge and understanding of the psychological processes involved, as well as the functional contextual explanatory model, can be acquired and the mechanisms of acquisition, maintenance and extinction (functional analysis of behaviour and principles of modification) can be established. For this purpose, all group interventions would have the sessions that we call wildcard, and in them the explanatory model of what is happening and the methodological characteristics are established, the why and what for purpose each clinical method is used and the selection of the components of the programme, adapting them to the reality of the people who conform the group. It is here that we use the graphs and metaphors that conceptualize the keys to the intervention (see Figs. 30.1 and 30.2).

In the psychotherapeutic process, the clinical methods of ACT are used, verbal modalities that stay distanced from language: metaphors, paradoxes, experiential exercises that allow exposure to the private events that they avoid. The aim is to break the fusion between the word and what it represents (deliteralization) (Wilson & Luciano, 2002). The Socratic method, guided discovery, functional analysis of ongoing behaviour, visualizations, behavioural rehearsals, experiential exercises, etc., and materials prepared for the group with the content of each session that are delivered in a manual at the end of the group as well as ACT components are part of the whole process: the therapeutic relationship, creative hopelessness, personal values, cognitive defusion, acceptance and distancing from private events, etc. (see Table 30.2).

The following are the contents developed by sessions in one of the groups:

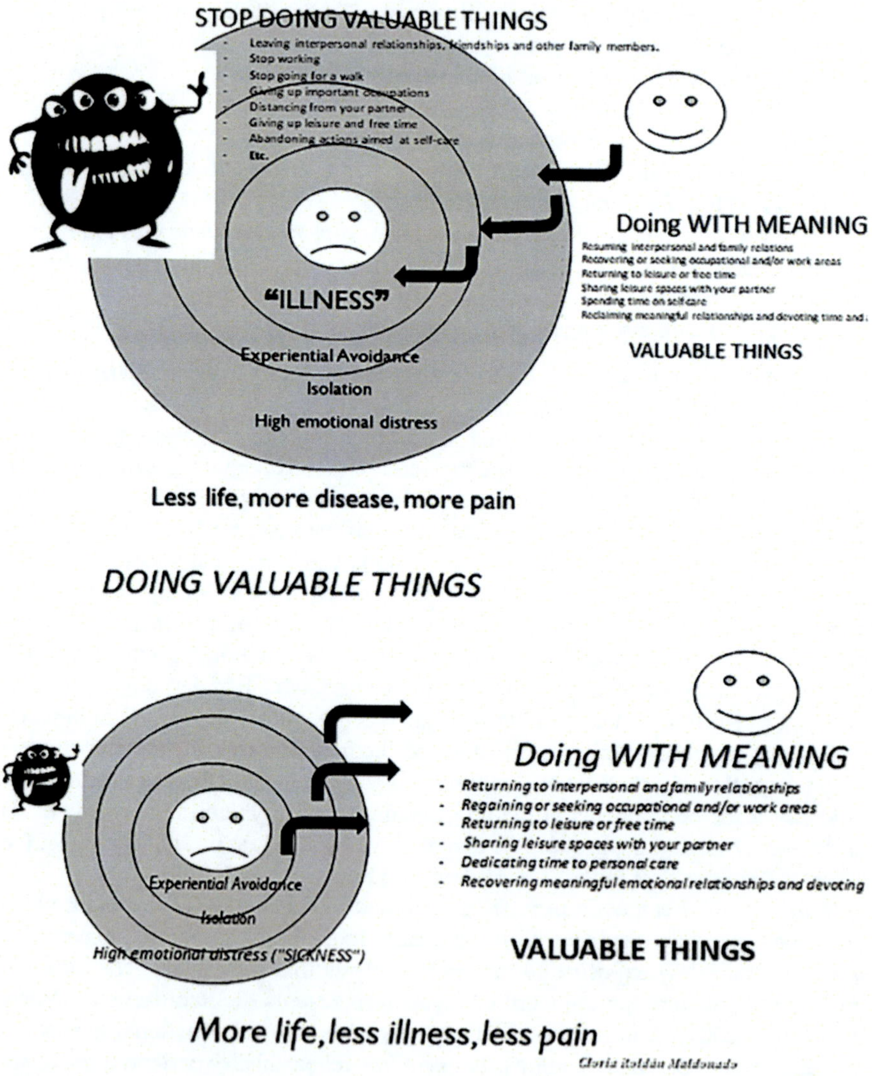

Fig. 30.1 Monster and experiential avoidance

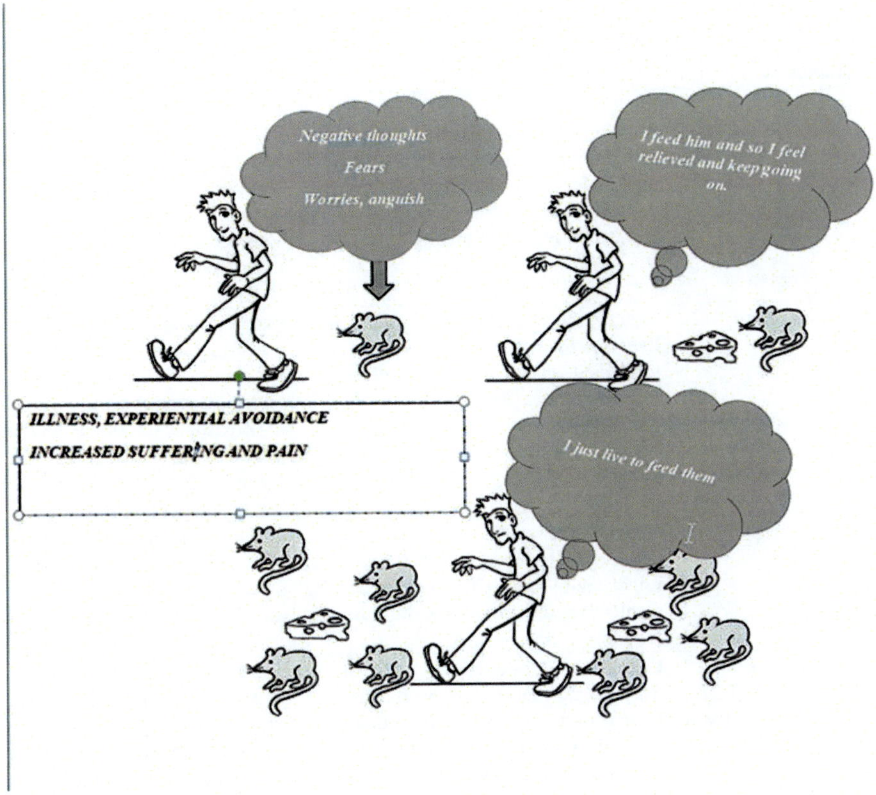

Fig. 30.2 Metaphor feeding the rats

Session 1

- Introduction of the therapist and group members.
- Explanation of frequency, duration, intervention objectives and rationale. The contextual model is conceptualized in terms of the images "feed the monster'.
- Work on orientation and clarification of values: 'Garden Metaphor' (see Fig. 30.3).

'Close your eyes and make yourselves comfortable.... We take a breath and release gently through the mouth. Let's concentrate only on our breathing. In this situation we will imagine that our life is like a garden and that we are the gardeners of our life. We are going to imagine that, as in any garden, weeds sometimes appear. The weeds are the worries, our fears, the negative thoughts, the negative things in each one of us. And each of you are the gardeners of your life. We are going to imagine what would happen if, every time I get up, I dedicate myself to cutting the weeds, just cutting the weeds, every time I get up I cut the weeds. Take a picture of what a garden would look like where I just weed, just weed.

Let's go for a walk in our garden. In it, there are also plants. These plants represent what is important to us in our life, they are our values. Let's see how the plants in our garden are doing.

Table 30.2 Diagram of the components and exercises of the integrated psychotherapeutic intervention

Components	Objectives	Exercises and techniques
Psychoeducation	Identification of the components and functioning of the different psychological processes involved, as well as functional and dysfunctional behaviour, acquisition, maintenance and extinction mechanisms.	Socratic method, visualization of a situation that generates negative and stressful emotions; components of the anxiety expression circuit. Representations of lived experiences. Functional analysis.
Clarification of values	Identify the valuable trajectories in their lives and the actions that direct them towards them, accepting the suffering inherent in that path.	Garden metaphor, funeral exercise, bus driver and passengers metaphor, boat and adversities metaphor; experiential exercise on how to please everyone and go nowhere; 'your last 10 min of life' visualization exercise
Creative despair	Generate the conditions for patients to experience and confront what is important to them, what they do and the results they obtain, both in the short and long term.	Metaphor of the man in the hole, metaphor of the farmer and the donkey; poetry 'you are the result of yourself'.
Distancing from private events (I). Control as a problem and acceptance as an alternative	Learning to distance themselves from the private events that prevent them from acting in the direction of their valuable areas, for which it is first necessary for them to realize that it is the control of these private events that has distanced them from their valuable trajectory and ultimately perpetuates and increases their suffering.	The fight with the monster, pink elephant exercise; experiential exercise 'the river'; metaphor of emotions as a wave; metaphor of the radio on; metaphor of the barking dog; pain visualization exercise.
Distancing from private events (II). Evaluating mind and observing mind	Take distance from your private events and differentiate between thought and who is having the thought, between emotion and who is having the emotion, between descriptive and evaluative, value judgments/reality and your subjective perception, etc.	Metaphor of house and furniture, autumn and leaves; describe behaviours behind value judgments. Evaluative labelling exercises, moving on to factual descriptions.
Deliteralization	Learning to break the fusion between words and their function.	Lemon exercise; repetition of thoughts with high negative charge for the patient. Singing.
Functional analysis of behaviour	Understand the functioning of behaviour and its relationship to context and consequences.	Observation, recording and relationship between thoughts, emotions, behaviours and consequences

(continued)

Table 30.2 (continued)

Components	Objectives	Exercises and techniques
Skills training (communication and problem solving).	Developing and strengthening of communication skills (communication obstacles and facilitators, 'I messages' [using the first person] vs. 'you messages' [using the second person], request for behaviour change, behavioural styles, assertive rights and socializing messages, ability to be reinforcing, making and responding to criticism, coping with emotional manipulation, etc.)	Instruction, modelling and role-playing; practice of skills in their daily life; fable of the oyster and the fish; 'listen to me' poem, etc.
Emotional regulation (identification, comprehension and expression of emotions)	Identify and discriminate emotions. Being able to establish the difference between feeling/thinking and doing in each of them, to experience how they work and to accept, manage and express emotions appropriately without abandoning the direction of the objectives based on values.	Breathing and relaxation exercises; work with specific situations that generate anxiety/hostility, associated responses (physical, emotional, behavioural and thought) and functional analysis. Use of fables, metaphors, deactivation and distancing exercises.
Mindfulness training	Learn to focus attention on the present moment in an intentional and non-judgmental way. Break with the rumination of the past and the anticipation of the future.	Meditations, breathing exercises, visualization of a daily activity with total fullness, exercises of compassion, self-compassion and loving kindness.

Now, imagine you are in front of the body plant (pause), how is this plant?, do I water it?, is it cared for?

Now you are going to imagine another plant in your garden, the leisure, free-time plant (pause), how is that plant?, did I forget that plant was there? Next, we stop in front of the couple plant (pause), how is this plant?, do I take care of it?, do I take care of it?, don't I take care of it?

Next, we walk into the family plant (pause), how is this plant?, is it big?, is it leafy?, have I watered it too much…?

The next floor is the work floor, my occupations' floor (pause), how is your work floor?

We continue walking and we arrive at the friends' plant (pause), how is your friends' plant?

Look at your garden and take a picture of it (pause). Now imagine that from the time you get up until the time you go to bed you dedicate yourself to cutting weeds, what would the garden look like?

Now I want you to imagine how you want your garden to be in five years, your body, your leisure, your family, your partner, your work, your friends. What would you like your garden to look like in five years?

Graphic: Garden metaphor

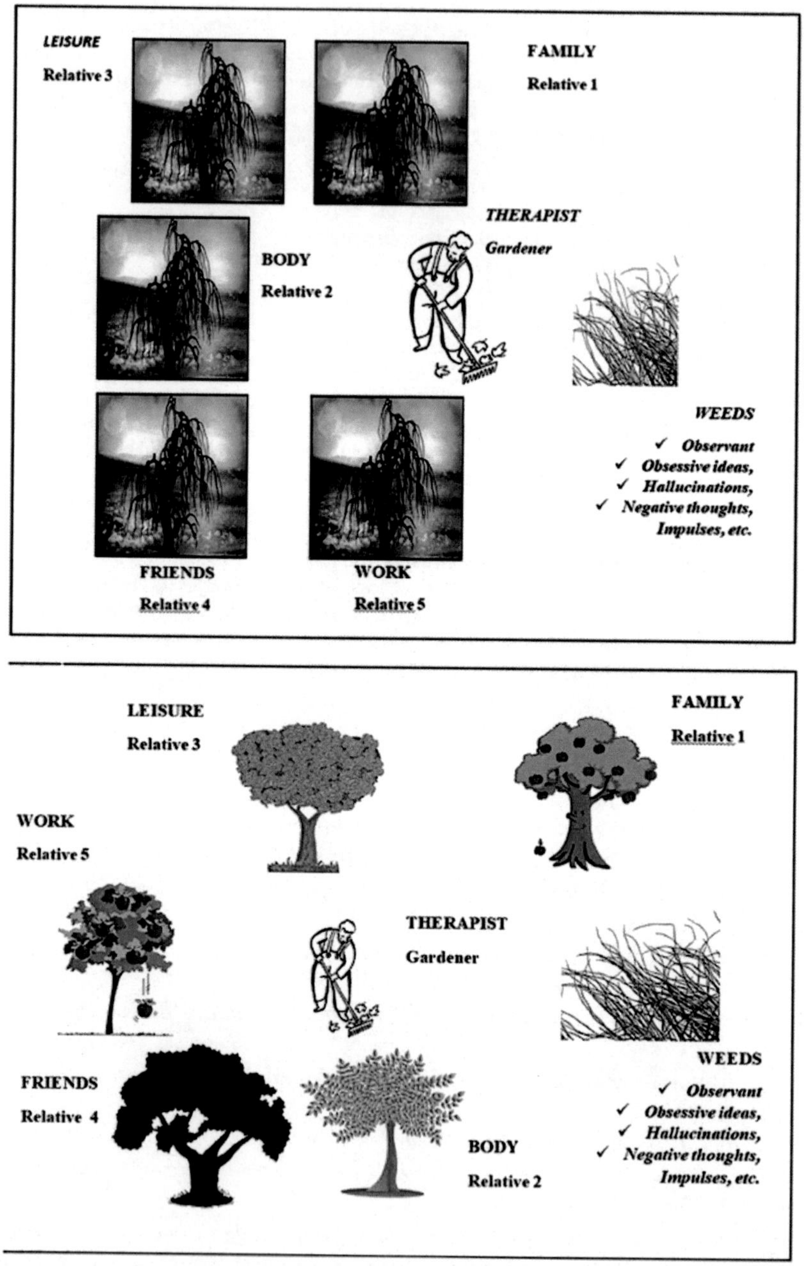

Fig. 30.3 Garden metaphor, dramatization of what happens if we take care of the weeds and neglect the care to the rest of the plants

Once you have the picture of your garden five years from now, keep it and open your eyes little by little'.

At the end of the exercise, each member of the group is asked about:

- What would happen if we just cut weeds, how is your garden looking now? What plants do you have in your garden? How do you see your garden in 5 years?
- They are invited to act out the metaphor. Act out as plants and think about if a plague occurs, what would happen if the rest of the plants are not taken care of.
- Tasks for the week:
  - Review the condition of the plants in your garden and the behaviours you are performing for caring for them.
  - Ask themselves what they are doing with what is important in their lives.
  - Set value-driven objectives. What to do for taking care of your plants.

Session 2

- Review the conclusions of the previous session and the assignments during the week (from now on, all sessions begin this way).
- Emotional regulation:
  - Psychoeducation on emotions and their function.
  - The relationship between thought, emotion, behaviour and consequences (use of functional analysis).
  - Strategies for emotional regulation (e.g. breathing, relaxation).
  - Strategies for the acceptance of private events – thoughts and emotions: Mindfulness exercises.
  - Mindfulness exercise:

'We close our eyes and focus on breathing…just how the air goes in and out…in this situation I want you to travel with your imagination to a place that you like…when you have the image of that place, raise your hand…place yourself in that place…you are going to look to the right and concentrate on everything that is on the right in that place…you are going to try to remember the smell of that place…you are going to pay attention to what is on your right…now you are going to do the same with what is on the left…now you are going to concentrate on what is in front of you…pay attention to all the details…now you are going to imagine that you are sitting in that place and that you have in your hand a piece of the fruit that you like the most…you are going to touch the touch of that piece of fruit…you are going to bring it to your nose and you are going to smell that fruit…we are going to take it away and we are going to look at it and we are going to look at the colours of that fruit…you are going to prepare to eat that fruit…you are going to take it to your mouth and you are going to feel the taste of that letter…you are going to feel the taste of that fruit mixing with your saliva…you are going to taste slowly that fruit…concentrating on the taste of that fruit in your mouth…and now we leave the piece of fruit and we are going to go to clean our teeth and we are going to remember how our toothpaste is…what colour it is…how your toothbrush is…now you are going to pour the toothpaste in the toothbrush and we are going to pour it

all over our mouth and feeling how the toothbrush rubs against our teeth what freshness it leaves in our mouth..., noticing the smell of the paste...concentrating on this action until you finish brushing and the water rinses our mouth...'

THERAPIST: These are examples of Mindfulness exercises, if we focus every moment on what we are doing and we are not aware of negative thoughts, we will not be feeding the monster. We live in an automated way and our mind is in the past or in the future, and the only thing we have escapes from me, which happens to be the present moment. One way to release distress is to focus on the present. As homework for next week, choose one activity, focus on that activity and become aware of it.

– Activities for the week:

  - Observe and record those situations in which they experienced some negative emotion. Describe the situation, what they feel, what they think, what they do and what happens next.
  - Practise, at least once a day, the Mindfulness meditation exercise.
  - Adopt concrete behaviours aimed at caring for the plants in your garden.

Session 3

– Through psychoeducation, the reaction to the diagnosis of their relative will be conceptualized as a major loss that in turn has led to other losses in important areas of their life (leisure, friends, partners, etc.). A dynamic and dialectic interactive relationship is established (Socratic method), to provide adequate information about grief, its characteristics, emotions and processes involved, normalizing the suffering and intense reactions of guilt, anger, worry, as well as confusion, the need to find out why and behaviours such as crying, isolation, etc. Emotions are validated and they are invited to expose what it has meant for each of them to have a relative diagnosed with psychosis.
– Anxiety management exercise.
– Activities for the week:

  - Practise, at least once a day, anxiety management exercises.
  - Identify emotions and continue with functional analysis.
  - What they stopped doing after their relative's diagnosis (losses, grief).

Session 4

– The reactions and interpersonal relationships maintained with the relative before, during and after the diagnosis up to the present time are explored and clarification of values is initiated. The following exercise is performed after closing the eyes and focusing on the breath by inducing the memory and images of the following biographical scenes:

'Place yourself in the day your child was born, how it was, how was the delivery, what did you feel when you saw it...place yourself in that moment and observe what you felt, what you thought, what you did after the birth of your baby.

Now you are going to take a leap to how it was before diagnosing the disease or observing any behaviour associated with it, how was your relationship, what were your illusions, your dreams, what fantasies did you have about your projects, etc. *Now focus on the moment when the disease starts to be noticed, the strange behaviours, what was changing up to the moment you were diagnosed?*

What was that moment like, what did you feel? Bring as vividly as possible your experience of the whole process of diagnosis and initiation of treatment. How did you see him/her? Remember how your relationship with him/her changed. What are the most relevant events that happened, how is the relationship now, how do you see your relative, how do you feel?

We imagine now that this is a novel, this chapter is written up to this point, the next one is written by you… What title would you give, what would happen or would you want to happen in the rest of the novel? Fantasize on an ending.

Group work promotes emotional expression and the identification of losses, suffering and what this has meant for them and the relationship with the relative.

Now begins the clarification of values by connecting it to the fantasies projected in the rest of the novel'.

– Activities for the week:

  • Identify during the week what they have lost in the grief after the diagnosis and what they would like to regain in the routine of daily life and in their relationships with their relative.

Session 5

– Working with potentialities: 'Fábula del Aguilucho' (Fable of the harrier) (in Costa & López, 2006).
– Brief anxiety management exercise.
– Working with self-empowerment: Poem 'No te rindas' (Don't give up) by Mario Benedetti.
– Tasks for the week:

  • Read and work on the Fable of the harrier: in order for them to realize when they are holding on to difficulties and to unleash their potential.
  • Practise, at least once a day, anxiety management exercises. Abdominal breathing training exercise. During the week perform the breathing exercises.
  • Perform a leisure and self-care-oriented activity every day.

Session 6

– Creative despair: metaphor of the 'Man in the Hole'. Digging behaviour is everything we do that aggravates the problem and increases our discomfort. Each group member identifies what behaviour would be for him/her to dig.

'You go down a road and there's a hole and you fall. You really want to go out, but because you're so overwhelmed you start digging, what happens?'

– Defusion, distancing: exercise 'The suitcases'.

'Let's take a deep breath by concentrating on the breath. Breathe deeply..., become aware of your breathing, and mentally say to yourself: calm, calm, calm. You are in the hall of the airport, in front of the baggage conveyor belt, it is a circular belt, they pass and disappear. When you have it, raise your right hand. Now I want you to take those thoughts that are an obstacle to the achievement of your goals, thoughts that bother you, and put them on the conveyor belt. Whenever an emotion or thought comes to you that is an obstacle to your goals, leave it on the belt without picking it up...I don't pick it up, but I keep going in the direction of my goals. He watches them go around, but does not catch them. You can contemplate your thoughts and/or feelings, but don't catch them...don't let them govern your behaviour. You are more than your feelings or thoughts'.

- Distancing exercise: we work with the vignette called what happens if we feed our fears, thoughts, worries, etc. We would make a simile as if they were rats that we want to keep away from us (see Fig. 30.4). But to distract them, we give them food, what would happen? It identifies with what happens in our lives when we get caught up in rumination, hyper-reflexivity, getting away from our path.
- Tasks for the week:
  - Identify and record which behaviours refer to 'digging'.
  - Practise, at least once a day, the distancing exercise.

Session 7

- Emotion management: the hostility curve.
- Working on psychological flexibility: the ability of the reeds through the fable. In order to emphasize the importance of being flexible and adapting to circumstances, the therapist can introduce the following fable to the group. At the end of the session, each member will receive a copy:

'On the bank of a river, an oak tree was felled by a storm and, swept away by the current, one of its branches met a rush grown in a reed bed near the bank. The impact produced a great bewilderment in the oak tree, which could not help but ask the reed how it had managed to stay safe and sound in the midst of a storm that, in its fury, had even been able to uproot an oak tree. The reason, said the reed, is that I achieve my security by an ability opposite to yours: instead of remaining inflexible and stubborn, I adapt to the gusts of wind and do not succumb'.

- Caring for the plants in our garden: learning to be loving to ourselves and others.
- Activities for the week:
  - Practise being loving to others and to oneself.
  - Practise, at least once a day, the distancing exercise.

Session 8

- Communication skills: 'Metaphor of the oyster and the fish (Costa & López, 2006)'. Obstacles and facilitators (I): characteristics of poor communication.
- Learning exercises aimed at distancing negative emotions: training in breath awareness, abdominal breathing training, tension relaxation exercise.

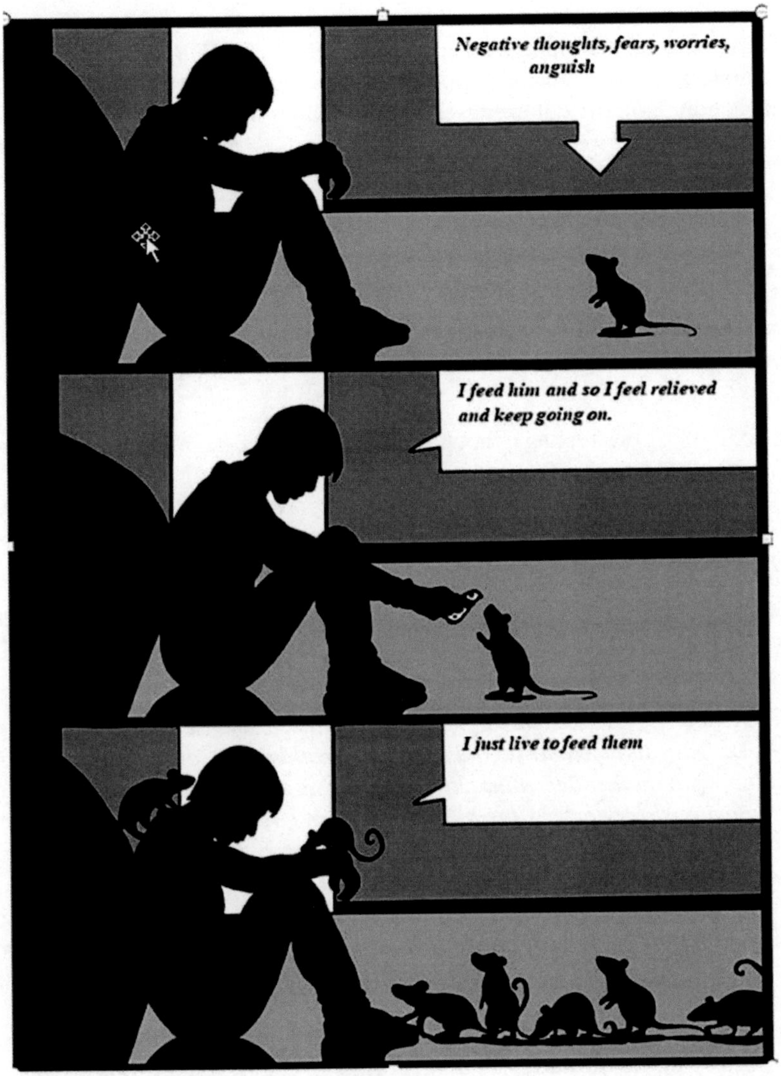

Fig. 30.4 Metaphor when we are only feeding mice

- Activities for the week:
  - Pay attention to obstacles and facilitators in the relationship with others.
  - Identify and record the most frequent obstacles and the effect it has on the relationship.

Session 9

- Taking care of the plants in our garden: communication skills (obstacles and facilitators of communication) (II) putting facilitators, listening, empathy, etc., into action. Experiential exercises and role-play.
- Activities for the week:
  - Evaluation of the obstacles that are preventing them from achieving the garden they want to achieve.
  - Practise listening and empathy.

Sessions 10 and 11

- Care for the plants in our garden: communication skills ('I' messages and request for behaviour change) as a method of caring for interpersonal relationships.
- Activities for the week:
  - Expressing our feelings, thoughts and opinions through the 'I' messages.
  - Detect a behaviour that bothers me and request a change.
  - Use 'I' messages in communication with your relatives during the week and bring an example for the next day of the behaviour change request.

Session 12

- Reinforcement of what has been learned: 'I' messages and request for behavioural change.
- Relaxation exercise: 'The cloud'.

'Close your eyes. Take in air through your nose and release it through your mouth. Let's try to concentrate only on our breathing. We are going to imagine a deep blue sky… on that deep blue sky, we are going to start to see a white, soft, fluffy cloud, moving slowly across the blue sky. We are going to imagine that this cloud can pass through our body from head to toe. You keep repeating to yourselves: "relax, relax," and I will tell you which part will go through…

The cloud goes up the feet, relax, relax; the cloud goes up the calves, relax, relax; the cloud goes up the thighs, relax, relax; the cloud goes up the belly, relax, relax; the cloud goes up the hands, relax, relax; the cloud goes up the chest, relax, relax; cloud goes up the shoulders, relax, relax; cloud goes up the back of the neck, relax, relax; cloud goes up the neck, relax, relax; cloud goes up the mouth, relax, relax; cloud goes up the nose, relax, relax; cloud goes up the eyes, relax, relax; cloud goes up the forehead, relax, relax, relax…

A wave of relaxation invades our body… your hands are heavy, your feet are heavy, your eyelids are heavy. Your eyelids are heavy as when you are about to plunge into a peaceful sleep. A wave of relaxation invades your body, relax, relax. We are going to feel relaxed, at ease with ourselves, we will feel how our body is more and more relaxed. I'm going to count from 5 to 1, and you would be feeling more and more relaxed and a little bit better'.

- Activities for the week:
  - Practise communication skills with relatives. Record them for presenting them to the group.

Session 13

- Work on communication skills: behavioural styles, assertive beliefs, assertive rights and socializing messages.
- Distancing exercise: 'the leaves of autumn and learning to be loving to ourselves', visualization of pain and practice in self-love.

'You have to stand up straight, with your feet flat on the floor, hands resting on your thighs...let's focus on how the air that goes in and out...let's focus only on our breath...feeling how the air goes in and how the air goes out.... we are going to imagine that it is autumn and we are going to imagine a river and a forest...we are going to bring to our mind thoughts and feelings that are barriers to get what we want...imagine now those thoughts and feelings that we have been talking about this afternoon... "I am thinking that....i am thinking that...", "I am feeling that...", take those thoughts, those emotions and build the sentence "I am thinking that...", "I am feeling that..."... and now we are going to imagine that those thoughts and those emotions that prevent us from getting out of the tangle we are going to write them on a piece of paper and we are going to throw them into the river and we see how they go away along the river... and we watch them go by... you take another thought, another emotion and let it go... imagine how they move away on the river...(pause) ... we are going to let the thoughts and emotions run along the river and now we are going to repeat to each other breathing deeply "come on, go ahead", "keep on the way", "if you change, maybe the others will change"... you are going to talk to each other with affection feeling great compassion towards your pain, being great companions in the journey of your life, giving love to yourselves, embracing those words, talking to each other in a loving way "calm", "quiet" and caressing each other with the words, "this then passes", "this life is the only one we have and it is worth living the here and now", "thoughts are words and the reality is outside"... take a second to love each other, to accept your defects and imperfections, with the whole package, the good and the bad and prepare to continue on the path with much more affection...you are going to pass your hands affectionately through your arms, caressing each other and you are going to transmit peace of mind with the caresses of your hands... (Pause)... you can go opening your eyes'.

- Activities for the week:
  - Reading the material (communication skills: behavioural styles, assertive beliefs, assertive rights and socializing messages).

Session 14

- Facilitating the mourning of the loss of the illusions and projects deposited in the children: accepting the limits and creating realistic expectations.
- Learning to be loving to ourselves and others.
- Training in expression of affection.
- Value orientation exercise: 'your last ten minutes of life'.

'We are going to close our eyes and concentrate on our breathing...we concentrate on how the air comes in and comes out... we do not hold on to anything that appears other than focusing on our breathing... you are going to concentrate on imagining that suddenly some terrorists come into the Day Hospital and tell us that we are going to die, but they give us ten minutes to spend and do whatever we want with those ten minutes. After ten minutes, they are going to gas the hospital and we are all going to die... I would like you to imagine what you would like to do in those ten minutes, what people you would like to see...what would you do in those ten minutes?...we are all going to die... but I ask you, what would you like to do in those ten minutes?... when you have been able to visualize it, open your eyes'.

- Activities for the week.
  - Put into practice the expression of positive emotions, affection and affection.

Session 15

- Through a guided recall, each one reproduces a situation in which they felt a great emotional charge that led them to explode doing/saying something that currently causes them pain and emotions of guilt and remorse. For example, threats of autolysis. Using the role-play technique, the scene is represented and the group works together, identifying when we have acted in the opposite direction to what we want because we are fused to negative emotions. The purpose of these techniques is to encourage full expression of thoughts and feelings related to loss, including remorse and disappointment.
- Activities for the week:
  - After the exercise, we should explain him how to keep a daily pain journal during the week in order to keep track of the suffering and become aware of the thoughts that normally go with the internal struggle. Anytime you find yourself struggling with emotional discomfort, difficult thoughts, painful memories, uncomfortable bodily sensations or unwelcome needs, you should write them down in the journal.

Session 16

- We continue with emotional regulation and distancing exercises: 'The river' metaphor and 'Pleasing everyone' exercise.

(1) *Experiential exercise of the river:* fusion and control attempts versus acceptance and distancing of private events. Aim of the exercise: how to separate what we feel from what we think and what we do.

In order to introduce the concepts of cognitive fusion, acceptance and control attempts and enable the understanding of these concepts, we propose performing the following exercise. The therapist stands in the centre of the room. His aim is crossing an imaginary river, as on the other side are valuable goals for him (each member of the group should place their own on that river side). Three participants are needed to represent their negative thoughts and to stand next to the therapist, just as thoughts that constantly accompany us. Each participant is instructed to repeat different messages to the therapist, e.g. *'this is worthless', 'don't do it', 'be careful!', 'you're going to have a hard time'.*

The therapist then depicts the different options for handling our negative self-talk:

- Cognitive fusion: the therapist does not cross over, but allies with your thoughts of helplessness, anxiety, worthlessness, etc.
- Acceptance and detachment: the therapist 'catches' all your thoughts and crosses over, moving towards your valued goals.
- Control attempts or give reasons: the therapist does not cross over, but stays on one side of the river listening to their thoughts and responding to them with arguments that refute them.

(2) *Experiential exercise of pleasing everyone, being carried away by impulses or how not to go anywhere.* Aim of the exercise: how trying to please everyone or letting ourselves be carried away by our impulses leads us away from our vital goals. This exercise is considered part of the work on value orientation.

The therapist stands in the centre of the room, and instructs the group members to call out to him or her, as his or her goal is to please everyone. The therapist will place a chair outside the group circle that represents your goals in relation to your values. The therapist will run in the direction of each participant as he/she is called. The aim of this exercise is getting participants to visualize what happens to our lives if we try to please others or let ourselves be driven by immediate impulses (e.g. *I'm hungry and I eat, I don't feel like going to work and don't go,* etc.*).*

After the exercise, the therapist can work with the group based on the following questions:

- What if I try to please other people?
- What happens to the goals I have in my life?
- Is life about doing what we want (e.g. eating when we are hungry, leaving when I feel like it, etc.?
- Activities for the week:
  - Exercises of distancing and including leisure and free time activities that had been abandoned.

Session 17

- Become aware of the danger of taking thoughts literally and getting caught up in them. For this purpose, the metaphor of 'The Ferris wheel' can be used: going *round and round, getting caught up in inner thoughts and feelings as life goes on.* They will be asked: What can we do to get off the Ferris wheel?
- Exercises of deliteralization to break the fusion of word and reality. Differentiate the I concept from the I content.
- Activities for the week:
  - Practise what was learned in the session.
  - Remember the plants of the garden metaphor and each one commits to carry out an activity aimed at the important vital areas during the week. To achieve

this aim, they will use the strategies learned (acceptance, deliteralization, defusion…).

Session 18

- Continue with emotional regulation by identifying an intense emotion. The goal is to acquire the habit of responding with kindness and caring when self-criticism and destructive emotions arise.
- We learn the exercise of softening, calming and enabling to manage difficult emotions (Germer, 2011). Explain them the use of the exercise, its meaning and its usefulness for destructive emotions.

'Again, begin this practice by finding a comfortable position, close your eyes and take three deep breaths.

Bring attention to your body and what you feel in the present moment. Then, focus the breath in the heart region and begin to follow each breath with Mindfulness. After a few minutes, stop paying attention to your breathing and bring your attention to that part of your body where you can feel the difficult emotion most strongly.

It softens that area of the body. Let the muscles relax without demanding softness from them. It is like applying heat to a sore muscle. You can silently say to yourself, "soft… soft… soft… soft…" to empower the process. Allow the discomfort to be there. Abandon the desire for the feeling to disappear. Let the nuisance come and go as it pleases, like a guest in your own home. You can repeat, "allow… allow… allow… allow…".

Now give yourself love for suffering this way. Place your hand over the heart area and breathe. You can also send love to the part of the body that is stressed. It can help to think of your body as that of a beloved child. You can repeat, "love… love… love… love…".

"Soften, allow and love". "Soften, allow and love". Use the three words as a mantra, remembering to send tenderness to your suffering.

If you experience too much discomfort with a particular emotion, keep breathing until you feel better. Slowly, open your eyes when you're done'.

- Mindfulness exercises, Mindfulness, living in the present, self-compassion and compassion, loving kindness, etc., are worked on and practised. Mindfulness exercises should be provided on a web page or on CD to be practised at home (Simón & Alonso, 2013).
- Activities for the week:
  - Practise the exercise of softening hard emotions every day.

Session 19

- Mindfulness exercise in daily life activities (awareness: brushing teeth, combing hair, etc.).
- Activities for home practice:
  - Choose an activity and focus on that activity and become aware of it.

Session 20

- Strategies for managing anger and expressing it.
- Acquire skills for emotion reduction.
- Activities for the week:
  - Implement emotion reduction strategies.

Session 21

- Identifying positive behaviours and expressing positive emotions by learning to be reinforcing, loving and kind to others, reducing hypercriticism and encouraging phrases that reflect unconditional love. Participants are invited to express qualities of their relatives with psychotic disorder and to identify behaviours they consider appropriate. Perform role-play work to express affection, kindness, etc. Some of them play the role of the relative and others play the role of the patient and are invited to put into practice the expression of love, affection and care.
- Activities for the week:
  - Practise the exercise 'catch your relative doing something you like and tell him/her'. In addition, they will practise the expression of love, affection and affection.

Session 22

- Work with psychoeducational material (most frequent self-protective attitudes and fears, their thoughts and feelings, management of some negative emotions and positive thoughts) (delivery of materials).
- Facilitate the distancing between the I context and the I content (move from focusing attention on the previous negative story to what I have now). Focus on the present, break with the past and the anticipation of the future. Attention focusing exercise: 'The air conditioner', metaphor for 'The radio on' and/or 'The furniture'.
- Work on value orientation (creating a life project apart from that of the parents, children and the sick person).
- Generation of creative hopelessness and acceptance of resentment: you are the master of your behaviour and you can create different responses towards whatever you want to achieve.

Sessions 23 and 24

- Work on specific difficulties.
- Delivery of the material 'Fables, songs, metaphors and poems'.
- Group conclusions ('what helped you the most?').
- Delivery of a certificate of participation in the group.
- Schedule follow-up sessions.
- Evaluation by each member of the group of what the experience has meant in terms of what they have changed, what has been most useful.
- Brief overview of the contents of the programme, exchange of experiences and analysis of the changes observed in the relationships.
- Assessment of the current state of your life project.

Follow-up Sessions

- In 6 months and 12 months.

30.5 Results and Discussion

After the psychotherapeutic intervention presented with relatives of people diagnosed with psychosis in a group, both the efficacy and maintenance of the results obtained over time were demonstrated.

The results obtained, in the investigations carried out in the Day Hospital from 2010 to date, confirmed our starting hypothesis, the observations in clinical practice and what was verbalized in the interviews we had with them. They were used to highlight the selected intervention programme components that constitute transdiagnostic psychological processes.

30.5.1 Psychological Variables Assessed in Relatives Which Enables the Group Intervention Development

Assertiveness was significantly related to anxiety, depression and perceived stress. Assertive relatives do not present clinical problems compared to non-assertive relatives. It was also significantly related to perceived health status. Those relatives who are assertive have a better assessment of physical role, vitality, mental health, social functioning, general health, bodily pain compared to those who are not. It is clear that the lack of assertiveness correlates with anxious-depressive problems, greater perceived stress and more health problems, constituting a risk factor for developing and maintaining it. Therefore, it supports the importance of assertive training within communication skills at the preventive level and in intervention programmes with relatives of patients diagnosed with psychosis.

The most commonly used coping strategies were desiderative thinking, social isolation and problem solving, and the least used were cognitive restructuring, self-criticism and emotional expression. After analysing the relationships with the health dimensions evaluated with the SF-36, it was observed that those who had less social isolation had a better physical role and emotional role and reported less body pain; those who used more problem solving had a better physical role and greater vitality; those who used more cognitive restructuring had a lower perception of body pain, greater vitality and better emotional role and those who used less self-criticism had greater vitality and better emotional role, all of these relationships being significant. The use of strategies aimed to solving problematic/difficult situations have the best positive impact on different aspects of health, while emotion-oriented strategies do not seem to have a significant impact, with the exception of self-criticism which, according to the results, its lower use is associated with better mental health.

A high incidence of emotional problems (depression, anxiety, stress and bereavement) was detected in relatives of patients with MGD and a high interference in their lives. 56.38% of them presented significant depressive symptoms, distributed according to sex, 53.9% for men and 63.3% for women. The effect is worse in women (21.1% severe depression and 21.1% moderate depression). The same occurs with anxiety in which we found that 53.14% of the relatives presented anxious symptoms (53.9% men, 57.6% women). Perceived stress in the last month was high, being medium (68.4%) and high (15.8%) for 84.2% of the women. 69.2% of the men presented medium stress. Therefore, stress constitutes a relevant clinical problem in relatives, having a higher impact on women. In terms of grief of caregivers, in 100% of men and 94.7% of women is high. In the feelings and emotions of grief after diagnosis (measured by the ITRD), 69.2% of men had a high level compared to 78.9% of women. Scores remain high at present, they have dropped a bit for men (61.5%) and remain the same for women.

Levels of depression correlate positively with levels of anxiety, perceived stress, caregiver grief and grief at diagnosis and present and negatively with resilience and post-traumatic growth. At the same time, post-traumatic growth and resilience correlate positively and, as expected, negatively with clinical and grief variables. In this sense, the same occurs with interference in vital areas, the more the interference (family, leisure, self-care, friendship, etc.) the higher the levels of depression, anxiety, sustained grief and stress, and of course, there is an inverse relationship with resilience. As previous studies have shown, the greater the interference in important life areas, the greater the risk of psychological distress and emotional disorders, as well as chronic or complicated grief areas, and there is a greater risk of psychological distress and emotional disorders, as well as chronic or complicated grief.

With regard to emotions, the following stood out as those experienced most intensely after the diagnosis of the relative: sadness, fear, pain, anxiety, helplessness and anger, and in lesser proportion resentment, injustice, resentment and shame. Resilience correlates significantly negatively with pain, resentment, anxiety, fear and helplessness. However, the significant positive correlation with rage, resentment, injustice and anger is curious. It seems that certain levels of anger are good for fighting and coping and not the experiential avoidance that is often linked to sadness, fear or hopelessness. Sadness, loneliness, fear, helplessness and pain correlate positively with grief, as expected. The positive correlation found between resentment and practically all other measures (anxiety, depression and grief) and resentment with grief is noteworthy. Destructive emotions can be considered facilitators of emotional problems, which, in turn, present an inverse correlation with the protective variable resilience, as shown in the studies carried out by the group that analysed destructive emotions and was included in Goleman's book (2003).

The relatives highlighted emotions of sadness and grief upon learning of the diagnosis of their relative with SMD. They also noted difficulty and disbelief and feeling very frightened about the future and the development of the disease. Some also felt guilt, rage and anger. In addition, their lives changed significantly, with time constraints (due to care of the relative) and a reduction of their social and leisure activities. Likewise, they expressed loss of illusion, peace of mind and freedom. Also, a subgroup pointed out how the family unit worsened, with an increase of the arguments and tension in family relationships.

30.5.2 Evaluation of Programme Effectiveness

There was a positive change in all psychological variables evaluated after the intervention, presenting significant differences in perceived stress, in all areas of perceived health (mental health, social functioning, bodily pain, emotional role, vitality and general health), in the two aspects of assertiveness (discomfort/anxiety and response probability), in post-traumatic growth, resilience and in five of the eight coping strategies (cognitive restructuring, problem solving, desiderative thinking, emotional expression and self-criticism), post-traumatic growth, resilience and in five of the eight coping strategies (cognitive restructuring, problem solving, desiderative thinking, emotional expression and self-criticism), in three coping strategies (problem avoidance, social isolation, and social support), and in depression, anxiety and grief.

Levels of depression and perceived stress significantly decreased and positive appraisal of three aspects of health improved: bodily pain, vitality and emotional role. Likewise, there was an increase in assertive behaviour and in the use of adaptive and problem-focused coping strategies (problem solving, cognitive restructuring and social support) and a decrease in less adaptive and mostly emotion-focused coping strategies (self-criticism, emotional expression, desiderative thinking).

According to the assessment made by the relatives about the programme, most of them report having achieved important changes in their lives, in the direction of the values they had abandoned due to their children's illness, and they carry out concrete actions in different areas of their lives (e.g. they now dedicate more time to themselves – self-care, leisure, resuming personal and occupational projects – to their partners –they have resumed joint activities, they have used strategies to communicate better – to the rest of the family –they pay more attention to the rest of the relatives, they share activities – to their friends – they have resumed contact and activities with friends). It significantly decreased experiential avoidance and increased psychological flexibility. In this regard, relatives reported behaviours aimed at everything that was important in their lives and the changes made in each area.

Group participants highlighted the following learning points applied to their lives and specific actions which showed their commitment to personal values. Below are some examples of each area:

- *Emotional regulation:* implementation of relaxation exercises, emotional deactivation and reduction of aggressive behaviours (shouting, disqualifications, etc.). Take distance and time to calm down. Distance yourself from negative thoughts. Know how to listen and lower the anger curve. Facing with more serenity the situations of conflicts and stress.
- *Communication*: use expressions with 'I messages'. Improve communication with listening and empathy. Increase expressions of affection and care. Avoid the use of labels, value judgments. Know how to make requests for behavioural change. Set limits and say no. Avoid blaming.

- *Acceptance and coping:* better understanding and accepting of the emotions of their relatives and themselves. Disarm unfounded fears and accept pain and discomfort in difficult situations. Focus on the present by distancing oneself from the past and not anticipating the future. Resume activities that I had stopped doing because of fear. Express what you feel and think that you used to repress because of fear of conflict.
- *Mindfulness:* increase the time to take care of oneself and enjoy (cultural) activities by distancing oneself from guilt. Living here and now. Appreciate and dedicate more time to little things. Live fully in other areas of your life that are not related to the diagnosed relative.
- *Leisure:* they resumed abandoned activities, such as reading, walking, resting, watching TV, having a cup of coffee and excursions.
- *Affective relationships:* a greater approach to abandoned friendships, an increase in contacts and communication. More time dedicated to the couple. They resumed and began to enjoy activities as a couple, increasing the expressions of affection. An increase in the relationships with the rest of the family significantly improved communication by implementing listening, empathy and timely withdrawal in high-stress situations. Increase in positive communication, caring phrases and expressions of affection.
- *With oneself:* significantly improved the relationship with oneself. They included personal self-care and rest. They learned to be kinder and gentler with themselves and less hypercritical. They acquired self-compassion skills.

Most of them highlighted the importance of what they learned for their lives in general, including different areas and interpersonal relationships. The skills improved extended beyond the home environment, for example, to the workplace.

The relatives also evaluated what had been most useful to them from the group work, specifying what they had learned and what had been most useful. In this sense, they highlighted the metaphor of the garden, which marked before and after in their lives and led them to be aware of and implement behaviours aimed at caring for the plants in their lives. The metaphor of the river, the suitcases and not falling into fusion through the exercises worked on were considered very relevant to reduce useless suffering and internalize a new philosophy of acceptance and commitment. They emphasized emotional regulation and the importance of decreasing violent reactions and increasing kind and caring ones. To feel more calm, comfort and peace, distance oneself from the inner world and put the behaviour in the direction of what is important. They also pointed out Mindfulness, living in the present with full intensity and relativizing. They emphasized the importance of communication training and becoming aware of and changing the ways of relationships.

Therefore, the selection of the components for the programme, which was adjusted to the needs observed and evaluated, showed the effectiveness and importance of carrying out integrative interventions oriented to the real needs of each person in his or her context. Most of the relatives rated the experience of participating in the programme as very useful and satisfactory.

30.6 Conclusion

Training in emotional competencies and regulation, integrated with ACT and Mindfulness, helps strengthen important skills for the achievement of life goals, such as adaptive coping strategies, and is aimed at actively modifying stressful situations.

After the experience, we can conclude that the relatives of patients with SMD present emotional disorders that require psychotherapeutic spaces that go beyond psychoeducation. The application of a psychotherapy programme (including ACT, Mindfulness and communication training) has been shown to be very useful in reducing psychological distress, emotional problems, increasing quality of life, acquiring coping styles, breaking the avoidant pattern of negative emotions and thoughts, learning communication and interpersonal relationship skills, and learning to live in the present moment with *Mindfulness*, in short, to learn to live more fully by following their existential goals.

All this highlights the importance of creating psychotherapeutic spaces for relatives who live with patients diagnosed with SMD, showing that psychoeducation is insufficient since they present a clear experiential avoidance and have abandoned valuable areas of their lives to dedicate themselves to the care of their children. This is facilitating the emergence of emotional responses of anxiety and depression that intensify suffering and interfere with family interactions.

In the words of some relatives,

'Because now I feel able to cross the river despite the fears. Because I have learned to live in the here and now and focus on the present moment. Because now when I get stressed I stop and imagine that a cloud caresses me while I breathe… For all this and much more that is impossible to compile in more lines: Thank you! Thank you from the bottom of my heart, I take with me a very valuable learning experience and the purpose of continuing to strive to improve. Thank you for allowing me to be part of this project and congratulations to all the professionals who have taught us so much' (sister).

'Everything we have learned has helped us to be able to make family and personal decisions to get back on track with our lives. During this time we have discovered our internal emotions and have better understood our external ones, something that had not occurred until now. Now I can distance myself and see what is important and valuable in my life, as well as diminish useless suffering. Fears and apprehensions now accompany us without preventing us from moving forward, and it is then that the darkness has turned into clarity' (mother).

'How different everything I learned about what was happening to us. What we have experienced here does not exist anywhere else, we discuss it in the associations, it is the opposite of what we thought before. Becoming aware of my viscerality and how I was distancing myself from what was important in my life has led me to change so much… my relationships have improved. Eternally grateful' (father).

References

Babacan, A. (2008). Health education needs of patients schizophrenia and their relatives. *Archives of Psychiatric Nursing, 22*, 156–165.

Barraca, J. (2004). Spanish adaptation of the Acceptance and Action Questionnaire (AAQ). *International Journal of Psychology and Psychological Therapy, 4*(3), 505–515.

Beck, A. T., Epstein, N., Brown, G., & Steer, R. A. (1988). An inventory for measuring clinical anxiety: The Beck anxiety inventory. *Journal of Consulting and Clinical Psychology, 56*, 893–897.

Beck, A. T., Steer, R. A., & Brown, G. K. (1996). Beck depression inventory-II. *San Antonio, 78*(2), 490–498.

Bonilla, G. (2018). *Duelo y alteraciones emocionales en familiares de pacientes con trastorno mental grave*. Master's dissertation, Universidad de Granada. Retrieved from https://digibug.ugr.es/handle/10481/192

Cano, F. J., Rodríguez, L., & García, J. (2007). Adaptación española del Inventario de Estrategias de Afrontamiento. *Actas Españolas de Psiquiatría, 35*(1), 29–39.

Cohen, S., Kamarck, T., & Mermelstein, R. (1983). A global measure of perceived stress. *Journal of Health and Social Behaviour*, 385–396.

Connor, K. M., & Davidson, J. R. (2003). Development of a new resilience scale: The Connor-Davidson resilience scale (CD-RISC). *Depression and Anxiety, 18*(2), 76–82.

Costa, M., & López, E. (2006). *Manual para la ayuda Psicológica. Dar poder para vivir. Más allá del counseling*. Pirámide.

Desviat, M. (2000). La asistencia de las psicosis en España o hacia dónde va la reforma psiquiátrica. *La Psicosis en la Comunidad*, 41–73.

Escalante, V., & Gavlovski, J. (2011). Tener un hijo con enfermedad mental: Vivencias de madres de pacientes con esquizofrenia/Having a son with mental illness experiences of mothers with schizophrenic patients. *Revista Anales, 11*(1).

European Federation of Associations of Families of People with Mental Illness. (2014). *Family careers of people with Schizophrenia are a hidden workforce at breaking point*. Retrieved from http://www.eufami.org/news/56-press-release-family-carers-ewith-schizophrenia-are-a-hidden-workforce-at-breaking-point2

Faschingbauer, T., Zisook, S., & DeVaul, R. (1987). *The Texas revised inventory of grief. Biopsychosocial aspects of bereavement*. American Psychiatric Press.

Gambrill, E., & Richey, C. (1975). An assertion inventory for use in assessment and research. *Behavior Therapy, 6*(4), 550–561. https://doi.org/10.1016/S0005-7894(75)80013-X

Germer, C. K. (2011). *El poder del mindfulness. Libérate de los pensamientos y las emociones autodestructivas*. Paidos.

Gilbert, P. (2015). *Terapia centrada en la compasión. Características distintivas*. Descleé De Brouwer.

Girón, M., Fernández, A., Mañá, S., Molina, A., Nolasco, A., & Gómez, M. (2010). Efficacy and effectiveness of individual family intervention on social and clinical functioning and family burden in severe schizophrenia: A 2-year randomized controlled study. *Psychological Medicine, 40*, 73–84.

Godress, J., Ozgul, S., Owen, C., & Foley-Evans, L. (2005). Grief experiences of parents whose children suffer from mental illness. *Australian & New Zealand Journal of Psychiatry, 39*(1), 88–94.

Goleman, D. (2003). *La práctica de la inteligencia emocional*. Kairós.

Guardia, J. (2010). *Ansiedad y afrontamiento en cuidadores de pacientes con esquizofrenia*. Tesis de licenciatura, Pontificia Universidad Católica del Perú. Retrieved from http://tesis.pucp.edu.pe/repositorio/bitstream/handle/123456789/665/GUARDIA_CANALES_JAVIER_ANSIEDAD.pdf

Gutiérrez-Maldonado, J., & Caqueo-Urízar, A. (2007). Effectiveness of a psycho-educational intervention for reducing burden in Latin American families of patients with schizophrenia. *Quality of Life Research, 16*, 739–747.

Hidalgo, M. (2013). *Sobrecarga y afrontamiento en familiares cuidadores de personas con esquizofrenia*. Unpublished doctoral thesis. Pontificia Universidad Católica.

Kabat-Zinn, J. (2016). *Vivir con plenitud las crisis: Cómo utilizar la sabiduría del cuerpo y de la mente para enfrentarnos al estrés, el dolor y la enfermedad*. Kairós, S.A.

López de Arróyabe, E., & Calvete, E. (2005). Síntomas de duelo en familiares de personas con daño cerebral adquirido. *Mapfre medicina, 16*(4), 266–276.

Magaña, M., Ramírez, I., Hernández, M., & Cortez, R. (2007). Psychological distress among Latino family caregivers of adults with schizophrenia: The roles of burden and stigma. *Psychiatric Services, 58*, 378–384.

Meichsner, F., Schinköthe, D., & Wilz, G. (2016). The caregiver grief scale: Development, exploratory and confirmatory factor analysis, and validation. *Clinical Gerontologist, 39*(4), 342–361.

Neff, K., & Germer, C. (2020). *Cuaderno de trabajo de Mindfulness y Autocompasión. Un método seguro para aumentar la fortaleza y el desarrollo interior y para aceptarse a uno mismo*. Bilbao.

Porcar, M., Guillamón, L., Pedraz, A., & Palmar, A. M. (2015). Cuidado familiar de la persona con trastorno mental grave: una revisión integradora. *Revista Latino-Americana de Enfermagem, 23*(2).

Rascón, M. L., Caraveo, J., & Valencia, M. (2010). Trastornos emocionales, físicos y psiquiátricos en los familiares de pacientes con esquizofrenia en México. *Revista de Investigación Clínica, 62*(6), 509–515.

Roldán, G. M., Salazar, I., Garrido, L., & Cuevas-Toro, A. M. (2015). Intervención psicológica grupal, basada en la aceptación y el entrenamiento en comunicación, familiares de personas con trastorno mental grave. *Anales de Psicología, 31*(3), 759–772.

Roldán, G. M., Garrido, L., & Bonilla, G. (2017). Psicoterapia en grupo para familiares de pacientes con Trastorno Mental Grave. In J. R. Sánchez (Ed.), *Terapia de Aceptación y Compromiso en grupo*. Ediciones Lulu.

Scheirs, J. G. M. (2007). Psychological distress in caregivers or relatives of patients with borderline personality disorder. *International Journal of Social Psychiatry, 53*, 195–203.

Simón, V., & Alonso, M. (2013). *Meditaciones de Minfulness y Autocompasión. Libro de CD*. Magrana Studios.

Society of Clinical Psychology, APA, Division 12. (2010). *Family psychoeducation for schizophrenia*. Retrieved on May 4, 2017, from http://www.psychology.sunysb.edu/eklonsky-/division12/treatments/schizophrenia_family.html

Steele, A., Maruyama, N., & Galynker, I. (2010). Psychiatric symptoms in caregivers of patients with bipolar disorder: A review. *Journal of Affective Disorders, 121*, 10–21.

Stengler-Wenzke, K., Trosbach, J., Dietrich, S., & Angermeyer, M. C. (2004). Experience of stigmatization by relatives of patients with obsessive compulsive disorder. *Archives of Psychiatric Nursing, 18*, 88–96.

Tartaglini, M., Feldberg, C., Hermida, P., & Stefani, D. (2011). Factores de riesgo de sobrecarga en el cuidador familiar: los problemas conductuales en pacientes con demencia. *Acta Psiquiátrica Psicológica América Latina, 57*(1), 4–10.

Thomen, M. (2020). *Relaciones Familiares Básicas en diferentes estructuras familiares con un hijo con Trastorno del Espectro Psicótico*. Master's dissertation, Universidad de Cataluña. Retrieved from https://www.recercat.cat/handle/2072/443448

Vallina, O., & Lemos, S. (2003). Guía de tratamientos psicológicos eficaces para la esquizofrenia. In M. Pérez, J. R. Fernández, C. Fernández, & I. Amigo (Eds.), *Guía de tratamientos psicológicos eficaces I*. Pirámide.

Vilagut, G., Ferrer, M., Rajmil, L., Rebollo, P., Permanyer-Miralda, G., Quintana, J. M., Santed, R., Valderas, J. M., Domingo-Salvany, A., & Alonso, J. (2005). El Cuestionario de Salud SF-36 español: una década de experiencia y nuevos desarrollos. *Gaceta Sanitaria, 19*(2), 135–150. Retrieved from 2022, from http://scielo.isciii.es/scielo.php?script=sci_arttext&pid=S0213-91112005000200007&lng=es&tlng=es

Wancata, J., Freidl, M., Krautgartner, M., Friedrich, F., Matschnig, T., Unger, A., Gössler, R., & Frühwald, S. (2008). Gender aspects of parents' needs of schizophrenia patients. *Social Psychiatry and Psychiatric Epidemiology, 43*, 968–974.
Weiss, T., & Berger, R. (2006). Reliability and validity of a Spanish version of the posttraumatic growth inventory. *Research on Social Work Practice, 16*(2), 191–199.
Wilson, K., & Luciano, M. C. (2002). *Terapia de aceptación y compromiso (ACT): un tratamiento conductual orientado a los valores*. Pirámide.
Wittmann, D., & Keshavan, M. (2007). Grief and mourning in schizophrenia. *Psychiatry: Interpersonal and Biological Processes, 70*(2), 154–166.

Chapter 31
Family Intervention in Psychosis: A Case

Ernesto Baena, Carol Harvey, Cristina Abelleira, Jaime A. Fernández, and José A. Sánchez

31.1 Introduction

This chapter is dedicated to a clinical case in which family intervention was provided. The patient is a young man living with a psychotic illness with significant symptoms, both positive and negative. From the outset, he experienced adverse impacts on his functioning, such as social withdrawal, and had difficulties in abstract thinking and self-reflection. His parents experienced many of the well-recognised negative effects of living with a relative experiencing mental ill-health (Harvey & O'Hanlon, 2013). These included their experiences of prolonged grief and difficulties with unrealistic expectations, as well as finding their daily lives constrained by their caring roles. However, the patient and his parents were able to participate in, and benefit from, a family intervention. This illustrates how family intervention can play an important role in recovery, even when patients and families are facing significant challenges. The benefits of family intervention for both the patient and the family are strong and have been repeatedly demonstrated through rigorous trials in many countries (Harvey, 2018; Lobban et al., 2013).

This case presents a range of formats that can be used in working with families such as single-family and multi-family approaches, as well as demonstrating the increasing use of the Internet. Both single-family and multi-family formats have an established evidence base (Harvey, 2018). Those aspects of a family's difficulties, which may be considered in deciding to transition from a multi-family to a

E. Baena (✉) · C. Abelleira · J. A. Fernández · J. A. Sánchez
Canary Health Service, Island Psychosocial Rehabilitation Program, Gran Canaria, Spain
e-mail: cabevid@gobiernodecanarias.org; jferferr@gobiernodecanarias.org; jsanpad@gobiernodecanarias.org

C. Harvey
University of Melbourne and NorthWestern Mental Health, Melbourne, Australia
e-mail: c.harvey@unimelb.edu.au

J. A. Díaz-Garrido et al. (eds.), *Psychological Interventions for Psychosis*,
https://doi.org/10.1007/978-3-031-27003-1_31

single-family approach, are helpfully set out for the reader in this case. These include working with a family where the situation appears "stuck". The development of an Internet-delivered multi-family format by the professionals, in this case, is understandable in the context of the COVID-19 pandemic and shows their flexibility in continuing to meet families' needs. This echoes wider developments in the delivery of family interventions, where there is emerging evidence for digital family interventions (Alvarez-Jimenez et al., 2014) and their acceptability to families. It has been recognised for some time that most family interventions, whatever their type and format, have many common features (Dixon et al., 2001; Harvey & O'Hanlon, 2013; Lobban et al., 2013). Two central features of all family interventions concern professionals showing positive and non-blaming attitudes towards families as well as involving families as respected partners in care. These are amply demonstrated in this clinical case. When families are respected as partners in care, it is easier for professionals to be responsive to the family's changing circumstances and needs, as this case illustrates.

Psychoeducation is recommended in most models of family intervention, as described here. Increasingly, this is conceptualised as sharing information with families in an environment of mutual support (Harvey, 2018). Recognition of the importance of this emphasis on sharing information (as opposed to providing psychoeducation) is reflected in this case through the professionals' decision to rename the psychoeducational module in the face-to-face multi-family format. It is likely that this module, renamed as "Sharing Information", was better understood by families and more coherent with the process and intervention described in the chapter.

Some strategies used in contextual therapies were incorporated in the multi-family approach described here, both for its face-to-face and Internet delivery. These included aspects of acceptance and commitment therapy (ACT), such as emotional coping, cognitive defusing and commitment making as well as strategies such as the use of metaphors and mindfulness practices.

Their contribution to promoting and supporting the family's self-care is described and emphasised here. This is an important but often overlooked aspect of working with families, who often report leading lives constrained by their role as carers. For example, a mother who was a participant in a single-family intervention reported that "*I just don't have a life at the moment*" (page 4, Coker et al., 2016). The percentage of carers reporting a need for assistance in "making time for themselves" reduced markedly after participation in the afore-mentioned single-family intervention (Coker et al., 2016).

Similarly, the parents, in this case, were able to improve their self-care and incorporate "spaces of personal Independence" into their lives following family intervention. It is perhaps surprising then that reduction in the burden experienced by this family after participation in the intervention was not demonstrated. A number of plausible explanations for this observation are suggested. Further, and as mentioned in this chapter, previous reviews of family interventions have tended to report less impact on reducing family burden. However, there is recent encouraging evidence that these interventions can result in decreased carer burden, including in similar settings, as shown in a trial conducted in Spain and Portugal (Martin-Carrasco et al., 2016).

This case also illustrates the use of various Cognitive-Behavioural Therapy (CBT) strategies within family intervention. CBT strategies incorporated in the multi-family intervention included coping strategies and problem-solving as well as modelling more assertive communication styles. Use of another CBT technique, the behavioural contract, also proved effective in the single-family session. Similarly, a recent systematic review noted that CBT strategies were incorporated in several of the family interventions evaluated in the included studies (Killaspy et al., 2022).

The work with this family was conducted within a well-established program of care for family members of people with severe mental disorders which, in turn, is part of a network of psychosocial rehabilitation programs. This reinforces how family interventions can be helpful, even for those significantly affected by mental health problems, as reported recently (Killaspy et al., 2022). It is a noteworthy feature of this family work that it is part of a well-established program. A significant global challenge is how to establish and sustain family intervention programs. The importance of a supportive organisational context is likely to be highly relevant (Harvey & O'Hanlon, 2013). However, the success in sustaining family intervention programs, with some exceptions (Maone et al., 2021), often goes unreported, due to the understandable emphasis on clinical work undertaken in such interventions, rather than more robust research and evaluation. This case usefully adds to our knowledge of how to develop, improve and maintain a family intervention program.

31.2 Family Intervention

In order to contextualise the family intervention carried out in the case presented, it is necessary to briefly describe the field of care in which it is carried out. For more than two decades, the Mental Health Network of Gran Canaria (Spain) has been developing a program of care for family members of people with severe mental disorders (SMD), called the "Family Support and Collaboration Program" (FSCP. The Spanish acronym, PACF, will be used in the chapter). The PACF is described in the work entitled, "Guide of Family Intervention in Schizophrenia": Touriño et al. (2004/2007); Baena et al. (2022, in press). The family intervention to be presented has been developed over an extended period. The intervention will be described for the period 2019/2021. The case described corresponds to a patient attending a Psychosocial Rehabilitation Centre. The Network of Psychosocial Rehabilitation Centres (NPRC. The Spanish acronym, CDRPS, will be used in the chapter) of Gran Canaria is made up of 10 services that are distributed throughout the island's geographic area. The number of patients treated is 373. The population of Gran Canaria is 855,520 inhabitants. The family intervention has been carried out in different formats: Multi-family Intervention (MFI) Face-to-Face; Single Family Intervention (SFI); MFI Online. They are described below.

31.2.1 Face-to-Face Multi-family Format

In 1998, the initial design of the PACF was carried out. For this purpose, a detailed review of the literature available at that time on family intervention models and programs was carried out: Goldstein et al. (1978); Leff et al. (1982); Kuipers et al. (1992); Falloon (1985); Falloon et al. (1982, 1985); Falloon and Pederson (1985); Falloon et al. (1993); Anderson et al. (1986, 1988); Tarrier and Turpin (1992); Barrowclough and Tarrier (1992); Goldstein (1994); Tarrier and Barrowclough (1995); Barrowclough and Tarrier (1995); McFarlane et al. (1995a, b). Subsequently, the model of Bloch et al. (2009) was reviewed. As a result of this review, some aspects of each model were selected that seemed essential for integration into the PACF. These were:

- Of the Anderson et al. model (1986, 1988): Its basic objective in the intervention, which is to favour an adequate family environment and climate.
- Of the Kuipers et al. model (1992), the following was selected: Their use of the vulnerability-stress explanatory model identified by Zubin and Spring (1977) as the element that should frame the intervention, and its principles. (1) The basic principle of collaboration with the family. (2) The principle of considering family intervention as part of the overall treatment strategy.
- Of the McFarlane et al. model (1995a, b): Their specific strategies for intervention with multi-family groups.
- Of the Bloch et al. model (2009): The principle pointed out by this group concerning the personal involvement of professionals in certain pacts or agreements. For example, in the multi-family sessions of the current PACF dedicated to family self-care, the professionals also commit themselves to carry out a pleasant activity that they have not done for a long time.

A detailed review of the main components of family intervention and the greater or lesser relevance assigned to each component was also carried out. Twenty years of experience in working with groups of families made it advisable to reflect in depth on the initial structure of the PACF, its approach, its contents and even the generic titles of the modules developed.

One of the issues observed was that families were aware of their competences, strengths and difficulties and that, in general, they had knowledge and experience of the patient's illness and the nature of their relapses. It is therefore necessary for family intervention to be carried out in a context of collaboration and mutual support between family members and professionals, given that an excessive focus of family intervention on the psychoeducational component may make it less effective. For the team of authors, the aim of psychoeducation should not be to "provide information" but to "share information", along the lines of Harvey (2018). Professionals and family members report what they know. This change of focus meant that the first module, entitled "Psychoeducational Module", was renamed "Sharing Information". The multi-family intervention, both in its face-to-face format and via the Internet, includes contributions from the cognitive-behavioural model. Among them, it is worth mentioning the session specifically dedicated to intrusive thoughts, where a tour of the most frequent types of thoughts is carried out, exemplifying each one and offering final suggestions for their management. Modelling is used extensively, as well as activation control techniques such as progressive muscle relaxation, which are included in the sessions dedicated to family self-care. Coping and problem-solving techniques are central elements in the multi-family intervention program.

In the latest revision of the PACF, some strategies used in contextual therapies are incorporated into MFI. The work carried out by some of the authors of this chapter (Abelleira et al., 2021), where the applicability of these strategies was explored, contributed to this. This work also elaborated a proposal for the integration of Acceptance and Commitment Therapy (ACT) in multi-family intervention. Some of the contributions and studies reviewed were particularly useful for the elaboration of this integration proposal. These include: Wilson and Luciano (2002); Luciano and Valdivia (2006); Barraca (2007); Navarro et al. (2012).

From the ACT model, the mental illness of a person in whom their families have placed high expectations can generate a breakdown of values and a loss of personal projects for the family members. This can lead to their main objective being the avoidance of crisis situations and conflicts (Roldán et al. 2015). It was considered that the basic components identified by ACT (emotional acceptance, cognitive defusion, value-directed action, commitment) and the therapeutic strategies used in this model could be particularly useful and could be integrated into MFI without any difficulty. For the new MFI format, a set of videos related to contents developed in some sessions were selected, incorporating different strategies: metaphors, experiential exercises, self-care practices, mindfulness practice. These included: the fable of the harrier to illustrate the importance of trusting in the possibilities of any person in spite of their difficulties, the metaphor of the man in the hole, the metaphor of the passengers on the bus, the metaphor of the garden, the metaphor of the unwanted guest, the metaphor of the jar full of things, the experiential exercise for the construction of one's own tree of values, the 1-min meditation exercise, and the practice of progressive muscle relaxation. These strategies have been collected in some works and contributions made by the ACT model: Wilson and Luciano (2002); Barraca (2007); Luciano and Valdivia (2006); Roldán et al. (2015). The characteristics of the multi-family intervention carried out in a face-to-face format are described in Table 31.1.

31.2.2 Single Family Format

In Psychosocial Rehabilitation, attention to families in any of its variants (single-family or multi-family) is considered a key element integrated, like others, in the rehabilitation programs as a whole. However, the single-family intervention (SFI) in the framework of the PACF, usually has a more precise and conjunctural scope. Its objective is usually to overcome specific difficulties defined in the MFI. The

Table 31.1 Characteristics of the MFI in face-to-face format

Group type	Closed group. $N = 6–8$ families. The group of relatives is maintained throughout the MFI.
Patient participation	For consent and authorisation of the integration of their family into the group. In joint family and patient single-family sessions to address problems selected by the multi-family group in the third module on coping with problems.
Professionals	2 (main and support) who do not swap roles in the same session.
Means and equipment	Adequate meeting room with sufficient space. Semi-circular or circular position allowing full eye contact. Projection equipment and whiteboard for annotations.
Structure of sessions	In modules 1 and 2: Prior socialisation. Review of previous session. Description of the objectives of the session. Development of content. Final socialization.
Structure of sessions	In module 3: Previous socialization. Review of previous session. Round of problems. Choice of the problem. Round of proposed solutions. Choice of solutions. Implementation of selected solutions. Final socialization.
Sessions and timing	Module 1: 6 sessions. 1 session/week (possible extension). Module 2: 4 sessions. 1 session/month (possible extension). Module 3: 5 sessions. 1 session/bimonthly (possible extension). Duration of the MFI: 2 years (approximately).
Modules	*Module titles and session contents*
Module 1	"SHARING INFORMATION" Session 1: What is schizophrenia? Session 2: What are the causes of schizophrenia? Session 3: What to do about schizophrenia? Session 4: The family and schizophrenia. Session 5: What more can the family do? Session 6: Basic concerns of families. Current resources.
Module 2	"IMPROVING PATIENT COMMUNICATION AND FAMILY SELF-CARE" Session 1: Improving communication and conflict management. Session 2: Family tension and stress. Intrusive thoughts. Session 3: Attitudes and actions that favour self-care. Session 4: Attitudes and actions that favour self-care. Review of covenants.
Module 3	"SUPPORTING RECOVERY. IMPROVING COPING" No content is developed. Specific family problems are addressed.

indication for SFI is carefully considered during the course of the PACF, based on the observations of the different professionals involved in the case, and on the family's own evolution during the third Module. Also, and as a general rule, the criteria established by Dixon et al. (2000) for all forms of family intervention are considered. The problems susceptible to single-family intervention in the course of psychosocial rehabilitation are very diverse: imbalances in the distribution of roles and tasks, management of residual symptoms, resistance of the patient to take over certain responsibilities, rearrangement of the intra- and extra-familial environment after a relapse, development of strategies against warning signs, various expressions of stigma and social isolation, persistent communication problems that could not be addressed in the framework of the multi-family intervention or have been addressed with little success, development of study or work habits, generational conflicts.

Single-family interventions will never be aimed at forcing more or less improbable or arduous agreements, but at strengthening the consensus of family and patient on certain issues that tend to "get stuck" in their day-to-day realisation. Cognitive-behavioural model techniques are often particularly useful, for example, the use of therapeutic contracts is one of the most widely used. With respect to the formal structure of the single-family sessions, the recommendations of Anderson et al. (1986) are followed quite strictly, except that it has been considered preferable to clearly differentiate the selection of priority problems, the discussion of possible solutions and the assignment of tasks. Each session is structured in different sections or segments and is developed in approximately 90 min. The formal structure of the single-family sessions in the care setting of the CDRPS Network is as follows:

- Section 1: Opening and previous socialization (5 min).
- Section 2: Review of the tasks agreed with each family member (15 min).
- Section 3: Selection and definition of priority problems (20 min).
- Section 4: Choosing solutions (30 min).
- Section 5: Distribution and assignment of tasks (20 min).

31.2.3 Multi-family Format Through the Internet

In 2021, this new format of multi-family intervention via the Internet was designed and implemented in the CDRPS Network. The exceptional and changing circumstances during the COVID-19 period led to significant readjustments in face-to-face care activity. It was necessary to open a new avenue for family care. In view of this, family intervention via the Internet was presented as an appropriate intervention strategy to complement face-to-face attention. The patient's family, who had been participating in the face-to-face MFI that was suspended due to the health crisis, was offered to continue with the MFI via the Internet. The patient's family showed their willingness and interest to participate in both the design of the intervention and their integration into the group.

For the design of this new format, a detailed review of the literature and research on the subject was carried out beforehand. This helped to outline the criteria that should guide the new format. The review focused on these main areas:

- E-mental health interventions: Álvarez-Jiménez et al. (2012); Lal and Adair (2014); Mateu-Mateu and Navarro (2015); Williams et al. (2019); Coumoundouros et al. (2020).
- Components and quality criteria for e-mental health interventions: Kerr et al. (2006); Guay et al. (2017); Sin et al. (2019).
- Systematic reviews and controlled studies of networked interventions for caregivers: Onwumere et al. (2018); Ploeg et al. (2018); Sherifali et al. (2018); Spencer et al. (2019); Yu et al. (2020); Lobban et al. (2020); Sin et al. (2020).
- Networked interventions for caregivers focusing on the provision of psychoeducation, stress-burden reduction and family self-care: Rotondi et al. (2010); Hu et al. (2015); Soto-Pérez and Franco (2014); Chan et al. (2016); Honary et al. (2018); Vaughan et al. (2018); Fitriani and Suryadi (2019); Fuller et al. (2020).
- Networked interventions for caregivers with a therapeutic goal: Stjernswärd and Hansson (2018); Semonella et al. (2020); Biliunaite et al. (2021).
- Networking interventions for carers of patients with various pathologies: Kaltenbaugh et al. (2015); Zheng et al. (2016); Leng et al. (2020); Cherak et al. (2020).

31.2.3.1 Objectives of the MFI Through the Internet

Overall Objective

- Implement an intervention aimed at users' families via the Internet, complementary to face-to-face family attention, where this is not possible, or for situations where families are not available to maintain a continuous commitment to face-to-face MFI.

Specific Objectives

- Improving the quality of life and resilience of family members.
- Contribute to the overall acceptability and satisfaction of family members with MFI through the Internet.

31.2.3.2 Criteria Used for the Design and Implementation of the New Intervention Format

The main elements and criteria used in the design and implementation of the new format were:

- Analysis and valuation of some of the conclusions drawn in the studies and contributions made in the literature and in the field of research.
- Professional experience with family groups.

- Attention to the opinions of the participating relatives. With regard to this aspect, it was considered essential to involve the participating relatives from the beginning and to sound out their opinions on the elements and contents that should be included in the intervention and on other questions related to logistics. A short survey was developed asking relatives for their opinions on these seven areas: themes and contents, presentation of contents, technological supports and skills, preferred technological means, time and contact preferences, inclusion-exclusion of patients in sessions, privacy.

31.2.3.3 Description of the New Internet-Based MFI Format

Considering the majority preferences of the families on the contents and themes to be dealt with, an intervention program was designed, structured in five modules with a total of 16 sessions. In Table 31.2, the characteristics and structure of the program are provided, in terms of modules, content of sessions, timing and frequency of sessions.

Table 31.2 Internet-Based Multi-family Intervention Program

Modules	Module titles and session contents
Module 1	"Information sharing" Session 1: The disease. Concept and causes. Session 2: The disease and its treatment. Session 3: The impact of the disease on family members. Session 4: What the family can do. Session 5: Basic concerns and current resources.
Module 2	"Improving communication" Session 1: Communication and communication styles. Session 2: Factors that can hinder communication. Session 3: Suggestions for improving communication. Session 4: Suggestions for the control of intrusive thoughts.
Module 3	"Improving family self-care" Session 1: Attitudes and actions that promote self-care. Session 2: Putting self-care into practice.
Module 4	"Improving coping" Session 1: Common problems in daily life together. Session 2: Suggestions for managing conflicts and everyday problems.
Module 5	"Supporting recovery" Session 1: Confidence in recovery and hope for the future. Session 2: Autonomy and empowerment of users and family members. Session 3: Closing and final evaluation.
	Frequency and timing
	Frequency of sessions: 1/every 3 weeks (longer periods during holidays). Duration of sessions: 60 min (approximately). Duration of the program: 1 year.

31.3 Presentation of the Case and Evaluation

The following is the case of Samuel, a 33-year-old male diagnosed with paranoid schizophrenia who attends a Psychosocial Rehabilitation Centre and whose family was selected to participate in the Multi-family Intervention Programme. In order to present the case and for the purpose of clarity in the presentation, the steps taken in the evaluation prior to the integration of the family in the programme will be followed. The family evaluation carried out has not been uniform, neither in the evaluation criteria chosen nor in the instruments selected. The reason for this difference is related to the different family intervention formats that have been used. In the face-to-face MFI format, the standard evaluation was carried out, as outlined in the PACF (Touriño et al., 2010). This evaluation is carried out by means of:

31.3.1 Semi-structured Family Interview

31.3.1.1 Onset and Course of the Disorder. Symptoms and Functioning

With regard to Samuel, there is no clear reference to the onset of the disorder. It seems to have been progressive. According to his family, from the age of 12, they began to observe a marked social withdrawal accompanied by what they defined as a great sense of ridicule that hindered his social interactions. He also abandoned the sporting activities he had been doing up to that time and his relationships became progressively more limited, until he focused exclusively on his family. As a possible triggering factor, the family reports that, at that time, he was bullied at school. It was at the age of 15 that they consulted a private psychologist for the first time. His academic performance had dropped considerably and his isolation and social withdrawal persisted. In the following years, he saw several psychologists and psychiatrists in this field. At that time, he had an intense fear of going out alone in the street, with hypervigilant behaviour, constantly looking backwards. According to the family, he "heard noises" that prevented him from concentrating, which seemed to be elementary hallucinatory phenomena. However, despite the family's statements, the patient denied the psychic origin of these difficulties, always alleging external causes, for example: "the neighbours make a lot of noise". He also presented obsessive ruminations in relation to orthodontic procedures carried out at puberty (it has never been clear whether this experience coincided with the onset of the symptoms) which interfered with his daily life and generated irritability at specific moments in the family environment, especially with his father. However, what was most striking at that time was his significant personal impoverishment and great social withdrawal, with evident difficulties in reflection beyond the concrete and specifically in self-reflection, presenting great difficulty in describing any issue related to his "inner world", as well as a minimisation or denial of symptoms. Shortly before his 18th birthday, a diagnosis of psychotic disorder was established and treatment with low-dose antipsychotic medication was initiated. He passively accepted the treatment despite the fact that he was not aware of needing it or of its benefit.

The enormous difficulties in putting into words what was happening to him, talking about himself and carrying out any exercise involving personal reflection, meant that the psychotherapeutic intervention carried out at that time was seriously limited, as reflected by the professionals who were attending him at that time, and so referral to a psychosocial rehabilitation resource was indicated. In spite of all the difficulties mentioned, the family and the patient maintained their efforts to continue his studies, making various unsuccessful attempts, as his academic performance was very poor and generated great personal and family frustration. Finally, they accepted a referral to the public mental health network and a psychosocial rehabilitation service. He was then 23 years old. The referral report confirms the diagnosis of psychosis and highlights the poor capacity for introspection and a high degree of personal vagueness. The symptomatology present at that time was mainly negative: social withdrawal, affective blunting, abandonment of activities, difficulties in abstract thinking, poor social skills, lack of initiative, difficulties in decision-making, personal insecurity, vague and empty discourse, although formally adequate. Referral to a rehabilitation service was proposed with the aim of establishing routines and habits, improving socialization, increasing activities and adjusting expectations.

On reception at the CDRPS, this personal impoverishment was noted as the main limitation, together with a lack of awareness of the illness and a lack of ability to describe his symptoms, tending to minimise or deny them outright. His expectations for the future in the area of training and employment were unrealistic, with no plans other than studying for a university degree. Acceptance of the intervention at the centre was initially passive and he found it difficult to comply with the timetable. The family reported irritability and aggressiveness in the family environment. However, at the centre his behaviour was precisely the opposite: a passive acceptance of decisions without taking a position at any time with his own discourse.

He valued his relationships with other colleagues positively, despite frequent complaints from them about Samuel's invasive behaviour (multiple phone calls in the afternoon) or inappropriate jokes. These situations occurred in informal relationships. In organised activities, his behaviour was more passive and conformed to the established rules. After a few months of attendance at the centre, the parents reported some improvement, although they pointed out that in the afternoons, he remained unoccupied. They also reported episodes of irritability when contradicted. These episodes only occurred in the family environment, although they could be managed without major complications. Despite the fact that all the agents involved, patient, family and professionals agreed on these objectives, the changes did not materialise. Guidelines for action, therapeutic contracts, self-registers and other intervention techniques were established, but the patient showed passive resistance. At the age of 26, he expressed for the first time the presence of commanding voices, which urged him to carry out tasks and if he did not do them, "bad things" happened (he tripped, some plan was truncated). He acknowledged at that time that the voices had always been present to a greater or lesser extent. At the age of 28, and given the stagnation in his clinical evolution, an attempt was made to introduce Clozapine, but this was withdrawn after a month, as he could not tolerate the necessary control tests associated with this drug, presenting anticipatory anguish before the injections, which generated a worsening of his psychopathology at a general level. In terms of his current symptomatology, the clinical situation described remains unchanged.

The psychotic anguish he presents in relation to his firm conviction of the damage caused by his parents when they took him to the dentist for orthodontics constitutes the core of his distress. He constantly reproaches his parents for this, in any space in the home (including his parents' bedroom) and at any time (even in the early hours of the morning), even behaving in a disruptive and threatening manner. His constant demands and requests are not only made in the family sphere, but also with his closest colleagues at the CDRPS, who are constantly approached by means of insistent phone calls made by the patient at any time. This behaviour causes great overload and tension in others, which has led to complaints from these colleagues and even from their families to the professional team of the CDRPS, requesting their mediation so that the patient limits this behaviour. His clinical history includes several episodes of intensified psychotic distress accompanied by intense irritability and exacerbation of his delusions of harm, for which he was transferred to the emergency department of the referral hospital, where he remained under observation without the need for admission. During the period of home confinement caused by the COVID-19 health crisis, the patient presented an episode of the same characteristics, at which time his family contacted the CDRPS team. During this period, it was also recommended that hospital emergency services should not be used. By telephone, various interventions were carried out with the patient and his family, in coordination with the referring Mental Health Unit. This acute episode resolved without the patient having to be transferred to hospital.

31.3.1.2 General Family Information. Genogram and Life Cycle

Samuel lives with his parents (Matilde and Carmelo), both are 70 years old. Samuel is the youngest in a family of three siblings. His older sisters are independent. The family genogram is shown in Fig. 31.1.

In relation to the family, Matilde is the one who initially accompanied Samuel to consultations with professionals and who spent the most time with him (his father was working). At first, she held out hope of an improvement or cure, although she gradually accepted the possibility that it was a chronic problem. Her attitude was sympathetic and uncritical, with low expressed emotion.

Her son's situation produced in her an intense feeling of grief that translated into a difficulty in setting limits, accepting the maladjusted behaviour in a passive way. She gradually lost authority and was sometimes afraid when the patient became irritated or made insistent demands, tending to avoid conflict and accepting all her son's requests. Until retirement, the father had a more limited involvement in the patient's treatment, although from the information provided by the mother, it was

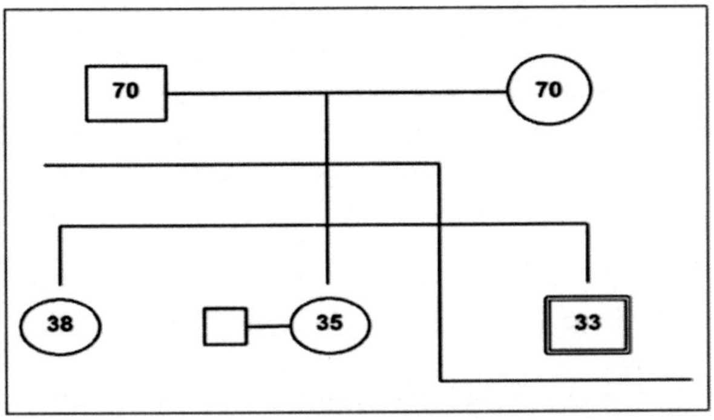

Fig. 31.1 Family genogram

difficult for him to accept the limitations and seriousness of the disease. In fact, when the patient was 21 years old, they asked for a second opinion, due to their perception that their son was not progressing adequately.

The professional consulted (psychiatrist) agreed with the referring professionals (psychologist and psychiatrist), recommending that he should be incorporated into a therapeutic environment such as a day hospital, which would allow some group activities to be carried out where he could work not only on social skills but also on the recognition of his difficulties. It was not until 2 years later that this recommendation was accepted by all. Initially, the patient's irritability and aggressiveness was directed almost exclusively at his father, who was the one who expected the most from him academically and socially. His father had a high level of expressed emotion (criticism). When the father joins the therapeutic process, the presence of unprocessed grief and his difficulties in managing his feelings about the loss become evident. The sisters, at the beginning of the illness, were a very important support by providing the patient with the possibility of leisure activities with their own groups of friends. However, this was progressively lost due to the difficulties in Samuel's social interaction and the ambivalent position of his sisters regarding the seriousness of the disease. His sisters also provided less support to Samuel as they progressively distanced themselves from the family due to their stage of life and their need for greater independence (due to their commitments and relationships). The parents' demands on the professionals have varied from the cure in the early stages to the current focus on improving coexistence, which was seriously complicated due to the patient's very demanding behaviour.

31.3.1.3 Family Communication Style

Frequent critical comments towards the patient, mainly paternal, were observed. This style hindered fluid communication with the patient.

31.3.1.4 Coping Strategies

Poor coping skills and competencies were observed. The patient's symptomatology and behaviours overwhelmed his family. Conflict avoidance and passive acceptance of Samuel's continuous requests were the coping strategies commonly used by his parents.

31.3.1.5 Family Psychopathological History

The parents reported that a paternal aunt had mental health problems, without being able to specify the psychotic nature of the disorder.

31.3.2 Standardised Evaluation

The load evaluation was carried out using the Zarit Scale (Zarit et al. 1980). This scale measures different dimensions: caregivers' quality of life, self-care capacity, social support network and caregivers' competences to cope with behavioural and clinical problems of the patient. It consists of 22 items with five response options. The total score (Minimum: 22. Maximum: 110) is assigned to one of the three levels assessed by the scale: intense overload, light overload or absence of burden. In the initial evaluation, after Samuel's integration in the CDRP, parents had high overload (Zarit = 87). In the subsequent evaluation prior to the face-to-face MFI, they maintained high overload (Zarit = 77). For the online MFI format initiated in 2021, the criteria that were to guide the new intervention format are modified. This decision followed a review of the literature on networked interventions for caregivers, and the lack of uniformity noted in some systematic reviews on the criteria and selection of key areas to measure as outcomes (Onwumere et al. 2018). It was felt, for example, that simply to evaluate the potential impact of the intervention on reducing potential family overburden was not sufficient. Family members do not experience or perceive the "burden of caregiving" in the same way. Some caregivers may even derive secondary benefits from caregiving (Bauer et al., 2013). For this reason, it was considered necessary to extend the evaluation to include a more global assessment of the "real situation" of the caregivers, which would allow us to investigate other areas such as: their psychological and physical well-being, family and couple relationships, relationship with the therapeutic team, social network and support from friends, and their perceived ability to overcome adversity and resilience. After a review of the available instruments, the following were selected:

- S-CGQol: Schizophrenia Caregiver Quality of Life Questionnaire (Richieri et al., 2011. Adapted).

- CD-RISC 21: Resilience Scale for Chronic Stress Situations (Crespo et al., 2014. Spanish adaptation-validation of the original version by Connor and Davidson (2003).

In Fig. 31.2, the overall results (%) of the quality of life evaluation (S-CGQoL), prior to the online MFI, are shown. The S-CGQoL instrument allows the evaluation of 7 dimensions related to the quality of life of caregivers of people with schizophrenia. These are: (1) psychological and physical well-being; (2) psychological burden and daily life; (3) relationship with partner; (4) relationship with therapeutic team; (5) relationship with family; (6) relationship with friends; (7) material burden. The valuation of the results indicated the following:

- The dimensions worst rated by both parents were: psychological-physical well-being and material burden.
- In the rest of the dimensions, some differences are observed between both parents, which may be justified by the different family tasks and roles, with the mother being the main caregiver.

In Fig. 31.3, the overall results (%) of the resilience evaluation (CD-RISC 21), prior to the online MFI, are shown. The CD-RISC 21 instrument assesses 4 factors related to resilience. These are: (1) coping skills; (2) ability to overcome and achieve goals; (3) positive appraisal of stressful situations; (4) relationships and self-confidence The valuation of the results indicated the following:

- In both parents, the factors: 2nd (ability to overcome/achievement of objectives) and 4th (relationships and self-confidence), are the best rated.
- In the first and third factors, partial differences are observed between both parents, with the mother showing a worse valuation of her coping skills and a more negative attitude towards stress.

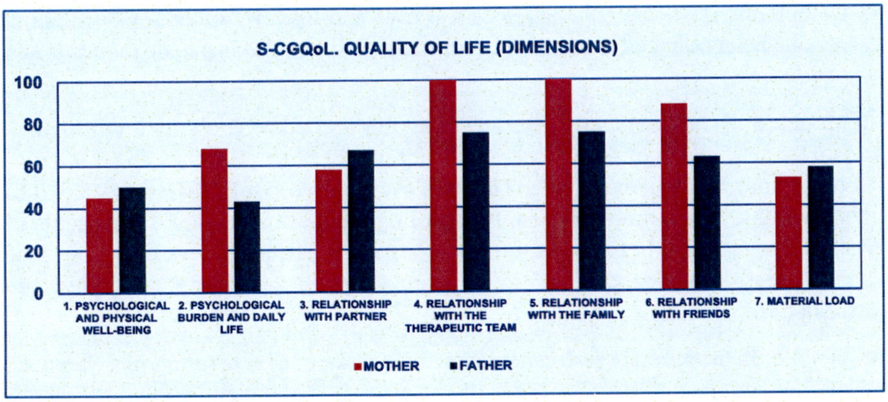

Fig. 31.2 S-CGQoL. Caregivers' Quality of Life questionnaire
Results of previous evaluation (%)

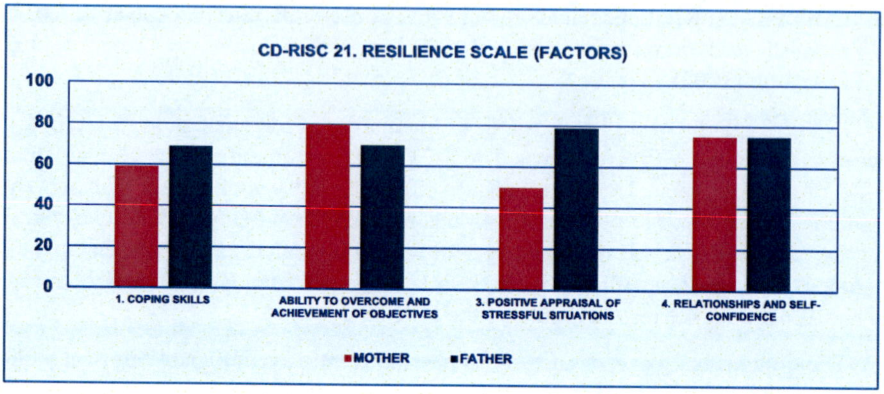

Fig. 31.3 CD-RISC 21. Resilience scale
Results of previous evaluation (%)

31.4 Interventions

The interventions carried out are described below.

31.4.1 Multi-family Intervention in Face-to-Face Format

The patient's family was selected to participate in a multi-family group that was to start at the CDRPS where their son was integrated. The clinical team selected this family according to the following criteria:

- Observed family difficulties in coping with the disease and patient behaviours.
- Presence of high family overload (Zarit Scale: $P = 77$).
- Complaints made by colleagues of the user and even by other relatives about certain behaviours of the patient (constant phone calls, insistent requests and petitions).

Matilde and Carmelo were informed of all this and asked about their willingness to join the new group of family members that was to begin. Both accepted the proposal without raising any doubts. The MFI was carried out from January 2019 to January 2021. Some central elements regarding the participation and comments of Matilde and Carmelo in the multi-family group are described below, throughout the different sessions and modules of the program, the main characteristics of which are described in Table 31.1.

1° Module: In the second session dedicated to the causes of schizophrenia, Samuel's mother commented that her older daughters had shown concern that their children, should they become pregnant, might be "just like their brother".

2° Module: In the third session dedicated to family self-care, Samuel's parents commented that it had been a long time since they had done any activity without the patient, due to the constant attention he required and his many phone calls, when they sometimes went out alone. Samuel's parents actively participated in the sessions by presenting the problems arising from living with their son. For this purpose, some of the problems were dramatised. For example, a situation related to the father's overload due to Samuel's continuous requests and demands was dramatised. The father was assigned the role of the patient and another father with low expressed emotion and an excellent relationship with his son was assigned the role of the affected parent. The group of relatives provided alternative solutions to those preferably used by the family (conflict avoidance and passive communication style), highlighting the need to be clearer and more assertive in their responses to the patient's requests and the need to remain calm and patient.

3° Module: In the first session, following the description of specific problems by the family members, the problem to be addressed was chosen. All the families unanimously selected the "multiple problem" raised by Matilde and Carmelo. No operational definition of the problem as a whole was made, given the multiplicity of elements it contained. And each of them was dealt with separately. The problem selected in this first session of the third Module contained the following elements:

- First Element: Current state of overload due to the patient's constant demands for attention and constant reproaches for the harm caused when he was taken to the dentist for orthodontics, and which the patient carries out in any space in the home (including his parents' bedroom) and at any time (including at night), even engaging in very disruptive behaviour with his mother (grabbing her violently by the arm or shaking her).
- Second Element: Excessive intake of cola drinks by the patient on a daily basis, and concern about the impact on his health.
- Third Element: Playing music and television at high volume, forcing his parents to retreat to other spaces in the house.

In the next phase of solution proposals, the rest of the family members suggested various strategies. After discussing the feasibility of the suggestions made by the group in the subsequent phase of choosing solutions, the family involved chose the following ones:

For the first element:

- In relation to overloading, the two solutions provided were: (1) That the parents (and above all Matilde) should engage in pleasant activities outside the home in the evening. (2) That Matilde did not have her mobile phone with her when she went out.
- In relation to complaints about orthodontic treatment, only one of the solutions provided, which was: To attend to him if he was observed to be distressed about this issue, but in the patient's room. The group of relatives

considered that such attention should consist of "accompanying and listening" to the patient, and that it was to be carried out by Carmelo and not Matilde, given Samuel's disruptive behaviour towards her.

For the second element (excessive intake of soft drinks):

- Impose economic restriction, justifying its decision on health grounds.

For the third element (loud music and television):

- Impose limits for reasons of cohabitation with parents and neighbours.

For the implementation of the solution strategies chosen for the 2nd (excessive intake of soft drinks) and 3rd (loud music and television) elements, a dramatization was performed. The mother involved and another assistant mother with low expressed emotion acted out a possible coping formula as a preliminary rehearsal. The firm and empathetic way in which the latter mother responds negatively to the patient's demand was helpful to Matilde. As an additional strategy and given the complexity of the problem due to its multiple elements and the need for patient collaboration, it was agreed in the group to transfer the problem to a single-family session with the family and patient, with the CDRP clinical team. On this point, it should be remembered that patients are not included in the multi-family sessions (See Table 31.1).

In the multi-family session, it was established that there was a need to:

- Inform Samuel that the problem raised by his family was chosen by the multi-family group.
- Gain the consent of Samuel for such an approach in a subsequent single-family session with the family and the patient.
- Gain the consent of Samuel for the covenants and agreements made in that joint session to be transferred back to the multi-family group.

In order to address the problem selected in the multi-family session described above, a subsequent single-family intervention was carried out jointly with the family and the patient. Beforehand, the following was carried out:

- To inform Samuel that in order to try to solve the problem raised by his parents in the family group, it was necessary for him to collaborate and give his consent. He showed a favourable disposition and agreed to carry out the interview.
- He also agreed that his therapeutic team at the mental health unit (MHU) should be informed.

It was felt that the time lapse from the multi-family session to the subsequent contact with the patient for consent to the joint interview and the conduct of the interview should not be extended. Therefore, it was set at 2 weeks after the multi-family session. In the subsequent joint family and patient interview, and in accordance with the requirements indicated for the single-family intervention carried out in the PACF (See Sect. 31.2.2), the following was carried out:

31.4.1.1 Dissection of the Problem

In this first part of the session, a detailed dissection of each of the elements of the problem was carried out. The patient's comments on each of these elements contributed to a better understanding and provided new data. They are as follows:

- Dental problem: The patient was not able to distinguish the exact reason for his discomfort. He acknowledged that when his parents took him to the dentist it was for his own good, but he also pointed out that when he thought about it, he was distressed because he thought he had been harmed.
- Excessive soft drink intake problem: The patient was able to admit that he had a very bad habit with it and that he sometimes travelled long distances to buy cans of soft drinks in the cheapest supermarkets, given the little money he usually had in his pocket. Finally, he reported (with the confirmation of his parents) that the total amount of liquids he drinks amounts to approximately 7–8 l per day (Soft drinks: 7 cans per day of 33 cl. Water: 3–4 bottles daily, of 1.5 l each).
- Problem of loud music: The patient recognised this behaviour. But he had not realised that it was so annoying for his parents that they even had to move to other areas of the house.

31.4.1.2 Problem-Solving and Implementation Strategies

- Dental problem: It was agreed that when he felt distressed about this issue, he should not go to his parents' room and that he should call his father (not his mother) to come to his room and talk to him. His father accepts such a strategy (coinciding with the one suggested in the multi-family group).
- Problem of excessive intake of soft drinks: Samuel was able to recognise that such behaviour could have serious health consequences, which were already manifesting themselves in some form in his overweight and dental deterioration. He showed some initial reluctance to propose not having any money as a solution but finally accepted it for these health reasons. It is specified: That he would not have any cash. That his mother would give him 1 can of soft drink (caffeine-free and sugar-free) every morning.
- Problem with loud music: It was agreed that he would use headphones (preferably) or earphones and in case of forgetting, his parents would remind him.

All these agreements were drafted in a therapeutic contract that included each of the elements of the problem and their solution strategies. The document was signed by all those attending the joint single-family session: Samuel, Matilde, Carmelo and CDRPS clinical team. Mechanisms were also established to monitor the evolution of the problem, its progress or possible difficulties. The CDRPS team offered its total availability to the family and patient to review or clarify any doubts or difficulties regarding the implementation of the agreed solution strategies as often as necessary. The agreements were:

- Family and patient accepted that the CDRPS clinical team would follow up on each of the agreements adopted, either in person with the patient and/or family (in consultation) or by telephone.
- A formal review was agreed after 3 months.

31.4.1.3 Return of Information to the Multi-family Group and Therapeutic Team of the MHU

Family and patient accepted that the agreements adopted in this joint session be passed on to the multi-family group and also to the referring MHU, given its central role in the patient's treatment and the need for it to be informed of the patient's evolution. As noted, (See Sect. 31.2.3), during the period of confinement due to the COVID-19 health crisis, the multi-family face-to-face intervention that had been taking place was suspended. Following this period, the patient restarted attending the CDRP. Likewise, the face-to-face MFI, which prior to the confinement was at the beginning of the third Module, is restarted. Some comments made by the patient's parents in the subsequent sessions and some observations by the clinical team are briefly described.

Second Session:

- In review of the previous session, the family recounts the difficulties they had during the period of confinement, related to the first element of the problem (orthodontic treatment): aggressive episodes, CDRP intervention, subsequent MHU intervention which finally indicated scheduled hospital admission (only one night).
- They also point out that the situation has now stabilised and that no new aggressive episodes have occurred.
- The family does not pay much attention to the other two elements of the problem, although they are adequately addressed.
- The rest of the family members reinforce that they have coped adequately with the problem.
- Some relatives especially emphasise the importance of the patient having reduced excessive intake of soft drinks.
- Professionals remind that coping strategies take time. A positive change in the father's critical communication style towards the patient is observed.

Third Session:

- The family reports that the situation remains stable and that there have been no new disruptive episodes or verbal threats.
- A substantial reduction in the level of emotion expressed by this family was observed, especially with regard to the usual critical comments towards the patient.

Fourth Session:

- Situation remains stabilised.
- The family reports that Samuel's requests related to his psychotic distress over the dental correction performed continue to occur on an occasional basis, but they also report that they are coping better.

31.4.2 Internet-Based Multi-family Intervention Format

The situation of the COVID-19 health crisis and domestic confinement were the origin of this new format of family intervention via the Internet. It was necessary to open a new way for the intervention that had been carried out in a face-to-face format. In Jan/2021, it was decided to tackle the design of the new format and its subsequent implementation in the CDRPS Network.

For the construction of the new design, it was considered necessary to involve family members in the process. This aspect has been recommended as a quality component associated with networked interventions for caregivers. In this regard, the contributions already cited by: Kerr et al. (2006); Guay et al. (2017); Sin et al. (2019). In addition, it is essential that family intervention (face-to-face or online) takes place in a context of collaboration and mutual support between family members and professionals. This aspect has been indicated in some works (Harvey, 2018). It was also necessary to adapt the support material used in the face-to-face MFI format that was being developed in the CDRPS network for this online MFI. Finally, an audiovisual support of 240 slides was developed, which covers a variety of contents.

The patient's parents are involved in the project and join a new online multi-family group held at the CDRPS that their son attends. The group is composed of 7 families and a total of 9 family members participate. The MFI via Internet starts in March/2021.

Tables 31.3 and 31.4 summarise some of the interventions and dynamics carried out in this new online MFI format, with regard to the participation and comments made by Samuel's family, extracted from the record of the following sessions:

Table 31.3 Family participation. Interventions and dynamics. Module 1. Session 3 (Impact of the illness on family members)

Patient's family participation: Observations	Interventions and dynamics
Mother: Following the development of content referring to the common feelings of the families in the face of the news of the diagnosis, the mother stresses the bewilderment it caused them.	It is highlighted that such confusion is very frequent and common in all families.
Father: After the development of content referring to the process and stages of grief, the patient's father reads the metaphor of the river and assesses its importance in the subsequent sharing with the group.	Samuel's father's appreciation of the importance of the metaphor and the message it symbolises is reinforced.

Table 31.4 Family participation. Interventions and dynamics. Module 2. Session 1 (The communication and communication styles)

Patient's family participation: Observations	Interventions and dynamics
Mother: In this session, secondary position with respect to the spouse who is the one who usually responds and participates.	Reads content on assertive communication style. Subsequent group discussion.
Father: Currently, he assesses the communication with the patient as adequate. He describes that the greatest difficulty is related to unidirectional communication, where the patient asks questions and requires answers, but does not respond when asked.	The adequate appreciation of the father is reinforced. Another mother in the group also points out that one-way communication is frequent and that her daughter does not usually respond either. Father also does content reading.

- Session 3 of Module 1, dedicated to the impact of the illness on family members.
- Session 1 of Module 2, dedicated to the communication and communicational styles.

31.5 Current Family and Patient Situation

The intervention was carried out over a period of approximately 2 years. During this time, multiple contacts were made both with the family and the patient jointly and individually. In the opinion of the team, this has been an important element in monitoring the case and the evolution of the family's coping strategies. The current situation of the case described below is offered as a balance of results. The results presented are not conclusive. They are based on clinical observation and some data from the evaluation carried out by the team of professionals involved in the case. They are broken down for the family and patient. Also presented is a summary of the last interview carried out, in which the opinions of Matilde, Carmelo and Samuel regarding the intervention carried out were explored.

31.5.1 Family

- *Current coping with the disease*: Favourable development. This has been influenced by the significant reduction of the patient's aggressive reactions and the parents' better knowledge that the psychotic distress experienced by their son and the aggressive reactions were related to his delusions and firm conviction of the damage caused by them when they took him to the dentist. In the present case, the information shared with the patient's relatives in the MFI has led to a change in their conception of the meaning of "psychotic distress". This has not reduced his state of overload, but it has contributed to a better coping with the illness.

- *Patient communication and family communication style*: Partially favourable development. On the one hand, parents have a negative perception of their communication with the patient. The greatest difficulty is related to what they call "one-way communication", where the patient asks questions and requires immediate answers, but does not respond when they ask him or try to communicate with him. On the other hand, there is a noticeable reduction in critical comments towards the patient (mainly from his father). The father's involvement in his son's therapeutic process has had a particular influence on this reduction in the level of emotion expressed.
- *Cognitive family restructuring*: In general, the observed development is favourable. This can be related to the diversity of strategies used for intervention in this area (psychoeducational, cognitive-behavioural, contextual strategies). It is therefore complex to assign the influence of each of them on the observed evolution. For example, in the face-to-face and Internet-based MFI, the importance of intrusive thoughts and how the continued presence of such thoughts can affect family competencies in coping with the disease is addressed. For this approach, suggestions are provided from a cognitive-behavioural approach, but also strategies from the ACT therapeutic model (metaphor of the unwanted guest or metaphor of the passengers on the bus) are used.
- *Influence of "group space"*: In multi-family groups, powerful synergies are established whose impact on families is often very positive. This has been recurrently pointed out in the literature. However, it is more complex to know the exact reasons for this impact. In evaluations of acceptability and satisfaction with family interventions, it is often noted how important it is for families to have a "group space" where they can share and express their concerns and worries with other families. However, this does not indicate exactly what the influence of the "group space" is. In the present case, it may have been influenced by: the involvement of the group of relatives in the resolution of the problem posed by the patient's parents, or the role-play rehearsals prior to the implementation of the strategies, or the comments made by other relatives about the importance of maintaining a calm attitude, or to see how another of the mothers participating in the group managed the illness and the daily life with her son and husband (both schizophrenics).
- *Emotional acceptance and coping with bereavement*: Favourable development. Observed in the decrease in family requests to the professional team, and in comments made in face-to-face and online multi-family sessions on the importance of accepting reality.
- *Adjusting family expectations*: Favourable development. The parents have lowered their expectations and are not worried or expectant about the patient's future at work, academically or emotionally. Currently, their basic concern is that the patient will be able to cope in life when they are absent.
- *Family self-care*: Parents have progressively improved their self-care and are incorporating "spaces of personal independence" into their lives where the patient is not included.

- *Family burden*: The family intervention has not contributed to reducing the family burden. Pre-evaluation (Zarit: 77) and post-evaluation (Zarit: 75) data are virtually unchanged. This may be related to several factors: lower energy and older age of parents, blurred intra-family boundaries, unsuccessful coping strategies in the past, very permissive family educational styles, little support from other family members (daughters). However, this is also in line with some outcome studies on the effectiveness of family interventions, indicating that such interventions are effective in reducing relapse rates and hospital readmissions, but have less impact on reducing family burden. In this regard: Pharoah et al. (2010); Sin and Norman (2013); Lyman et al. (2014).
- *Quality of life*: In Fig. 31.4, the overall results (%) of the subsequent quality of life evaluation (S-CGQoL) are shown. The comparative evaluation with the results of the previous evaluation (See Sect. 31.3) indicates that: The dimension of psychological-physical well-being is still the worst rated by both parents in the post-evaluation. The dimension "psychological burden and daily life" shows less favourable results in both parents with respect to the previous evaluation, however, the dimension "material burden" offers better results in the subsequent evaluation. The dimensions "relationship with the partner" and "relationship with the therapeutic team" show favourable results similar to the previous evaluation. In the rest of the dimensions, partial differences are maintained between both parents, with a worse evaluation of the father with respect to the previous evaluation of the dimensions, relationship with family and relationship with friends.
- *Resilience*: In Fig. 31.5, the overall results (%) of the subsequent resilience evaluation (CD-RISC 21) are shown. The comparative evaluation with the results of the pre-evaluation (See Sect. 31.3) indicates that: The subsequent evaluation of resilience in both parents offers less favourable results for all factors. For the team of authors, it is not possible to determine with precision the elements or

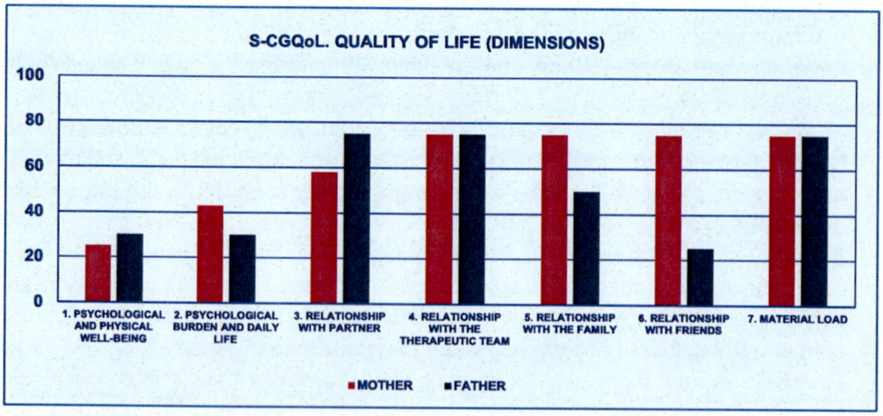

Fig. 31.4 S-CGQoL. Caregivers' Quality of Life questionnaire
Results of subsequent evaluation (%)

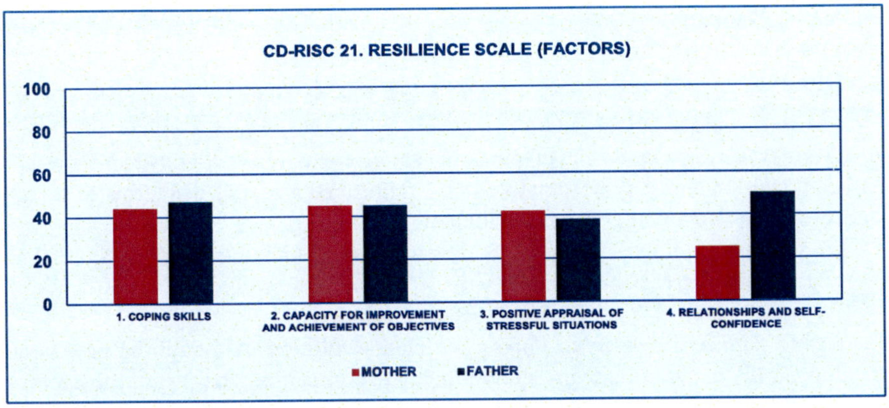

Fig. 31.5 CD-RISC 21. Resilience scale
Results of subsequent evaluation (%)

variables that may have influenced the worse results obtained in this area. It has been estimated that the impact of the COVID-19 period with regard to the increase in family contact time and the restrictions on being able to carry out activities outside the home, first totally (confinement) and then partially, may have had an influence. It has also been estimated that the high family burden and the advanced age of both parents may have had an influence. The ability of family members to cope with adversity may be weakened when energies wane due to the passage of time and the family burden has been and continues to be high. For the team of authors, it cannot be inferred either, that the family intervention carried out has contributed to worsening the resilience capacity of both parents.

- *Perspective and current family narrative on the intervention*: In the last follow-up interview, Samuel's parents make the following observations about the intervention carried out: (1) They consider that the professional support received has been adequate and sufficient. (2) As the main benefit they point out the decrease in Samuel's disruptive episodes. (3) They consider that the involvement of Samuel's father in the patient's recovery process has also been beneficial. Matilde refers to this as a greater "feeling" between the patient and his father. (4) They consider that the intervention has contributed to the improvement of their own self-care, being able to carry out specific activities where the patient is not included. (5) They point out that Samuel's requests and complaints related to his dental problem are still present, but that they are facing them from a position of greater understanding and "resignation". At this point, they point out that Samuel warns them and asks them beforehand if he can come to them at night if he is in distress. The parents replied in the affirmative.

31.5.2 Patient

- *Illness awareness*: Favourable development. The patient now recognises his illness and is able to talk about his symptoms, without minimising or denying them.
- *Changes in symptomatology*: Delusional activity remains very active and crystallised. Hallucinatory symptomatology has improved markedly, in terms of intensity and frequency of auditory hallucinations.
- *Behavioural changes*: Favourable development. Fundamentally, a significant reduction in aggressive episodes.
- *Communication with the family*: No clear evolution.
- *Coping with and managing illness*: No clear evolution. Although he now goes alone to his therapeutic team without being accompanied, the rest of the aspects related to his treatment (medication intake and dosage, acquisition of drugs) continue to be managed by the mother.
- *Autonomy and competences*: Partial improvement, but still requires support.
- *Functioning in daily activities*: No clear evolution. No domestic collaboration.
- *Social functioning*: Partial improvement is observed. Less demanding and insistent behaviour towards peers.
- *Perspective and current patient narrative on the intervention*: In the last follow-up interview, Samuel makes the following observations about the intervention carried out: (1) He considers that his complaints and requests to his parents about his dental problem must be stressful for them. (2) He believes that he and his parents understand the disease better nowadays. (3) He considers that the different interventions carried out (single-family, face-to-face multi-family, network multi-family) are adequate and that they are aimed at supporting him in his recovery process.

31.6 Conclusions

There are new times for family interventions that imply new challenges. These challenges, and along the lines of the present work, are also shaping a paradigm shift in the attention of family members of people with psychotic spectrum disorders. They are the following:

- Incorporate into family interventions, the techniques and strategies indicated by more comprehensive current models of attention to severe mental disorder (ACT, Open Dialogue, Dialectical-Behavioural Therapy), maintaining the general framework of these interventions in the model of community attention and person-centred recovery, in accordance with the current focus on user empowerment.
- Involve caregivers in family interventions, through their co-participation in the construction of new family intervention designs.

The main conclusions of the family intervention carried out, in this case, are as follows:

- The integration in the family intervention of an action on the main components of the ACT model (cognitive restructuring, emotional acceptance, value-directed action, commitment setting) and the use of techniques indicated by this model (metaphors, experiential exercises, mindfulness) has proved to be an appropriate strategy with beneficial repercussions, but whose real impact and effectiveness should be the subject of future research.
- It is difficult for a family member to cope with day-to-day problems if your communication or communication style with the patient is an obstacle to it. Family stress and overload add to this difficulty. Finally, the importance of family self-care, often forgotten or considered irrelevant by the relatives themselves, and not always encouraged by professionals. In the present case, the intervention carried out in these areas has meant a new form of "approach" and family conceptualization of the patient's psychotic experience and of their communication with the patient. Similarly, the implementation of commitments to improve self-care has been beneficial for parents.
- The family intervention carried out was not intended to turn the parents of the patient into "expert and effective problem solvers", but rather to provide them with strategies and tools that they could use to cope with daily coexistence, regardless of the speed or degree of success obtained in solving the problem. The temporal extension of the intervention allowed for a more adequate monitoring of the implementation of family coping strategies for the resolution of problems and conflicts in daily cohabitation.
- It is not possible to determine exactly what the possible benefits and repercussions of the family intervention have been for the patient. It can only be affirmed that the patient accepts and values positively the participation of his parents in the multi-family group.
- The participation of the patient's family in the construction of the new multi-family intervention format via the Internet has contributed to strengthening their commitment to the intervention and the link with the professionals involved.
- The use of the Internet-based multi-family intervention format has proved to be an appropriate intervention strategy to complement face-to-face multi-family intervention, but not to replace it. In the opinion of the authors, this should be considered by the assistance services.
- Careful selection of evaluation criteria and instruments, beyond simple indices of acceptability and family satisfaction with the intervention, is considered a key element.
- The evaluation of family satisfaction with the intervention has allowed a first approximation of its acceptability but does not indicate anything at all about its effectiveness. This will require future research studies and randomised controlled trials with control groups.

Disclaimer Clinical cases presented in this chapter do not include real names or personal information of real persons.

References

Abelleira, C., Baena, E., Sánchez, J. A., & Touriño, R. (2021). Integración de ACT en la Intervención Multifamiliar. In J. A. Díaz, H. Laffite, & R. Zúñiga (Coord.), *Terapia de Aceptación y Compromiso en Psicosis: Aceptación y Recuperación por Niveles (ART)* (pp. 287–309). Ed. Pirámide.

Álvarez-Jiménez, M., Gleeson, J. F., Bendall, S., Lederman, R., Wadley, G., Killackey, E., & McGorry, P. D. (2012). Internet-based interventions for psychosis: A sneak-peek into the future. *The Psychiatric Clinics of North America, 35*(3), 735–747. https://doi.org/10.1016/j.psc.2012.06.011

Alvarez-Jimenez, M., Alcazar-Corcoles, M. A., González-Blanch, C., Bendall, S., McGorry, P. D., & Gleeson, J. F. (2014). Online, social media and mobile technologies for psychosis treatment: A systematic review on novel user-led interventions. *Schizophrenia Research, 156*(1), 96–106. https://doi.org/10.1016/j.schres.2014.03.021

Anderson, C. M., Griffin, S., Rossi, A., Pagonis, I., Holder, D. P., & Treiber, R. (1986). A comparative study of the impact of education vs. process groups for families of patients with affective disorders. *Family Process, 25*(2), 185–205. https://doi.org/10.1111/j.1545-5300.1986.00185.x

Anderson, C., Reiss, D., & Hogarty, G. (1988). *Esquizofrenia y familia. Guía práctica de psicoeducación*. Amorrortu (original publication 1986).

Baena, E., Fernández, J. A., Sánchez, J. A. Touriño, R., Abelleira, C., Benítez, N., Álvarez, J., Giráldez, A., García, M., & Quintana, F. C. (2022, in press). *Guía de Intervención Familiar en la Esquizofrenia*. Federación Española de Asociaciones de Rehabilitación Psicosocial (FEARP).

Barraca, J. (2007). La terapia de aceptación y compromiso (ACT). Fundamentos, aplicación en el contexto clínico y áreas de desarrollo. *Miscelánea Comillas, 65*(127), 761–781.

Barrowclough, C., & Tarrier, N. (1992). *Families of schizophrenic patients: Cognitive behavioural intervention*. Chapman & Hall/CRC.

Barrowclough, C., & Tarrier, N. (1995). Intervenciones con las familias. In M. Birchwood & N. Tarrier (Eds.), *El tratamiento psicológico de la esquizofrenia* (pp. 69–99). Ariel.

Bauer, R., Sterzinger, L., Koepke, F., & Spiessl, H. (2013). Rewards of caregiving and coping strategies of caregivers of Patients with mental illness. *Psychiatric Services (Washington, D.C.), 64*(2), 185–188.

Biliunaite, I., Dumarkaite, A., Kazlauskas, E., Sanderman, R., & Andersson, G. (2021). ICBT program for improving informal caregiver well-being: A qualitative study. *Internet Interventions, 23*, 100361. https://doi.org/10.1016/j.invent.2021.100361

Bloch, G. R., Gronnestad, T., & Oxnevad, A. L. (2009). *Trabajo familiar y multifamiliar en las psicosis. Una guía para profesionales*. Herder.

Chan, S. K., Tse, S., Sit, H. L., Hui, C. L., Lee, E. H., Chang, W. C., & Chen, E. Y. (2016). Web-based psychoeducation program for caregivers of first-episode of psychosis: An experience of Chinese population in Hong Kong. *Frontiers in Psychology, 7*, 2006. https://doi.org/10.3389/fpsyg.2016.02006

Cherak, S. J., Rosgen, B. K., Amarbayan, M., Plotnikoff, K., Wollny, K., Stelfox, H. T., & Fiest, K. M. (2020). Impact of social media interventions and tools among informal caregivers of critically ill patients after patient admission to the intensive care unit: A scoping review. *PLoS One, 15*(9), e0238803. https://doi.org/10.1371/journal.pone.0238803

Coker, F., Williams, A., Hayes, L., Hamann, J., & Harvey, C. (2016). Exploring the needs of diverse consumers experiencing mental illness and their families through family psychoeducation. *Journal of Mental Health (Abingdon, England), 25*(3), 197–203. https://doi.org/10.3109/09638237.2015.1057323

Connor, K. M., & Davidson, J. R. (2003). Development of a new resilience scale: The Connor-Davidson Resilience Scale (CD-RISC). *Depression and Anxiety, 18*(2), 76–82. https://doi.org/10.1002/da.10113

Coumoundouros, C., von Essen, L., Sanderman, R., & Woodford, J. (2020). Implementation of e-mental health interventions for informal caregivers of adults with chronic diseases: A protocol for a mixed-methods systematic review with a qualitative comparative analysis. *BMJ Open, 10*(6), e035406. https://doi.org/10.1136/bmjopen-2019-035406

Crespo, M., Fernández-Lansac, V., & Soberón, C. (2014). Spanish version of the CD-RISC resilience scale for chronic stress situations. *Behavioral Psychology/Psicologia Conductual, 22*, 219–238.

Dixon, L. B., Adams, C., & Lucksted, A. (2000). Update on family psychoeducation for schizophrenia. *Schizophrenia Bulletin, 26*(1), 5–20. https://doi.org/10.1093/oxfordjournals.schbul.a033446

Dixon, L. B., McFarlane, W. R., Lefley, H., Lucksted, A., Cohen, M., Falloon, I., Mueser, K., Miklowitz, D., Solomon, P., & Sondheimer, D. (2001). Evidence-based practices for services to families of people with psychiatric disabilities. *Psychiatric Services, 52*(7), 903–910. https://doi.org/10.1176/appi.ps.52.7.903

Falloon, I. R. (1985). Behavioural family therapy. In J. Leff & C. Vaughn (Eds.), *Expressed emotion in families: Its significance for mental illness*. The Guilford Press.

Falloon, I. R., & Pederson, J. (1985). Family management in the prevention of morbidity of schizophrenia: The adjustment of the family unit. *The British Journal of Psychiatry: The Journal of Mental Science, 147*, 156–163. https://doi.org/10.1192/bjp.147.2.156

Falloon, I. R., Boyd, J. L., McGill, C. W., Razani, J., Moss, H. B., & Gilderman, A. M. (1982). Family management in the prevention of exacerbations of schizophrenia: A controlled study. *The New England Journal of Medicine, 306*(24), 1437–1440. https://doi.org/10.1056/NEJM198206173062401

Falloon, I. R., Boyd, J. L., McGill, C. W., Williamson, M., Razani, J., Moss, H. B., Gilderman, A. M., & Simpson, G. M. (1985). Family management in the prevention of morbidity of schizophrenia. Clinical outcome of a two-year longitudinal study. *Archives of General Psychiatry, 42*(9), 887–896. https://doi.org/10.1001/archpsyc.1985.01790320059008

Falloon, I. R., Laporta, M., Fadden, G., & Graham-Hole, V. (1993). *Managing stress in families: Cognitive and behavioural strategies for enhancing coping skills*. Routledge.

Fitriani, N., & Suryadi, I. (2019). A review study on online psycho-education for the bipolar disorder patient and their caregivers. *Humanities & Social Sciences Reviews, 6*, 84–89. https://doi.org/10.18510/hssr.2018.6210

Fuller-Tyszkiewicz, M., Richardson, B., Little, K., Teague, S., Hartley-Clark, L., Capic, T., Khor, S., Cummins, R. A., Olsson, C. A., & Hutchinson, D. (2020). Efficacy of a smartphone app intervention for reducing caregiver stress: Randomized controlled trial. *JMIR Mental Health, 7*(7), e17541. https://doi.org/10.2196/17541

Goldstein, M. J. (1994). Psychoeducational and family therapy in relapse prevention. *Acta Psychiatrica Scandinavica, 382*, 54–57. https://doi.org/10.1111/j.1600-0447.1994.tb05866.x

Goldstein, M. J., Rodnick, E. H., Evans, J. R., May, P. R., & Steinberg, M. R. (1978). Drug and family therapy in the aftercare of acute schizophrenics. *Archives of General Psychiatry, 35*(10), 1169–1177. https://doi.org/10.1001/archpsyc.1978.01770340019001

Guay, C., Auger, C., Demers, L., Mortenson, W. B., Miller, W. C., Gélinas-Bronsard, D., & Ahmed, S. (2017). Components and outcomes of internet-based interventions for caregivers of older adults: Systematic review. *Journal of Medical Internet Research, 19*(9), e313. https://doi.org/10.2196/jmir.7896

Harvey, C. (2018). Family psychoeducation for people living with schizophrenia and their families. *British Journal Psychiatric Advances, 24*(1), 9–19.

Harvey, C., & O'Hanlon, B. (2013). Family psycho-education for people with schizophrenia and other psychotic disorders and their families. *The Australian and New Zealand Journal of Psychiatry, 47*(6), 516–520. https://doi.org/10.1177/0004867413476754

Honary, M., Fisher, N. R., McNaney, R., & Lobban, F. (2018). A web-based intervention for relatives of people experiencing psychosis or bipolar disorder: Design study using a user-centered approach. *JMIR Mental Health, 5*(4), e11473. https://doi.org/10.2196/11473

Hu, C., Kung, S., Rummans, T. A., Clark, M. M., & Lapid, M. I. (2015). Reducing caregiver stress with internet-based interventions: A systematic review of open-label and randomized controlled trials. *Journal of the American Medical Informatics Association: JAMIA, 22*(e1), e194–e209. https://doi.org/10.1136/amiajnl-2014-002817

Kaltenbaugh, D. J., Klem, M. L., Hu, L., Turi, E., Haines, A. J., & Hagerty Lingler, J. (2015). Using web-based interventions to support caregivers of patients with cancer: A systematic review. *Oncology Nursing Forum, 42*(2), 156–164. https://doi.org/10.1188/15.ONF.156-164

Kerr, C., Murray, E., Stevenson, F., Gore, C., & Nazareth, I. (2006). Internet interventions for long-term conditions: Patient and caregiver quality criteria. *Journal of Medical Internet Research, 8*(3), e13. https://doi.org/10.2196/jmir.8.3.e13

Killaspy, H., Harvey, C., Brasier, C., Brophy, L., Ennals, P., Fletcher, J., & Hamilton, B. (2022). Community-based social interventions for people with severe mental illness: A systematic review and narrative synthesis of recent evidence. *World Psychiatry: Official Journal of the World Psychiatric Association (WPA), 21*(1), 96–123. https://doi.org/10.1002/wps.20940

Kuipers, L., Leff, J., & Lam, D. (1992). *Family work for schizophrenia: A practical guide*. Gaskell/Royal College of Psychiatrists.

Lal, S., & Adair, C. E. (2014). E-mental health: A rapid review of the literature. *Psychiatric Services (Washington, DC), 65*(1), 24–32. https://doi.org/10.1176/appi.ps.201300009

Leff, J. P., Kuipers, L., Berkowitz, R., Eberlein-Vries, R., & Sturgeon, D. (1982). A controlled trial of social intervention in the families of schizophrenic patients. *The British Journal of Psychiatry: the Journal of Mental Science, 141*, 121–134. https://doi.org/10.1192/bjp.141.2.121

Leng, M., Zhao, Y., Xiao, H., Li, C., & Wang, Z. (2020). Internet-based supportive interventions for family caregivers of people with dementia: Systematic review and meta-analysis. *Journal of Medical Internet Research, 22*(9), e19468. https://doi.org/10.2196/19468

Lobban, F., Postlethwaite, A., Glentworth, D., Pinfold, V., Wainwright, L., Dunn, G., Clancy, A., & Haddock, G. (2013). A systematic review of randomised controlled trials of interventions reporting outcomes for relatives of people with psychosis. *Clinical Psychology Review, 33*(3), 372–382. https://doi.org/10.1016/j.cpr.2012.12.004

Lobban, F., et al. (2020). Clinical effectiveness of a web-based peer-supported self-management intervention for relatives of people with psychosis or bipolar (REACT): Online, observer-blind, randomised controlled superiority trial. *BMC Psychiatry, 20*(1), 160. https://doi.org/10.1186/s12888-020-02545-9

Luciano, M. C., & Valdivia, M. S. (2006). La terapia de aceptación y compromiso (ACT). Fundamentos, características y evidencia. *Papeles del psicólogo, 27*(2), 79–79.

Lyman, D. R., Braude, L., George, P., Dougherty, R. H., Daniels, A. S., Ghose, S. S., & Delphin-Rittmon, M. E. (2014). Consumer and family psychoeducation: Assessing the evidence. *Psychiatric Services (Washington, DC), 65*(4), 416–428.

Maone, A., D'Avanzo, B., Russo, F., Esposito, R. M., Goldos, B. L., Antonucci, A., Ducci, G., & Narracci, A. (2021). Implementation of psychodynamic multifamily groups for severe mental illness: A recovery-oriented approach. *Frontiers in Psychiatry, 12*, 646925. https://doi.org/10.3389/fpsyt.2021.646925

Martín-Carrasco, M., Fernández-Catalina, P., Domínguez-Panchón, A. I., Gonçalves-Pereira, M., González-Fraile, E., Muñoz-Hermoso, P., Ballesteros, J., & EDUCA-III group. (2016). A randomized trial to assess the efficacy of a psychoeducational intervention on caregiver burden in schizophrenia. *European Psychiatry: The Journal of the Association of European Psychiatrists, 33*, 9–17. https://doi.org/10.1016/j.eurpsy.2016.01.003

Mateu-Mateu, J., & Navarro, N. (2015). Claves y evidencias del uso de las TIC en trastorno mental. *Psychology, Society, & Education, 7*, 85. https://doi.org/10.25115/psyev7i1.542

McFarlane, W. R., Link, B., Dushay, R., Marchal, J., & Crilly, J. (1995a). Psychoeducational multiple family groups: Four-year relapse outcome in schizophrenia. *Family Process, 34*(2), 127–144. https://doi.org/10.1111/j.1545-5300.1995.00127.x

McFarlane, W. R., Lukens, E., Link, B., Dushay, R., Deakins, S. A., Newmark, M., Dunne, E. J., Horen, B., & Toran, J. (1995b). Multiple-family groups and psychoeducation in the treatment of schizophrenia. *Archives of General Psychiatry, 52*(8), 679–687. https://doi.org/10.1001/archpsyc.1995.03950200069016

Navarro, N., Martín-Murcia, F., & Carmona-Torres, J. (2012). Posibilidades de la terapia de aceptación y compromiso en la intervención familiar en esquizofrenia. 13° Congreso Virtual de Psiquiatria.com. *Interpsiquis*. https://www.researchgate.net/publication/233951838

Onwumere, J., Amaral, F., & Valmaggia, L. R. (2018). Digital technology for caregivers of people with psychosis: Systematic review. *JMIR Mental Health, 5*(3), e55. https://doi.org/10.2196/mental.9857

Pharoah, F., Mari, J., Rathbone, J., & Wong, W. (2010). Family intervention for schizophrenia. *The Cochrane Database of Systematic Reviews, 12*, CD000088.

Ploeg, J., Ali, M. U., Markle-Reid, M., Valaitis, R., Bartholomew, A., Fitzpatrick-Lewis, D., McAiney, C., & Sherifali, D. (2018). Caregiver-focused, web-based interventions: Systematic review and meta-analysis (Part 2). *Journal of Medical Internet Research, 20*(10), e11247. https://doi.org/10.2196/11247

Richieri, R., Boyer, L., Reine, G., Loundou, A., Auquier, P., Lançon, C., & Simeoni, M. C. (2011). The Schizophrenia Caregiver Quality of Life questionnaire (S-CGQoL): Development and validation of an instrument to measure quality of life of caregivers of individuals with schizophrenia. *Schizophrenia Research, 126*(1–3), 192–201. https://doi.org/10.1016/j.schres.2010.08.037

Roldán, G. M., Salazar, I. C., Garrido, L., & Cuevas-Toro, A. M. (2015). Intervención psicológica grupal, basada en la aceptación y el entrenamiento en comunicación, con familiares de personas con trastorno mental grave. *Anales de Psicología, 31*(3), 759–772.

Rotondi, A. J., Anderson, C. M., Haas, G. L., Eack, S. M., Spring, M. B., Ganguli, R., Newhill, C., & Rosenstock, J. (2010). Web-based psychoeducational intervention for persons with schizophrenia and their supporters: One-year outcomes. *Psychiatric Services, 61*(11), 1099–1105. https://doi.org/10.1176/ps.2010.61.11.1099

Semonella, M., Vilchinsky, N., Dakel, R., Biliunaite, I., Pietrabissa, G., & Andersson, G. (2020). *SOSteniamoci: An internet-based intervention to support informal caregivers*. PSYCHOBIT. Second symposium on psychology-based technologies.

Sherifali, D., Ali, M. U., Ploeg, J., Markle-Reid, M., Valaitis, R., Bartholomew, A., Fitzpatrick-Lewis, D., & McAiney, C. (2018). Impact of internet-based interventions on caregiver mental health: Systematic review and meta-analysis. *Journal of Medical Internet Research, 20*(7), e10668. https://doi.org/10.2196/10668

Sin, J., & Norman, I. (2013). Psychoeducational interventions for family members of people with schizophrenia: A mixed-method systematic review. *The Journal of Clinical Psychiatry, 74*(12), e1145–e1162. https://doi.org/10.4088/JCP.12r08308

Sin, J., Henderson, C., Woodham, L., Sesé, A., & Gillard, S. (2019). A multicomponent eHealth intervention for family carers for people affected by psychosis: A coproduced design and build study. *Journal of Medical Internet Research., 21*, e14374. https://doi.org/10.2196/14374

Sin, J., Henderson, C., Cornelius, V., Chen, T., Elkes, J., Woodham, L., Sesé, A., Spence-Polin, D., Batchelor, R., & Gillard, S. (2020). COPe-support- A multi-component digital intervention for family carers for people affected by psychosis: Study protocol for a randomized controlled trial. *BMC Psychiatry, 20*. https://doi.org/10.1186/s12888-020-02528-w

Soto-Pérez, F., & Franco, M. (2014). PsicoED: Una alternativa online y comunitaria para la psicoeducación en esquizofrenia. *Psicoperspectivas, 13*(3), 118–129. https://doi.org/10.5027/psicoperspectivas-Vol13-Issue3-fulltext-416

Spencer, L., Potterton, R., Allen, K., Musiat, P., & Schmidt, U. (2019). Internet-based interventions for carers of individuals with psychiatric disorders, neurological disorders, or brain injuries: Systematic review. *Journal of Medical Internet Research, 21*(7), e10876. https://doi.org/10.2196/10876

Stjernswärd, S., & Hansson, L. (2018). Effectiveness and usability of a web-based mindfulness intervention for caregivers of people with mental or somatic illness. A randomized controlled trial. *Internet Interventions, 12*, 46–56. https://doi.org/10.1016/j.invent.2018.03.004

Tarrier, N., & Barrowclough, C. (1995). Family interventions in schizophrenia and their long-term outcomes. *International Journal of Mental Health, 24*(3), 38–53. https://doi.org/10.1080/00207411.1995.11449318

Tarrier, N., & Turpin, G. (1992). Psychosocial factors, arousal and schizophrenic relapse: The psychophysiological data. *British Journal of Psychiatry, 161*(1), 3–11. https://doi.org/10.1192/bjp.161.1.3

Touriño, R., Inglott, R., Baena, E., & Fernández, J. (2004/2007). *Guía de Intervención Familiar en la Esquizofrenia*. Editorial Glosa.

Touriño, R., Baena, E., Benítez, N., Abelleira, C., & Fernández, J. A. (2010). Evaluación familiar en Rehabilitación Psicosocial. In J. A. Fernández, R. Touriño, N. Benítez, & C. Abelleira (Eds.), *Evaluación en Rehabilitación Psicosocial* (pp. 125–134). FEARP.

Vaughan, C., Trail, T. E., Mahmud, A., Dellva, S., Tanielian, T., & Friedman, E. (2018). Informal caregivers' experiences and perceptions of a web-based peer support network: Mixed-methods study. *Journal of Medical Internet Research, 20*(8), e257. https://doi.org/10.2196/jmir.9895

Williams, A., Farhall, J., Fossey, E., & Thomas, N. (2019). Internet-based interventions to support recovery and self-management: A scoping review of their use by mental health service users and providers together. *BMC Psychiatry, 19*(1), 191. https://doi.org/10.1186/s12888-019-2153-0

Wilson, K. G., & Luciano, C. (2002). *Terapia de aceptación y compromiso. Un tratamiento conductual orientado a los valores*. Ed. Pirámide.

Yu, Y., Li, T., Xi, S., Li, Y., Xiao, X., Yang, M., Ge, X., Xiao, S., & Tebes, J. (2020). Assessing a WeChat-based integrative family intervention (WIFI) for schizophrenia: Protocol for a stepped-wedge cluster randomized trial. *JMIR Research Protocols, 9*(8), e18538. https://doi.org/10.2196/18538

Zarit, S. H., Reever, K. E., & Bach-Peterson, J. (1980). Relatives of the impaired elderly: Correlates of feelings of burden. *The Gerontologist, 20*(6), 649–655. https://doi.org/10.1093/geront/20.6.649

Zheng, Y., Head, B. A., & Schapmire, T. J. (2016). A systematic review of telehealth in palliative care: Caregiver outcomes. *Telemedicine Journal and e-Health: The Official Journal of the American Telemedicine Association, 22*(4), 288–294. https://doi.org/10.1089/tmj.2015.0090

Zubin, J., & Spring, B. (1977). Vulnerability: A new view of schizophrenia. *Journal of Abnormal Psychology, 86*(2), 103–126. https://doi.org/10.1037/0021-843x.86.2.103

Chapter 32
The Transformative Power of the Open Dialogue Approach in the Mental Health Field

Teresa Abad-Sierra and Sara Toledano-Márquez

32.1 Introduction

In recent years, there has been a resurgence around the world of movements of service users and psychiatrized persons demanding a different type of care and requesting—among other issues—the introduction of social factors and material living conditions in mental health analysis and treatment.

Recently, relevant events such as the global pandemic caused by COVID-19 have shown that the context has a determining influence on our lives and that anyone can have mental health problems. However, the organization of mental health care is based on an individualistic conception of the phenomena it deals with. In the framework of the public care system, mental suffering is still considered as something exceptional that happens only to some people, which must be treated by experts in places intended for this purpose (hospitals and mental health centers), using specific techniques and products (drugs, psychotherapy, rehabilitation), with the support of policies focused on the number of professionals and care infrastructures, and under the protection of laws that support the idea of exceptionality, which is a decrease of rights and increase of abuses (Rotelli, 2015).

For our part, as therapists, we still find it difficult, at least in practice, to abandon the individualistic perspective to which most schools of psychology adhere. The idealistic and subjectivist legacies on which our discipline rests connect well with current neoliberal thinking and lead us to study people in an isolated and abstract way, disconnected from the concrete situations of their lives. Experience shows that these conceptions produce practices that chronify people who come to services for help, especially those who present what we consider to be severe symptoms, and turn them into indefinite consumers of drugs and resources.

T. Abad-Sierra (✉) · S. Toledano-Márquez
Fundación Manantial, Madrid, Spain
e-mail: tabad@fundacionmanantial.org; stoledano@fundacionmanantial.org

J. A. Díaz-Garrido et al. (eds.), *Psychological Interventions for Psychosis*,
https://doi.org/10.1007/978-3-031-27003-1_32

This chapter aims to provide a situated perspective of Open Dialogue, the approach with the best results in the world in the treatment of people going through moments of intense psychic suffering. In our opinion, the Open Dialogue approach provides some clues that we can follow to imagine other ways of dealing with mental suffering.

Through Open Dialogue, we want to draw attention to the urgency of integrating the context in its material dimension in our professional practice and to deepen the need to adopt a crisis perspective in the care models we develop. With this in mind, we are going to share reflections on some of the characteristics of the approach that we believe are very useful when thinking about possible futures. To this end, we will focus on:

- The importance of Open Dialogue as an approach and not as a theoretical model.
- The work it does with the context on a material and linguistic level.
- The crisis perspective it maintains in understanding the discomfort of people seeking help.

32.2 Open Dialogue as an Approach

Each theoretical model in the field of mental health expresses a position in the world, a way of understanding and relating to human problems. That is why no theory, hypothesis, or therapeutic proposal lacks ideology. Since in our profession there is an unavoidable link between the interpretation we give to phenomena and the way we intervene on them, we can say that ideology permeates therapeutic practice.

Ideology is understood as the set of fundamental ideas that underpin the thinking of a person, group, or culture. An ideology is composed by a system of practices, relationships, and discourses that can acquire a dominant character at a given moment. All the aspects that make up the field of mental health—the hegemonic scientific paradigm, professionals, techniques, policies, laws, the industry and the structures and facilities intended for care—are determined by and coherently related to the ideology that sustains them at a given time, and materialize that ideology in practice.

However, the fact that one configuration acquires a dominant character at a given moment does not mean that it is the only one. Simultaneously, in the same social system, other ideas, other positions, and other practices coexist.

In the face of complex phenomena such as mental health problems, different approaches can be adopted, or, in other words, different viewpoints through which to analyze and observe them. For example, when speaking of psychic suffering, we can adopt a biological approach that looks at how organic processes influence emotional-cognitive states and what kind of actions modulate their effect. Or we can adopt a cross-cultural approach that studies the same phenomenon by observing the influence of different cultures on the understanding of these problems and the way they manifest themselves.

In contrast to an approach, the theoretical model is an abstract mental representation for understanding the structure and functioning of a phenomenon that it is intended to represent accurately. Theoretical models include hypotheses of the causes and functioning of phenomena with the intention of making predictions. "Psy" models attempt to establish the causes of individuals' behaviors in order to predict future behaviors. The model is a conceptual development that seeks to fit the facts.

What we find interesting about Open Dialogue is that it is not a theoretical model of mental health problems, but an approach, a phenomenological look at what happens in terms of material, linguistic, and relational contexts. It is not concerned with causes nor does it pretend to make predictions. Its theoretical and practical development remains open-ended, alive. It does not dispute the truth in the explanation of what happens when we go through situations of intense suffering, but focuses on establishing contexts that facilitate dialogues that leave room for the possibility of integrating multiple perspectives. It does not propose hypotheses about what happens or has happened to people who seek help, but leaves the meanings open to the construction that can be made by those who participate in the treatment meetings in each encounter. By focusing on contexts, the question that guides the exploration is not why what is happening is happening, but what it is in response to.

The origin of Open Dialogue dates back to the 1980s, when a group of mental health professionals working in the Finnish region of Western Lapland dared to organize the entire public care system in a way that was radically different from how it continues to be organized today in most countries of the developed world. This reorganization unfolded in a way that was consistent with the results they were obtaining from the research they were doing on their own practice. Research to theorize about the factors that proved to work, rather than developing a theoretical framework to apply, is a major feature of the approach and is a major departure from the usual way of proceeding in psychotherapy. In this way, it is theorized what is shown to be useful in practice.

From the research, they identified seven fundamental principles of the approach which are the factors that were present in all the success stories. On the one hand, these principles allude to the organization of the treatment and, on the other hand, to the dialogic process that is stimulated in the encounters with the social network. The principles are as follows[1]:

- Immediate help
- Flexibility and mobility
- Working from a social network perspective
- Assuming responsibility
- Ensuring psychological continuity

[1]A comprehensive description of the seven principles of Open Dialogue can be found in Seikkula and Olson (2003), Seikkula and Arnkil (2016), and Abad and Toledano (2019).

- Tolerance of insecurity
- Dialogism

These principles are neither a therapeutic model nor an intervention methodology with phases and tools. They are a system of contextual rules and procedural factors that have proven to be effective in facilitating crisis resolution.

Within the context they promote, therapists focus on what is relevant to the social network and adapt, through the course of conversation, to their own language. This implies an ethical attitude of recognizing the other as other and unconditionally accepting and respecting their experience without trying to change it (Galbusera & Kyselo, 2017).

32.3 Working with the Context in Open Dialogue

Context is the material, social, cultural, and/or political environment in which a fact is considered. It is also the linguistic environment on which depends the meaning of a statement. Likewise, context is considered to be the composition or content of a story and the entanglement or union of things that are linked and interwoven (Real Academia Española de la Lengua[2]).

The peculiarity of working with the context from Open Dialogue approach has to do with the fact that it takes the material and linguistic dimensions of the context to intervene directly on them. Thus, Open Dialogue:

- *Intervenes on material contextual aspects* that had not been taken into account in other models, such as the places where to meet, the people who can be involved in the treatment, and other elements of the setting included in the seven principles.
- *Intervene on linguistic aspects* through professionals themselves, who are part of the context. They listen, speak, and respond in a specific way to facilitate the emergence of dialogues.

In Open Dialogue, context is considered a basic element in the understanding of psychic suffering and a main factor in dealing with crisis situations.

The purpose of intervention is not behavioral, intrapsychic, or relational change of the people consulting. The work of therapists in this approach consists in ensuring that certain contextual conditions—material and linguistic—are present in treatment meetings, so that the emergence of dialogues is possible. It will be the dialogues themselves that will generate intersubjective and intrapsychic changes in all the participants of the meeting, including the professionals. This way of intervening requires a radical trust in people's capacity to develop their own personal resources in the contextual conditions proposed.

[2]Translator's note (TN): Real Academia de la Lengua Española dictionary is the official in the Spanish Language

The role of professionals is to ensure that certain material contextual conditions are met and to develop a particular way of listening, responding, and speaking.

Let's take a closer look at the material and linguistic dimensions of the context in which Open Dialogue intervenes.

32.3.1 *Working with the Material Dimension of the Context*

By the material dimension of the context in Open Dialogue, we refer to the aspects of treatment organization that have to do with the physical environment, which is embedded in the seven principles of the approach. This is the case of flexibility and mobility of the team, the work with the social network, or responsibility and psychological continuity. These principles are related to the meeting places, the people called to participate in the meetings, the specific way of contacting the team, and the professional follow-up over time.

The organization of treatment in Open Dialogue is based on the availability and flexibility of a non-hierarchical professional team. In what would be the equivalent of mental health centers, they have a telephone open 24 h a day, which anyone can call. When someone calls, they are attended by a professional from the team, who asks where they would like to be attended and what other people would be interesting or important for them to attend the meeting. In this way, meetings of two or three members of the therapeutic team are convened with the person in crisis, his relatives, and other important people in his social network, who meet in the place that has been thought to be the most accessible or most comfortable for them, generally their own home. The first meeting also means the constitution of what is called the "treatment system," which is made up of the professionals who have attended, the person in crisis, and his or her social network. From that moment on, all treatment decisions—from the taking of drugs, to the indication of individual and/or family psychotherapy, or referral to other resources—are made at the meetings held by the system. At the beginning, the meetings may be daily, until the crisis situation subsides and may be spaced out over time. In this way, people are attended from the beginning in their own context and admission to a psychiatric ward in a crisis situation is no longer the first option (Abad & Toledano, 2019).

The proposals of different perspectives in psychotherapy are usually based on theoretical elaborations that guide clinicians in their practice when establishing hypotheses, interpreting what happens to patients, providing therapeutic tools and strategies, or establishing languages with which to shape realities and experiences. They are proposals for intervention on what happens in the encounter between therapist and patient. Aspects of the setting such as the place where therapy takes place, the therapist's agenda as a point of reference for setting appointments, the establishment of a certain frequency of sessions, or referral to other professionals when certain problems arise are not usually the object of theorization or direct professional intervention.

Open Dialogue intervenes precisely on this material dimension of the context. What it proposes is a restructuring of the way in which we professionals organize ourselves and our assistance.

These organizational aspects are fundamental, since they determine the structure of the discursive situation and the internal orientation of the speaker. That is, both the meaning of what is said and the mental context of the speaker in a given situation depend on the physical, material context in which utterances are produced. Thus, the way in which the material contexts of treatment are organized determines the possible conversations.

A statement is always directed to a listener and, therefore, does not have a unique meaning, but is related to the concrete circumstances of its enunciation, which point to the sociohistorical and material context in which the discursive communication is carried out.

The construction of meaning happens not as a static process that is established once and for ever on, but is something in continuous transformation and movement. The speaker's context-dependent internal structure is a process always open to the influences of the present. In its speech, the speaker constructs its words according to its bodily emotional situation, which is directly affected by the immediate environment (Bakhtin, 1986). All contextual details present become internal parts of the speaker, which may change with each new response he receives.

Therefore, a conversation in different social contexts generates different meanings. Even if the same type of conversation takes place with the same participants, if the material context is different, the conversation will be different as well. Each conversation creates its own social language, which is not a firmly established and static code, but is carried out differently compared to previous conversations. Meanings emerge with new nuances in each concrete interaction.

As we explained elsewhere (Abad & Toledano, 2019), when a person goes to a health center, a consultation, or a hospital ward, they receive some messages from the context itself, such as that they are a sick person, for example, or that they should put themselves in the hands of experts to solve their situation. The fact of caring for people in these places also makes it difficult for professionals to step outside the roles imposed by the context (role of expert who has to solve the situation of the patient who comes for help) and can be an obstacle to the participation of other people in the social network besides the family, who are often excluded from the places of professional intervention. The material context has a very decisive influence on the relationships between the actors involved and the possibilities for dialogue.

The way treatment is organized provides the fundamental structure for the co-creation. Moment by moment, in the encounter with the people of the social network that requested help, new relational and intrapsychic contexts that will emerge as people make progress in their dialogues.

As we have pointed out above, the material organization of the treatment is based on the results of research on the practice itself and is consistent with essential aspects of Bakhtin's dialogism, which is part of the epistemological basis of the approach.

Following the Bakhtinian proposal, it is understood that relationships that constitute us from the beginning of life take place in historically determined material contexts. The objective conditions of life are the pillars on which we build our discourses and our universes of meaning (Ponzio, 1998).

Open Dialogue seeks to leave our classic and known contexts and establishes, through research, that this change operated by professionals on the material context is one of the keys to the success of the treatment.

32.3.2 *Intervention in the Linguistic Dimension of the Context*

Classical communication models conceive communication as an exchange of messages between a sender and a receiver. The meaning and purpose of what is said is located in the content of the individual messages.

In contrast to this conception, dialogic communication is understood as an interactive, generative process through which people create, maintain, negotiate, and transform their social realities. There is no pre-established meaning in language, but rather a meaning that emerges in a given context. The meaning and purpose of language is ongoing and the focus is on the dialogical process.

Language, therefore, is understood not only as a system of signs, but also as a material reality that supports certain ideological values (Hernández, 2011). Language is not only an instrument for the transmission of already configured experiences, but also an instrument for the constitution of individual and collective experiences and mental processes that are, at the same time, social. The grammatical rules of a language arise from specific historical contexts and determine the way in which speakers can reproduce social discourse and relate to it (Hernández, 2011).

If, as we have pointed out, the meanings of things are not something static, but can change depending on the people who emit them and the context in which they are found, what we call reality is not something that pre-exists us, but something that is created, that is continually being constructed through the interactions we have with others.

For Open Dialogue, it is fundamental to take into account this condition of participation of individuals in the construction of social reality and to work so that all voices are heard. The members of a social network, or of a community, can only feel that they belong to the shared reality of that community if they are treated as legitimate participants in its authorship, when they are not excluded from it in one way or another. For only then will they feel that the reality in which they live is theirs as well as everyone else's (Shotter, 1994).

Therapists in Open Dialogue consider themselves part of the treatment context, on the same level as the other participants and features that make up the meeting settings. The intervention on the linguistic context has to do with the change that therapists operate on their own ways of listening, speaking, and responding to facilitate dialogues to take place. It is useful to review dialogic epistemology and review what dialogue means to understand how they do this.

32.3.3 Dialogism

We call dialogue a particular kind of conversation in which participants engage in processes of understanding and learning about how others make sense of something and what it means to each other (Anderson, 2012). Through this process, new understandings and meanings emerge as a result of shared inquiry.

Working with a dialogic methodology implies that the therapists' task is not to make sense of what happens from their own frames of reference, but to prioritize the perspectives of the people they serve. The most important thing is to learn more about people's experiences and the way they understand them.

In order to do this, attentive and respectful listening must be developed, without preconceived ideas about what is important to talk about or how to talk about it. In this act of open, non-interpretative listening, the therapist may make comments or ask questions aimed at clarifying understanding. There are no interpretations of what is heard or veiled assumptions. The questions are not tools to introduce information, propose a new meaning, or pass judgment on what is said. All the expressions of therapists working from this approach are an attempt to better understand people from their own points of view and not to misunderstand them.

In groups of people, families, or social networks, there is no single language, but each member has his or her own, with his or her own words and particular way of expressing himself or herself. The dialogic technique invites all the voices present to express themselves and all perspectives to have a voice in a process of shared inquiry. The objective is to deepen the understanding of what is happening through the multiple voices that are brought into play through dialogue.

In situations of intense psychic suffering, it is difficult to find words to convey complex and painful experiences. Given that the universe of shared meanings is socially constructed, when this type of experience cannot circulate within the social network or nourished by the reflection of others, painful experiences run out of words to be transmitted. The result is that people undergoing such experiences become increasingly isolated as their monologues become more silent and opaque (Anderson et al., 1986). In these circumstances, there is a crisis of shared communicative patterns (Seikkula & Olson, 2003). The possibilities for joint meaning making and dialogue fade away. The question then is, as we have been explaining throughout this chapter, how to create contexts and relationships that invite dialogue.

The power of dialogue lies in the fact that it deeply connects people, and allows, through the creation of new languages that will be shared by a community, to find words for experiences that until now had no name.

32.4 The Crisis Perspective in Open Dialogue

The concept of mental health is diffuse and confusing. When we talk about *the mental health field,* we refer to the set of practices, discourses, and devices that make up the assistance to people who have been diagnosed with some psychic problem.

In our opinion, diagnosis is a main organizer of this field, since it determines who will be included as patients and receive therapeutic care (Abad & Toledano, 2017). Diagnosis in mental health is a translation of diagnosis in the medical field and comprises the set of observations and tests that lead to the identification of pathological processes underlying a series of symptoms and signs of alterations in normal functioning. This idea of "normal functioning," which should define what good mental health is, is problematic and has been questioned for decades (Pérez, 2021). It is not clear what constitutes normal emotional, psychological, cognitive, and behavioral functioning. In the end, considerations about what mental health is are made in terms of subjective well-being and active adaptation to the environment.[3] Regardless of this, psychopathological-diagnostic models in mental health are still in force and continue to organize the whole system.

This situation is generating difficulties when deciding, for example, which population is susceptible to being attended by the public mental health system. Mental health is associated with well-being and at the same time the mental health field is organized on the basis of pathology diagnosis. So, who should be attended by the specialized mental health services: anyone who presents suffering or only those whose malaise can be categorized within what is known in the diagnostic systems as mental disorder? The social demand arising from the COVID-19 pandemic for "more professionals, more resources for mental health" is, in our opinion, related to this confusion.

The Open Dialogue approach does not work with diagnostic models. It is more akin to the idea of subjective well-being and active adaptation to the environment. It proposes an approach to psychic suffering based on the concept of crisis and the recognition of diversity in the way people express their emotional and mental states.

From the psychopathological-diagnostic models, crisis is understood as a situation of acute stress caused by an exacerbation or emergency of a basic pathology. It is something that happens to an individual and that impels the intervention systems to resolve urgently, with whatever means, because it is considered an extremely serious situation. Based on this way of understanding and attending to crises, it is easier to generate situations of violence against people, since priority is given to what is understood as the protection of health[4] rather than the right to self-determination.

[3] For example, the World Health Organization"s definition of mental health can be found at https://www.who.int/es/news-room/fact-sheets/detail/mental-health-strengthening-our-response

[4] On many occasions, the danger to one"s own physical integrity or to the integrity of others is referred to in order to implement actions that restrict the freedom of individuals in their mental

From the Open Dialogue approach, crisis is understood as an unstable and transitory condition, which arises from different types of interruptions in life and relational processes, and which implies the inevitability of a transformation (González de Rivera, 2001). These aspects of interruption, instability, and need for transformation are accompanied by high levels of uncertainty, incomprehension, and suffering, which often lead people to ask for help.

Crises do not occur to a person in isolation from his or her relational context. In fact, on many occasions, the initial idea that there is a problem usually comes from the people closest to the "designated patient," when they notice some behavior that does not conform to their expectations (Seikkula & Arnkil, 2016). Those who observe a problem are also part of the social system that defines it. Therefore, from a social network perspective, all the people involved must be included in the process, since the problem will cease to be a problem when this system stops defining it as such and the situation of instability disappears (Anderson et al., 1986).

The Open Dialogue intervention involves responding to all the people or networks that request professional help, because they are all going through a crisis situation, not just the person who manifests what we call symptoms. That is why it is important to give an immediate response, which consists of enabling contexts for dialogue within the entire network, to deepen the understanding of the crisis and mobilize the resources and tools that the community has.

The locations where to meet are carefully selected. The professional team is available to go wherever it is most convenient for the people involved. Natural settings, such as the patient's home, are usually preferred. This is the place that research has revealed to be the most suitable, as people's resources are most available in their own environment (Seikkula & Arnkil, 2016), hence the importance of flexibility and mobility of the professional team.

From a social network perspective, all people for whom the crisis situation that is occurring is relevant and who are willing to collaborate are invited to the meetings that are organized. Usually, the family participates, but also other close people such as friends, co-workers, and neighbors and professionals of other services involved. This system remains open so that people can join it or leave it throughout the duration of the process.

In a critical situation, the levels of uncertainty are very high and, with them, the need to find answers quickly. The approach in therapeutic encounters is to postpone decision-making until dialogue produces answers that dissolve the need to act. The first challenge of a crisis intervention is to increase the security. This is achieved by building a sense of trust in a shared process aimed at mobilizing the psychological resources of the patient and his or her social network. This process implies working with a certain amount of anxiety at the beginning, which is mitigated by making decisions about the frequency of the meetings and assuming among all the people involved the uncertainty of the process and the responsibility for the decisions taken.

---

health treatment: forced medication, involuntary hospitalization, mechanical restraint, etc. This aspect is one of the most important denunciations of the first-person movements.

Crisis situations can become opportunities to generate new narratives, in which experiences that emerge in the form of symptoms are clothed in words and find a place in a specific relational context. Dialogue facilitates the connection of ideas previously experienced as unconnected, allowing a narrative to develop and become meaningful. The therapeutic team creates an atmosphere and a disposition in which any kind of utterance is valued and made possible, including psychotic forms of expression, which become part of the general conversation. Thus, it becomes possible to talk about experiences considered horrible and/or strange, and all voices are welcome in the construction of meaning about what is happening.

Working with this idea of crisis distances mental health problems from pathological conceptions that imply the dysfunctionality of individuals, and places them alongside the challenges of life and relationships. Attending crises implies attending to issues that are problematic for the people of a given network and seeking how to understand their essence in order to find solutions or new perspectives (Pérez, 2021).

The results of Open Dialogue research demonstrate that this approach is an effective way to limit the use of drugs, decrease the use of services, and reduce the incidence of mental health problems (von Peter et al., 2021). The literature describes numerous benefits and positive effects on the people served, but above all it points out that promoting a contextual and relational understanding of psychic suffering is a way of respecting human rights (Arnkil & Seikkula, 2015).

32.5 Conclusions

Since 2013, the authors of this chapter have shared the interest and commitment to contribute to making the Open Dialogue approach known and widespread, because in our opinion it has great potential for transforming the mental health system.

The results of all the research carried out since the beginning of the approach in the 1980s have attracted the attention of professionals and users of mental health services all over the world (von Peter et al., 2021). Since the first decade of the twenty-first century, the effort of the creators of the model to transmit their knowledge through training in different countries, added to the growing dissatisfaction with the care we provide from the professional sphere, has led to the multiplication of experiences of adoption of this approach in different parts of the world, such as the United Kingdom, Australia, the United States, Italy, Denmark, Ireland, Japan, the Czech Republic, Spain, Portugal, Germany, Hungary, and the Netherlands.[5]

One of the issues that is most often argued when investigating the application of this approach is the difficulty of doing it as it was done in Western Lapland: modifying the entire care system. The experiences that are emerging in other countries are, for the most part, limited projects, from public and private spheres, and have not so

[5] Countries participating in the HOPENDIALOGUE project, an international collaborative study designed to connect emerging Open Dialogue research projects around the world.

far involved the reorganization of care systems in a global way. In most of our contexts, laboral, institutional, and cultural conditions make it too demanding, if not impossible, to develop the seven principles set out in the approach.

However, until organizational policies can be modified, adopting the approach we have tried to explain in this chapter can introduce fundamental changes in the way mental health care is provided, which are also respectful of human rights and respond to the demands of people who have experienced the effects of the current mental health system as patients. In this chapter, we have tried to give an account of some of them.

It is fundamental to consider that the meanings of what happens are socially constructed and that the same phenomenon can be understood from multiple perspectives, in order to place ourselves on a horizontal plane in our relationship with the people we serve. Focusing on how to respond to people who need help, rather than hypothesizing the causes of what is happening to them, may be a way to begin repositioning ourselves.

Another key aspect is working directly with contexts rather than seeking to intervene on people. Trying to create contexts in which it is easier for feelings of connection to appear between people. Introducing the materiality of environments in the conceptualization of treatments is a first step to operate a necessary shift from the causes of emotional and psychic suffering in the individual to the extent to which the material conditions of life influence our mental health.

It is essential to maintain a crisis perspetive when we approach mental suffering and to avoid psychiatric diagnoses. Crises are natural responses to contextual challenges, and do not happen to someone in isolation, but affect a whole group of people and their material environments.

Open Dialogue has great potential to transform the mental health system. The analysis of the aspects presented here is only a starting point that proposes a cultural and practice change at the micro level.

Open Dialogue also provides, as we have pointed out, a model for producing knowledge from direct research on practice. Instead of focusing on confirming preestablished hypotheses or explanatory models, the proposal of this approach is to use qualitative research techniques to detect which elements are vital for making treatment processes work. In our opinion, it is necessary to produce theory from practice, a practice that is inevitably linked to specific cultural contexts.

The same opportunities that came together in the Finnish region of Lapland that gave birth to the Open Dialogue approach may not be repeated in another context or at another historical moment. But we have full confidence that we have more and more clues on how to operate, as political actors, the necessary transformation in mental health care that we are waiting for.

References

Abad, T., & Toledano, S. (2017). Power relations and psychic suffering. The influence of diagnosis in mental health. *e-Átopos, 3*, 129–142.

Abad, T., & Toledano, S. (2019). *Open dialogue in psychosis*. In E. F. Pedrero (Ed.), *Psychological treatments for psychosis* (pp. 551–574). Pirámide. ISBN 978-84-368-4133-6.

Anderson, H. (2012). *Conversation, language, and possibilities. A postmodern approach to therapy* (2nd ed.). Amorrortu.

Anderson, H., Goolishian, H., & Winderman, I. (1986). Problem determined systems: Towards transformation in family therapy. *Journal of Strategic and Systemic Therapies, 5*, 1–14.

Arnkil, T., & Seikkula, J. (2015). Developing dialogicity in relational practices: Reflecting on experiences from open dialogues. *Australian and New Zealand Journal of Family Therapy, 36*, 142–154.

Bakhtin, M. (1986). *Problemas de la poética de Dostoievski*. Fondo de Cultura Económica.

Galbusera, L., & Kyselo, M. (2017). The difference that makes the difference: A conceptual analysis of the Open Dialogue Approach. *Psychosis (Psychological, Social and Integrative Approaches), 10*.

González de Rivera, J. L. (2001). Crisis psychotherapy. *Revista de la Asociación Española de Neuropsiquiatría, 21*(79), 35–53. ISSN 0211-5735.

Hernández, S. M. (2011). Dialogism and otherness in Bakhtin. *Contributions from Coatepee, 21*, 11–32.

Pérez, M. (2021). *Science and pseudoscience in psychology and psychiatry: Beyond the mainstream*. Alianza Editorial.

Ponzio, A. (1998). *The Bakhtinian revolution: Bakhtin's thought and contemporary ideology*. Frónesis. Cátedra Universitat de Valencia.

Rotelli, F. (2015). *Living without asylums. The Trieste experience*. Editorial Topía.

Seikkula, J., & Arnkil, T. (2016). *Therapeutic dialogues in the social network*. Herder Editorial.

Seikkula, J., & Olson, M. (2003). The Open Dialogue Approach to acute psychosis: Its poetics and micropolitics. *Family Process, 42*(3), 403–418.

Shotter, J. (1994). *Conversational realities: Constructing life through language*. SAGE.

von Peter, S., Bergstrøm, T., Nenoff-Herchenbach, I., Hopfenbeck, M. S., Pocobello, R., Aderhold, V., Alvarez-Monjaras, M., Seikkula, J., & Heumann, K. (2021). Dialogue as a response to the psychiatrization of society? Potentials of the Open Dialogue approach. *Frontiers in Sociology, 6*, 806437.

Chapter 33
Raúl, Be Noise Amidst the Din, and Silence in the Murmur: Open Dialogue and First Episodes of Psychosis

Silvia Parrabera-Garcia and María Chico González

33.1 Open Dialogue

In Western society, we have been witnessing for years a process of pathologization of everyday life that seems to be advancing in a determined manner. A new syndrome or disorder labels every suffering. Every visit to the doctor, fruit of the anguish generated by the complex life we lead, results in pharmacological treatment. In the face of this unstoppable trend, the OD approach offers a way of accompanying psychic suffering with excellent potential for depsychiatrization (von Peter et al., 2019): limited use of medication, the response through the collectivization of suffering, and dialogue in the affective network, professionals "letting go" of their position of expertise, using non-psychiatrizing language, and the results of research, show a decrease in the incidence of mental health diagnoses and the use of psychiatric services. This framework is a valuable tool in the paradigm shift in mental health that citizens and professionals have been asking for, for a long time.

33.1.1 Introduction to Open Dialogue

OD is the organizational system initially used in the Western Lapland region's Mental Health and Social Services Network (Finland). It is a way of organizing care for people with mental health problems and a philosophical and therapeutic approach that rethinks how to accompany efficiently and responsibly, responding to people's needs within their environment (Putman, 2021).

During those years, intending to improve care in the mental health system and within the Finnish National Schizophrenia Project framework, Jaakko Seikkula

S. Parrabera-Garcia (✉) · M. C. González
Psychosis Early Attention Unit, Hospital Universitario Príncipe de Asturias, Madrid, Spain

J. A. Díaz-Garrido et al. (eds.), *Psychological Interventions for Psychosis*,
https://doi.org/10.1007/978-3-031-27003-1_33

(University of Jayväskylä) and his team at Keropudas hospital started working based on the Treatment Adapted to Needs (TAN). Initially developed by the psychoanalyst Jork Alanel and his collaborators in the Finnish city of Turku between the 1960s and 1980s (Haarakangas et al., 2016), the TAN framework was developed to respond to the high incidence of schizophrenia in the Länsi-Pohja mental health area, with an annual average of 35 new cases per 100,000 inhabitants in the 1980s.

When dealing with psychosis, TAN emphasizes treatment as an ongoing process, planned according to the person's needs and family, which are both included in the treatment from the beginning. It should offer immediate care and integrate different forms of intervention, employ a minimum use of medication, and continuously evaluate results. Moreover, it emphasizes an evident psychotherapeutic attitude of the professionals, both in the initial assessment and treatment stages (Alanel, 1997).

Seikkula's team started using the TAN approach by introducing the patient and family to treatment coordination meetings where decisions were made about whether or not to admit the patient to psychiatric care. In addition, it expanded the network involved in the treatment to include the closest community. In terms of therapeutic skills, it introduced the tool of Tom Andersen's Reflective Team in the meetings (Tromso, Norway), the way of understanding reality as a typical construction through the shared language of Social Constructionism and the concept of dialogue inspired by the philosophical theory of the Russian linguist Mikhail Bakhtin. It progressively added mobile teams to travel to homes, starting home-based accompaniment to avoid hospitalizations (Birgitta & Seikkula, 2021).

Today, OD is not solely used to treat psychosis. The basic organizational principles of the framework have restructured the entire mental health and social services system in the region, involving other institutions such as education and employment in the transformation process. This new approach to mental health, the relational context understood as an integral part of the person, has generated a significant cultural change in the community with an increase in dialogue and a new way of understanding the family and the social environment from a more collaborative perspective. In a region of no more than 70,000 inhabitants, over the last 40 years, a significant proportion of citizens and community organizations have, sooner or later, participated in network meetings in one or other settings (Seikkula & Arnkil, 2019).

The starting point in this mental health system is that anyone who asks for help, for themselves or for someone else in their environment, defines a situation of crisis that needs to be dealt with immediately. The goal is to talk as soon as possible about what has happened and what is needed, get the socio-affective network involved, listen to all participants equally, and take decisions in a consensual way.

A phone call due to an extreme situation (from the person in crisis, the family, or an institution) can be received at any time and will trigger the established protocols. The professional who receives the call organizes a mobile team of two or three professionals who, within 24 h, will travel to hold an initial meeting with the person requesting care and their social and emotional network at the designated place. From this first meeting, it is decided by all involved, which people can help and accompany the process of open meetings, on-demand, for an indefinite period, at the place where they feel most comfortable—trying at all times to avoid hasty decisions about psychiatric admission and medication. Resources such as the "24h crisis team" to accompany the most distressed people are available, including the possibility of the professional team staying at the person's home overnight.

Although OD is currently at the core of all psychiatric interventions in the Western Lapland region, research has focused exclusively on people with experiences of psychosis. The results so far show a 90% decrease in the incidence of schizophrenia diagnosis in the Western Lapland region (from 33 to 3 diagnoses of schizophrenia per 100,000 inhabitants) (Seikkula, 2019).

A recently published article by Sebastian von Peter and colleagues on the potential of this framework summarizes the most important results of the five studies conducted so far in the Western Lapland region with people facing first episodes of psychosis:

> [...] a significant reduction in hospital stays (i.e., inpatient days and readmissions) as well as lower relapse rates over time in all cohorts (Seikkula et al., 2003, 2006; Bergström et al., 2018). Furthermore, results show reintegration into work and education of up to 84% of participants and the considerably low and infrequent use of neuroleptic medication both initially (28–50%) and during the intervention (11–29) (Seikkula et al., 2006; Bergström et al., 2018). In comparing the individual cohorts, shorter and less severe psychotic episodes were described, and a drastic reduction (up to 82%) of participants with residual symptomatology. In addition, a decrease in the use of psychiatric services and frequency of network meetings was reported (Seikkula et al., 2006; Aaltonen et al., 2011; Bergström et al., 2018). Moreover, significantly fewer disability pensions were allocated compared to historical control groups (Seikkula et al., 2006; Bergström et al., 2018). Overall, in all cohorts from 1992 to 2005, the evidence showed that the treatment outcomes achieved in each case remained reasonably stable over the entire period or even increased over time (Bergström et al., 2018). (Von Peter et al., 2019, pp. 3.2)

Also of interest is the rigorous review by Freeman and colleagues of all qualitative and quantitative research to date on OD (Freeman et al., 2019).

Concerning the global impact that OD is having, it is clear that there is a growing development worldwide. Currently, OD is being implemented in more than 30 countries adapted to their particular cultural and social contexts. There is considerable research related to the training programs offered in countries such as the UK, USA, Italy, Germany, Denmark, Norway, Australia, and Japan.

The ODDESSI trial titled *Open Dialogue: Development and Evaluation of a Social Network Intervention for Severe Mental Illness* stands out. (https://www.ucl.ac.uk/pals/research/clinical-educational-and-healthpsychology/research-groups/oddessi). This research program, led by Professor Stephen Pilling of the University of London on crisis and continuing mental health care in the NHS, aims to evaluate the clinical and cost effectiveness of OD interventions compared to current treatments. Furthermore, the international HOPEnDialogue project (www.hopendialogue.net), linked to the ODDESSI trial and based in Rome, with more than 20 advisors, is designed to connect emerging OD research projects worldwide.

33.1.2 Mental Health in Open Dialogue

Information collected in the Finnish region of Lapland correlated economic, political, and social circumstances of the 1980s (transition from rural to a service economy, high unemployment rate (50%), geographical dispersion, etc.) to the high incidence of schizophrenia diagnoses. OD contemplates psychosis as an adaptive response to very severe stressful situations (Seikkula, 2019). This is based on the idea that people develop their personality and emotional life in interrelationship with others and that what causes severe suffering are traumatic, one-off, or accumulated, relational, and emotional experiences. In the case of psychosis, these traumatic experiences reappear in delirium and unusual ideas due to a radical and temporary alienation of communication (Seikkula & Olsen, 2003), preventing the necessary accompaniment and elaboration for their assimilation.

More broadly, OD, like other humanitarian approaches, posits that emotional distress has a natural meaning and is related to the person's lived experiences, history, and environment. It recognizes that people develop and live in a web of affective relationships with others. Emotional problems are understood as something that emerges from the social and family network rather than as individual deficits. In this line of thought, symptoms are forms of adapting to the suffering and the circumstances. Removed from their context, the person and their affective network define the symptoms as a problem, and consequently, the professionals present a diagnosis. According to the framework, through language and the shared understanding that dialogue generates, we can construct new interpretations that offer a meaning to the appearance of symptoms, describe the suffering with words that sustain it, and define ways of dealing with it.

Thus, the OD focuses on affective and social relationships and communication as the primary focus for defining the problem and finding solutions. This relational understanding of mental health problems considers other vital factors in the development and recovery from psychosis. This way of working is based on the belief that everyone can recover and take back the reigns of their lives, indistinctly from the problem which originated the consultation. Moreover, it allows each person to be seen as the protagonist of their own story, emphasizing subjective knowledge about oneself.

This understanding of mental health, which affirms the value of the knowledge gained from the experience of the people we care for, should be expanded to include an image of the present-day individual with psychosis. In the EAU's journey so far, we have learned that the majority of people facing first episodes do not want to be labeled. They do not want to take on a disability or depend on psychiatric services that imply that their condition will require them to be monitored and medicated for life. Throughout these past years, the EAU has had the opportunity of accompanying primarily young people in crisis with experiences of psychosis who had a voice of their own and who wanted to make decisions about the treatment and support they preferred. They also showed us that they can live with their psychotic experiences, add meaning to them, participate in the community, and create support networks.

33.1.3 The Foundations of Open Dialogue

The term “Open Dialogue” first appeared in 1995 with seven basic defining principles that organize the care processes within the framework (Seikkula et al., 1995). “Dialogue” as in the use of dialogue as a therapeutic tool, employing polyphony within the social-affective network and ensuring that the participants’ voices (including the voice of psychosis) are all heard equally. And “Open” as in the transparency of the process in terms of the treatment’s planning and decision-making (Olson et al., 2014), authenticity in communication, and continuity in dialogue as a dynamic and shared living act, without a planned end.

The main element that structures the process in OD is the use of network meetings (Dialogic Meetings). A meeting place for the person, their closest socio-affective environment, and the professionals who accompany the process (sometimes for years). The aim is to develop a form of therapeutic dialogue within the same meeting, re-establish open and sincere communication between the attendees about the experiences surrounding the crisis, and thus produce a mutual and deeper understanding of the moment they are facing. Consistent with a relational approach to mental health problems, the goal is to create a network of support from the outset and harness all participants’ creativity and resources to plan and make treatment decisions together. Per the agreements, all the support elements decided upon for the particular treatment, such as individual psychotherapy, pharmacological support, groups, and others, are integrated throughout the process.

The foundations for the development of these meetings are built from the seven fundamental principles that organize the process and the twelve key elements that define “dialogic practice” as a form of communication that transforms the dialogue of the meeting into a therapeutic experience.

33.1.4 The 7 Basic Principles and 12 Key Elements for the Practice of Dialogism

In the following section, we will briefly describe the seven fundamental principles followed by the twelve key elements for the practice of OD. This summary aims to frame and guide the reader to the final two sections: Raúl’s experience with psychosis, and Reflections. [Multiple publications are readily available for those interested in the study of the basic principle and the key elements (e.g., Haarakangas et al., 2016; Olson et al., 2014; Putman, 2021; Seikkula et al., 2006; Seikkula & Arnkil, 2016).]

The Dialogic Meetings in the Western Lapland mental health system are integrated in the specific organization of the treatment system according to seven basic principles obtained from research on the framework’s effectiveness (Aaltonen et al., 2011; Seikkula et al., 1995). Five organizational principles are as follows: (1) immediate care; (2) flexibility and mobility of the team; (3) social network perspective and support systems; (4) teamwork and shared responsibility; and (5) continuity in the link with professionals. And two therapeutic principles are as follows: (6) Tolerance of uncertainty and (7) dialogism as a form of communication.

1. **Immediate Attention**: The first meeting is set up within 24 h following the initial contact. This way of responding allows the team to take advantage of the opportunity offered by the crisis to mobilize the social support network of the person and their family as well as to mobilize the psychic resources of the attendees. A window of opportunity opens to deal with contents that are difficult to share, now in a context of greater emotional stability.
2. **Mobility and Flexibility**: The treatment design, being highly flexible, integrates different forms of intervention according to the particular needs of each environment and at each stage of the process. The meeting place is decided upon by consensus, where people will feel safer. The meetings are held on-demand, allowing for an increase in meetings when the need is greater.
3. **Social Network Perspective and Support Systems**: All those social and family network people who have something to say about the crisis and who can be supportive throughout the process are invited to the meetings. Professionals from the institutions involved at some stage of the treatment (social worker, psychotherapist, psychiatrist) are also invited to attend. Lastly, the network perspective of two or more is also applied to the team of professionals in charge of the process from the beginning to the end. Together, they form a support network that provides a variety of resources and points of view that will sustain the crisis environment throughout the process.
4. **Teamwork and Responsibility**: In Finland, the professional who picks up the first call organizes the team responsible for accompanying the process. From the outpatient or inpatient setting, the colleagues are chosen according to the nature of the problem for which help is sought. Shared responsibility is built through the search for consensus in the decision-making regarding the treatment. This way of working leads, naturally, to a responsible involvement of all those attending the meetings.
5. **Continuity in the Link**: The same team accompanies the process regardless of whether the person in crisis is at home or in the hospital and regardless of the duration of the treatment. If the same environment requests care again toward the end of the process, it will be the same team that responds to the request. Continuity also refers to the integration of the different forms of intervention in the treatment through dialogue, which is established with the professionals of the different therapeutic models who participate in the network meetings as guests, whenever it is considered necessary.
6. **Tolerance of Uncertainty**: Time is needed to reflect, together with the person and his or her environment, to avoid hasty conclusions regarding admission or neuroleptic medication issues. This possibility depends on the capacity of the whole network to tolerate uncertainty. Moreover, it develops in the process of joint learning guided by professionals who show confidence in the resources of the whole network and bear hope gained from previous experiences. This

requires facilitating meetings in a climate of safety built through multiple considerations explained in the section on EAU.

7. **Dialogism**: The central role of practitioners is to ensure that dialogue is generated among those attending the meeting. This requires equal time for all voices to be heard, openness and careful listening, and taking all contributions seriously. In such a way, through the creation of new meanings, new possibilities for understanding the nature of the crisis are accessed.

The 12 key elements of fidelity were established in 2014 concerning the practice of Dialogism, defining and differentiating how dialogue is used as a therapeutic tool within the framework of OD.

These key elements are as follows: (1) including two or more therapists in the meetings; (2) including the affective network in the dialogue; (3) responding to what is verbalized; (8) transparency; (9) responding in an accurate and meaningful way; (10) focusing on the life story rather than symptoms; (11) employing reflective dialogue between therapists; and (12) developing the affective network's tolerance for uncertainty (Olson et al., 2014).

1. **Employing Two or More Therapists**: The therapists (also called facilitators to emphasize their task of ensuring dialogue) attend the meetings as a team. Firstly, to facilitate communication within the network. And secondly, to conduct dialogues among themselves in which they reflect on what they have heard out loud, contributing their own ideas in an open and genuine way.
2. **Involvement of the Emotional and Social Network in the Dialogue**: With permission of the person assisted, the affective and social network is included from the beginning of the process. In this way, the intervention is carried out upon the environment and not so much on a sole person. Even if working with the network is not possible, the network is present via the person assisted, as they work on the internal dialogue with the most important people in their present and past reality.
3. **Use of Open Questions**: Questions are addressed to all attendees to allow them to be involved from the very first meeting of the process. Open-ended questions are an opportunity for each attendee to speak from their point of view regarding their concerns, needs, and intentions in relation to the request for assistance. For example, at the beginning of the first meeting, you might ask how the idea for this meeting came about; what is the reason for attending; how they would like to spend the time to be shared today; or how are they doing since we last met. Moreover, open-ended questions addressing the content being shared during the meetings are used throughout the dialogue facilitation process to go deeper into the different points of view.
4. **Emphasize the Current Moment of the Conversation**: Therapists prioritize the shared moment in the present rather than the content of the stories, responding sensitively to the immediate emotional reactions of the participants and giving space for their expressions (without interpreting).
5. **Providing Multiple Points of View**: Facilitators ensure that all participants have the opportunity to speak out and have a similar amount of time to express

their points of view on the shared topics, thus ensuring polyphony (versus a dominant voice). Participants feel heard, acknowledged, and respected, as much so if they choose not to participate in the dialogue. The principle of polyphony also applies to the internal dialogue of each person. It is a very useful tool for expressing contradictory or conflicting voices that help shape a richer and more complex reality.

6. **Relational Approach to Dialogue**: Therapists use questions about relationships in response to what has been heard (when they consider that a unique opportunity has been given to explore relationships between participants), showing interest in the context of the problem being addressed in the meeting (e.g., circular questions from the Milan systemic school).
7. **Responding to What Is Verbalized**Von Peter et al., 2019Facilitators respond by listening sensitively to the emotional load conveyed by the speaker's words, manner of being in the meeting, and body language. They use the exact words the network uses without resorting to professional language. In addition, they allow the silences that facilitate a prelude that will help find moments to talk about what is difficult to talk about, which sometimes facilitates the telling of stories that have not been told so far.
8. **Responding with Transparency**: Everything that is discussed regarding the treatment is done so in the presence of all the attendees, which means that all treatment decisions are made in the presence and with the participation of all. After listening, the professionals contribute their reflections in a personal, genuine, and authentic way, with absolute transparency. Transparency is paramount concerning any other issues raised in the meetings. For example, when facilitators explore the risks faced by the network due to the crisis situation, the safety of each participant, the invitees for the next meeting, or the decision of when to meet again.
9. **Responding Meaningfully to Problems**: Normalizing versus pathologizing: The therapists listen to the participants' different experiences to understand the context in which the symptoms develop, to understand how they appear and the meaning that emerges in them by recontextualizing them within the stressful or traumatic circumstances to which the person is adapting.
10. **Focusing on the Life Story rather than Symptoms**: Therapists facilitate the space where participants can express themselves and talk about their experiences, feelings, and thoughts to put words to what they have experienced in a narrative about their suffering. It is a shared process enriched by the contribution of the other participants and their own experiences, feelings, and thoughts. In this way, an understanding of suffering is built, enriched by the multiple points of view and a unique common language among the network, leaving diagnosis and symptoms in the background.
11. **Using Reflective Dialogue between Therapists**: Therapists facilitating the dialogue reflect aloud in conversation with each other in the presence of the people attending the meeting and contribute tentative, genuine, and personal input about what they associate and feel in relation to what they have heard (Andersen, 1994). In this way, practitioners can listen to themselves and access

their internal dialogue, and attendees can listen to the therapists without feeling obliged to respond.

12. **Developing Tolerance for Uncertainty in the Affective Network**: The development of tolerance for uncertainty and dialogue will facilitate the opening of space for the creativity of the participants and the building of a necessary collaborative attitude before making decisions about the supports included in the treatment, especially when it comes to potentially distressing measures such as the use of medication or psychiatric admissions. These are indispensable elements for the progress of the process. It generates from the support network's trust in the therapists' attitude who knows from experience the importance of allowing dialogue to build understanding together.

33.2 The Early Attention Unit (EAU)

33.2.1 Introduction to the EAU

The EAU is an early attention unit pioneer in adopting the OD framework within the Spanish public mental health system. The unit belongs to the Hospital Universitario Príncipe de Asturias (Madrid). The Area's First Episodes Process is defined as a specialized Mental Health Centre (MHC) program that attends to people over 16 years of age within a population of approximately 250,000 inhabitants. The team is dedicated to accompanying people who report unusual experiences (classified as psychotic) for the first time and who request care in the Mental Health Network of Alcalá de Henares.

Since 2017, the EAU has been working to adapt the OD framework to the social, cultural, and economic circumstances of the unique context of Alcalá de Henares. Moreover, in these five years of journey, the EAU team has accompanied more than 100 processes (mostly people diagnosed with first-episode psychosis and their socio-family networks) and has conducted more than 2600 Dialogical Meetings. Network meetings are the central element of each process and facilitate the particular construction of each treatment, responding to the unique needs of the people we attend.

Working within the OD framework in the EAU is a choice based on many reasons such as the way of being with and accompanying people, the way of understanding mental health and psychosis, the way of including and being in the community, and the results of previous research with early episode psychosis. However, it is an aspect of the OD framework that determined the choice to carry out early care in the EAU in this manner: The treatment it offers to people, especially those undergoing severe suffering.

On studying the framework, we realized that, shaped by the organizing principles of the treatment system and the key elements of the practice of dialogism, OD legitimizes and protects the positioning of the subject, including his history and that of all those attending the meetings, but especially of the person carrying the psychosis. We could say that, based on our experience, if we cannot guarantee the positioning of the subject in treatment (as well as that of each participant in the network), it is not possible for any of the practices we carry out to be therapeutic.

OD is an approach developed primarily in the community with an understanding of health through the affective and relational context of people that opens up a space of equality, respect, and democracy in which all attendees can express themselves equally, and which results in the empowerment and agency of each participant in the process. OD has been identified as one of the most highly valued psychiatric practices in mental health for its respect for human rights (Von Peter et al., 2019).

The current EAU team made up of a clinical psychologist, a mental health nurse, a psychiatrist, and an occupational therapist (at an earlier stage, the team included a peer worker), is organized as a mobile team and travels wherever people feel more comfortable and safe to talk. Usually, it is at home, though sometimes they prefer a park, a café, or the EAU itself or wherever they are at [the Short Stay Hospital Unit (SSHU), the Hospital Emergency Room (ER), Interconsultation, the Drug Dependency Care Centre (DDCC).]

The idea is to attend to the psychosis wherever the experience takes place (the community) and whenever it occurs; to assist the crisis by being within reach of the people as quickly as possible; to accompany the suffering in the moments of greatest severity; to take the opportunity that the openness of the moment offers to establish a bond of trust, proceeding to talk about the experiences that have triggered it.

We must bear in mind that the EAU is part of the mental health system and that a professional from another service, generally the ER or the SSHU, assigns our team (sometimes, they come from other services in the area, or relatives come directly to the EAU to request treatment, and we tend to them while facilitating the administrative process.) That same day, within a maximum of 48 h, we set up the first meeting. The person, their affective network, and the professional requesting the intervention (on some occasions, the network has given us a later date, and on others, the team has not been able to meet the deadline) are invited to attend.

When we start a process, we ask the person coping with psychosis, which other people in their emotional network they think may be of help. We explore with questions such as: Who knows what is happening? Who has something to say? Who could help at this time? The intention is to create a support network from the beginning that includes the people closest to them emotionally as well as the professionals who will be part of the process.

The EAU professionals attend in pairs, generally together with a resident. We try to ensure that they are always the same (we name the therapists who will attend). In addition, in agreement with the network, we invite other professionals who are involved in any of the stages of recovery of the environment to specific meetings to talk about what they need to address [colleagues from the ER, SSHU, MHC, and Social Services (SS.SS)]. The person in crisis and their affective network are always present, and the idea is to reach agreements upon the treatment. In this way, we incorporate one of the most valued maximums of this approach: Transparency. We do not talk about people if they are not present.

In this process of necessary cooperation, the aim is to activate the personal resources of each attendee, family member, and the community before offering the specialized resources of the mental health network. We believe that everyone has their own resources and is specially willing to use them in times of great suffering or need, not encouraging dependence on professional resources beyond what is necessary.

Supports arise from the creativity generated in the dialogue between all the participants, decided upon by consensus. We reach agreements that, in principle, serve to contain the crisis, avoiding admission and over-medication as far as possible, and that will later serve to build the path that we will walk together until the situation that the network is experiencing around psychosis dissolves.

33.2.2 The Dialogue Meetings at the EAU

Network meetings or Dialogue Meetings are requested on-demand by any of the people involved in the process.

At this point, it is perhaps important to note that at the EAU, at the beginning of the treatment process, we spend time on all aspects of the setting so that the treated person and their network understand its importance and give us their consent. Meetings may be requested by anyone involved, always after an initial agreement on how we will work together going forward.

The meetings, as mentioned in the introduction, have three functions: To obtain information about the problems that have precipitated the crisis, to organize the necessary supports to sustain it, and to develop a therapeutic dialogue that facilitates understanding (Alanel, 1997), so that communication, in a necessarily collaborative process, allows all attendees to recover from the situation they are facing.

It is essential to clarify that the content of these meetings, which are at the heart of treatment, is not planned, and therefore professionals cannot anticipate a standard response. The goal is to reach support agreements according to the needs of the moment after listening to the contributions of all involved (mental health experts and experts in their own lives). A therapeutic process develops in parallel through communication within the treatment system itself.

Regarding this way of communicating, the aim is to help the person with psychosis make sense of their behavior and delirium and dilute situations of risk and isolation. Throughout the process, a story will emerge from listening to the experiences of the participants (memories of family history and personal and shared experiences), which generally can help understand the most enigmatic parts of the delirious discourse, and from which a recontextualization appears, giving meaning to the unusual experience of the person with psychosis. In this way, the person and his or her affective network gradually cease to feel in crisis.

In this sense, we take as a criterion the steps taken by all members of the affective network (not only the person assisted) in the recovery of their lives and personal projects. In the EAU, we have learned to leave the diagnosis and the reduction of symptomatology in the background. These seem not to consider the needs of people with experiences of psychosis, and most people we have attended tell us that when they understand the meaning of their symptoms, these are no longer more important than building or rebuilding their life project.

33.2.3 The Sense of Security

The facilitators of the network meetings, the EAU professionals, are the guarantors of this dialogue. Their primary function is to generate and maintain the climate of security and trust necessary for all participants to find the time to talk about things that are difficult to share. These things need to be discussed in depth because, one way or another, they are experiences of the crisis they are facing.

Developing an emotional climate of safety involves paying attention to the needs of all of the participants. To do this, the facilitators start with the concerns brought to the meeting, ensuring that the members of the network speak without interruptions and that the contributions to the dialogue are in the first person. In other words, each person talks about themselves, and about how they are affected by the experiences they describe concerning the crisis. Respecting the pace at which each person can express themselves and the pace at which others can reflect is important. As is, ensuring that all participants have a similar amount of time to say what they need to say before the end of the meeting, including the voice of the person with the psychosis. Of course, it is possible that someone may not want to speak, in which case we respect their decision to attend and remain in silence, listening.

Taking care of the framing elements of each meeting is also a way of helping to create the necessary climate of security. At the beginning of each meeting, the EAU professionals pay attention to the introductions and acknowledgments, give the floor to the person who called the meeting and allowing each participant to express his or her concerns. Then, by consensus, we decide the topic with which we will start. In the same way, when the meeting is coming to an end (generally, an hour and a half is usually enough), we ask the network if they want to share anything else before finishing. We set a date for the next meeting, agreeing who will be the people invited according to the reason for the new meeting. If there is still no clear idea, this can be fixed later by phone. The EAU professionals each have a mobile phone (which includes an instant messaging application) to respond to the needs that may arise in the day-to-day environments, with a commitment to respond as soon as possible during the day. It is a handy tool that can help contain crises.

Finally, we recall the agreements we have reached during the dialogue, if any, to know what we are committing to. Furthermore, before saying goodbye, we check that everyone is feeling safe enough concerning the risks involved at the moment, in anticipation of the next meeting.

Another key element that helps develop a climate of safety is flexibility in the frequency of meetings. At the beginning of treatment, meetings may be held daily or every other day. Over time, the development of everyone's capacity to tolerate uncertainty, and the support of working together, can be spaced out according to the needs of the moment.

At certain moments, we may disagree when someone approaches psychosis as an organic illness, and as often happens with the voice of psychosis, we may not understand them, but even then, the facilitators of the Dialogical Meetings listen to and take all contributions seriously. The EAU professionals convey the importance of respecting all points of view, trying to deepen, without judging, in each one of them until each person believes that all understand what they mean. To achieve this, we use the language of the environment as a common thread, open questions, express our interest in the words the person and their network members choose when explaining themselves, pay attention to those words that are emotionally charged or seem to have a special meaning, and borrow their words when the emotions are intense (they appear in non-verbal language) or are not easy to communicate.

The conversation leads us to put ourselves in place of the person who is speaking, so that time and again we re-establish the positioning of the subject with their history, who has something unique to say about what happened. Part of our work is to ensure that the dialogue does not get bogged down in a confrontation of forces about who is right about what happened. Sometimes we need to explain to those around us that, although the experience they are talking about is shared, the emotional experience is personal and may differ. It also helps to respect the difference and uniqueness of each person, to see professionals emphasize sensitive listening through genuine interest, genuine curiosity, and a search for transparency and understanding in communication with each of the participants.

33.2.4 Dialogical Reflections

During the meeting, part of the work of the EAU professionals is to carry out the so-called Dialogical Reflections (based on the concept of the Reflective Team of T. Andersen, 1994). Dialogical Reflecting consists on finding the right moment in the meeting to interrupt the surrounding dialogue and open a space for reflection among the professionals about what has been heard so far from the different participants.

Dialogical Reflections can occur between facilitators or between professionals attending the meeting as a Reflective Team specifically, with the task of reflecting on what has been heard in the dialogue. In the case of the EAU, this is most often between the facilitators and the resident attending the meeting.

Facilitators look at each other, and for no more than five or ten minutes of dialogue, they establish a conversation in which they reflect on how they have emotionally resonated with what they have heard so far and what it has led them to think. To do this, they always use the same language as the environment, making their internal dialogue explicit and explaining how they have been associating their particular ideas and emotions so that personal reflection prevails over expert knowledge. In addition, they take care to recontextualize what they have heard from a positive and constructive point of view, intending to transmit hope through a perspective that considers each participant's contribution. Finally, they leave new open questions that will help the participants to continue deepening in the dialogue that they will resume after the interruption.

At the end of the Dialogic Reflection, the facilitators look back at the network and ask the participants if they want to comment on what they have heard in the conversation taking place between the professionals. The intention is that they continue the dialogue based on the questions raised in the conversation or any comments that they have just heard and that have made them think.

33.2.5 Change in Communication

As the meetings follow one after the other and are linked together to form a single process, the person and the affective network tend to incorporate the OD framework. It seems that they internalize the way of talking and listening, at the same time as they are deepening in their own feelings and thoughts, in order to understand the crisis they are facing. As time goes by, they feel that the crisis is shared, even if each story is personal.

In fact, most people broaden their view beyond diagnosis and medication and find it easier to talk about their personal needs. In this process, almost all attendees take some responsibility for the communication problems in the network while at the same time feeling more able to rely on their personal resources. We often witness them providing other forms of support, forms they did not offer at the beginning of the treatment. For example, the environment helps the person in crisis by changing the way of accompanying or communicating with them; the person with psychosis changes their ways of being to smoothen the cohabitation with the people with whom they live. At this point, we realize a dialogue is developing that leads to cooperation in resolving the crisis.

At the EAU, on following the philosophy of the OD framework, we have confirmed that the change needed for the crisis environment to improve does not come from a professional intervention aimed at change. It comes as a consequence of the re-establishment of authentic communication among all.

In the encounters, facilitators strive for a shared emotional experience. We do this by listening so that each individual feels recognized and accepted through the emotional resonance produced in others. In other words, what changes is the mode of communication resulting from introducing a dialogue that opens a space for each individual as a person, with their unique way of feeling and expressing their suffering. A place that recognizes him as a subject with the full right to feel the way he feels and to interpret reality in a unique way, which happens when he feels accepted and legitimized through the emotional resonance that he awakens in the facilitators (as well as in others) who are witnesses to his story.

This form of communication allows each participant to perceive themselves as active and ask themselves what they can change to improve the situation. In other words, each person, feeling listened to in their suffering and needs, being recognized as unique and with their own capacities, can ask themselves, "how can I contribute?"

It is necessary to point out, at this point, that this way of listening and contributing to the dialogue that is developing requires sensitive respect for each person's discourse. It demands that professionals participate with extreme care and do not make value judgments, either verbal or non-verbal (gestures, body posture, tone of voice). Otherwise, we risk leaving out voices that do not concur with our vision that we do not seem to understand, which prevents the person in question from experiencing the needed acceptance in order to take on responsibility, and contribute and participate in the path of recovery. In addition, our attitude reinforces the communication problems in the environment.

33.2.6 The Internal Transformation of Professionals

Reflecting on the journey of the EAU team, I believe that one of the most valuable aspects of this framework is the personal nurturing and continuous learning experience it offers to practitioners. In the OD and in the EAU, facilitators are primarily tasked with establishing a horizontality that enables dialogue and genuine, personal contributions. For this to happen, they need to participate in the dialogue as people who offer a particular knowledge according to their experience and their own history. Thanks to their primary role as guarantors of dialogue, therapists have the privilege of attending meetings as human beings (rather than professionals) and of removing themselves from the position of the expert with extraordinary knowledge, a position which I believe is impossible to sustain when the task consists of accompanying experiences as severe as psychosis on a daily basis.

In the meetings, there is a shared emotional experience with great transformative power for all participants, including the facilitators. The EAU professionals know that they are included in the process of change in each environment they serve. They participate by accompanying the emotional experiences that emerge with each person's story and contribute unique insights through what resonates with them according to their own story. In other words, intending to make the process authentic, facilitators allow themselves to be led through a process of continuous learning about themselves and psychosis in particular. By their attitude, they recognize how little we still know about psychosis and the uniqueness of psychosis according to the environment they are working with.

This framework allows us to work without the pressure of having to occupy over and over again the position of supposed knowledge that the biologicist paradigm and the mental health system usually demands of us. This is an excessive responsibility for professionals who feel that they must manage the lives of the people in their care, rushing their decisions about treatment, for fear of what might happen, when they should, instead, be making decisions about the best way to accompany them in moments of serious suffering. This does not mean that we are exempt from responsibility, but sharing it with the team and the support network allows us to reflect more calmly on the best of accompanying the crisis.

As the OD professionals in Finland say, we at the EAU have become experts in saying that we are not experts, not only because each experience of psychosis is unique, as are the people and circumstances around them, but also because it is necessary to make authentic contributions associated with personal reflections in line with the moment we are sharing, so that the affective network we accompany feels our involvement. And so that, thanks to the climate of horizontality that this manner of intervention provides, the network can use its own resources and sense of responsibility when facing the crisis.

33.2.7 Other EAU Tools

On the other hand, in the Dialogic Meetings, in addition to using personal, family, and community resources, other specific mental health activities are offered, such as Pharmacological Support, Therapeutic Accompaniment (Dozza de Mendoça, 2018) in the community, and different Groups (depending on the stage of the EAU, Multifamily, Sports). All of this, according to the needs of each setting and after reaching agreements regarding treatment planning.

Regarding the prescription of psychiatric medication, we offer the possibility of inviting the psychiatrist of the EAU team to the network meetings or to the personal consultation for the person in crisis, accompanied or not, according to their preferences. During the medication consultation time, following the drug-centered model (Moncrieff, 2013), we try to ensure that the person assisted, and their affective network, receive the necessary information about the possible beneficial effects of the drugs, as well as the possible side effects so that they can make an informed and responsible decision. (A bibliography is offered if requested.) Following the recommendation of the OD framework, our psychiatrist tries to address the most basic needs first, such as being able to sleep, eat, and contain the most intense distress, leaving neuroleptics to be used at minimal doses and in more extreme scenarios, always in agreement with the subject.

In addition, the EAU team can articulate support with referrals to other MHC activities, as we have done so far with individual psychotherapy or the Mindfulness group if the person so decides. Other devices of the mental health network are the Psychosocial Rehabilitation, the DDCC, or the Psychiatric Residence (Mental Health Network has more resources that can help), which occasionally has been especially useful to avoid psychiatric admissions when the family relationship is affected by serious misunderstandings or violence.

33.2.8 Non-coercion at UAT

The non-coercive commitment of the EAU team is a cross-cutting tool that has proved very useful. We have used it in all stages of the process. The people we treat have to agree at the beginning to receive treatment, voluntarily attend network meetings, and can decide whether or not to be referred to other mental health resources, whether or not to take medication, or ask for psychiatric admission. This element that defines the EAU as a coercion-free unit has dramatically impacted all those involved: people in crisis, socio-affective networks, clinical management, and our own team.

The EAU team has been building up this commitment through experience, walking the path, and at the same time developing its capacity to tolerate uncertainty. Nonetheless, in reviewing our learning process, we have sometimes, at some point, found ourselves insisting (out of fear) on using measures such as neuroleptic medication. However, we have always respected the individual's final decision.

It has helped us realize that when we do not force people in crisis, they are more inclined to trust the bond created with the EAU professionals. Furthermore, when people know that we will respect and support their decisions concerning medication, it is often easier for them to listen to the information we provide about the benefits, side effects, risks, different families of medications, and different options. This facilitates informed decisions as they reflect on whether or not to take medication at a determined moment. Moreover, in the case of wishing to end medication, they seem to be more willing to listen to the professionals on how to carry out a discontinuation process responsibly, in the most careful way possible. In consequence, they do not need to do it in solitude or lying, with the consequences on their physical and mental health that this entails.

Concerning admissions, what we have done so far has been that if the person, the team, or the socio-affective network considers it necessary, we go further into the point of view of each attendee during the necessary meetings until we reach an agreement. We might agree on a scheduled admission; or propose a way of relating at home that reduces tension; the use of some medication; a temporary separation that helps the people who live together to feel better; or the inclusion of other people in the process to accompany the person who feels worse. Indeed, it can happen that sometimes we do not reach an agreement during the week, and the crisis can lead to admission after a request for help from the family to the ER during the weekend. It is essential to clarify that the EAU team can only accompany the crisis from Monday to Friday from 9:00 am to 4:00 pm.

In any case, the feedback we have received so far from the people we care for is that the programmed admissions have been helpful for them instead of the involuntary ones, which have sometimes been traumatic. Involuntary admissions add the difficulty of re-traumatization, and the mistrust instilled in them prevents them from asking for help in case of need (from family, friends, or professionals).

We think it is important to point out that one of the experiences that we have to deal with in the processes of the people we accompany in the EAU is related to the circumstances in which involuntary admissions occur. The severe suffering involved in the crisis situation is compounded by the protocol used in psychiatric ambulances (people are tied up) and the protocol used in hospital ER and in the SSHU (where they are sometimes also tied up and forced to take medication). Many of the people we have cared for, who have faced coercion, have traumatic memories imprinted in their memory in a way that prevents them from trusting mental health professionals, and in consequence, our team, as we are part of the system. (In fact, some have refused to receive care, and we have had to respect their decision in coherence with our commitment). To repair in as much as possible, the damage and suffering caused by this experience, a significant amount of time is spent throughout the process on the elaboration of memories, a slow and meticulous task of exquisite respect and bonding, for the subject to regain confidence in the family trying to understand why they requested admission.

Regarding the socio-affective networks, we believe that belonging to a network committed to the process and not feeling alone with the risk or responsibility has helped the team not use coercion. It also seems to have helped request as many meetings as necessary and include other people or professionals in the meetings and the network to accompany them or consult them about the crisis.

From what we have been told, it has been very helpful for them to have the possibility of calling the mobile phone of the EAU professionals for consultation during the day. We always offer this support to those around us after asking their permission and respecting their decision. They generally say yes because they know that sometimes family and friends need to talk about what is happening to them, that it is needed to cope with the situation they are facing, or simply to be able to think about how to move forward. This entails the difficulty of reminding callers that they should talk to us about what is happening *to them* concerning the experience they are sharing with the person with psychotic experiences, and not so much about what is happening *to the other* person.

Regarding the mental health service professionals with whom we work in coordination, it seems that accepting non-coercion in the EAU is not easy. It might seem that the sense of responsibility for people's lives and the care of families about the suffering generated by uncertainty due to the risk are the central arguments against the need to prioritize accompanying the process of people in crisis in the most therapeutic way possible. These are legitimate drawbacks brought forth by our colleagues in the coordination meetings that lead us to reflect over and over again (every time we encounter a situation of risk) on how to avert the use violence (which has permanent consequence on people's lives as we know per the stories they share with us), without generating greater suffering in their environment and without putting the integrity of any of the members of the network at risk.

The experience developed so far in our unit has made us reflect on the need to have other resources available so that involuntary admission is no longer the only resource that families can access when cohabitation is unsustainable, or they feel at risk. Other resources could be (1) availability of spaces where people can go through the most difficult moments of the crisis without having to be hospitalized, and (2) availability of teams that can accompany the processes and offer the necessary support outside the usual hours of the EAU, similar to the crisis intervention teams that work 24/7 in the health area of Länsi-Pohja in Finland.

33.2.9 *The Exit Process at the EAU*

The EAU has a two-year limit time frame to accompany each process as agreed with the area's first-episode process. This is a flexible time frame that we have been able to extend in cases in which it was clearly harmful to interrupt the link with the professionals of the EAU. It is a major limitation of our unit because not all environments recover in two years. However, taking into account the inhabitants of the area and that it is a team of four professionals, limiting treatment to 2 years, seems the only way to offer immediate care at the moment.

When the process that we have been accompanying comes to an end, we make a referral to the general adult program at MHC. Depending on the person, they will attend or not. Some prefer to end their treatment when their process in the EAU comes to an end and do not accept the follow-up in the MHC as they do not want to take medication. Some have started their work or training and prefer to receive treatment in the private network. Some do not want to continue within the mental health system. If the person decides to continue treatment at the MHC, then, if the professional who receives them agrees, we hold one or more Dialogic Meetings with the network and the professional to facilitate the commitment and the continuity. In the presence of the person and their environment, we have the opportunity to explain how we see their process in the EAU. The person can also tell them how they feel, what they think has happened to them, and what they feel is needed going forward in the presence of the EAU support network that has accompanied them so far.

33.3 Raul's Experience with Psychosis

In this section, we would like to share with readers that Raúl has supervised this recounting of his process at the EAU himself. Throughout the joint revision of the text, we agreed on which parts of his story would appear and which would not. Some parts of the story were critical, and he agreed to their publication, such as his experience with medication. Whereas other parts, some of his delusional ideas, he did not want to share in a book.

Raúl, Ana, and Víctor (pseudonyms) have given us their consent and contributed to this chapter by reviewing the story and participating in a network meeting to reflect on the imprint left on them by the OD process at the EAU. Some of the phrases taken from this meeting appear in the final reflections of the chapter.

Finally, we would like to point out that throughout the text, there are annotations that refer to the 7 basic principles of the organization of the process (Pp.) and the 12 key elements of dialogic practice (Cl.) to serve as small examples and facilitate a didactic reading of the story.

33.3.1 Introduction

I met Raúl on the acute ward of the hospital in a standard room while waiting to attend a Dialogic Meeting with another admitted patient and his family. Raúl introduced himself in a friendly way, and we talked about his tattoos. While we talked, he explained very sympathetically what each of them meant to him. When the time came to join the pending meeting, Raúl said goodbye, saying: "you and I will get along very well." Little did we know that we would soon start working together.

Two days later, as head coordinator of the EAU, I received a phone call from Raúl's psychiatrist of reference, asking for the support of the EAU team for his patient. He informed us that this 24-year-old man had been admitted to the SSHU and was suffering from an episode of mania with psychotic symptoms. I tried to keep him from telling me his story in that call, explaining that he could inform us of what was necessary at the meeting we would set up to get to know him (Cl. 8. Transparency). I then asked to speak to Raúl on the phone. I introduced myself, and we agreed to meet on Monday at the SSHU. Friday was over, and it was no longer possible to meet that same day at such short notice (Pp. 1. Immediate attention). The Monday meeting was attended by Raúl, who invited his father and mother. I explained to him that my partner in the EAU team, María, would accompany me (Cl. 1. Two or more therapists), and that he could bring whomever he preferred (Pp. 3. Social network and support system).

33.3.2 First Dialogue Meeting

It was the first network meeting of the process that we would do together in the EAU, and it took place in the SSHU, where Raúl had been temporarily admitted (Pp. 2. Flexibility and mobility). We intended to start the accompaniment from the beginning because we knew from experience that it is easier to talk about the experiences that have precipitated the crisis (Pp. 1. Immediate attention) during its most acute phases.

When we arrived at the meeting, María and I briefly introduced ourselves and shook hands with each attendee. In addition to Raúl and his parents, his psychiatrist and a psychiatric resident involved in Raúl's treatment were in the room (Pp. 3. Social network and support system). Taking the floor, I thanked all the participants for attending the meeting. I explained briefly that my team accompanied people going through unusual and difficult experiences, which professionals often described as psychosis (Raúl was aware of the diagnosis). I then asked the rest of the participants to introduce themselves and say something regarding why we had gathered or what the problem we were meeting was about.

My colleague commented that we had an hour and a half for the meeting and confirmed that the attendees were available for that time. She explained that in these meetings, it was important that each person speaks in the first person, presenting their point of view with a willingness to listen to the point of view of the others (Pp. 7. Dialogism). We also asked, if at some point in the meeting, it would be all right to interrupt the dialogue to reflect among ourselves about what we had heard so far (Cl. 11. Reflective Dialogue). Without further ado, we set about listening to each person about the reason for the meeting. The psychiatrist opened the dialogue since he was the person who had called us together (Pp. 7. Dialogism) and spoke of his concern for Raúl.

He recounted Raúl's arrival at the hospital ER, at the request of his parents, following a suicide threat that culminated in an involuntary admission. He also described how he perceived Raúl as per his observations during the previous days spent in the SSHU: His irritable behavior; the speed at which he spoke; his failure to adapt to the rules of the ward; his insistence on not taking neuroleptics; his difficulties in sleeping; his relationship with drugs; and his unusual ideas about himself. The psychiatrist was concerned about his progress. Raúl had been admitted for 20 days for a similar manic episode two years earlier, and he had faced two depressive periods when he was younger. His psychiatrist was concerned about how Raul's mental health could be affected in the future.

Raúl took the floor and explained what he thought was his current problem. He disagreed with the admission; he did not think it was necessary. Nevertheless, he did think he was having a bad time. He told us about his relationship with the world of drugs; he said he had tried many of them. He also talked about the violence he had suffered in the village where it had been difficult for him to fit in and the violence he had used to defend himself and make himself respected. Some of the experiences he shared had to do with the bullying he suffered from age fourteen. Many of these experiences he had never told his family, and his mother, Ana, seemed genuinely surprised.

He was able to talk about the lack of recognition he felt from his father, how he suffered when he realized how proud his father was of his older brother, and how nothing he did made him pay attention to him. He mentioned his father's words: *whatever you do, be the best.* He said that somehow, he had been the best in a marginal world.

Ana was shocked to hear this and said she could not recognize her son. The polite and considerate person he was with her at home could not be the same person Raúl described through his experiences with drugs and violence. *I knew he smoked hashish, but everything else...* according to her, he was sick. That could be the explanation for everything that was going on. Besides, he had a cousin on his father's side diagnosed with bipolar disorder. *It must be hereditary, right?*

Víctor, Raúl's father, talked about mental illness but focused more on addictions. *The problem are the drugs; if he got off the drugs, he would recover. He needs a detox center, and then everything will be fine, right?*

However, Raúl did not want to be seen as a madman. He thought that they would not listen to him, that in fact, they no longer listened to him. That his parents did not want to know the things he had lived through, the things he had had to do in that marginal world to get ahead. That they thought he was mentally ill. He said he would rather go to prison than stay locked up in a hospital.

It was a very tough meeting. Raúl was honest and full of guilt about his experiences. He reflected a lot upon how painful it was for him to see the suffering he was inflicting on his mother and to not meet his father's approval. His parents had to listen to things they could never have imagined happening in Raúl's life. The other two sons were adults with families of their own, but their youngest son presented them with a new challenge, a situation they had never experienced before.

This part of the meeting took place while my colleague and I facilitated the dialogue with questions interested in going deeper into what each person was recounting (Cl. 3. Use of open questions); repeating some phrases and words that seemed more significant to us, and; giving time for the expression of the emotions that were rising up in each one of them as they told their story (Cl. 4. Emphasising the current moment of the conversation). In this way, we encouraged each speaker to continue explaining themselves.

At the same time, we were trying to stop Raúl from continually interrupting and confronting his father. I had to intervene, looking directly at Raúl, to explain how important it was for us to listen to each person's point of view and to allow time for each person to tell the group how they had felt during the experiences they had shared (Cl. 5. Providing multiple points of view). I also pointed out the need for my partner and me to think while talking and the difficulty of interruptions in the reflection process. Raúl understood this but found it difficult not to respond continuously to his father's statements. At different times, we reminded him that we would have time to talk about it later.

After allowing Raúl and his parents to share their impressions of the problem they were facing, we asked for permission to talk to each other about the dialogue we had facilitated for about 40 min (Cl. 11. Employing Reflective Dialogue).

Using the Reflective Team technique (Andersen, 1994), the facilitators began a conversation looking at each other, about what each participant's story had made us feel and think, and how they related to each other. We struggled to put into words the emotions that resonated within us as we listened to their words, gestures, and body language. We reflected on the emotionally charged phrases in each story that had touched us. Anguish, guilt, anger, and pain emerged in the conversation between us, but also Raúl's determination to move forward, the energy he transmitted, his honesty, courage, and his decision to rescue himself as a person beyond the diagnosis. We put in words the parent's strength and constant support that came from the experiences shared with their son since he began to show signs of depression when he was younger. Finally, after allowing ourselves a few seconds of silence before continuing in a more hopeful way, we asked ourselves some questions that came to mind as we reflected and tried to recontextualize some of the issues that stood out in Raúl's and his parents' stories (mental illness and drug addiction). (Cl. 9. Respond in a meaningful way). (Cl. 10. Focus on the story rather than the symptoms).

After our reflections, we gave the floor to the other participants in the case that they might want to comment on what they had heard in our conversation (Cl. 11. Employing Reflective Dialogue). Raúl identified with the pain and the guilt he felt for causing his mother to suffer, but he did not leave much room for others to reflect.

He could not seem to stop interrupting his father and entering into an escalation of mutual corrections that had no end.

My partner and I continued to listen attentively to the emotion that accompanied the moment, trying to connect with the frustration that Raúl was conveying for not understanding his father (Cl. 4. Emphasising the present moment). Between the interruptions, I found the opportunity to point out that I thought that what Raul was saying was very important. I paraphrased part of what he said (Cl. 7. Responding to what verbalizations) and reminded him that we would have time to talk about what he needed to share in the following meetings. This crisis offered the possibility of setting up as many meetings as necessary in order to, together, understand what had happened: He had only to ask, and if the parents agreed to accompany him, we could all meet as many times as they thought necessary (Pp. 2. Flexibility and mobility).

My colleague added that we could meet where they chose to meet to feel more comfortable. That we were at present attending them in the SSHU because that was the place where Raúl was at the moment. However, when he left the SSHU, if they wanted to, we could meet at their house or anywhere else where they felt safe and we could talk peacefully. All three agreed that meetings at home would be best (Pp. 2. Flexibility and mobility).

I informed the family that we would accompany them for the duration of the process till emerging from the crisis, with a duration of about two years. (Pp. 5. Continuity in the link). And that, if they agreed, they could invite other people to the meetings to talk about what they deemed necessary. For example, Raúl's older brother seemed to be an essential person in his life because of the doubts he had raised about drug use. (Pp. 3. Social network and support system) (Cl. 2. Involvement of the network in the dialogue).

We also told them that it was important to remember that everything we talked about other people should be in their presence. If Raúl wanted to talk about his brother, inviting him would be the best way to avoid misunderstandings in the family and clarify what he needed. And, if his parents or we wanted to talk about Raúl, we would do it in his presence. We know from experience that it is easy to worry about what others talk about behind our backs (Cl. 8. Transparency). Raúl commented that he would like to invite his older brother because he wanted him to confirm some of the things he had explained to his father and which his father did not believe.

At that moment, I took the opportunity to go a little deeper into what we had requested at the beginning of the meeting about how to talk in the meetings. Upon meeting, we should approach the subject by talking about ourselves, how we feel about it, and not as much about what happens to others (Cl. 5. Contribution of multiple points of view). I pointed out that in this first meeting, it seemed that the conversation about who was right between Raúl and Víctor had provoked moments of confrontation that prevented reflection. I tried to convey the idea that things happen to all of us when we face a crisis like the one they were going through, and that if they talked about themselves it would be easier for everyone to understand their personal experiences and try to address what each one needed to feel better (Pp. 7. Dialogism).

The psychiatrist took the floor and commented on Raúl's progress on admission and the possibility of getting permission to go home now that the EAU team would accompany him. In the SSHU of our hospital, it is possible to have permission to leave, which helps assess the appropriateness of discharge and to resume daily life progressively.

After all these exchanges, I asked the SSHU psychiatry resident if he wanted to say anything about what had been discussed so far during this first meeting. My intention was that all attendees would have the opportunity to contribute somehow and say what was on their minds (Cl 5. Contribution of multiple points of view). Also to help the resident be a part of the support network (Pp.3. Social network and support systems). (Cl.2 Involvement of the affective and social network in the dialogue), avoiding that his reflections emerge in other spaces outside the meeting and not in the presence of the network (Cl. 8. Transparency).

As we approached the end of the time as agreed, Ana and Víctor looked exhausted. I asked them how they were feeling (Cl. 4. Responding to the present moment) and they talked about how hard it was being. Ana said she was exhausted: She realized that hearing about Raúl's experiences with drugs repulsed her, and that she was starting to understand how complicated the relationship and the communication between Raul and his father was. It had always been like that, but the misunderstanding seemed much more serious these days.

My partner asked Raúl, Ana, and Víctor if they wanted to meet again and when they thought would be best time (Pp. 2. Flexibility and mobility). All three agreed to see each other as soon as possible. The psychiatrist also asked to participate in the next meeting to further discuss Raul's possible discharge, but he finally did not have time the next day. Looking at everyone's agenda, we agreed to meet in two days to continue going deeper into the issues raised in this first meeting. The next meeting convened in the interest of all would be held again at the SSHU (Pp. 4. Teamwork and shared responsibility).

33.3.3 Raúl's Process

We met for 15 days, three times a week after that first meeting. Every two days, we had a Dialogue Meeting and continued talking about the critical issues to each of us. We decided together which one we would start with, and at the end of the meeting, we agreed on a new date for the next meeting (Pp. 4. Teamwork and shared responsibility). In the beginning, the meetings were held at the SSHU. Two weeks later, after Raúl was discharged, at his home.

Ana and Víctor would welcome us with a cup of tea or coffee, and Raúl would show us the music and lyrics he was writing. Afterward, we would sit for an hour and fifteen minutes in the living room chatting while they delved into the topics, they had mentioned in the first meeting and others that came up.

In this initial stage, my partner and I focused on using the same language as the family. If a new word came up (for example, because of the diagnosis or the hospital admission), we asked the person who introduced it to explain what it meant to them. The rest of us also said what it meant to us (Cl. 7. Responding to what was verbalized). I think this care was critical in helping to establish the bond with Raúl, Ana, and Víctor, to explore the meanings of their stories, and to build a common language that inaugurated the universe of the support network that was beginning to arise among all of us.

In addition, as these were the first meetings of the process, we spent some time reaching agreements on the framework with which we would work in the meetings. (How to see each other on-demand, how to contact each other, the objective of the meetings, how to talk in order to achieve a therapeutic dialogue, how to make decisions by consensus).

We also talked about possible resources and support depending on the moment they were going through, such as, how to accompany each other at home so that the three of them felt at ease until the next meeting. For example, I remember that we reached some agreements about Raúl's need to go out while taking into account the concern of the parents who needed to set the time for him to return and with the condition that he would not use drugs as not to be too worried. Raúl negotiated this because he did not feel capable of not using hashish again; he could reduce his use, but he could not give it up entirely (Pp. 5. Teamwork and shared responsibility).

As the network meetings progressed, Raúl became less anxious and more stable. So we began to see each other twice a week. In the meantime, we discussed topics such as Raúl's recent separation from his partner, his relationship with his siblings, his drug use, his experience with medication and the side effects of other treatments and his current treatment, experiences of hospital coercion, going out with his friends, his past in the village and his return to work. Now and then, the idea came up of whether to invite other people to the meetings and involve them in the process. Sometimes we agreed to invite a family member or a close friend (Cl. 2. Involvement of the social network in the dialogue).

During the course of these conversations, the difficulty in understanding each other between Raúl and Víctor became particularly apparent. The dynamic in the relationship was invariably repeated. It was difficult for them to listen to each other. It seemed like a duel between opponents in which Ana felt she had to mediate to lower the intensity of the confrontations. Raúl would say something about the experiences he had lived through; Víctor would focus on some collateral detail of the story to correct Raúl; his son would rebut him seeking recognition of his emotions; Víctor would again correct some fact instead of listening to him; and finally, Raúl would burst out of the room frustrated at not being able to communicate with his father.

Gradually, we were able to put into words the difficulties the two of them had in talking to each other and the lack of space they left for Ana to talk about herself (Cl. 6. Relational approach to dialogue.). One of the situations that helped us understand in greater depth was that Víctor needed to continually check the two mobile phones he had at hand while we were talking. It infuriated Raúl because Víctor gave the impression of being disconnected from the dialogue, of not wanting to listen. This circumstance, which exploded in one of the confrontations between Raúl and Víctor, helped us talk about the anguish that the dialogue aroused in each of them because of what it implied in reliving emotions that were difficult to tolerate and express. By understanding the situation, we accepted that each one did different things to regulate the anxiety. Perhaps these supports helped them be present at the meeting. For example, Raúl would leave the room and smoke, Víctor would check mobiles or eat biscuits, and Ana would mediate and hold back crying when she could not stand the discomfort of being in the middle of a battle.

During the first few months, we learned together to talk more slowly and calmly. Ana was able to talk about her sadness about Raúl's life experiences, which she was coming to terms with, and about the rivalry between her husband and her son. Víctor tried to be aware of how he disrupted the dialogue with his non-dialogue and his difficulties in talking about feelings, and Raúl had the opportunity to be recognized and accepted, gradually integrating the two lives he led, one inside, the other outside the home (Pp. 7. Dialogism).

As time went by, Raúl seemed to feel better, he no longer felt so much anguish or anger, but he decided to stop the drug treatment unilaterally. He later told us that he felt increasingly sad and wanted to change something.

When he was admitted to the SSHU, he had refused to take neuroleptics and antidepressants because his experience in the previous crisis had left him with the memory of a severe blockage, of not being able to feel, of perceiving himself as a doll, of having low spirits and feeling isolated. He remembered the past drug treatments in a traumatic way, showing great mistrust because of the coercion he had suffered. However, he had agreed to take a mood stabilizer and anxiolytics on admission. Although he had not been able to follow the regimen completely, he had tried to do so.

33.3.4 A New Crisis

One day Raúl announced to all of us that he had completely stopped taking his medication, alone, in secret. Víctor was not at the meeting; he had decided not to attend because he could not find a way not to argue with his son over and over again as in the previous meeting. Ana heard the news, surprised and affected. She was scared, and Raúl had been lying to her: He had not taken medication for a week, and she had not known it. My partner and I thanked her for her transparency and the courage to share it in the meeting (Cl. 9. Responding in a meaningful way.) We talked to her about our concern regarding facing the change alone with the effects of radical and abrupt medication withdrawal if he had not followed a careful discontinuation process (Cl. 8. Transparency).

After our recommendation, she agreed to see the team's psychiatrist, whom she already knew since she was following the pharmacological treatment. We offered the possibility of inviting the team's psychiatrist to one of the Dialogue Meetings at her home or attending the EAU for an individual consultation. However, she chose to see her alone, where she was informed on how to withdraw the mediation safely. I explained to him that I could accompany his withdrawal process, carefully and responsibly, examining the side effects, assessing other strategies to deal with the discomfort (sport, shared activities, sleep care), and giving the body time to adapt, but Raúl was in a hurry.

On the same days, we looked for other supports that could help, and all three agreed that Raúl should do a Therapeutic Accompaniment (Dozza de Mendoça, 2018). So, at the same time as we continued with the network meetings, I started to see Raúl alone while we were walking in the countryside, and we talked about whatever was on his mind.

The accompaniment we had just begun would continue throughout the whole process. Not only with me, but later with my partner María. It depended on our availability and the frequency with which he asked to see us. From what Raúl told us when we went through the process together for this report, these walks were helpful to him at all times. Especially in the isolation stage caused by the insecurities that emerged when he was so affected by the new crisis.

Back to how it was triggered. In the meetings, Raúl talked about how he was actively seeking to change his mood as soon as possible to get back to being "high." He could not stand being sad, let alone the state he was left in by the antidepressants he had taken in the past and did not want to take again. Moreover, he was certain that when the psychiatrist had prescribed them, it was for fear that he would start to feel euphoric. Eventually, we were also able to talk about how he tried to alleviate the discomfort he felt when coming off his medication by going back to smoking hashish more frequently at home. So the meetings started to revolve around drugs again. Ana, in an attempt to control his drug use, Víctor, in an attempt to reaffirm that what Raúl needed was to go to a detox center.

Raúl was able to talk about how he perceived that what his father desired was for him to leave home because he proposed a detoxification center and other residential resources to keep him away. These dialogues precipitated the parents being able to talk about their relationship as a couple, the disagreements, and the rift that had opened up between them in recent years. In the course of these conversations, the need for a change of residence grew in the family. Thus, they decided to leave the village and return to where they had come before they moved in Raúl's adolescence (Cl. 6. Relational approach to dialogue).

In any case, Raúl's mood swings were becoming frequent and sharper. He seemed irritable, sometimes aggressive, and unhappy with himself and others. He conveyed, or we sensed, guilt and, at the same time, determination about his hashish use. He told us honestly that he sometimes went out at night and used other drugs.

Ana spoke at the meetings about her suffering for Raúl while he was away and at the same time tried to help him at home. She made sure he was well-fed, chatted with him whenever he asked for it and stayed awake with him when he could not sleep. The whole network had meetings every two days, and in the meantime, we met alone with Raúl in Therapeutic Accompaniment. (Pp. 2. Flexibility and mobility).

Even so, the crisis precipitated, and Raúl's mind seemed to become disorganized. He began to share ideas of feeling very big. Along with this self-perception came fear for his life and the certainty that he had been threatened with death. The delirium was progressing to such an extent that he could not go out in the street and he did not feel protected at home either, unable to sleep because of what might happen.

In this context, it was challenging to go deeper into the situation shared by the family. The confrontation with Víctor went so far as to be included in the delirium as a threat. Ana, exhausted, once again did not recognize her son. Moreover, Raúl no longer counted on her to calm him down; he saw her as a control figure because of her insistence that he retake medication. He could not trust her.

In the meetings, the parents raised the need for a temporary income, and during several meetings, we elaborated on the proposal. Víctor and Ana were able to talk about why they thought an admission might help at this time. Although Raúl was doubtful, he did not think he would feel safe in hospital (Pp. 5. Tolerance of uncertainty.) (Cl. 12. Tolerance of uncertainty.)

As we discussed the possibility of admission with him, Raul's father seemed to be going through a process of inner transformation. He was beginning to understand the severe suffering his son was undergoing. He gradually stopped confronting him and began to offer his support, clearly taking the fatherly role that Raúl had been demanding for so long (Cl. 6. Relational approach). Thus, the two began to spend more time together. Raúl managed to go out in the street with Víctor to play pool, have a drink, or tend to some unfinished business.

At the weekends, the situation became extreme for the parents; they called the ER for help, and following the protocol, they called a psychiatric ambulance and the police to the house. The encounter with the agents resulted in a violent confrontation and Raul being tied up and taken to hospital. The beginning of a new involuntary admission and a new episode of institutional violence added to his story: A record that has been difficult to elaborate.

During the admission, which lasted a month and a half, we carried out accompaniment and some Dialogic Meetings with Raúl's family and reference professionals at the SSHU. The meetings became even more complicated due to Raúl's refusal to remain in the hospital and take pharmacological treatment and the lack of mutual trust and dialogue between the SSHU's and the EAU's professionals.

In this context, I would visit the SSHU to continue the accompaniment. Raúl, post permission, would go out with me into the streets where we would talk about his concerns, which gradually shifted from fear for his life to traumatic experiences from the past which he had not yet shared in the meetings.

Later, whenever he was allowed to go home for a night or a weekend, he refused to return to the hospital. Our accompaniment during his permits helped him think about his reasons for returning or not (where he felt safer, how to negotiate medication with his psychiatrist, leaving, having to remain in the room). Some Mondays, we would spend more than two hours together before he decided to return.

While accompanying Raul, I was very shocked at the suffering that arose from his delirium, and at certain moments, I felt very distressed and powerless. When Raúl explained to me the arguments he used to make sense of his delirium, he asked me if I believed what he was telling me I had not had such an experience; I wished to understand, but I told him it was difficult to put myself in his shoes (Cl. 7. Responding to verbalized). I also told him that I was grateful for his trust in sharing his experiences with me, highly challenging experiences, and that if he wanted to tell me more, we could try understanding them together (Cl. 9. Responding meaningfully).

In these conversations, I could resonate with the suffering buried under layers of drugs and hyperactivity. His constant need to be "high" made sense. He could not to risk becoming depressed or having to take drugs for relief. I understood why Raúl chose to stop the medication and return to the drugs when, in the process of coming out of the first crisis, a series of traumatic experiences he would have to deal with began to emerge. These experiences later helped us to understand the second crisis' delirium.

I would say it was the most emotionally intense time for everyone in the network. Raúl was again involuntarily admitted, and we knew the suffering that this type of admission had entailed in the past. On the other hand, the parents had a chance to somewhat recover themselves from the intensity of the previous weeks, although the confirmation of a diagnosis of severe mental disorder would bring about added suffering.

After being discharged from the hospital, Raúl continued to be delirium, felt threatened, and had problems giving up hashish. Shortly afterward, on one of the outings with his father, Raúl felt in danger and reacted by defending himself against Víctor. A police officer was nearby, and his father called for help. Raúl returned to the ER, which initiated a second involuntary admission.

When the COVID-19 pandemic hit, the SSHU was being reorganized, and Raúl was transferred from the ER to another hospital. While in the new hospital, he fell ill and had to be transferred in a severe condition to the Intensive Care Unit of a third hospital, where he managed to recover and end his psychiatric admission. Doctors told Raúl that the incident was related to an excess of neuroleptics and this experience further strengthened his mistrust of the mental health system.

With Raul's permission (Cl. 8. Transparency), during all of this second admission, my partner and I met with his parents at home to help them deepen their understanding of how they were feeling and assist them in assimilating their experiences so far. Also, to help them think about what they needed before Raúl came home. When the parents' meetings began to discuss drug use and what to do about it, Raúl (who had been hospitalized away from his referral hospital) would participate via videoconference or on a hands-free call. A few weeks later, Raúl returned home.

As the months went by, slowly, the delirium was left behind, and his personal story started to take its place. Meeting in a network a couple of times a week, Ana and Víctor would tell bits and pieces of Raúl's story that, in their view, related to what he was expressing in a way that was not very comprehensible. With the story interwoven in the meetings, Raúl showed himself to be less and less confident, expressing doubts about his delirium and recognizing his memories in his parents' story (Cl. 10. Focusing on the life story instead of the symptoms).

After returning home, Raúl integrated one of his SSHU buddies into the Dialogue Meetings. The input from this friend regarding his particular mental health journey seems to have helped him accept his problems. Moreover, his company helped him feel less alone once he decided to stop associating with the friends with whom he had used drugs in the past (Cl. 2. Involvement of the social network in the dialogue).

At the same time, he began to demand Dialogue Meetings without the network, using them to talk about more personal issues, addressing them, and deepening in the changes he was experiencing internally.

After been recently diagnosed with a severe mental disorder, some of the content revolved around the obsessions and insecurities that surfaced in response to the transformation he felt in his identity due to the change he had undergone when abandoning the world of drugs. He also dealt with other issues of his emotional life and personal projects. The meetings included the network through his internal dialogues about the contradictions he felt between the different voices in his reflective process (Cl. 2. Network perspective on dialogue). And we continued to do the work of the reflective team, contributing genuine input (Cl. 11. Reflective Dialogue).

All this was happening while on the day-to-day basis Raúl was drifting away from the friendships of the past, feeling increasingly isolated and at the same time closer to a necessary change. For the first time, fruit of his own decision, he stopped smoking hashish.

Thus, in the final stage of his process at the UAT, Raul attended Dialogical Network Meetings, individual Dialogical Meetings, Pharmacological Support consultations for treatment review and undertook Therapeutic Accompaniment in the community that facilitated his exposure to social life in an environment other than that of drugs (Pp. 2. Flexibility).

After two years of treatment at the EAU, we agreed, together with Raul and his parents, to extend the process for another six months. The aim was to facilitate an attentive farewell that would give him some leeway and give him time to work through the aggravation he experienced before recovering, and thus consolidate his achievements. In the course of the first extension, we agreed on a second 6-month extension. In the end, the treatment lasted three years (Pp. 5. Continuity).

Raúl is currently in the process of being discharged from the EAU. With regard to continuing his treatment, he told us: *I am hesitant to return to the CSM because I had a very bad time there, I felt ignored, and I don't trust the way they treated me.* Raúl still talks about the lack of trust in the public health system due to experiences of coercion in hospital settings at times of great suffering. He takes a minimal dose of a mood stabilizer. He does not use drugs except hashish, which he takes up intermittently as part of his process (by personal decision) while giving it up completely. In the last year, he has considered individual psychotherapy in the private circuit with a professional he trusts and attends online classes to prepare for university entrance.

33.3.5 *Reflections by María Chico González. Opportunities, Difficulties, Limits, and Challenges: What Has Happened to Me?*

I want to begin by communicating the intention of being attentive and respectful with Raúl, Ana, Víctor, and all the people who have participated in some way in this process. I feel that their intervention was essential, so the following lines are interspersed with some of my reflections and fragments of a conversation we had in a network meeting convened for this purpose. I thank you for your generosity and courage in accepting the proposal.

I desire to speak in the first person, tentatively, and from the "stance of not knowing" (Anderson, 2012). I hope to write with honesty and transparency, being aware of the privilege that comes with being able to use this space and to "have my voice heard." I hope to convey that it is possible to work in different ways when accompanying people going through psychotic crises, in that those who are going through it feel less alone, that my internal dialogue helps us reflect, and that it is helpful.

As Silvia has narrated above, I met Raúl and his family in a hospital unit. Throughout almost three years of sharing, the learning and challenges have been continuous. Writing this text has offered me multiple opportunities, difficulties, limitations, and internal challenges.

On thinking upon my experiences, it was difficult for me to differentiate between them, feeling that they were all intertwined (a ball of wool of different colors and threads I could not separate), which led me to think that maybe it wasn't necessary to separate them. I am aware of the possibility that for the rest of the people who were part of this chapter of Raúl's life, the colors or the thickness of the threads may be different. Each of us will have added different threads to the jumper, made to measure, throughout the process.

In order to show part of my addition to the design of my jumper, I will use the OD principles as a guide, as threads that are linked together.

33.3.5.1 Immediate Attention

Maintaining immediacy with 4 people in the team, working Monday to Friday from 9 am to 4 pm, is sometimes very difficult. I felt that being able to take a phone call from Raúl when he needed to or to call a meeting the next day allowed for less rushed and more consensual decisions to be made.

However, I recall feeling very uneasy about turning off my mobile phone on Friday afternoon and turning it back on, on Monday morning. On the other hand, I think that these limits also allowed us to think about possible options and to consider what to do if the distress increased: Which people they wanted to and could count on and which ones not; the time limit of each one of them before calling the ER; being able to strengthen the mutual care and "care pacts" (Pérez, 2016).

- *Raúl: I felt safe in the knowledge that you were there if I needed you, that I have a phone number I can call. It was reassuring to write to you and know that you would read me and that I would get an answer at some point.*
- *Ana: "It's a wonderful thing. Feeling less lonely, knowing that you could call and they would lend you a hand, feeling attached to something." "But at weekends... the last two times he went in at the weekend. At those times we felt that there was no other option, knowing what it means to call 112."*

33.3.5.2 Flexibility and Mobility

Throughout almost three years, I have been able to accompany Raúl in his daily life (Dozza de Mendoça, 2018), holding meetings in the hospital, at the round table in the living room of his old house with his family, having a coffee together in a shopping mall while he was staying in a hotel while moving houses, or, while Ana offered us tea, in his new house. We strolled through a street market when it seemed that his spirits were very high, we were able to take the countryside air in and walk around his neighborhood when he felt very sad, and it was hard for him to leave the house. We also managed to go back inside a supermarket, after months, and sit down to drink the refreshment he bought with a taste of victory.

On the other hand, I remember going to Raúl's house when it was very difficult for him to get out of bed. At a Dialogue Meeting, we agreed that he would give us permission to call his room if this happened. This made it easier for him to attend the Dialogue Meetings in the living room of his home. During the meetings, such agreements were made. For me, it was essential to have his consent and to have worked at the decision-making together.

I feel that Raúl and his family have opened the doors of their home and their world to us. The fact that we are the guests in their home—and in his life—entails even more delicacy on our part, extreme respect, asking permission to enter, where to sit, and so forth. At the end of the day, we have to adapt to his rules as good guests. I think there is a strong parallel with the position that we, as professionals, should maintain in the dialogue: attentiveness toward the doors that can be opened, or not. In the same way, he can decide whether to eat, get up, and dress. Nevertheless, I think that our sole presence modifies the way of being. I find it endearing how a "practice of mutual collaboration" was created in which Raúl asked us if we were bothered if he smoked or where we preferred to meet, at the table or in the living area.

It was interesting to see how not being able to be with him physically when he was hospitalized far from Alcalá, at the beginning of the pandemic, led us to think of other ways of being present, such as phone calls. When it was difficult to leave the house, Raúl would ask us to hold meetings at the EAU to force himself to get out. Together we came up with alternatives to the limitations.

- *Raúl: It made it easier. Closer. The fact that they can come to your house to help you is great when it's hard to get out of the house and you're feeling unwell. You can't get close to them, but they can get close to you. (...) It is very important, a great relief to know that professionals can reach you when you can't reach them.*
- *Ana: It facilitates trust. It is warmer.*
- *Víctor: It represents more support, more protection. It was like knowing that if something happened, they could come.*

33.3.5.3 The Social Network and Support Systems

As already mentioned, inviting friends, family, and professionals into the crisis situation helps define and dissolve the problem. Not only does the person define the problem, but the unique listening of each person allows us to enrich the vision of what is happening and not simplify it. The fact that Raúl's entourage was present helped us to understand a little more about the meaning of unusual experiences, which, until then, made little sense (Seikkula & Arnkil, 2016). An example of this occurred in a Dialogical Meeting when Ana mentioned that the distress she thought Raúl felt regarding these unusual ideas could be related to the two crucial moments in his life. It was a challenge, and we had to delve carefully, more profoundly, so that all participants were as comfortable as possible. Eventually, Raúl commented on the relationship between these delusional experiences and painful moments in his life.

On another occasion, Raúl, amid a crisis, was able to invite one of his brothers to have a conversation that he had not been able to have until then, and clarify an issue that was hurting them very much. Addressing it was both exciting and painful at the same time. At one meeting, he invited two friends, wanting to have other points of view about what was happening to him. And yet at another one, Raúl said he wanted to address what was troubling his mother rather than focus on what was happening to him. I remember meetings during which Ana and Víctor talked about their childhood, parents, and marriage, and how this influenced them to be who they are today, and how they related with Raúl.

It was important to provide a caring space for all people experiencing crises and consider their needs.

- *Ana: I felt accompanied and understood. You were with us. Nobody understands what really happens to you. To understand how to live it, you have to be there.*

  The first time, of course, it is not easy to open up. I did not seen myself being able to do so. Then, of course, opening up and telling your story and him his... That was a before and after in my life.
- *Raúl: When my brother came, things became clear to me that I might have been fuzzy in my head. He clarified things for me. And I said: OK, that's it. It was a dialogue that we needed. We needed it. We had a pending dialogue because some things were very diffused, right?*

The more participation around you, the better because different points of view can be given and other possible conclusions can be reached. Including friends is great. Another opinion, another person who can help. Another point of view.

This is not just a crisis for me, there are several of us involved, and my family also needed to talk.

33.3.5.4 Teamwork and Shared Responsibility

For reasons beyond our control, I have had to facilitate more than one meeting this year without a partner or with someone new to the unit. When I was alone as a professional, at times I felt a stronger need to lead and make decisions. The commitment to offer an answer weighed much more heavily on me. When working in a team, I feel that pressure dilutes, which allows you to think more carefully (like carrying a suitcase and sharing the weight with another person). I believe that the same thing can happen to someone in a distressing situation. If they feel accompanied, they may not feel the need to react and can wait to think more carefully about handling the distress, avoiding hasty decisions that may be dangerous. In the same way, the family or environment of the person "carrying the symptom," feeling accompanied, may have less need to impose a solution.

I can think of the management and decision-making around drug treatment. Raúl was able to participate in the process of adjusting medication, having been informed of the possible effects and knowing that his opinion and needs were fundamental in adjusting the treatment. It was possible to have these conversations with the psychiatrist in the unit with and without his environment. In addition, we provided him with various first-person collective guides and talked to him about the different approaches to mental health that currently exist (Moncrieff, 2013) in order for him to decide with which one he felt most connected.

The horizontality also made it easier for the family and for Raúl to express criticism and what they disagreed with. To integrate the collaboration, I had to be willing to listen to what did not help them, as well as what did help them. Listening to criticism is not always easy. I believe that shared responsibility and teamwork are key to tolerating and managing uncertainty.

I remember how Raúl shared his decision to stop the medication abruptly. I remember my fears about the effects of abrupt discontinuation, and I remember being able to go deeper with Raúl and his family into the reasons for that decision. I remember sharing with Silvia (my dialogue partner) the feelings that this decision generated in each of us, and I remember Raúl listening to us and taking us into account. I remember planning together to see each other more often during the following weeks. I remember how important it was for me to support him in his decision, even if I did not share the chosen way or moment. I remember feeling grateful toward Raúl for sharing this with us.

This makes me connect with a naïve idea I had years ago: If I tell someone to take medication, they will do it. I recall many who have told us they were hesitant to share their desire to discontinue medication with the professionals for fear of not being allowed to do so. I think about how finally they did it alone, in secrecy, without support, without talking about the effects of discontinuing the medication. I did not want that to happen to Raúl; I did not want him to have to lie to me. What kind of trusting relationship would we be building?

- *Raúl: When I was bad, they (Víctor and Ana) may have told you in the meeting how they felt, they wanted something to be done, but I did not want (to be forced). Being able to talk about it helps.*

  Being taken into account and having my opinion respected made me feel more confident.
- *Ana: Yes, all the fears you have… and we asked what should do because we wanted to know. Sometimes, finding the answer is complicated.*

33.3.5.5 Continuity of the Bond

Since the beginning, Silvia and I have been the EAU referents for Raúl and his environment (together with the psychiatrist of the EAU for the Pharmacological Support.). For almost three years, we have seen each other every week in different places and situations. Due to circumstances beyond the EAU's control, I was accompanied by different professionals during this past year, instead of my original partner, Silvia, in the meetings with Raúl. I believe that these continuous changes have been both a difficulty and an opportunity. Raúl said so himself.

It was imperative that I not tell his story to the professionals joining the process: He needed to tell them whatever he wanted to tell them and felt they needed to know. If I thought it could be helpful to share certain information, I did so in front of him. Before going to the meeting, I would ask his permission and let him know who was available to accompany me. On specific days, he thanked me for listening to him and taking into account that he preferred not to interact with a person he did not know, that it was not a good day for him. Subsequently, Raúl authorized me to share what I esteemed important with the professional who was going to meet him, whether he was present or not. He trusted me, and I spoke as if he were present. This decision to speak in front of the people we attend is not a trivial act: It is the opposite of what usually happens in the traditional system. In my opinion, some professionals have not yet understood its importance.

It is worth mentioning that Raúl also understood and accepted that it was important and necessary for me to be accompanied by another member of the team.

The limited time frame during which we can attend the people also produces internal shifts and emotions in the participants of the process, as the date of farewell approaches. In addition, I recognize that being the person who had to maintain the psychological continuity of Raúl's process represented a great deal of pressure, given the responsibility that this entailed.

- *Víctor: If you go to the doctor for a problem and you arrive at a consultation, and the next day you are seen by someone else and the next day you are seen by someone else… It's like a "capea." It's annoying, it's important to be seen by someone who knows you and even more so when it comes to this type of issue.*
- *Ana: When someone already knows you, you don't think about it, it just comes out, you don't have to think about it. Otherwise, you withdraw a bit.*
- *Raúl: If you know the person you open up more, it's more natural. (…) You go to other services and they may read your report, they know your diagnosis, your label… but they don't know you or what you are going through.*

  It's like when you change psychiatrists. Telling your story to so many people is tiring. It's the same for me. Although seeing so many people at the EAU this year has also been good, it has opened up different approaches for me.

  When he introduced me to a new person, the way he treated me, the way he introduced me and all of that… I felt very comfortable because he did it with a lot of tact and respect for me. In other words, asking me and telling me what he thinks I would want. It's the feeling that the other person takes you into account.

  I have only seen professionals asking permission at the EAU and residents showing up at the Dialogue Meetings, instead of standing quietly and observing as in other places where they come in without asking and stand there just observing. You have to have respect for the patient.

33.3.5.6 Tolerance of Uncertainty

On many occasions during a Dialogue Meeting, the cover of "Navigating in Crises" (Distri Afecto, 2017) comes to mind, in which there is a ship at sea I find it interesting to think that the people who participate in the process are in that boat. Everyone may want to go at a different pace; some people are more tired and find it hard to row, and others prefer to row faster because they are in a hurry to get somewhere. In those moments when uncertainty increases, I think it is more important than ever to listen to everyone's rhythm. To be able to tune in, speed up, or wait. That is to say, to keep in step so that the boat stops turning and goes somewhere (with the possibility that the destinations may be different). To row together, even if you cannot see land, forging the way as you row.

I think learning to tolerate uncertainty was a very intense exercise for all of us. At the same time, however, it generated the desire to come together, reach agreements, and feel closer to each other when there was more anguish and violence. Precisely, the uncertainty and the commitment not to act against Raúl's will, made it easier to have more dialogue. It was personally reassuring to know that we were in the same boat when the sea was rough and that there would soon be another meeting.

With many of my colleagues and friends with whom I had the pleasure of coinciding at the EAU, I have talked about what this principle entails. It could be that we connect with fears, responsibility, and power in very difficult moments. In those moments, the need may arise to want to control the actions of the other to mitigate our anxiety because we connect with fear, and the feeling of being in control calms us down. We want the other person to do what we think they should do (stop smoking joints, take their medication, or go into hospital for a few days), but to be able to talk about it as a possibility, not as an imposition, is a liberation and a paradigm shift. Power is assigned to you by the institution and by society, the question is: What do you do with that power? Do you give it back to the people you serve*?*

The truth is that when these fears arise, we tend to look for answers in expert knowledge that tells us what to do. This has happened to me when I have visited my doctor and it also happened to Ana and Víctor. It is complex to sustain the idea that the professionals who facilitated the meetings are not experts in their lives, we don't know what the best decision would be, but we can help them find those answers by collaborating. In my opinion, as we got to know each other, what we were addressing became clear. One of my fears may be that this position is not understood, that they feel alone and end up losing confidence in us. In those days, reading different authors, Sylvia London, Irma Rodríguez, Harlene Andersen, Tom Andersen, and Jaakko Seikkula, helped me to remember my duty and role in the meetings.

Due to the timetable of the unit and the current resources, we were able to talk about how far we could tolerate certain risks, about fears, about each person's needs. Both the parents and Raúl himself were able to generate their own resources to manage the anguish: playing sports, talking to his granddaughter, or listening to certain music. For my part, working as a team is an essential part of sustaining it and being able to think about the small changes that are taking place, even if they are sometimes imperceptible.

- *Ana: You have other weapons, you panic less. You say: well I'm going to do this, or I'm going to do that. You have built other resources. To be more trusting in that you can control something. That has much merit. It's not easy.*
- *Raúl: Not even the most mentally knowledgeable person can heal himself. You can have the tools in theory, but sometimes it's difficult to put them into practice.*

33.3.5.7 Dialogism

The premise of "not talking about people without people" is revolutionary. It sounds simple, but to practice it is a continuous challenge. To convey this idea and to ensure it is fulfilled, is not easy. So what do we talk about? We can talk about what happens to each one of us who is present at the moment. In our culture, we are so accustomed to talking about others that we are not connected to what is happening to ourselves, what happens to us when the other speaks, what we resonate with, why we are saying what we are saying, and to whom we are saying it. Keeping in mind this way of communicating, that is, talking about *ourselves* and what we resonate with, and not the other, allows for deeper listening and an openness to new possibilities, to the multiverse (Bateson, 1972, Maturana, 1978 as cited in Andersen, 1994). *A phenomenon, e.g., a problem, can be described and understood in different ways, none of which is right or wrong, and our task is as far as possible to engage in a dialogue to understand how different people created their descriptions or explanations* (Andersen, 1994, p. 58). There is not just one way of looking at things; such an idea allows us to listen to other visions that can coexist simultaneously. I recognize the effort it can take to listen when another person is not being dialogical, when their view of things is very different from mine, or when what someone thinks or feels is denied and invalidated.

- *Ana: The first time, of course, it's not easy to open up. I hadn't seen myself in such a situation. Then, of course, to open up about your things and for him to tell you his, to find out things. That was a before and after in my life. (...) Listening to how a person feels. You're going to see that maybe it's a person who feels bad and you haven't heard that before from that person, so all of that has an impact on you.*
- *Raúl: I am grateful that people always spoke in front of me because that way I didn't feel pushed around (...). I remember you saying that when we first met and I thought whether it wasn't a manipulation of the person, like when you are admitted, when you turn your back on a lot of things. I have also seen the damage it has done to other friends of mine in psychiatry, who had others decided for them.*

  It's great, it's a different way of working, it gives you more confidence. It's a different thing. It has made me see psychiatry from a different perspective. Before I was very reluctant, I couldn't see psychiatrists. But with you now I go to another one and I don't. You don't feel tied down and you appreciate that.

In my opinion, being dialogical is a philosophy that you decide to integrate into your life. However, at least in my case, I don't always succeed. Working in a team, in pairs, allows us to let each other know when we are being monologic, when we are taking up more space, when we are not speaking tentatively. This allows us to express our different points of view. For this, the bonds of union and security are identified as fundamental. If we could talk about our different visions of things, then so could Raúl, Víctor, and Ana.

On the other hand, we had to remind Víctor and Raúl of the commitment to speak in the first person in many of the meetings. This slowed down the pace of some discussions and changed the focus: Finding out who was right was not significant. In our last meetings, it was exciting to hear phrases like: *I see it this way, even if you don't* or *that's your point of view, mine is different*.

During Raúl's admissions, we had to be more flexible in the way we attended meetings because while he was in the hospital, his reference professionals were different, and the work model was also different. In these meetings, it was difficult for me to express a different vision from the prevailing one, even if I had one.

At this point, I ask myself how to make this section on dialogue less monologic. I think of the various conversations with Silvia, with Raúl, his parents, my colleagues and friends, my learning community, and other mental health professionals. I think of "their voices," which I carry with me, and which are present in me, both inside and outside the Dialogical Meetings. All these people are present even when

I don't want them to be, as they influence what I say and why I say it. Making explicit my internal dialogue and what I connect with has led me to work on my vulnerability. I live with an internal struggle, as different models in mental health inhabit me, and there are times when I feel that exposing myself (as I am doing) means "being a bad professional." That voice I also hear.

I think the polyphony (that all voices count equally) made it possible to respect Raúl's wish not to take neuroleptics, to hear about his experience with them in the past, him feeling *like a soulless, blocked doll.* It was difficult for everyone to agree. It was very hard to facilitate communication in moments of extreme distress, suffering, and violence, and listening was difficult. However, I suppose it was then that the most intense, unspoken issues came up: The traumatic experiences in Raúl's past which he had not shared before and what it meant for his father not to recognize or understand him.

I remember a scene around the round table of the living room when Raúl was talking about his suffering and his hashish consumption. It was difficult for his father to listen without interrupting, and he seemed to be restraining himself from using his two cell phones. We had agreed that everyone should be in the meeting as present as possible. Raúl got up angrily and threw his father's work phone on the floor while saying, *first it's work and then it's me.* After taking a breath and giving each of us the necessary space, we were able to go deeper into what this scene meant for each of us.

In Raúl's process, something happened to me that has also happened in other processes. His brother, his parents, and Raúl were able to talk about what Raúl needed to clarify. Raúl pointed out what nobody wanted to hear, he referred to explicit events from the past that seemed to be the fruit of his imagination but that, after delving more profound, we found out really happened. What seemed crazy was no longer crazy. It is essential to create a safe and nonjudgmental space to address those events that have not been acknowledged before.

Not wanting to lead the conversation and being prepared to be carried along by the tide means embarking on an adventure with the other, where we create a common language, "a language of our own." When repeated in the meetings, there were phrases that made us laugh, and there were also moments when words such as "joints" came up, which made us look at each other and take a deep breath because they were loaded with emotion and meaning.

When I think of Ana I connect with generosity, gentleness, strength, and care. When I think of Víctor I connect with his drive, action, perseverance, and humor. When I think of Raúl, I connect with his intelligence, ability to connect with others, sensitivity, his gift for noticing things before the rest of us do, great creativity, capacity for introspection, authenticity, and transparency.

Sharing part of this journey with Raúl, Ana, and Víctor, has been an incredible and valuable adventure. I am delighted to have "rowed" with them and to feel part of the crew. It has been a process of mutual transformation where I have felt I was learning in listening, not taking my hypotheses as truths, allowing myself to be led and surprised by others.

I would like to end this account with Ana words:

– *Ana: The EAU has been a cane to lean on in the tortuous path of darkness and the unknown.*

And with a final reflection sent by Raul to us when we were finishing the edition of this chapter:

– *Raúl: Yesterday I had a conversation with my father, I felt listened to. What came up took the weight off my shoulders. So I wrote these words:*

Sometimes you just need to be heard.
And feel that they understand your pain,
At the usual Round Table
The look of a gentleman at last proved it to me.

Ethical Statement For confidentiality reasons, the identifying information and names of the family members have been changed. All members gave their consent for their words to be included in the above account. The transcription of the fragments of the conversation has been as faithful as possible. For this reason, in some segments, the language may not be grammatically correct.

References

Aaltonen, J., Seikkula, J., & Lehtinen, K. (2011). The comprehensive Open Dialogue approach in Western Lapland: The incidence of non-affective psychosis and prodromal states. *Psychosis, 3*(3), 179–119.

Alanel, Y. (1997). *Schizophrenia. Its origins and need-adapted treatment*. Karnac.

Andersen, T. (1994). *El Equipo Reflexivo. Diálogos y diálogos sobre diálogos*. Gedisa.

Anderson, H. (2012). Relaciones de colaboración y conversaciones dialógicas: Ideas para una Práctica Sensible a lo Relacional. *Family Process, 51*(1), 1–20.

Bergström, T., Seikkula, J., Alakare, B., Mäki, P., Köngäs-Saviaro, P., Taskila, J. J., Tolvanen, A., & Alantonen, J. (2018). The family-oriented Open Dialogue approach in the treatment of first-episode psychosis: Nineteen-year outcomes. *Psychiatry Research, 270*, 168–175.

Birgitta, A., & Seikkula, J. (2021). The historical development of open dialogue in Western Lapland. Putman y B. Martndale (Eds.), *Open dialogue for psychosis. Organising mental health services to prioritise dialogue, relationship and meaning*. Routledge.

Distri Afecto. (2017). Navegando en las crisis: Autocuidados y apoyo entre iguales en momentos difíciles. *Portada* (Painting). https://primeravocal.org/wpcontent/uploads/2017/05/navegando-en-las-crisis_primera-vocal.pdf

Dozza de Mendoça, L. (2018). *Acompañamiento Terapéutico y clínica de lo cotidiano*. Amazing Books.

Freeman, A., Tribe, R., Stott, J., & Pilling, S. (2019). Open dialogue: A review of the evidence. *Psychiatric Services, 70*(1), 46–59.

Haarakangas, K., Seikkula, J., Alakare, B., & Aaltonen, J. (2016). Diálogo Abierto: Una aproximación al tratamiento psicoterapéutico de la psicosis en Finlandia del Norte. In A. G. García (Ed.), *Terapia Colaborativa. Relaciones y conversaciones que hacen una diferencia*. A Taos Institute Publication.

HOPENDIALOGUE. https://www.hopendialogue.net/

Moncrieff, J. (2013) *Hablando claro. Una introducción a los fármacos psiquiátricos*. .

ODDESSI. Open dialogue: Development and evaluation of a social network intervention for severe mental illness. https://www.ucl.ac.uk/pals/research/clinical-educational-and-health-psychology/research-groups/oddessi

Olson, M., Seikkula, J., & Ziedonis, D. (2014). *The key elements of dialogic practice in open dialogue: Fidelity criteria.* http://umassmed.edu/psychiatry/globalinitiatives/opendialogue/. V 1.1.

Pérez, E. J. (2016). *Saldremos de esta*. Primera Vocal.

Putman, N. (2021). What is open dialogue? En N. Putman y B. Martndale (Eds.), *Open dialogue for psychosis. Organising mental health services to prioritise dialogue, relationship and meaning*. Routledge.

Seikkula, J. (2019). Psychosis is not illness but a survival strategy in severe stress: A proposal for an addition to a phenomenological point of view. *Psychopathology, 52*(2), 1–8.

Seikkula, J., & Arnkil, T. E. (2016). *Diálogos terapéuticos en la red social.* Herder.

Seikkula, J., & Arnkil, T. E. (2019). *Diálogos abiertos y anticipaciones terapéuticas. Respetando La alteridad en el momento presente*. Herder.

Seikkula, J., & Olsen, M. (2003). The open dialogue approach to acute psychosis: Its poetics and micropolitics. *Family Process, 42*(3), 403–418.

Seikkula, J., Aalantonen, J., Alakare, B., Haarakangas, K., Keranen, J., & Dutela, M. (1995). Treating psychosis by means of open dialogue. En S. Friedman (Ed.), *The Reflecting Team in action: collaborative practice in family therapy*. The Guilford Press.

Seikkula, J., Alakare, B., Aalantonen, J., Holman, J., Rasinkangas, A., & Lelithinen, V. (2003). Open Dialogue approach: Treatment principles and preliminary results of a 2 year follow up on first episode schizophrenia. *Ethical Human Sciences and Services, 5*(4), 163 182.

Seikkula, J., Alakare, B., Aalantonen, J., Haarakangas, K., Keranen, J., & Lehtinen, K. (2006). Five-year experience of first episode nonaffective psychosis in Open Dialogue approach: Treatment principles follow up outcomes, and two case studies. *Psychotherapy Research, 16*(2), 214–228.

Von Peter, S., Aderhold, V., Cubellis, L., Bergström, T., Stastny, P., Seikkula, J., Stastny, P., Seikkula, J., & Puras, D. (2019). Open dialogue as a human rights-aligned approach. *Frontiers in Psychiatry, 10*, (387). https://doi.org/10.3389/fpsyt.2019.00387

Chapter 34
Conflicted Stories: A Case of Expanded Reality

Isabel Clarke and Tilda

As human beings, we have experience and we have story. We tend to shape the experience with story into a form that makes sense, is comfortable for ourselves, and presents us in the best light to others. In the case of psychosis, and other exceptional and anomalous experiences, the experience threatens to overwhelm story. In these circumstances, the obvious recourse is to go to the "experts," perhaps the doctor, who has a ready story based on the medical model. You are ill. We can treat you. Cognitive Behaviour Therapy for psychosis (and other psychotherapies) has a different story, based more on what has happened to you and emotional overload, but in judicious deference to superior power, this story tends to slot neatly into the medical model. There are of course other relevant stories: Spiritual emergence/emergency (Grof & Grof, 1991), Shamanism, Power, Threat Meaning Framework (PTMF) (Johnstone & Boyle, 2018). Tilda, the experiencer whose story is featured in this chapter, was bounced between stories, and her history is instructive for all of us who assist travellers accessing the further reaches of the mind.

Introductions are in order. I am a therapist—I trained as a clinical psychologist in mid-life; my career change was driven by a passion to find a more helpful story for mental breakdown. I have worked in the UK National Health Service (NHS) for 30 years, with a focus on people with complex problems. However, Tilda is not "a case": she is not my patient. She is a colleague in the core, managing, group, of the Spiritual Crisis Network UK. I am a founder member of this organization that offers a more hopeful story than the medical one to anyone who recognizes the spiritual dimension to their struggles with alternate realities, and provides sensible but

Tilda is a pseudonym. The real name of the second author has not been disclosed to protect her identity since the case presented in this chapter is based on her personal story.

I. Clarke (✉) · Tilda
Southern Health NHS Foundation Trust, Southampton, UK
e-mail: isabel@scispirit.com

J. A. Díaz-Garrido et al. (eds.), *Psychological Interventions for Psychosis*,
https://doi.org/10.1007/978-3-031-27003-1_34

optimistic support. Tilda has agreed to collaborate with me in presenting her account of a resilient individual, a single Mum who has pursued a successful career (in mental health), despite a number of excursions into alternate realities that have also taken her into the heart of the psychiatric system; the inpatient unit; more than once.

34.1 Tilda's Early Journeys in Expanded Reality

Tilda's first experiences of alternative realities; anomalous experiencing—however you would like to describe it, came through engaging with the 1990s party scene. This partying was fuelled by a variety of substances such as ecstasy and MDMA. Tilda emphasized that this was a leisure pursuit. Her career as a young mental health nurse took precedence, and she saw herself as a well-grounded individual, with no dependency or unhealthy relationship with the substances she enjoyed as part of the social scene she engaged with. It was a magic mushroom omelette ingested when on holiday in an idyllic beach location in Thailand that really "opened a gateway" to a "God-like experience," enveloped in and enhancing perception of the beauty of the natural surroundings. That experience, and another where she experienced effective spiritual healing in India, opened doors to a new interest in things spiritual and in spiritual healing such as Reiki.

Tilda emphasized her natural scepticism and indeed the groundedness that enabled her to engage in unusual experiences and then come back to the normal world. Where she began to explore spiritual healing and Reiki, learning to become a healer herself, she started to experience a clash of stories. For 7 years, she had been working in mental health nursing and achieved the transition from wards to community work, which she loved. Professionally, she was steeped in the medical story, but was now encountering an alternative both at the level of theory (story) and experience—she had received and was delivering spiritual healing. So far, she had maintained balance between the two, but it is at this point, in 1999, when things got out of hand and the venture into new conceptual realms landed her in the psychiatric hospital—as a patient, not a member of staff.

34.2 A New Scientific Story

Studying psychology in mid-life, I had been keen to make psychological sense of two areas I had identified as being incompletely understood; spirituality and mental health, and my explorations led me to a common source for both, which I have written about extensively elsewhere (Clarke, 2008, 2010, 2021). What follows is informed by the Interacting Cognitive Subsystems model of cognitive architecture (Teasdale & Barnard, 1993), which is solidly grounded in the findings of cognitive science about pathways in the brain; what is connected and not connected to what, and where there are bottlenecks; in short, the limitations and idiosyncrasies of human processing that are screened out of awareness as we cannot know in any other way.

In summary, our two ways of knowing—experience and story, or being and thinking about, are rooted in our having two separate circuits in the brain. The sophisticated, verbal one developed as we needed more specific communication to manage living in larger groups, and finer tuned tool use with the development of the hand and fingers (Barnard, 2010). This new capability was bolted onto the original processing capacity, which was focused on survival, as our evolution progressed from animal to human. Working together, these two networks in the brain give us a great degree of control over a considerable, but ultimately limited range, and filter our experience. The two circuits will loosen and separate in specific circumstances—high or low arousal; taking substances, etc. This opens the individual to that expanded consciousness that is sought in drug and in spiritual experiences. However, it takes the person away from their groundedness in their individual self-consciousness and boundedness within their skin. This is fine for a short time, but if allowed to take over too far, or where the route back is lost and the person is stranded in this state, it can quickly become unmanageable and even dangerous. This view recognizes the positives associated with such states—the way they can open an individual up to new creative possibilities, as Tilda was opened to the spiritual and to healing. However, it also recognizes the dangers and the need to learn to manage the threshold between the two states, by remaining grounded in current physical reality and the shared world. This is what SCN teaches.

34.3 Tilda's Breakthrough, Breakdown, Experience

By 1999, Tilda's earlier party, drug induced, experiences were giving way to a deeper appreciation of spiritual states and the powers, particularly of healing, that went with these. Time in India where she experienced effective Reiki healing on an ankle injury, and went on to learn Reiki herself, chimed in with a friendship group taken up with new age spiritual exploration through reading and workshops. This new story about healing was pursued in parallel with the medical model dominated environment of her profession as a psychiatric nurse. However, moving from working in a hospital into the community gave this work a freer and more therapeutic character.

Tilda managed to keep these two worlds in balance until one memorable weekend when, in her terminology, she experienced a popping open to a spiritual awakening—I see "popping" as crossing the threshold between the two processing capacities, the two ways of knowing; crossing from sharing control, so keeping things manageable but limited, into the place of expanded consciousness, where that safety is left behind. I am handing over to Tilda to relate what followed

> The healer that I was following was doing a weekend workshop, and I was looking forward to it. I had been feeling in the flow, and experiencing synchronicities. The breakthrough came while doing distant healing with someone I met in the pub – the healing I had been

taught to do. I met by chance whilst with friends, having a couple of drinks, (no drugs). While doing the agreed distant healing later, alone, I had the experience. I initially entered into a very peaceful state, contented. I then experienced a time warp in from a traumatic incident when I was 10; I had been resuscitated following having been run over by a car. From that time onwards all my life flashed before me, even the minutia: a near death experience displaced. Arriving back in the present, I felt enveloped by all-encompassing love, beginning with myself onwards to all humankind which spread out to all sentient beings, raising above earthly matters to the universe beyond, making me at one with the universe. I received insight that my healing was true. Before that, I had been sceptical and in two minds about it, though people had been giving me feedback that they had results. The peak experience came to an end when my rational mind kicked in and I became consumed by the idea that this was an initiation into becoming the/a messiah. From there it dissolved as my rational mind became scared of the implications of that. 22 years later my only regret around this experience, was that I did not sit with the peak for a little longer.

After that profound experience, I remained awake through the night, absorbing the enormity of what had occurred, whilst I was relatively calm until the morning. Getting up for the day, I found myself now filled with excitement and arousal at the possibilities. I was experiencing my thoughts as never before, seeming linear, all lying there together as if I could think all things all at the same time, whilst feeling really calm about that. Amongst that was a feeling of 3: there would be 3 events. I also had what appeared to be a download of information. I had been staying at the house of spiritually attuned people, who were accepting of it being a spiritual experience. In an experiment, an encyclopaedia was brought out, and I could answer any question posed to me from the broad range of material.

I should have stayed at their house. My mistake was to phone my Mum and say I was going to heal the world. She organised for me to be taken to hers to be seen by an out of hours GP. In my innocence, I told him my framework and told him I really needed something to help me sleep, and was hoping to get into my comfortable bed as I instinctively knew I needed calm time. Instead of which, he told my family I needed to go to Accident and Emergency (A&E) as I was psychotic and could turn violent at any moment. Manipulated into appeasing the family against my better judgement, I went along with it. A&E made things worse as there was a 4 h wait in what was a far too stimulating environment, given the experience I had been through.

By the time I was seen and was undergoing Mental State Examination, my brain was completely scattered. My need to go home to sleep was overridden. I was persuaded to take Haloperidol, and was put in a side room. It was half an hour after consuming this that my peace came crashing down and I experienced unbearably loud screaming in my ears and could not get up to seek assistance, instead seeing black ghost/shadow figures until unconsciousness took over. I woke up in the Acute Psychiatric Ward. W In the morning, I was dumfounded, so shocked at now residing in a room rather than being on duty as staff. However, by the evening I had, as the medication wore off, been able to gain clarity and the insight that they considered mine a mental health presentation. It seemed I could not then go home, I was in disbelief how easily the powers of detainment and medication against your will was do-able. I had the misfortune to meet the ward manager from hell.

I was in hospital for 10 days until a Tribunal released me, after which I went to Ireland, where I had family, to settle and chill out. I felt highly traumatised. I had been injected against my will, being surrounded by men and given Acuphase in my backside; an awful drug mostly used in the case of potential for violence. It annihilated me physically but I learned then it gives no relief to the mind, just prevents you from moving effectively or to be able to string together sentences. I couldn't cope. I was dribbling and suffering inside. I had a realization around what my patients had been through, all those years I had been working in Acute. They had told me, however I had only a limited ability prior to my own experience to fully understand.

At this point I had fallen out with Mum. Because I didn't want to speak to her because of her failure to recognize the abuse, I was undergoing in hospital, preferring the view that the professionals know best, she phoned the services describing me as in breakdown. I had a near panic attack when they arrived unannounced at my door. This led to me being sectioned and brought straight back to the traumatic ward scenario, that I was trying to escape.

I shifted strategies and realised it was best to go with it. I accepted I needed their medication and subsequently proceeded to give appearance of compliance with the prescribed Olanzapine. Only in Northern Ireland can it be that when you phone a solicitor would they give you the advice to get over the border. A work colleague I phoned advised I did not sound drowsy enough, so it was unlikely I would be getting the early discharge I was hoping for, one where I could get back to enjoying nature, and indeed enjoying this new found expansion, within which I never did lose touch with reality, provided I was in an environment of my own choosing. So, with careful planning, I managed to escape.

I got to Dublin, where I stayed with my uncle and his family. I had sought him out, knowing him to be my wise uncle. I was right, and in doing so I made much more progress. For a man with no actual experience in psychiatric matters. he was the first who was able to assist me in seeing what others' concerns were in a comprehensible way, by being respectful of my experience, whilst pointing why other people were worried. Unlike myself at that point, he could see what others could see.

I moved on from him to the family farm, now with another uncle who had lived there all his life. The simplicity of his life was the grounding that I had instinctively known I needed. I was still in an altered state, whilst, as from the beginning, I felt quite in control of it, and could experience it in this sanctuary. My uncle, who had known me all my life, was easy going and offered me the space to do so.

Unfortunately, my peace was again shattered following my father having used the ability to have me sectioned yet again, on the grounds of my escape. I was hoodwinked into entering outpatients quite sure I was not detainable: however, papers had already been signed. I was surrounded by numerous nurses, walked down to a bed; told to lie down with no information as to what was occurring and was injected. I subsequently found out I was on section, and there was no right to appeal; no right what so ever to object to medication and no advocacy, and the nurses were dreadful. Southern Ireland psychiatric services were in the dark ages.

I came home as a shadow of my former self, experiencing panic attacks for the first time in my life. I was defeated by the meds and accepted the medical model. I was so traumatised from my experiences, that my actual life had turned into a living nightmare, whilst my internal world had experienced so much discovery that was being so interrupted, and ultimately repressed. It left me feeling I had let myself down when the drugs crushed me: for instance, how stupid I had been to believe that my experience was valid. I carried on with the meds for 6 months, and they had disturbing side effects. I was detached from myself; I just loved going to sleep at night, thankful I now had easy access to Valium in addition to the anti-psychotics. I did continue to be out with friends at all opportunities, as I found it not so easy to sit with myself. However, I was not responding in social situations, rather just becoming a quiet bystander, the opposite of the way anyone had ever known me to be. I was informed afterwards by people who had known me before, how upset they were at this apparent loss of the friend they had known. Having heard I'd had a "breakdown" people assumed that my side effects from the drugs was it.

34.4 A Clash of Stories

Tilda's account nicely illustrates three different positions that can be taken in relation to such experiences, and the difference in outcome for each. To start with there was the spiritual and transformative experience, going with the flow, at one with the universe, synchronicities abounding, access to new powers of knowledge and healing that worked well for quite a while. A social environment that was supportive of the spiritual world view combined with staying grounded in employment helped to sustain the peak experiences safely. However, there came a time when it went over the top, and telling other people such as mother about special mission and abilities raised alarm bells.

According to the medical story what was happening was simple. Tilda was ill, probably with bipolar disorder, and this needed to be crushed as quickly as possible using powerful drugs and legal coercion. Her viewpoint was not to be heeded as she was "out of her mind." According to my, spiritual, understanding, she had for some time been managing the threshold between the two ways of experiencing: the ordinary, everyday one and what I call "the transliminal," following Claridge (1997) (which is the Latin for across the threshold). Because crossing this line means leaving behind individual self-consciousness and moving into relationship with the whole, it leaves behind the sharp distinctions we are accustomed to in our everyday life. Things feel connected—hence the synchronicities. The sense of self becomes fluid—hence the new messiah feeling. Clearly all this has its dangers, but it did summon real powers of healing for Tilda and was life enhancing without the artificial assistance of drugs. The existence of a supportive social milieu, accepting of this potential of human experience as something positive and to be pursued, was important for its remaining in balance.

The effect of the medical establishment taking charge was to shut down, side line, and devalue all the positives that went with the spiritual perspective. All agency was taken away from Tilda. She was confined in a frightening environment and forcibly given powerful drugs with side effects more disabling than the original imbalance. Moreover, in removing the positive story she was given a new perception of herself as defective and unstable, defeated by the system, whereas her first instinct had been to rebel. Again, the importance of the social milieu can be noted. Tilda's mother, sister, and father were all indoctrinated into the medical perspective, which teaches fear of anomalous experiencing, leading to coercion and not listening to Tilda's point of view.

The third perspective is the balanced one represented by the wise Irish uncles. They accepted that Tilda was not fully functional and so needed temporary support and protection until she regained her balance and was able to operate efficiently in the ordinary world. Her Dublin uncle helped her to see things from the other side of the threshold in terms of her impact on others. The calm atmosphere provided by her rural uncle was enabling her to get back together, when her father's intervention, instructed by mother and sister, disrupted the slow healing and plunged her back into the medical story.

34.5 Schizotypy

The entitlement of the medical world to take charge and coerce in these circumstances rests on the assumption that this is the scientific approach. Our society's unquestioning deference to science is soundly based on the material benefits it has brought in terms of control over the environment and progress in physical medicine. However, it has been pointed out that Psychiatry's claim to this status is flimsy. The concept of distinct mental "illnesses" has been effectively challenged (e.g. Bentall, 2003, 2009; Boyle, 2002), and the operation of psychiatric medication has been shown to be miss-sold as "cure" for these fictitious conditions (Moncrieff, 2008). It is undeniable that these medicines do have an effect and have a place where someone is in overwhelming distress or a danger to themselves and others, but they operate more simply by modulating state of arousal etc. Whitaker (2010) and others have uncovered how the research on which the inflated claims are based is seriously unreliable, as overwhelmingly funded by pharmaceutical companies benefitting from the exaggeration.

There is a sounder strand of science that has been investigating this area thoroughly for decades in an unbiased atmosphere, and this is Schizotypy research conducted by Claridge and his collaborators (1997). Unfortunately, this has been a predominantly academic exercise with little overlap, until recently, with clinical application. Schizotypy accepts anomalous experiencing as on a continuum with ordinary experience, and as a potential open to all human beings, but more accessible to some than to others. It examines the neural correlates of these experiences, and the life circumstances creating greater susceptibility, as well as looking even-handedly at the effects for the individual of high Schizotypy (or openness to anomalous experiences—i.e. crossing the threshold).

The results of this research strand offer a very different story to the medical one. High Schizotypy does indeed correlate with vulnerability to psychotic breakdown, but equally with high creativity, sensitivity, and spirituality—attributes that are highly prised in our society. I use this to rebalance the direly stigmatizing effect of the medical story on self-image in my approach to psychosis within psychiatric services—to be covered later.

High Schizotypy has been shown to be associated with both genetic predisposition and trauma, so I explored with Tilda where her susceptibility might have come from. On the one hand, she declared that, "if it happens to me, it could happen to anyone" as she was a singularly well-grounded, pragmatic, individual. She also has a ready sense of humour, on hand to debunk anything over solemn and pretentious. However, there were also relevant factors in her background. Her extensive Irish family roots contributed both Celtic spirituality and Catholicism. She recounted a particular mountain she often climbed as a child where she felt a strong Celtic feminine memory; having a psychic dream from the Celtic world when her Granny died; a meaningful experience of spiritual healing in a church with an aunt. On the trauma aspect, there was the near-death experience of being run over age 10, and her most recent episode, which will be related next, came in the context of extreme stress and personal threat to herself and her son. All these experiences will have helped to prepare Tilda to cross that threshold.

34.6 Bringing the Narrative Up to Date

Tilda did indeed have two more episodes following the one narrated; one she could attribute to smoking cannabis, and the second, with no apparent trigger, but once the experience had taken hold, she did consume cannabis, leading to what she could more easily view as psychosis. This included a very humorous and enjoyable experience, witnessing the A&E doctors turning into fully grown farm animals, leading to the realization that "I'm clearly out of my head here." Following a relatively brief admission to a private hospital and allowed to remain psychiatric drug free, she was recovered and back at work within 3 weeks. After that she was essentially stable for about 20 years. Ten years later, she had her son, with no ill effects. She had delayed pregnancy fearing it might produce a relapse, until she felt confident that all that was behind her.

Though this episode was acute and she had found herself temporarily trapped in a nightmare hospital experience, she came through it determined to work for a truly therapeutic mental health system. The difference was that Tilda's alternative story had developed considerably in the interval.

When going through the earlier episodes, Tilda had two separate stories that did not connect. One was about enlightenment and spiritual awakening, and the other was about mental illness. As a result, she yo-yoed between the two, with the damaging medical one essentially winning in the end. Encountering first Emma Bragdon (e.g. Bragdon, 2013) and then the Spiritual Crisis Network changed that, and provided a narrative that embraced both poles, along with techniques to manage imbalance. At the SCN conference in Mundesley, Norfolk in 2015, she said she met her peer group—people who recognized mental breakdown as, potentially, a stage in the process of spiritual growth and development. This process can be managed by grounding in the physical present and staying in touch with the normal, social, world, even though the mind might be in a completely different place. This is not about obliterating the experience as the medical approach dictates, but managing it, while aware of the potential risks and dangers that might ultimately make recourse to the mental health services unavoidable. Having a supportive social milieu is crucial for successful navigation of crisis. This is well illustrated by Tilda's history so far. She was making good progress at finding the balance when she was supported by her Irish uncles, before her immediate family, with their fear and adherence to a purely medical solution, weighed in. SCN provides precisely this alternative context through its responses to emails and its peer groups.

Tilda threw herself into SCN, undertaking the training and joining the team of volunteers who compose responses to crisis emails. This entitled her to join the Core Group and participate in the running of the organization. Consequently, when the intolerable stress of a situation with child protection catapulted her into another episode, she entered the system with a more elaborated and helpful story to counter the medical one, and bounced back relatively quickly and successfully as a result.

34.7 Tilda Resumes; The Next Instalment

As mentioned above, the background to my latest episode was a result of the intolerable strain of being placed incorrectly under child protection and monitored by social services through misinterpretations and incompetence, just as the Covid pandemic lockdown commenced. Despite being subjected to intolerable stress, I continued to work as an NHS frontline responder. A few months in, with the previous records of "mental illness" also being cited as a problem, I had no option but to be signed off work. I soldiered on, joining a weekly women's development group which used archetypes, accessing a bespoke counselling by an ex-colleague who had created her own consultancy, with a spell in Ireland and using SCN grounding techniques, alongside their support group. At this point I hadn't actually figured that I might be heading into another peak experience. I was more consumed with the miscarriage of justice, and ruminating unwanted thoughts. Finding it impossible to relax, I lost appetite, and resorted to chain smoking. All the while I was in lockdown and having to prioritise my son's wellbeing. In the initial phase, whilst I had been able to offload on the phone to a trusted set of work colleagues, I put up a front around the neighbourhood, concealing the stress I was enduring, due to the apparent shame (it transpired that was incorrect as it was later revealed they had become my greatest supporters).

Six months into this stress condition, a letter from a solicitor that was a breakthrough, set the ball in motion in the other direction. It started with subtle experiences and coincidences that signified to me that we are aligned with the global emergency created by COVID. I identified with Demeter in the Persephone myth, and the Bat out of Hell album that I had sung my heart out to as a teenager in front of what had become my sacred mountain years later. I connected this with COVID and was aware of the presence of my deceased father and uncles, as well as the presence of my best friend from school who had died young.

This new episode began as before with a relatively euphoric phase. I knew I had "popped" again. While this was something I had avoided for over the 20 years, once it took hold, it was addictive. I was aware of what was happening and of the need to stay grounded. I had some emergency meds, Lorazepam, that I had requested. I took that one night, and very unusually, had disturbing side effects that I had never experienced before with that drug.

The psychedelic experiences started to go faster. A fateful weekend, involving time in the pub and some alcohol, tipped things over the edge, leading to a trip in the back of a police van to a seclusion room, while experiencing that I was going to "burst into god." I had lined up a safely held space with my trusted friend and was looking to make my way home to take more Lorazepam at the point when the police van arrived.

The mental health services became heavily involved. I consider that I was sectioned too early and really one should not be sectioned whilst intoxicated. Whilst the peak experience lasted a few more days, in the hospital environment, I would rather have had that within an environment of my choosing. However, I spent

14 days in an extremely unsympathetic hospital environment, where the nurses wandered around with clipboards, making no effort at communication. The ward round and tribunal (that failed to release me from my section despite the fact I had settled) were particularly invalidating experiences, taking more notice of my son's social worker and other professionals than of me. I was treated as a person who had no rights, and they failed to recognize my realistic worries around care for my son while I was in hospital.

I was not given the opportunity to discuss my medication options with the doctors, rather given high doses of what it became apparent all the patients were prescribed. Whilst still holding on to the powerful experience I had just been through, I was not disclosing this to anyone within the ward, but palmed the meds as I didn't want them to steal the magic realm. I found my grounding by supporting the peer group on the ward, who similarly were being ignored by the nursing staff, using my working knowledge to make the ward a bit more therapeutic, to the annoyance of the awful nurses and the amazement of the few more dynamic nurses. Not taking medication covertly was a dangerous strategy in this particular establishment as I was aware that they were very quick to administer the long-lasting depot injection, which brought much fear.

Once out of hospital, I was able to clear up misperceptions and so resolve matters with Social Services, resume normal life, return to work, and in fact, soon, secure a more senior position.

I have emerged from this experience if anything stronger and more determined to fight for a revolution in mental health services. Collaborating over this chapter is one element of that fight.

34.8 Transforming the Ward Environment

Tilda's experiences well illustrate what can be wrong with the mental health services. The Comprehend, Cope, and Connect (CCC) approach that I have developed within acute mental health services is an attempt to remedy precisely this situation by taking a person-centred, individual formulation, based approach and applying it to the entire ward culture. This is covered extensively elsewhere (Durrant et al., 2007; Clarke & Wilson, 2008; Araci & Clarke, 2017), so what follows is a brief summary.

CCC meets the individual presenting to the acute mental health service as someone whose coping capacity has been overwhelmed by events and experiences. They are coping in ways that make sense at the time, but when persisted with, simply reinforce the problem. For instance, when things feel intolerable, withdrawal and self-neglect, or attempting to escape through suicide, make sense, but do not ultimately solve anything and in fact make things worse. In cases like Tilda's, where there is a tendency to cross that threshold, referred to above, into altered states of reality, this other dimension can offer a welcome escape, but one with inherent dangers.

For a significant proportion of people accessing mental health services, past trauma or adversity plays a role in producing the intolerable internal state. This phenomenon can be understood by reference to the two processing systems described earlier that have been labelled experience and story here. Essentially, when the emotional, experience based, processing becomes divorced from the "thinking about," story, system, contextual information held by the story side is lost. Crucially, this includes time, so that earlier threat experiences are added to current issues. There is also evidence that such experiences facilitate crossing the threshold (i.e. high Schizotypy). In Tilda's case, it is probable that the near-death experience she had as a child contributed to her vulnerability here.

Ideally, each person accessing the service will be engaged to collaborate on a formulation that draws on these factors, in the form of a diagram that brings it to life (Fig. 34.1). The overwhelming feeling is identified in the centre, along with immediate circumstances leading to breakdown and any past circumstances feeding into it. The person's strengths, potential, values, and, if any, faith or sense of spiritual connection are then explored and named. The individual is met as a whole person, not just a problem. Then, their current ways of coping, with short-term gains these bring, along with the disadvantages in the longer term, are tracked. These form the vicious cycles keeping the person trapped. Breaking these cycles can then inform the agenda for the admission, whether by programmes delivered in the hospital or other forms of support and intervention.

It is not always possible to coproduce an individual formulation with everyone; lack of someone qualified to provide a formulation when needed, and the capacity of the person at a difficult time can all impact here. However, the team can think about them together using this structure—but always staying with everyday,

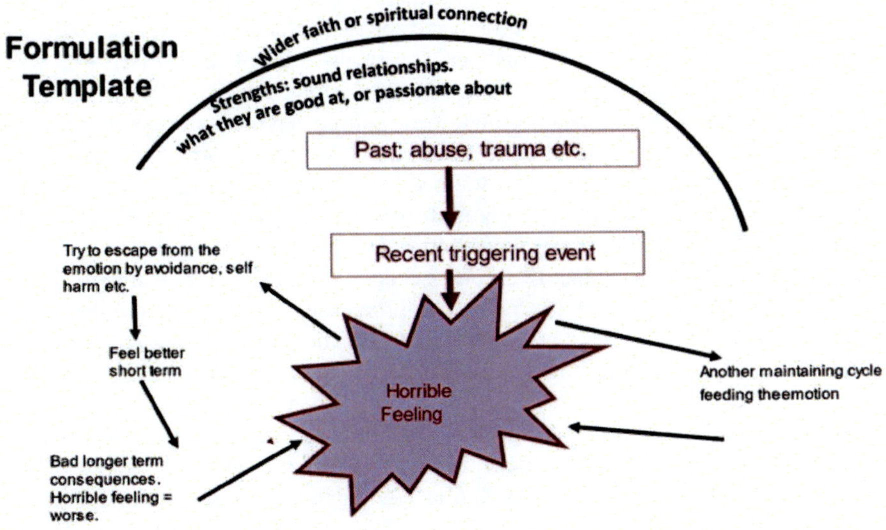

Fig. 34.1 Formulation template

respectful, language that would be appropriate if coproduced. This thinking can then inform goals and structure for the admission. Programmes that fit naturally with this approach are often quite simple: arousal management both up and down, to help keep the two processing systems together; emotional coping skills so that the emotion can be faced and expressed rather than drive behaviour; self-compassion skills, and psychotic symptom management approached in a way that normalizes anomalous experiencing and counters stigma (Clarke, 2010, 2013). Crucially, all staff members are involved in this programme. Even if they do not coproduce formulations or run groups, they know enough to see their patients as suffering individuals trying to cope, and can help coach them in new skills using the available programmes.

There are a number of acute (and other) services employing this CCC approach in England, Scotland, and Northern Ireland, and there are a few evaluation studies, though more are needed (Bullock et al., 2020; Araci & Clarke, 2017; Paterson et al., 2018; Durrant et al., 2007).

34.9 Conclusion

The account given by Tilda of her experiences will hopefully enable the reader to appreciate mental health breakdown more from the inside. From the outside, conventional, medical point of view, Tilda had a number of bipolar episodes requiring admission under the mental health act as she was non-compliant and lacked "insight"—i.e. she did not agree with the psychiatrist. From the inside, exploration "across the threshold," whether through spiritual healing or substances, was a valued part of her life, but did sometimes have a tendency to spiral out of control. At such times, her behaviour became erratic and she made disturbingly grandiose statements. Through much of these episodes, she retained an observing self—as witnessed by the fact that she was able to plan and effect escape with considerable efficiency. She was aware when things were getting beyond her and she needed help, but unfortunately, the help offered failed to take into account her preferences and was blunt and coercive. She was trapped between the two, conflicted, stories.

However, there is research that demonstrates that the scientific, medical, world needs to take account of the other story; research showing that how someone makes sense of their experiences has real consequences for health and recovery. Peters et al. (1999), Peters (2010) looked at the significance of context for the impact of unusual beliefs and experiences. More recently, in the work of Brett et al. (2007), Brett (2010) and Heriot-Maitland et al. (2012), comparable experiences for people in different contexts (clinical or non-clinical) have been shown to result in significantly different life adaptation. Spiritual and religious ways of making sense of anomalous experiences figure alongside mediumship and new age beliefs in the group being favourably compared with those seeing their episode in medical terms. Taken together with robust epidemiological findings (Warner, 2007), these data point to the uncomfortable conclusion that much routine health service practice is producing iatrogenic harm.

I have long been only too conscious of this situation and have attempted to remedy it through my work within the mental health services, e.g. Clarke (2021), Araci and Clarke (2017), and beyond them, through SCN. Tilda joins me in this agenda in both these arenas, bringing with her the unique advantage of deep immersion in both.

References

Araci, D., & Clarke, I. (2017). Investigating the efficacy of a whole team, psychologically informed, acute mental health service approach. *Journal of Mental Health Journal, 26*, 307–311. https://doi.org/10.3109/09638237.2016.1139065

Barnard, P. J. (2010). Current developments in inferring cognitive capabilities from the archaeological traces left by stone tools: Caught between a rock and a hard inference. In A. Nowell & I. Davidson (Eds.), *Stone tools and the evolution of human cognition* (pp. 207–226). University Press of Colorado.

Bentall, R. P. (2003). *Madness explained. Psychosis and human nature*. Allen Lane.

Bentall, R. P. (2009). *Doctoring the mind: Why psychiatric treatments fail*. Allen Lane.

Boyle, M. (2002). *Schizophrenia: A scientific delusion?* Routledge.

Bragdon, E. (2013). *The call of spiritual emergency: From personal crisis to personal transformation*. Lightening Up Press.

Brett, C. M. C. (2010). Transformative crises. In I. Clarke (Ed.) *Psychosis and spirituality: Consolidating the new paradigm (2nd Edition)*. Wiley.

Brett, C. M. C., Peters, E. P., Johns, L. C., Tabraham, P., Valmaggia, L. R., & Mcguire, P. K. (2007). Appraisals of anomalous experiences interview (AANEX): A multidimensional measure of psychological responses to anomalies associated with psychosis. *The British Journal of Psychiatry, 191*, 23–30.

Bullock, J., Whiteley, C., Moakes, K., Clarke, I., & Riches, S. (2020). Single-session comprehend, cope, and connect intervention in acute and crisis psychology: A feasibility and acceptability study. *The Journal of Clinical Psychology and Psychotherapy, 28*, 219. https://doi.org/10.1002/cpp.2505

Claridge, G. S. (Ed.). (1997). *Schizotypy. Relations to illness and health*. Oxford University Press.

Clarke, I. (2008). *Madness, mystery and the survival of God*. 'O' Books.

Clarke, I. (Ed.). (2010). *Psychosis and spirituality: Consolidating the new paradigm*. Wiley.

Clarke, I. (2013). Spirituality: A new way into understanding psychosis. In E. M. J. Morris, L. C. Johns, & J. E. Oliver (Eds.), *Acceptance and commitment therapy and mindfulness for psychosis* (pp. 160–171). Wiley-Blackwell.

Clarke, I. (2021). *Meeting mental breakdown mindfully – How to help the comprehend, cope and connect way*. Routledge.

Clarke, I., & Wilson, H. (Eds.). (2008). *Cognitive Behaviour Therapy for acute inpatient mental health units; working with clients, staff and the milieu*. Routledge.

Durrant, C., Clarke, I., Tolland, A., & Wilson, H. (2007). Designing a CBT service for an acute inpatient setting: A pilot evaluation study. *Clinical Psychology and Psychotherapy, 14*, 117–125.

Grof, C., & Grof, S. (1991). *The stormy search for the self*. Mandala.

Heriot-Maitland, C., Knight, M., & Peters, E. (2012). A qualitative comparison of psychotic-like phenomena in clinical and non-clinical populations. *British Journal of Clinical Psychology, 51*, 37–53. https://doi.org/10.1111/j.2044-8260.2011.02011.x

Johnstone, L., & Boyle, M. with Cromby, J., Dillon, J., Harper, D., Kinderman, P., Longden, E., Pilgrim, D., & Read, J. (2018). *The Power Threat Meaning Framework: Towards the identification of patterns in emotional distress, unusual experiences and troubled or troubling behaviour, as an alternative to functional psychiatric diagnosis*. British Psychological Society.
Moncrieff, J. (2008). *The myth of the chemical cure: A critique of psychiatric drug treatment*. Palgrave Macmillan.
Peters, E. R. (2010). Are delusions on a continuum. The case of religious and delusional beliefs. In I. Clarke (Ed.) *Psychosis and spirituality: Consolidating the new paradigm (2nd Edition)*. Wiley.
Peters, E. R., Day, S., McKenna, J., & Orbach, G. (1999). The incidence of delusional ideation in religious and psychotic populations. *British Journal of Clinical Psychology, 38*, 83–96.
Paterson, C., Karatzias, T., Harper, S., Dougall, N., Dickson, A., & Hutton, P. (2018). A feasibility study of a cross-diagnostic, CBT-based psychological intervention for acute mental health inpatients: Results, challenges, and methodological implications. *British Journal of Clinical Psychology, 58*, 211–230. https://doi.org/10.1111/bjc.12209
Teasdale, J. D., & Barnard, P. J. (1993). *Affect, cognition and change: Remodelling depressive thought*. Lawrence Erlbaum Associates.
Warner, R. (2007). Review of recovery from Schizophrenia: An international perspective. A report from the WHO collaborative project, the international study of Schizophrenia. *American Journal of Psychiatry, 164*, 1444–1445.
Whitaker, R. (2010). *Anatomy of an epidemic*. Broadway Paperbacks.

Relevant Websites

Isabel Clarke's Website. http://www.isabelclarke.org
Spiritual Crisis Network. https://spiritualcrisisnetwork.uk

Chapter 35
Epilogue: Overcoming Adversities

Emilio Gotera-Sosa

I am a survivor with more than 40 years of lived experiences and today I work as a mental health professional.

I was born in a family made up of my parents and six siblings. I am the youngest of those. My parents gave us love, assistance, and education. They were involved at a social and political level, for a regime change toward democracy.

From a very young age, I got involved in social and political organizations, for rights, freedoms, and democracy. At that time, compulsory military service was carried out for all young people. Rebellious, I considered not doing military service because I heard the stories and experiences lived by my father. After a civil war, where brothers fought against brothers and later the very traumatic post-war, they advised me to do military service, so as not to be discriminated against. I ignored those advices due to my anti-militarist idea, and did not receive support with that attitude. I grew up in a political environment where anti-militarism prevailed, motivating me to alter public order and social peace, which made me restless and distressed, making my mind go off. I blamed the SYSTEM and my family. All aggravated by the death of a close friend, this further exacerbated the loss of control of my life and my mind. My family, advised by professionals, decided to admit me to a center, where they mechanically restrained my hands and feet, medicating me and depriving me of all freedom, and only gave me food and psychiatric treatment; that agony and lack of freedom made my mind race even more.

After a few days, the psychiatrist and paramedics untied me, allowing me access to the entire building and assigning me another, more comfortable room. The conclusion I had with this action was, if this is psychiatry, "God come and bring

E. Gotera-Sosa (✉)
Canarian Association for the Integration of Mental Health ESPIRAL, Las Palmas de Gran Canaria, Spain

J. A. Díaz-Garrido et al. (eds.), *Psychological Interventions for Psychosis*,
https://doi.org/10.1007/978-3-031-27003-1_35

justice." They continued with the same trend of locking us up at noon and at night in the room, letting me leave the room, the rest of the day per building. I saw the occasional electroshock given to the admitted people. They left the door open to intimidate and coerce other patients. I thought I would not escape, but rather I would go out through the door through which I was admitted and someday I would share my lived experience.

Since this admission at the age of twenty-one, I have had about twenty more admissions to private clinics, in the current psychiatric units. My last admission was more than 17 years ago. Today, I am aware that I have to take my treatment with total responsibility, as one more illness and continue fighting to mature, train, and collaborate in overcoming others, where today in those isolation units, they continue to practice the same containment protocols already described.

In the first stage of my life as a patient, I had a struggle within myself, not having information and training about what mental health was. I isolated myself at home for years, I lost all my friends, I dropped out of school, and all I wanted was to lie in bed without thinking about anything; fear and insecurity took hold of me. I didn't understand my new diagnostic label and professionals who attended me did not channel my anguish, but limited themselves to their upload and lower the treatment, under their criteria, I came to deify them, I consulted and was treated by many psychiatrists, changing from one to another. I did not understand that I had to structure and organize my mind. Also, in that stage of youth, I reflected and thought saying to myself, if a professional came to my home, he would accompany me to get out of this isolation and loneliness to help me overcome that circumstance. I thought that speaking with my family, health professionals and friends would make me see that the ideas of social and political changes do not change overnight, but rather by creating awareness in the citizen, in addition to the deaths of the loved ones, it is the law of life, and there is a grieving process that all people suffer.

With the help of my family, I began to develop mature ideas, to recover and remember the skills of daily life, instrumental and developmental, and they motivated me to acquire social responsibilities again.

In 2006, I decided to live alone, look for work to survive, and take charge of my life on my own initiative.

As we know, the evolution of the care of people with psychosocial problems, in my country, began with the ecclesiastics, and somewhat later, the users were endorsed by the professionals, and around the 60s, 70s and 80s, the relatives took sides claiming and fighting in the street for a more dignified care for their children and improve the quality of care, whereas in this decade, those affected are taking the initiative and making ourselves known in everything related to care, that they treat us and respect our decisions.

In 2009, with other colleagues affected by the same problems, we founded and legalized the Canarian Association for the Integration of Spiral Mental Health, with the objectives of showing our worth, working to break and end with the social, health, judicial, labor stigma, and work to achieve equal conditions. In short words, empower ourselves. We also fight for improvements, changes, and transformation of a new paradigm and mentality. In this association, I learned to channel my concern to live in a world where freedoms, justice, equality, in conclusion, human rights are respected.

We self-manage our own human resources. Our few resources are financial, technical, and material. We decided that in a democratic assembly we should resolve our incidents and conflicts among equals, with respect and empathy. We provide help, support, accompaniment, guide and orient other colleagues who request it and who need it to address their suffering.

Mental health user associations set an example for society, our families, professionals, and institutions that we know how we like to be treated, and mental health must be treated naturally. Anyone at some point in their life can have a mental health problem; misinformation, lack of training, and lack of personal maturity in vital life processes, such as trauma, heartbreak, conflict, personal relationships, poverty, loss of a job or work, lack of housing, drugs, addictions, etc., are all causes that can make one suffer from a psychosocial illness.

My overcoming and return to normality and social integration was due to the family support that I have always had. They transmitted me patience, kindness, tolerance, responsibility, occupation, and activity. Also with our association, I learned to channel my rebellion, and understood that it is necessary to have the ability to accept and adapt to reality, to achieve goals without confrontation, but with knowing how to be. Another formula was to resume studies as a Higher Technician in Social Integration. Currently I work in Service for the Promotion of Personal Autonomy in Mental Health, it also greatly influenced my life, sharing all my concerns with my partner. I owe all these achievements and personal goals to my effort, commitment, the spirit of fighting for life and to the people who have loved me, love me, and have always been by my side.

Today, I am being cared by a professional who continues to use the old techniques. They do not ask or question that everything evolves and changes. I have defendant the causes that they motivated the loss of the reins of my life I have defendant them. That suffering psychosocial I have overcome suffering for 20 years. I have learned to have my inner peace again, I am happy with the life I lead, I am a spirited fighter and I solve personal problems and conflicts without worrying, without losing emotional control. I have a life project, I have given meaning to life, I occupy my social role. Some professionals continue to treat you like a patient, without taking into account the evolution achieved. Legislation in my country continues to maintain by law that a person with a mental health diagnosis has that diagnosis for life, preventing in most of the cases their full integration, without respecting that we are citizens as any other, although they enact very nice laws, which are not enforced.

With great perseverance, an instinct to overcome, we will overcome adversity and achieve full integration into society.

Index

A

Acceptance and commitment therapy (ACT), ix, 17, 31, 94, 225–246, 249–281, 285–304, 307–317, 323–342, 347, 349, 350, 357–359, 361, 362, 364, 370, 373, 382, 383, 385–390, 395, 403, 405, 423, 425, 433, 439, 446–451, 467, 468, 488, 500, 560, 659, 660, 662, 666, 670, 671, 673, 674, 694, 700, 703, 721, 724, 725

Acceptance and recovery therapy by levels for psychosis (ART), 31, 347–374, 381–419, 423–451

Adaptation, 25, 88, 93, 126–130, 134, 171, 194, 252, 253, 326, 347–350, 355–364, 374, 381, 388, 390, 393, 399, 405, 410–419, 424, 428, 433, 439, 531, 575, 597, 669, 670, 739, 798

Adolescent, 6, 297, 485, 486, 488–490, 493–502

Antipsychotics, 1, 4, 14, 23–25, 28, 37–53, 59, 61, 83, 86, 87, 146, 149, 203, 235, 274, 276, 288, 348, 357, 360, 383, 391, 406, 435, 479, 493, 542, 596, 655, 709

B

Behavior analysis, 3

Behaviors, 8, 17, 28, 47, 71, 77–84, 86, 88–97, 105–121, 126, 131, 145, 156, 157, 172, 176, 180, 183, 184, 191, 203, 205, 211, 213–214, 226, 227, 230–233, 235–238, 240, 241, 250–252, 254–256, 262, 267–275, 280, 288, 289, 291–294, 296, 298–300, 302, 303, 309–312, 317, 324, 325, 330, 332–334, 338, 339, 349–355, 360, 365, 366, 369, 370, 372, 373, 382, 388, 392, 396, 399, 401, 425–434, 436, 438, 442, 445, 449, 466, 467, 469, 470, 474, 481, 486–489, 491, 493–495, 497, 498, 503, 509, 511, 513–516, 518, 519, 521, 528–531, 534, 536, 560, 566, 593, 594, 599, 605, 607, 616, 622, 623, 625, 626, 647, 663, 667, 669–671, 673, 676, 677, 679–682, 684, 689, 692, 693, 708–712, 714–717, 724, 733, 740, 755, 765, 798

C

Case study, 3, 17, 312–316, 372, 469–480, 559, 560, 562

Clinical cases, 186, 200, 202, 219, 246, 281, 304, 317, 342, 374, 381–419, 423–451, 482, 486, 489–493, 504, 522, 525, 540, 551, 555, 587–609, 699, 700, 726

Clinical practice, 7, 17, 26, 50, 200, 308, 425, 540, 622, 663, 668, 690

Clinical trial, 37, 41, 63, 172, 218, 228, 606

Cognitive, 1, 3, 9, 25, 29, 43, 44, 47–50, 83, 86, 88, 89, 106, 110, 112, 113, 125, 132, 147, 149, 153, 154, 171, 172, 174, 179, 180, 186, 205–207, 212, 217, 229, 233, 250–252, 254, 256, 262, 267–270, 276, 279, 286, 288, 295, 308, 311, 312, 324, 347–351, 355–357, 359, 360, 362, 364–369, 373, 374, 381–383, 385, 387–390, 392, 395, 397, 399, 404–407, 416, 427–429, 431, 433, 435, 436, 439–441, 446, 447, 450, 460, 469, 479, 486, 511, 554, 562, 588, 589, 593, 604,

J. A. Díaz-Garrido et al. (eds.), *Psychological Interventions for Psychosis*,
https://doi.org/10.1007/978-3-031-27003-1

659, 662, 664, 670, 672–674, 686, 687, 690, 692, 700, 703, 721, 725, 739, 788
Cognitive behaviour therapy (CBT), 88, 117, 119, 126–134, 171–186, 192, 193, 202, 249–250, 252, 272, 288, 323 , 370, 389, 511, 539, 560, 563, 629, 701, 787
Cognitive therapy, 172, 174, 191, 309
Compassion, 253, 254, 271, 370, 390, 401, 442, 530, 540, 542–546, 551–556, 561, 565, 566, 568, 571, 572, 574, 577–580, 584, 589, 592, 593, 597, 599–604, 606, 607, 609, 648, 659, 673, 677, 685, 688
Compassion focused therapy (CFT), 31, 309, 540, 542, 544–548, 550, 552–554, 559–562, 564–567, 569–579, 584, 587–609
Compassionate mind training, 544, 560, 571, 572, 575, 576, 578–580, 597, 601, 606
Consciousness in relation to sanity and madness, 613, 616
Context, x, xi, 3, 4, 6–16, 18, 25, 31, 61, 78–82, 86, 87, 91–96, 106–111, 113–115, 118, 120, 130, 132, 133, 143, 155, 159, 160, 162, 163, 174, 186, 202–205, 208, 210, 211, 215, 219, 226, 227, 232, 234–236, 238–241, 245, 246, 250, 252, 254, 267–269, 272, 274, 277, 278, 280, 281, 285–304, 309, 313, 324, 331, 338, 348, 350, 352, 354, 360–363, 365, 366, 369, 370, 382, 383, 389–391, 393, 394, 399, 400, 403–407, 423–426, 428–430, 435, 438, 439, 442, 446, 447, 461, 466, 467, 469, 478, 480, 481, 485–490, 494–498, 500–504, 513, 530, 531, 535, 540, 545, 546, 553, 554, 556, 590, 592, 605, 606, 608, 609, 616, 618, 620–622, 632, 639, 642, 644, 645, 657, 659, 663, 671–673, 676, 693, 700–702, 719, 731–738, 740–742, 746–748, 750, 752–754, 772, 793, 794, 798
Contextual analyses, 106, 108, 112, 113
Contextual behavioral science (CBS), 225–228, 487, 489
Contextual phenomenological approach, 1, 2, 17, 18
Contextual therapy, 94, 97, 225–246, 374, 446, 660, 700, 703
Culture, 3, 12, 79, 84, 125–127, 130–134, 143, 144, 147, 150, 154, 156, 161, 163, 204, 286, 341, 367, 437, 454, 475, 476, 561, 563, 567, 568, 575, 578, 619, 622, 624, 662, 732, 733, 781, 796

D
Day hospital, 485, 486, 489, 490, 493–502, 659, 660, 686, 690, 711
DBT for psychosis, 509–522
DBT skills, 510, 511, 518, 522, 531, 535
Dialectical behavior therapy (DBT), 31, 509–522, 529–536
Dialogism, 353–354, 361, 363, 389, 390, 418, 438, 734, 736, 738, 749–753, 765, 768, 770, 781–784
Disclosure, 327–334, 336, 338–342, 618
Disorders of thought and perception, 659

E
Early attention unit (EAU), 748, 751, 753–764, 768, 771, 772, 774, 776, 779, 780, 784
Early intervention, 61, 175, 360, 383, 562, 564, 639
Emotion regulation, 71, 515, 516, 518–521, 534–535, 588
Empowerment, 30, 31, 161, 164, 255, 256, 326, 381, 442, 458, 461, 465, 468, 469, 472, 473, 477, 480, 535, 555, 591, 597, 605, 607, 608, 707, 724, 754
Ethno, 126
Evidence-based medicine, 27
Evidence based treatment, 509

F
Family interventions, 88–90, 95, 202, 361, 382, 388–391, 405, 407, 699–725
First-episode, 39, 40, 43, 45, 51, 61, 62, 66, 72, 98, 172, 260, 274, 275, 445, 465–482, 540, 541, 552, 555, 590, 594, 604
First episodes of psychosis, 745–783
Functional analysis, 93, 239, 240, 270, 277, 293, 307–317, 371, 372, 402, 428–429, 431–434, 487, 494, 673, 676, 677, 679, 680
Functional analytic psychotherapy (FAP), 31, 293, 354–355, 372, 425, 426, 428, 430, 434, 468, 485–489, 494, 495, 497, 502–504
Functional contextualism, 225–226, 251, 324, 347, 349, 469, 671, 672

H
Hallucinations, 4, 6, 8, 9, 25, 79, 85, 88, 94, 97, 113–116, 143, 152, 172, 174, 176, 177, 208, 219, 226, 232, 233, 238, 252,

254, 272, 287, 297, 307, 308, 311, 312, 325, 338, 348, 351, 353, 357, 361, 365–373, 388, 389, 391, 399, 405, 435, 436, 441, 442, 512, 527, 528, 532, 534–536, 541, 561, 562, 590, 591, 596, 659, 724
Hearing voices, ix, 17, 31, 78, 115, 116, 143, 144, 146, 149, 152, 157, 158, 160, 164, 175, 177, 183, 203, 259, 260, 280, 307–317, 392, 424, 444, 447, 514, 561, 617–619, 629, 634, 637–657
Holistic-contextual approach, 16

I
Informed therapy, 307–317
Inpatient treatment, 285–304
Integrated therapy, 77–99

L
Leveled acceptance and recovery therapy for psychosis (ART), 31
Life contexts, 107, 109–111, 118
Lived experience
of psychosis, 561

M
Mental health, x, 2, 5, 24, 26–29, 40–41, 63, 67, 68, 78–80, 82, 85, 87, 92, 93, 98, 105–107, 109, 116–118, 127, 129, 132, 142–146, 149–153, 155, 156, 159, 162–164, 182, 196, 201, 203, 212, 218, 228, 235, 244, 253–255, 264, 267, 270, 276, 280, 307, 326, 328, 353, 373, 384, 388, 390–392, 404, 435, 445, 453–463, 466, 467, 487, 488, 490, 504, 509, 510, 512, 513, 520, 536, 546, 547, 563, 564, 583, 584, 609, 613, 659, 660, 663–666, 690, 692, 701, 709, 710, 712, 716, 731–742, 745–749, 753–755, 759–763, 765, 773, 774, 778, 782, 783, 788, 790, 794–799, 801–803
Metacognition, 202, 204–207, 209–212, 218, 219, 349, 351, 358, 359, 440, 486
Mindfulness, x, 88, 191, 193–195, 250, 256, 258, 309, 310, 314, 315, 324, 326, 329, 340, 341, 355–358, 361, 362, 364, 369–372, 383, 389, 399–402, 417, 431, 433, 439, 440, 516–518, 521, 529, 531–533, 539–556, 560, 571, 576, 592, 596–598, 606, 607, 648, 659, 660, 662, 666, 670–673, 677, 679, 680, 688, 693, 694, 700, 703, 725, 760

N
Narrative development, 143, 145, 160, 161, 164

O
Open dialogue, ix, x, 14, 15, 17, 29, 31, 47, 72, 94, 98, 202, 353, 363, 373, 382, 383, 389, 391, 629, 724, 731–742, 745–783

P
Paranoia, 15, 98, 142, 173, 191, 192, 200, 254, 326, 339, 520, 562, 590–592, 606, 608
Personality, 6, 9, 82, 83, 307, 437, 475, 491, 493, 509, 525–536, 632, 647, 664, 666, 748
Person-based cognitive therapy (PBCT), 31, 191–200
Phenomenology, 2, 7, 8, 10, 12, 14, 16, 25, 31, 125, 203, 204, 208, 209, 220, 307, 356, 366, 392, 399, 431, 621
Postpsychiatry, 620–623
Power, 17, 27, 69, 85, 128, 143, 172, 235, 266, 295, 308, 334, 410, 556, 562, 620, 640, 663, 738, 759, 787
Power threat meaning framework (PTMF), x, 28, 142–164, 787
Psychiatric drug, 24, 47, 60, 61, 63–65, 70–72, 117, 142, 151, 153, 164, 627, 634, 794
Psychiatric hospitalization, 512
Psychiatry, x, 3–7, 18, 23, 25, 27, 37, 39, 40, 43, 47–50, 52, 59, 66–70, 72, 73, 86, 92, 98, 99, 110, 117, 149, 152, 201, 203, 233, 286, 348, 384, 391, 405, 435, 471, 478, 511, 613, 615–628, 632–634, 768, 782, 793, 801
Psychic suffering, 732, 734, 738, 739, 741, 742, 745
Psychological flexibility, 94, 228, 231–233, 237, 239, 246, 250, 251, 254–256, 258, 273, 289, 293, 324, 326, 330, 331, 342, 353, 354, 360, 362, 382, 383, 388, 390, 391, 403, 439, 440, 468, 504, 662, 670–672, 682, 692
Psychological treatment, 60, 71, 87–91, 93, 202, 236, 287, 308, 486, 560
Psychology, x, 3, 4, 7, 17, 28, 77, 90–92, 98, 117, 144, 149, 154, 201, 208, 384, 391, 405, 406, 435, 470, 540, 575, 578, 579, 590, 597, 600, 603, 621, 639, 662, 672, 731, 788
Psychosis, ix–xi, 1–4, 6, 11, 15–18, 23, 24, 26–32, 37, 39, 42, 46, 49, 59–73, 77,

78, 80–82, 84, 89, 90, 92, 95, 105–121, 125, 126, 128, 131, 133, 134, 142–164, 171–186, 191–202, 204–206, 208–212, 217, 219, 220, 232–245, 249–281, 285–304, 309–311, 323–342, 347–352, 355–359, 361, 364, 367, 368, 372–374, 381–383, 385, 389, 410, 413, 423–435, 437, 443, 448, 450, 451, 465–482, 485–504, 509–522, 525–536, 539, 541, 553, 555, 560–564, 571, 584, 588–590, 592, 594, 597, 599, 601, 604–609, 619, 624, 629, 633, 638, 639, 659, 661, 666, 680, 690, 699–725, 746–749, 753–760, 763–784, 787, 793, 794
Psychosocial rehabilitation, 364, 405, 423–451, 467, 481, 701, 703, 705, 708, 709, 760
Psychotherapy, xi, 8, 14–17, 27, 29, 41, 71–73, 126, 127, 129, 162, 201, 202, 206–210, 212, 219, 220, 285, 288, 293, 297, 323, 328, 349, 350, 355, 374, 382, 389, 425–427, 433, 487, 488, 504, 509–511, 521, 562, 587, 589, 592–605, 694, 731, 733, 735, 749, 760, 774, 787
Psychotherapy groups, 659
Psychotic behaviors, 84, 86, 88, 92–94, 108, 110
Psychotic disorders, 12, 14, 15, 43–45, 47, 48, 50, 51, 83, 110, 202, 208, 210, 308, 470, 493, 591, 660, 661, 663–666, 668, 689, 708
Psychotic spectrum disorder (PSD), x, xi, 2, 15, 78, 81, 347, 401, 423, 425, 428, 450, 451, 485, 509–511, 517, 519–522, 724
Public health system, 97, 531, 774

Q

Qualitative methodology, 3, 8, 17, 128

R

Recovery, ix, xi, 6, 26, 29, 31, 37, 44, 45, 53, 66, 83, 87, 96, 108, 142, 159, 164, 171, 186, 204–206, 209–211, 219, 249–281, 316, 323, 325, 326, 342, 348–350, 352, 353, 363, 364, 385, 388, 389, 404, 417, 423, 427, 432, 433, 439, 442, 444, 448, 451, 454, 460, 461, 497, 501, 510, 534–536, 546, 551, 556, 559, 560, 576, 584, 588, 589, 597, 606–609, 618, 620, 633, 638, 655, 656, 659, 662, 699, 704, 707, 723, 724, 748, 754, 755, 759, 798
Relational frame theory (RFT), 226–227, 241, 324, 330–332, 672

S

Schizophrenia, x, 1–15, 17, 18, 24–26, 37–53, 61–67, 77–99, 105, 107, 108, 110, 111, 113, 125, 127, 128, 131, 142, 149–151, 155, 162, 171, 172, 182, 183, 201–204, 208, 209, 218, 260, 295, 307, 348, 349, 388, 391, 405, 425, 430, 435, 445, 453, 486, 489, 509, 512, 520, 527–529, 534, 536, 540, 541, 545, 546, 551, 552, 554–556, 560, 563, 584, 592, 618, 623, 626, 630, 633, 638, 655, 661, 664, 701, 704, 708, 712–714, 745–748
Service users movements, 731
Seven principles, 734, 735, 742
Severe mental disorder (SMD), 28, 31, 78, 353, 424, 660, 662–668, 691, 694, 701, 724, 773, 774
Shamanism, 787
Social activism
Social inclusion, 89, 453–463
Social integration, 89, 99, 364, 453–455, 803
Social interventions, ix, 92, 95, 98
Stigma, 6, 8, 26, 28–30, 32, 90, 96, 130, 133, 146, 149, 159, 255, 277, 280, 326, 352, 353, 383, 385, 388, 392, 453–455, 458, 460–462, 465, 466, 503, 511, 601, 630, 661, 662, 705, 798, 802
Supporting people in psychosis, 161

T

Talking with voices, 639, 641, 646–653
Therapeutic relationship, 8, 31, 174, 175, 181, 186, 204, 206, 208, 210, 211, 215, 218, 293, 327, 328, 331–335, 342, 351–353, 367, 385, 393, 394, 407, 430, 438, 486–488, 493–504, 560, 572, 592–595, 671, 674
Therapy, ix, 1, 4, 11, 25, 31, 45, 47, 59, 71, 72, 77–99, 108, 109, 116–120, 125–127, 129–134, 150, 171–181, 183, 185, 186, 191, 192, 194, 196, 199, 202, 209–212, 214–219, 233, 235, 240, 244, 250, 251, 261, 263, 273, 275, 279, 285, 288, 293–296, 303, 304, 308, 310–312, 316, 317, 325, 327–332, 334, 339–342, 347, 352, 355, 364, 366, 383, 385, 389, 407,

415, 418, 423, 426, 427, 429, 430, 435, 445–448, 450, 456, 460, 468, 485, 486, 489, 494, 496, 500, 503, 504, 511, 521, 529, 530, 532, 534, 539–541, 544, 546, 548, 553, 559–584, 592, 593, 600, 602, 604, 620, 639, 646, 657, 662, 670–672, 724, 735
Third-wave, 249, 288, 293, 308, 309, 311, 323, 487
Threat Meaning Framework, 17, 28, 141–164, 787
Transdiagnostic models, x, 31, 250, 385, 526–529, 533

U
Unusual beliefs, 143, 146–150, 152, 155–157, 159, 162, 164, 798

V
Values, x, xi, 2, 9, 11, 31, 79, 88, 94, 126, 127, 153, 160, 162, 227–229, 232, 233, 237, 238, 241–245, 250, 251, 253–256, 258, 259, 264, 266, 270, 271, 273, 279, 289, 291, 292, 296, 297, 300–303, 310, 311, 314, 316, 317, 324, 326, 327, 329, 331, 333, 334, 336–339, 350–353, 355, 360–362, 364–366, 368, 371, 373, 382, 383, 387–390, 393, 399, 401–404, 408, 409, 411, 412, 414–415, 417, 427, 432, 433, 438–443, 446–450, 453, 466–469, 471, 472, 475, 476, 481, 488, 494, 497, 500, 503, 510, 519, 535, 536, 565, 583, 605, 619, 621, 622, 642, 643, 647, 650, 651, 659, 662, 670–677, 680, 681, 687, 689, 692, 703, 725, 737, 748, 759, 797
Voice dialogue, 576, 577, 647–657
Voice hearing, 114, 115, 144, 146, 148, 149, 152, 155–157, 162, 164, 176, 182, 307, 309, 311–314, 316, 571, 582, 583, 638–641, 643–645, 655